Dental Caries

Dental Caries

Vimal K Sikri

MDS, DOOP (PU), DEME (AIU), FICD

Professor and Head
Department of Conservative Dentistry and Endodontics

and

Principal/Dean
Punjab Government Dental College and Hospital
Amritsar, Punjab
India

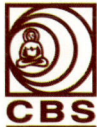

CBS

CBS Publishers & Distributors Pvt Ltd

New Delhi • Bengaluru • Chennai • Kochi • Kolkata • Mumbai
Hyderabad • Nagpur • Patna • Pune • Vijayawada

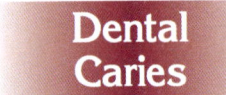

Dental Caries

ISBN: 978-81-239-2499-1

First Edition: 2016

Published by Satish Kumar Jain and produced by Varun Jain for
CBS Publishers & Distributors Pvt Ltd
4819/XI Prahlad Street, 24 Ansari Road, Daryaganj, New Delhi 110 002, India.
Ph: 23289259, 23266861, 23266867   Fax: 011-23243014   Website: www.cbspd.com
                                                         e-mail: delhi@cbspd.com; cbspubs@airtelmail.in.
Corporate Office: 204 FIE, Industrial Area, Patparganj, Delhi 110 092
Ph: 4934 4934   Fax: 4934 4935   e-mail: publishing@cbspd.com; publicity@cbspd.com

Branches

- **Bengaluru:** Seema House 2975, 17th Cross, K.R. Road, Banasankari 2nd Stage, Bengaluru 560 070, Karnataka
  Ph: +91-80-26771678/79   Fax: +91-80-26771680   e-mail: bangalore@cbspd.com
- **Chennai:** No. 7, Subbaraya Street, Shenoy Nagar, Chennai 600 030, Tamil Nadu
  Ph: +91-44-26680620, 26681266   Fax: +91-44-42032115   e-mail: chennai@cbspd.com
- **Kochi:** Ashana House, 39/1904, AM Thomas Road, Valanjambalam, Ernakulam 682 016, Kochi, Kerala
  Ph: +91-484-4059061–65,67   Fax: +91-484-4059065   e-mail: kochi@cbspd.com
- **Kolkata:** No. 6/B, Ground Floor, Rameswar Shaw Road, Kolkata-700014 (West Bengal), India
  Ph: +91-33-2289-1126, 2289-1127, 2289-1128   e-mail: kolkata@cbspd.com
- **Mumbai:** 83-C, Dr E Moses Road, Worli, Mumbai-400018, Maharashtra
  Ph: +91-22-24902340/41   Fax: +91-22-24902342   e-mail: mumbai@cbspd.com

Representatives

- **Hyderabad** 0-9885175004   • **Nagpur** 0-9021734563   • **Patna**   0-9334159340
- **Pune**   0-9623451994   • **Vijayawada** 0-9000660880

Printed at: HT Media Ltd., Noida

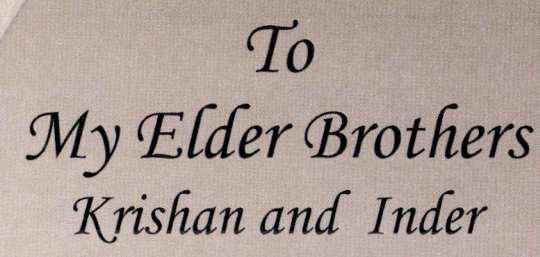

To
My Elder Brothers
Krishan and Inder

Will always be for me,
no matter how life gets tougher

...Growing with them to lean on...
Yesterday, Today and Tomorrow

Contributors

Abhishek Mehta
Assoc. Professor and Incharge
Dept. of Public Health Dentistry
Faculty of Dentistry
Jamia Millia Islamia
New Delhi Ph. 09971209069

Abi M Thomas
Professor and Head, Dept. of Pedodontics, and
Principal, Christian Dental College
CMC, Brown Road
Ludhiana-141008 Ph. 09417300473

Annupriya Sikri
Senior Lecturer, Dept. of Pedodontics
National Dental College
Derabassi (Punjab) Ph. 08727014177

Baljit Sidhu
Asstt. Professor
Dept. of Conservative Dentistry and Endodontics
Punjab Govt. Dental College and Hospital
Amritsar-143001 Ph. 09872205712

G. Kayalvizhi
Reader, Dept. of Pedodontics
MR Ambedkar Dental College and Hospital
Cooke Town, Bangalore-560005
Ph. 09886120559

Neeraj Gugnani
Professor and Head
Dept. of Pedodontics
DAV Dental College and Hospital
Yamunanagar (Haryana) Ph. 09416061087

Nidhi Gupta
Professor and Head
Dept.of Public Health Dentistry
Swami Devi Dyal Dental College and Hospital,
Barwala, Panchkula (Haryana)
Ph. 09876136514

Nirapjit Kaur
Asstt. Professor
Dept. of Pedodontics
Punjab Govt. Dental College and Hospital
Amritsar-143001 Ph. 09814815177

Nutan Tyagi
Senior Lecturer, Dept. of Oral Pathology
IDST Dental College,
Kadrabad, Modinagar
Ghaziabad-201201
Ph. 09968232567

Priyanka Setia
Senior Lecturer
Dept. of Conservative Dentistry and Endodontics
Chaudhary Devi Lal Dental College
Barnala Road, Sirsa-125055
Ph. 07027413977

Rakesh Mittal
Professor and Head,
Dept. of Conservative Dentistry and Endodontics
Sudha Rastogi College of Dental Sciences and
Research
Faridabad (Haryana) Ph. 09813172742

Rishi Tyagi
Assoc. Professor
Dept. of Pedodontics
UCMS & GTBH
Dilshad Garden
Delhi-95 Ph. 09868575552

S Balagopal
Vice Principal, Professor and Head,
Dept. of Conservative Dentistry and Endodontics
Tagore Dental College
Chennai – 600127 Ph. 09444039411

Simarpreet Virk Sandhu
Professor and Head
Dept. of Oral Pathology
Genesis Institute of Dental Sciences and Research
Firozpur (Punjab)
Ph. 09888887438

Viresh Teginmanni
Professor and Head
Dept. of Conservative Dentistry and Endodontics
AME'S Dental College and Hospital Bijangere Road,
Raichur-584103
Ph. 09448379305

Foreword

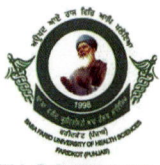

BABA FARID UNIVERSITY OF HEALTH SCIENCES
Sadiq Road, Faridkot - 151203 (Pb)
Tel : 01639-256756 & 256232, Fax : 01639-257886
www.bfuhs.ac.in
E-mail : officebfuhs@gmail.com, rajbahadur9@gmail.com

Prevalence of dental caries in human population is recorded since ages. Archeological evidences show that tooth decay is an ancient disease dating far into pre-history. The World Health Organization estimates that nearly all adults have dental caries at some point of time. Epidemiological data from many countries indicate a marked increase in the prevalence of dental caries. These global trends in dental caries prevalence signals a pending public health crisis. The concept of cariology has been transformed in recent years and the old philosophy of 'drill and fill' and 'extension for prevention' need to be updated keeping in view advances in reversal of caries process and also the regeneration of tooth tissues. The exciting innovation in the field of caries is 'resin infiltration' along with newer diagnostic gadgets and protocols, role of plasma and biotene in caries prevention and also the probability of utilizing biomimetic remineralization.

The book *Dental Caries*, the first of its kind by an Indian author, will develop core concepts on directions of epidemiology, microbiology and clinical cariology. As new research and clinical experience broaden our knowledge, changes in treatment and drug therapy are required. This book gives interest and zest to stimulate new thinking and changes in clinical practice. It could be beneficial to all practitioners, students and teachers as a valuable guide to development in the rapidly developing field of modern cariology. It will enlighten and encourage to explore new horizons in their clinical practice. Hopefully, this book will serve as a recipe which pleases and satisfies the appetite to learn and apply a modern approach for managing caries efficiently and effectively.

With my profound faith and professional respect for Dr Sikri, who has vast teaching experience and is a popular teacher, I wish him excel in the field of teaching and learning. Simultaneously I wish that this book should become treasure of knowledge with students and all libraries of the country.

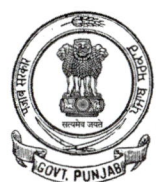

Prof. Raj Bahadur
PHF, MS Orth, FRCS (Glasg), FAMS, FIMSA, FICA, FPASc
Vice Chancellor

Preface

I vividly remember, when I asked my guru, Sir, I want to write a book. After a long pause, he replied; my dear son, for writing a book, you need a long deep patience saturated with your arterial blood. If you sincerely want to write a book, then read in abundance, breathe through your ideas, cry out making words, keep editing and continue updating yourself. The book before you is the outcome of my guru's diktat.

Dental Caries is ubiquitous in all population; the lesion development being continuous throughout life. A comprehensive book covering all aspects of dental caries and written in a simple and lucid language is presented before you. The book includes the concept of caries from ancient times to 'near future' describing the text along with photographs, diagrams, tables and flowcharts. All advancements in diagnostic tools, methodology in risk assessment, preventive regimes, microbiological aspects and the immunological influences have been added. A chapter on 'resin infiltration' describes caries therapy for initial lesions. I hope the book will appeal to dental students, teachers, educators, therapists and clinicians who wish to update their knowledge in the field of cariology.

I sincerely thank the Almighty God and my revered guru for giving me courage, patience and temperament for selecting, arranging and organizing appropriate text along with befitting photographs for this book. I am grateful to all the contributors for sharing their knowledge and expertise for the betterment of the manuscript writing. I am thankful to my colleagues, Dr Renu Sroa, Professor and Dr Baljit Sidhu, Assistant Professor for their constant help in evaluating the text. I am indebted to my students Dr Shikha Sharma, Dr Ibadat Preet Kaur, Dr Nidhi Gupta, Dr Niyetee Saraf, Dr Ashish Karode, Dr Meghna Mittal, Dr Shaveta Seth, Dr Tejinderpal Singh, Dr Komalgeet Kaur, Dr Jasbir Kaur, Dr Neha Mengi, Dr Nidhi Dhamija and Dr Navita Budhiraja for assisting me in organizing the manuscript.

I acknowledge with pride the understanding and patience of my dear wife, Dr Poonam, my sons, Dr Ankit, Dr Arpit and my sweet bitiya, Dr Annupriya. Last but not the least, I put on record my gratitude to all those great souls who shared their ideas for the betterment of the book.

I request all students as well as the teachers to go through the book and suggest areas of improvement, which can be incorporated in the next edition. I remember my Guru's words, 'your life is your dreams; write well, edit well and ...'

Vimal K Sikri

Prologue

The concept of cariology has been transformed in recent years and is expected to undergo far-reaching changes in future. The exciting innovation in the field of caries is 'resin infiltration' along with newer diagnostic gadgets and protocols, role of plasma and biotene in caries prevention and also the probability of utilizing biomimetic remineralization. The old philosophies of managing caries should be re-analyzed keeping in view advances in reversal of caries process and also the regeneration of tooth tissues.

The book *Dental Caries*, the first of its kind by an Indian author, comprehensively deals with all aspects of cariology including the clinical ones. Author's emphasis on the originality and the language of the subject matter is clearly evident in the book. The vast experience of Dr Vimal Sikri, a renowned teacher, coupled with his aptitude for writing, has conceived a nice way of presenting his vision in the book.

The book is recommended to all students, teachers and practitioners keen in updating their knowledge in the developing field of cariology. It is advisable to consider Dr Sikri's book for application in your routine teaching and practice.

I wish Dr Sikri a healthy life and hope he will keep guiding the youngsters through his writings in future also.

D Kandaswamy
Dean, Faculty of Dental Sciences
Sri Ramachandra University
Porur, Chennai-600116

Contents

Dental Caries: An Introduction

The word 'Caries' (Latin meaning 'dry rot') implies slow disintegration of any biological hard tissue as a result of bacterial action. The caries of spine or any other bone is a common finding associated with certain degenerative systemic diseases.

Dental caries is also the slow disintegration of hard tissues of the tooth. Dental caries is peculiarly a local disease, which involves destruction of hard tissues of the teeth by metabolites produced by oral micro-organisms. Dental caries has affected humans since prehistoric times; however; the documented reference of tooth decay and toothache appeared around the century BC, when oracle bone inscriptions excavated from the ruins of Ying Dynasty showed the character meaning 'caries'. The association of systemic disease and teeth was probably obtained from writings of a physician around 660 BC. The physician had mentioned that the inflammation in his arms and legs was due to tooth and that it must be extracted. Tooth loss resulting in diminished chewing ability, which can lead to nutritional disorders, was a significant problem especially in lower socio-economic groups. In addition, caries results in other significant problems in the form of pain and cosmetic defects. Dental caries and periodontal diseases are the most common chronic diseases in the world. Walter

Loesche (1986) described caries and perio-dontal disease as "perhaps the most expensive infections that most individuals have to contend with during a lifetime." In view of unique characteristics of tooth and caries, the caries does not fall into any of the pathological lesions of oral cavity. The caries is not inflammatory in origin nor is it degenerative in nature and neither it is a neoplasm. The cost of managing caries is enormous. While it is difficult to eradicate caries on a population level; individuals under professional supervision may minimize caries incidence. The knowledge of the factors affecting caries provides a general idea about the progression of the carious process and the susceptibility of other teeth in the oral cavity.

When acids are produced by bacteria interacting with local substrate, they diffuse into tooth enamel, partially dissolving the minerals from crystals and subsequently invading the tooth. The minerals are termed as carbonated hydroxyapatite. This is calcium phosphate with numerous inclusions (carbonated ions), which makes the mineral more acid soluble than pure hydroxyapatite. If the dissolution of minerals is not stopped or reversed, the early demineralization areas become a cavity.

Dental caries occur in deciduous and permanent teeth regardless of the age, sex, creed, etc. of the individual. Although caries were prevalent at the time of pre-neolithic humans (10,000 BC), it was not until fourteenth and fifteenth century when a sharp increase in caries prevalence was noted.

DEFINITIONS OF DENTAL CARIES

At the 1948 conference on caries, dental caries was considered as a disease of the calcified tissues of the teeth, caused by acids resulting from the action of micro-organisms on carbohydrates, characterized by decalcification of the inorganic portion, followed by disintegration of the organic substance of the tooth. The lesions predominantly occur in particular regions of the tooth and their type is determined by the morphologic nature of the tissue in which they appear.

WHO defined caries as a *localized post-eruptive, pathological process of external origin involving softening of the hard tooth tissue and proceeding to the formation of a cavity.*

Various authors have defined 'Caries' in different forms; however, not a single definition is universally accepted. The commonly used definitions are:

GV Black: Dental caries is defined as the chemical dissolution of the calcium salts, first of the enamel then of the dentin by lactic acid.

Shafer: Dental caries is defined as irreversible microbial disease of the calcified tissues of the teeth characterized by demineralization of the inorganic portion and destruction of organic substance of the tooth.

Kess and Ash: Dental caries is a disease involving hard portions of the teeth which are exposed in oral cavity and is characterized by disintegration of enamel, dentin and cementum forming open cavities.

Last: Dental caries is an illness due to specific infectious agent or its toxic products that arises through transmission of that agent or its products from an infected person, animal or reservoir to a susceptible host.

Sturdevant: Dental caries is an infectious microbiologic disease of the teeth that results in localized dissolution and destruction of calcified tissues.

GJ Mount: Caries is perceived to be a prolonged imbalance in the oral cavity such that the factors favoring demineralization of enamel and dentin overwhelm the factors that favor remineralization and repair of those tissues.

Cawson: Dental caries can be defined as progressive, irreversible bacterial damage to teeth exposed to the oral environment.

Kidd and Smith: Caries is a disease of the calcified tissues of the teeth caused by the action of micro-organisms on fermentable carbohydrates.

Lundeen: Dental caries is an infectious microbiological disease that results in localized dissolution and destruction of the calcified tissues of the teeth and progresses as a series of exacerbations and remissions.

Ernest Newburn: Dental caries or tooth decay, is a pathological process of localized destruction of tooth tissues by micro-organisms.

Ostrom: Dental caries is a process of enamel or dentin dissolution that is caused by microbial action at the tooth surface and is mediated by physiochemical flow of water dissolved ions.

Hume: Dental caries is essentially a progressive loss by acid dissolution of the apatite (mineral) component of the enamel then the dentin, or of the cementum, then dentin.

Fejerskov and Nyvad: The dental caries is a complex disease caused by an imbalance in physiologic equilibrium between tooth mineral and biofilm fluid.

Selwitz: Dental caries is a multifactorial disease that starts with microbiological shifts within the complex biofilm and is affected by salivary flow and composition, exposure to fluoride, consumption of dietary sugars and by preventive behaviours (cleaning teeth). However, it is mainly a disease that dates back to antiquity and has also occurred in populations that have never used sugar or processed foods.

Sikri: Dental caries is an infectious disease caused by imbalance of oral micro-organisms leading to acid production and subsequently dissolving the hard tissues of tooth.

Certain earlier definition of dental caries by unidentified authors:

- Dental caries, also known as tooth decay/cavity, is a disease where bacterial processes damage hard tooth structure (enamel, dentin and cementum). These tissues progressively breakdown, producing dental cavities (holes in the teeth).
- A disease of the teeth resulting in damage to tooth structure.
- The bacterial disease known as tooth decay/cavities that causes demineralization of teeth through exposure to sugars and starches.
- The disease processes leading to tooth decay.
- An infectious disease caused by the interaction of bacteria (which reside in plaque on the surface of the teeth) with retained food particles especially carbohydrates. This interaction produces organic acids which attack the enamel of the teeth.
- Decay of teeth due to penetration of bacteria through the enamel to the dentin.
- A disease of teeth in which micro-organisms convert sugar in the mouth to an acid that erodes the tooth, commonly called a cavity.
- A destructive process causing decalcification of tooth enamel and leading to continued destruction of enamel and dentin.

Certain terms whereby tooth tissue is lost due to factors other than caries:

a. *Attrition:* Attrition is the physiologic wearing away of hard tissue of teeth due to tooth-to-tooth contact in functional occlusion (no foreign object involved).

b. *Abrasion:* Abrasion is the pathologic wearing away of hard tissues of teeth because of abnormal and mechanical forces, viz. foreign objects repeatedly contacting the teeth.

c. *Abfraction:* Abfraction is a wedge shaped defect at the cement-enamel junction caused by deviated occlusal forces leading to tooth flexure, subsequently microfracture of cervical enamel and dentin.

d. *Demastication:* It implies wearing away of tooth tissues during mastication of food (wear is influenced by abrasiveness of the food).

e. *Erosion:* Erosion is described as the loss of dental hard tissues which are etched away by acids or chelation without bacterial involvement. Acids stem from dietary, occupational or intrinsic factors and not the products of intraoral bacteria.

The caries process and the associated terms used:

a. *Caries process:* The demineralization and remineralization is a continuous process. A shift in the balance between protective factors (remineralization) and the destructive factors (demineralization) is the caries process.

b. *Arrest:* The demineralization process is stopped with no further loss of minerals from the active caries process.

c. *Caries lesion/carious lesion:* This is a clinical manifestation of caries process; a detectable change in the tooth structure resulting from bacteria–tooth interactions due to caries.

d. *Caries lesion severity:* The extent of progress of caries lesion towards pulp.

e. *Non-cavitated lesion:* A non-cavitated caries lesion is one whose surface appears macroscopically intact (lesion without evidence of cavitation). It is also referred to as incipient lesion or initial lesion.

f. *Cavitated lesion:* The surface that is not intact macroscopically with distinct discontinuity or break in surface integrity (visual cavitation).

g. *Active caries lesion:* The continuation of mineral loss over a period of time; that is the lesion is progressing.

h. *Inactive caries lesion (arrested caries):* The lesion is no longer progressing; that is, the mineral loss is stopped after sometime.

i. *Caries lesion regression:* Replacing the loss of minerals affected during demineralization. The local surface shear is increased as compared to previous surface texture.

j. *Hidden caries lesion:* Lesions which are missed on visual examination, but are sufficiently demineralised to be viewed radiographically or detected by optical means.

k. *White spot lesion:* Initial, non-cavitated caries lesion, seen as white appearance on enamel surface.

l. *Brown spot lesion:* White lesions when acquire intrinsic or exogenous pigments appear as brown surface over the enamel.

m. *Monitoring of caries lesion:* Assessing caries lesion over a period of time. Earlier the term 'watch' was used to monitor the lesion and to note the changes, if any.

n. *Risk:* Risk is the probability that a disease process or any other harmful event may occur.

o. *Risk factors:* Risk factors are the biological reasons or the factors which have caused or liable to cause the disease. The presence of these factors increases the probability of the disease and if removed, the probability decreases. Once the disease occurs, the removal of factors is not helpful in cure.

p. *Risk indicator:* Risk indicators are indirectly related with the disease. A risk indicator or the combination of risk indicators may be associated as risk factors.

CLASSIFICATIONS OF DENTAL CARIES

I. Based on Location

1. Pits and fissure caries.
2. Smooth surface caries.
3. Root surface caries (senile caries).

II. Based on Rapidity of Caries

1. Acute dental caries (rampant caries).

2. Chronic dental caries.
3. Arrested dental caries.

III. Based on Extent of Caries

1. Incipient caries (reversible).
2. Cavitated caries (non-reversible).

IV. Based on whether it is a New or Recurrent Carious Lesion

1. Primary caries.
2. Secondary caries/recurrent caries.

V. Based on the Number of Surfaces Involved

1. *Simple caries:* Caries involving only one surface of the tooth.
2. *Compound caries:* Caries involving two surfaces of the tooth.
3. *Complex caries:* Caries involving three or more surfaces of the tooth.

VI. Based on the Age of the Patient

1. *Nursing bottle caries:* During early infancy, bottle-fed babies develop rapidly spreading caries usually on maxillary incisors.
2. *Adolescent caries:* Caries seen in the teenage population due to dietary habits.
3. *Root caries:* Caries of cementum; seen in older age patients.

VII. Based on the Treatment and Restorative Design (GV Black)

Class I: Caries in structural defects of teeth like pits and fissures and some defective grooves and occlusal surface of molars and premolars, occlusal 2/3rd of buccal and lingual surfaces of molars and lingual surface of anterior teeth.

Class II: Caries on the proximal surfaces of molars and premolars.

Class III: Caries on the proximal surface of anterior teeth without involving incisal edge.

Class IV: Caries on the proximal surface of anterior teeth with involvement of incisal edge.

Class V: Caries seen at the gingival third of facial and lingual surfaces of anterior and posterior teeth.

Simon later added a sixth category-Class VI: Caries seen on incisal edges and cuspal tips of molars and premolars, axial angles of teeth or any highly cleansable surface.

VIII. Bite Wing Radiograph Classification of Dental Caries (Grondahl, modified from Moller and Poulsen)

0: Sound on the bitewing.

1: Radiolucency confined to enamel.

2: Radiolucency in enamel up to dentino-enamel junction.

3: Radiolucency in enamel and outer half of dentin.

4: Radiolucency in enamel and reaching to inner half of dentin.

IX. Based on Clinical Scoring of Proximal Lesion at the Base of Approximal Box (by Bille and Thylstrup)

Scores 1 and 2: Progressive changes in the enamel.

Score 3: Changes in dentin, without cavitation in the enamel.

Scores 4 and 5: Changes in dentin and progressive cavitation in the enamel (i.e., at this stage no bacterial invasion of the dentinal tubules has occurred and there is no indication for operative intervention).

Score 6: Cavitation involving dentin (possible indication for operative intervention).

X. According to the World Health Organization (WHO) System

The shape and the depth of the caries lesion can be scored on a four point scale.

D1: Clinically detectable enamel lesions with intact (non-cavitated) surfaces.

D2: Clinically detectable cavities limited to the enamel.

D3: Clinically detectable lesions in dentin (with and without cavitation of dentin).

D4: Lesions into pulp.

XI. Based on Visual Examination and Radiographs (Epelid, et al and Tveit, et al)

Grade 1: Non-cavitated white spot or slightly discolored carious lesion in enamel (no lesion detectable on the radiograph).

Grade 2: Some superficial cavitation on the entrance of the fissures, some non-cavitated mineral loss in the surfaces of the enamel surrounding the fissures and/or a carious lesion in enamel (detectable on the radiograph).

Grade 3: Moderate mineral loss with limited cavitation in the entrance of the fissure and / or a lesion extended into the outer third of the dentin (detectable on the radiograph).

Grade 4: Considerable mineral loss with cavitation and/or lesion extended into middle third of the dentin (detectable on the radiograph).

Grade 5: Advanced cavitation and/or a lesion extended into the inner third of the dentin (detectable on the radiograph).

XII. Sturdevant Classification

Sturdevant divided dental caries mainly in three criteria:

a. *Location*
   - Primary caries.
     – Caries of pit and fissure origin.
     – Caries of smooth surface origin.
   - Backward caries.
   - Forward caries.
   - Residual caries.
   - Root surface caries.
   - Secondary (recurrent) caries.

b. *Extent*
   - Incipient caries (reversible).
   - Cavitated caries (irreversible).

c. *Rate*
   - Acute (rampant) caries.
   - Chronic (slow or arrested) caries.

XIII. According to Dental Clinics of North America

a. *According to tooth type*
  - Deciduous (A-T).
  - Permanent (1–32).

b. *According to anatomic site*
  - Pit and fissure.
  - Smooth surface-interproximal, cervical.
  - Root surface.

c. *According to hard tissue affected*
  - Enamel.
  - Dentin.
  - Cementum.

d. *Others*
  - Primary, secondary.
  - Nursing caries.
  - Radiation caries.
  - Rampant caries.

XIV. Classification by GJ Mount

Caries lesions occur in three main sites and are of four different sizes (Table 1.1):
- *Site 1:* Pits and fissures, enamel defects on occlusal surfaces of posterior teeth or other smooth surfaces.
- *Site 2:* Approximal enamel in relation to areas in contact with adjacent teeth.
- *Site 3:* The cervical one-third of the crown or following gingival recession, the exposed root.

Each site is further categorized according to the size:
- *Size 0:* Small and early enough to be remineralized or a remineralized lesion with only residual stain.
- *Size 1:* Minimal dentinal spread, can be remineralized.
- *Size 2:* Moderate involvement of dentin.
- *Size 3:* Enlarged with weakened cusps or incisal edges (need protection from occlusal load).
- *Size 4:* Extensive loss of tooth structure.

The explanations of sizes are:
1. Minimal involvement of dentin just beyond treatment by remineralization alone.
2. Moderate involvement of dentin following cavity preparation, remaining enamel is sound, well supported by dentin and not likely to fail under normal occlusal load. That is, the remaining tooth structure is sufficiently strong to support the restoration.
3. The cavity is enlarged beyond moderate. The remaining tooth structure is weakened to the extent that cusps and incisal edges are split, or are likely to fail or left exposed to occlusal or incisal load. The cavity needs to be further enlarged so that the restoration can be designed to provide support and protection to the remaining structure.
4. Extensive caries with bulk loss of tooth structure has already occurred.

This classification was proposed providing options for treatment planning, keeping in mind the treatment by adhesive restorative materials. Though the concept is not entirely unfair; however, there is always an element of subjectivity in deciding the size of the lesion. It may become difficult, especially for the beginners, to differentiate between different sizes; a few may decide it as size 3, whereas others may designate the same as

Site	Size			
	Minimal (1)	Moderate (2)	Enlarged (3)	Extensive (4)
Pit/fissure 1	1.1	1.2	1.3	1.4
Contact areas 2	2.1	2.2	2.3	2.4
Cervical 3	3.1	3.2	3.3	3.4

Table 1.1: GJ Mount classification

size 4. Secondly, treatment planning varies with operator to operator. Thirdly, the sites mentioned earlier which are missing in Black's classification are also missing in this classification. Contact caries (site 2) whether on one side or two sides is taken as one which is always misleading. And also clubbing root caries with crown caries creates confusion amongst readers. Because of the above mentioned reasons the Mount's classification was not accepted worldwide.

Keeping in view the simplicity and acceptability of Black's classification, the author is of the view that it should not be totally changed; however, little modification will cover the areas left by Black. The classification as proposed by the author is as follows:

XV. Dr. Sikri's Classification

Class I
Division I: Cavities involving pits and fissures of occlusal surfaces.
Division II: Cavities involving buccal and lingual pits of posterior and anterior teeth.

Class II
Division I: Cavities involving one proximal surface of posterior teeth.
Division II: Cavities involving both proximal surfaces of posterior teeth.

Class III
Division I: Cavities involving one proximal surface of anterior teeth.
Division II: Cavities involving both proximal surfaces of anterior teeth.

Class IV
Division I: Cavities on cervical one-third of labial and lingual surfaces of all the teeth.
Division II: Cavities on labial and lingual line angles of all the teeth.

Class V
Division I: Cavities on labial surfaces of anterior teeth other than cervical one-third.

Division II: Cavities on lingual surfaces of anterior teeth other than pits and cervical one-third.

Class VI
Division I: Cavities on incisal tips.
Division II: Cavities on occlusal cusp tips.

XVI. ADA Caries Classification System

American Dental Association Caries Classification System (ADA-CCS) categorized extent of carious lesion as initial, moderate and severe based on clinical findings regarding the progress of the lesion. The ADA-CCS has also characterized the site of origin of lesion as pit and fissure, proximal, cervical/smooth surface and root caries.

Initial caries is defined as visibly non-cavitated or micro-cavitated lesion limited to the enamel.

Moderate caries infers breakdown of enamel with non-cavitated carious dentin or loss of root cementum with non-cavitated carious dentin.

Severe caries are the lesions extending into dentin.

Pit and fissure caries refers to the caries of the anatomical pits and fissures of all the teeth.

Proximal caries refers to caries at the immediate proximity to the contact area of adjacent tooth surface (may be any tooth).

Cervical/smooth surface caries refers to the caries at the cervical area or any other smooth enamel surface of the anatomical crown (may exist anywhere around the full circumference of the tooth).

Root surface caries refers to the caries of the root surface (apical to the anatomical crown).

XVII. Classification of Root Caries by Billings
Grade I (incipient)
- **Surface texture:** Soft, can be penetrated with dental explorer.
- **Surface defect:** No.
- **Pigmentation:** Variable; light tan to brown.

Grade II (shallow)

- *Surface texture:* Soft, irregular, rough, can be penetrated with dental explorer.
- *Surface defect:* <0.5 mm in depth.
- *Pigmentation:* Variable; tan to dark brown.

Grade III (cavitation)

- *Surface texture:* Soft, can be penetrated with dental explorer.
- *Surface defect:* Cavitation present, >0.5 mm in depth, no pulpal involvement.
- *Pigmentation:* Variable; light brown to dark brown.

Grade IV (pulpal)

- *Surface defect:* Deeply penetrating lesion with pulpal or root canal involvement.
- *Pigmentation:* Variable; brown to dark brown.

XVIII. Classification of Root Caries by Nyvad and Fejerskov

1. Active or inactive.
2. With or without cavitation.
3. According to texture (soft, leathery, hard) and color (yellow, light brown, dark brown-black).

Bibliography

1. Abbott F. Caries of human teeth. Dental Cosmos. 1879;21:57–184.
2. Anjomshoaa I, Cooper ME and Vieira AR. Caries is associated with asthma and epilepsy. Eur. J. Dent. 2009;3:297–303.
3. Bartlett DW and Shah P. A critical review of non-carious cervical (wear) lesions and the role of abfraction, erosion and abrasion. J. Dent. Res. 2006;85:306–12.
4. Baum BJ. Will dentistry be left behind at the healthcare station? HJ. Am. Coll. Dent.2004;71: 27–30.
5. Bowen WH. Do we need to be concerned about dental caries in the coming millennium? Crit. Rev. Oral Biol. Med. 2002;13:126–31.
6. Bowen WH. Rodent model in caries research. Odontology: 2013;101:9–14.
7. Bratthall D. Dental caries: intervened-interrupted-interpreted. Eur. J. Oral Sci. 1996;104, 486–91.
8. Burt BA. Definitions of risk. J. Dent. Educ. 2001; 65:1007–8.
9. Clarkson BH. Introduction to cariology. Dent. Clinic North Am 1999;43:569–78.
10. Dulgergil CT and Colak H. Rural Dentistry: Is it an imagination or obligation in Community Dental Health Education. Niger. Med. J. 2012;53: 1–8.
11. Fejerskov O. Changing paradigms in concepts on dental caries: consequences for oral health care. Caries Res.: 2004;38:182–91.
12. Fisher J and Glick M. A new model for caries classification and management. JADA. 2012;14: 546–51.
13. Fontana M, Young DA, Wolff MS, Pitts NB and Longbottom C. Defining dental caries for 2010 and Beyond. Dent. Clin. North Am. 2010;54:423–40.
14. Glick M, Monteiro da Silva O, Seeberger GK, Xu T, Pucca G and Williams DM. FDI Vision 2020: shaping the future of oral health. Int. Dent. J. 2012;62:278–91.
15. Gower LB. Biomimetic model systems for investigating the amorphous precursor pathway and its role in biomineralization. Chem. Rev. 2008;108:4551–627.
16. Jenkin GN. Recent changes in dental caries. Br. Med. J. 1985;291:1297–8.
17. Kay EJ and Locker D: Is dental health education effective: A systematic review of current evidence. Com. Dent. Oral Epidemiol. 1996;59: 376–88.
18. Keyes PH. Research in dental caries. J. Am. Dent. Assoc.: 1968;76:1357–73.
19. Kunin AA, Evdokimova AY and Moiseeva NS. Age-related differences of tooth enamel morphochemistry in health and dental caries. The EPMA Journal. 2015, 6:3.
20. Longbottom C, Huysmans MC and Pitts NB. Glossary of key terms. Monogr. Oral Sci.: 2009;21: 209–16.
21. Lorber MF, Heyman RE and Dasanayake AP. Noxious family environments in relation to adult and childhood caries. JADA: 2014;145:924–30.
22. Macek MD, Heller KE and Selwitz RH, et al. Is 75 percent of dental caries really found in 25 percent of the population? J. Public Health Dent. 2004;64:20–5.

23. Makhija SK, Gilbert GH, Funkhouser E, Bader JD, Gordan VV, Rindal BD, Qvist V, Norrisgaard P. Twenty-month follow-up of occlusal caries lesions deemed questionable at baseline. JADA 2014;145:1112–8.

24. Maltz M, Jardim JJ and Alves LS. Health promotion and dental caries. Braz. Oral Res. 2010;24:18–25.

25. Meurman PK and Pienihakkinen K. Factors associated with caries increment: a longitudinal study from 18 months to 5 years of age. Caries Res.: 2010;44:519–24.

26. Mount GJ and Hume WR. A new cavity classification. Aust. Dent. J. 1998;43:153–9.

27. Mount GJ, Tyas MJ, Duke ES, Hume WR, Lafargues JJ and Kaleka R. A proposal for a new classification of lesions of exposed tooth surfaces. Int. Dent. J.: 2006;56:82–91.

28. Petersen PE, Bourgeois D, Ogawa H, Estupinan-Day S and Ndiaye C. The global burden of oral diseases and risks to oral health. Bull. World Health Organization: 2005;83:661–9.

29. Pitts NB. Modern concepts of caries measurement. J. Dent. Res.: 2004;83:43–7.

30. Pretty IA and Ellwood RP. The caries continuum: opportunities to detect, treat and monitor the re-mineralization of early caries lesions. J. Dent. 2013;41:S12–S21.

31. Ruby JD, Cox CF, Akimoto N, Meada N and Momoi Y. The caries phenomenon: A timeline from witchcraft and superstition to opinions of the 1500s to today's science. Int. J. Dent.: 2010;1–11.

32. Thompson VP, Watson TF, Marshall GW, Blackman BRK, Stansbury JW and Schandler LS. Outside-the-(cavity-prep)-box-thinking. Adv. Dent. Res. 2013;25:24–32.

33. Young DA, Novy BB, Zeller GG, Hale R, Hart TC Truelove EL: American Dental Association Caries Classification System for Clinical Practice. JADA, 2015;146:79–86.

34. Sikri V. Is it necessary to change Black's classification? J. Conservat. Dent. 1999;2:35–40.

35. Vieira AR, Gibson CW, Deeley K, Xue H and Li Y. Weaker Dental enamel explains dental decay. PLoS ONE. 2015,10: e0124236. doi:10:1371/journal.pone.0124236

36. Warren JA. Coming to terms with terminology. Oper. Dent.: 1998;23:105–7.

2

History of
Dental Caries

The study of human remains deriving information about the lifestyle of the population is referred to as Bioanthropology. A few authors do refer the same as Bioarchaeology. Tooth decay has been present throughout human history, from early hominids to modern humans. The study of dental diseases is being referred from oral Paleopathology (Paleopathology is the study of diseases in the past societies through human remains and ancient text). The teeth tend to resist destruction and taphonomic conditions better than any other body tissue. From a population perspective this phenomenon is a valuable element for the study of individual's diet, coupled with social and cultural factors related to it. Because infectious diseases result from the interaction between host and agent, supported by ecological environments, the comparative study of the prevalence of diseases in past populations may provide significant information about the etiology and the associated factors.

Out of dental diseases, caries is easily observable in human remains retrieved from archaeological excavations. Because of non-lethal nature and long time in the development, the caries presented at the time of the death remain recognizable indefinitely. And also the types of food consumed, the cooking technology, the relative frequency of consumption, etc. can also be analyzed from these archaeological and ecological data.

After thorough scrutinizing the available data, it is hypothesized that the rate and distribution of caries observed nowadays are the result of the change in dietary habits which can be linked to the western civilization. The routinely used terms in caries are explained for convenience. Caries prevalence is defined as the number of individuals in a population affected by caries in a specific time span, whereas Caries frequency is defined as the number of teeth affected for caries divided by the total number of teeth observed in an individual or population.

Caries is a very old disease of the human species. Evidences of lesions compatible with caries have been observed in creatures as old as Paleozoic fishes (570–250 million years), Mesozoic herbivores dinosaurs (245–65 million years), pre-hominines of the Eocene (60–25 million years) and Miocenic (25–5 million years), Pliocenic (5–1.6 million years), Australo-pithecines (1.6–0.01 million years) and Neolithic (since 10,000 years). Caries has also been detected in domestic animals. Caries was most common in great apes, particularly in Chimpanzees (the diet of chimpanzee is similar to humans). Gorillas which were primarily leaf eaters had a much lower rate of dental caries. The orangutan is intermediate between chimpanzee and gorillas.

Paleodietary could provide substantial data as regards presence of caries in ancestral generations. A proximal groove located in the cemento-enamel junction of bicuspids and molars has been noticed in fossil hominines like *Paranthropus robustus*, *Homo habilis*, *Homo erectus*, etc. In a specimen of *Homo erectus* from Olduvai George (1.87 million years BP), it is observed that the caries lesion could be an erosion produced by the habitual/therapeutic use of toothpicks.

The chronological dating methods use some conventional parameters. BP (before present) refers to a non-calibrated C14 date, calculated assuming 1950 as year zero. The figure is based on the proportion of radiocarbon found in the sample. It is calculated on the assumption that the atmospheric radiocarbon concentration has been the same as it was in 1950 and also the half life of radiocarbon is 5568 years. BC and AD (Before Christ and Anno Domini respectively) refers to a calibrated C14 date (calculated from accurate historical or geological data) in calendar years maintaining the year one of our era.

Interestingly, 75-year-old tooth was found in Malaysian digging. Approximately one inch long, this tooth belonged to a fish eating predator—a member of the Spinosaurid family of Dinosaurs. In another hominine fossil of Western Europe (1.3 million years BP), numerous lesions such as hypercementosis, calculus deposits and wear facet were observed without caries.

The discovery of fire by *Homo erectus*-like species, around 800 years ago, was a biologically significant step. It led to cooking of raw meat and vegetables. The patterns of chewing also changed. The process of cooking made the food safer, juicier and easy to digest. The calories/energy so produced was used to develop the brain. It is hypothesized that people at that time received approximately 50% of its calories from carbohydrates and caries should have been present much earlier in the fossil record. However, caries appeared much later. It is presumed that in the beginning, fire might have been used for cooking meat only and not carbohydrate/starch, etc.

The oldest evidence of caries was observed from a fossil found in Broken Hill, Northern Rhodesia (Zambia) during the exploration of a zinc mine in 1921. It showed extensive dental caries (except for the five teeth, all the rest were affected by caries). The extensive damage was attributed to a diet rich in vegetables. Later it was established that natural sources of carbohydrates could produce carious lesions. Caries have been reported in prime-age individuals of *Pongo pygmaeus* (4.1%), *Gorilla gorilla* (2.7%), *Hylobates* (0.9%) and *Pan troglodytes* (12.7% in juveniles versus 30.6% in older animals).

The Neanderthals (230,000–30,000 BP) showed a high prevalence of enamel hypoplasias and antemortem tooth loss; however, dental caries was rare. The presence of even small number of carious teeth in Neanderthals suggested the consumption of cariogenic carbohydrates despite the hunter-gatherer lifestyle and cold climate existing during the Middle Paleolithic. The Paleolithic or Antique Stone Age was the longest period of human prehistory ranging from 2.8 millions of years to 10,000 BP [The Paleolithic is divided in three periods: Lower Paleolithic (2.8 million years to 200,000 years: the epoch of the hominines and our first ancestors), Middle Paleolithic (the epoch of Neanderthals, from approximately 200,000 to 30,000 BP) and Upper Paleolithic (30,000 to 10,000 BP—the epoch of the earliest modern humans)]. The phase of transition between the Paleolithic and Neolithic is known as Mesolithic. Dental caries were present but still rare among early modern humans. Caries were found among more recent Eurasian foraging people, but caries frequencies remained below 10%.

CARIES AND DIETARY HABITS

The history of dental caries is associated with the rise of civilization and the dietary changes that occurred during industrial revolution. Several archeological studies have confirmed the relationship between high caries incidence and the increase of carbohydrates intake in human populations from the agriculture produce prevalent at that time.

It is reported that in the North America, the number of carious teeth in farmers were three times the number of carious teeth in foragers of prior epochs. The same tendencies have been observed amongst people those who replaced their traditional diets by western ones, during the process of globalization.

Caselitz (1998) analyzed the historical evolution of caries in 518 human populations of European, Asian and American from the Paleolithic era to the present. He observed that during Paleolithic and Mesolithic periods, the hunter-gatherers had less caries and also the lesions progress was slow. Caries indices increased gradually from Mesolithic times to date. He observed that the low indices at Mesolithic times remained relatively constant during the Early Neolithic era (between the 9th and 5th millennium BC). A dramatic increase of 75% in a span of few centuries (4500 BC) has been reported. This phenomenon has been attributed to the change in dietary habits of the population.

The Mediterranean region showed increase of caries between the 7th and 5th millennium BC. In the Indian region, the caries frequency ranged between 1.4 and 1.8%; however, in Harappa (Pakistan—5000 BP), the caries frequency was 12% and the Iron Age skeletal sample from Oman showed 32.4%. During the Chinese Neolithic, the initial phase Yangshao (7000–5000 BP) showed rare evidence of 0.04% caries (mostly on posterior teeth). The Longshan period (4500–4000 BP) presented caries frequencies of 0.30% (mostly on anterior teeth).

The antique reference of caries (dated 5000 BC) noted the existence of a "worm" responsible for tooth pain. More than 3000 years later, written literature was found in Egypt, correlating existence of pulpitis with dental pain. In antique civilizations, caries and other diseases seemed to have caused the same physical and psychological suffering it causes nowadays. The first attempt of restoration was recorded in Egyptians, Phoenicians, Etruscans and Romans.

In Europe, caries rates were almost stable during the Middle Bronze Age (1600–1200 BC) and increased continuously between 1200 BC and 500 AD. It was observed that during the fifth millennium BC, around one-third of individuals were affected with caries. In the Middle and Late Bronze Age (1500–300 BC) the affected proportion of individuals decreased relatively and then rose to 56% in the 7th century AD. This condition remained constant until around 1300 AD, it reached a new peak.

In the American continent, high indices of caries had been recorded around 7000 BC that decreased around 5000 BC. In this continent, the consumption of starchy food leads to the oral pathological profiles. The increase of caries frequency has been attributed to maize consumption, specifically to popcorn. There might be some other potentially cariogenic products such as wild and cultivated tubercles along with sticky fruits.

Late Antique and Early Medieval populations in Europe when analyzed showed high frequencies of caries and overall health deterioration.

During the Roman Age (1st–4th centuries AD), caries affected 71.6% of the individuals. Posterior teeth were mostly affected. The cervical caries was more frequent than occlusal ones. Moreover, occlusal caries decreased with age while cervical ones increased. Caries in Antique populations ranged between 4 and 15%, whereas in the Early Medieval the range was 11.7–17.5%. These changes suggested a significant increase of carbohydrates consumption in the Early Medieval times. The diet of that era included: bread, cereals, pulses, vegetables, fruits and wine, as well as goats and sheep.

In Britain, the diet included wheat, barley, oats, beans, milk, cheese, eggs, etc. In Scandinavia, the medieval diet basically composed of high amounts of dried fish; however barley porridge, cabbages, milk products, meat and beer were also a part of diet. In Spain, Muslims introduced higher consumption of sugarcane and rice during almost eight centuries of Iberia occupation. In that era the cooking techniques using ashes, or consumption of preparations made with unclean flour or non-dehusked grain cereals were common.

The domestic use of sugarcane (8000 BC) was reported from New Guinea (South-east Asia), from there it spread to southern China and India. Sugarcane was taken to Persia during Dario's epoch in the 4th century BC. Greeks and Romans knew it as a "salt from India" and imported it only for medicinal purposes due to its high cost. The crystallized sugar was discovered in India during the Gupta dynasty, around 350 AD. Muslims later spread its consumption in Western Europe after they conquered Iberia in the 8th century AD. In the 12th century, Venice built some colonies near Lebanon and began to export sugar to Europe. Sugar was taken to America in the late 14th century.

During 13th–14th centuries individuals showed caries frequencies of 17.5% (mainly occlusal and proximal caries). For medieval populations of England and Scotland from the 13th–15th centuries, the caries frequency varied between 6.0 and 7.4%, whereas in Croatia the prevalence of caries was 45%. It was observed that Late Medieval populations did not present frequencies significantly higher than Early Medieval populations. It suggested that in a time span of eight centuries, no significant changes in diet occurred.

Several studies have concluded that the most common locations of caries during medieval era were occlusal and cervical; whereas, proximal caries were rare. In 10th–11th century, some changes in the pattern of caries as regard to location were noted.

The transition from Middle Age to Modern Age in Europe was characterized by a remarked increase of bread and sugarcane consumption. The purchasing power might have contributed to the increase of caries and other oral diseases during that time. In the first half of the 17th century, caries prevalence of about 60% was observed in the Scandinavian populations. By the end of the 17th century, many kinds of foods such as maize, beans, potatoes, tomatoes, cocoa, coffee and sugar were brought to Europe. The sugar and sugarcane came to the West from India also. Carious lesions were most common in the molars (occlusal and proximal). In these populations, lesions were uncommon in children but appeared earlier in young adults. The increase in the production of refined sugar and the introduction of flour mills lead to the increase in caries in 18th century.

The North American diet included meat, bread, vegetables and sweet-baked goods. Maple sugar, maize, pumpkins and fruits were also used. People used to consume three meals a day. The diet used was having cariogenic potential (A cariogenic diet implies frequent intake of meals with a high content of carbohydrates quickly fermentable (mainly sucrose) with retentive and sticky consistency that may lower pH values and changes the ecology of dental plaque).

The remarkable increase in caries, occurred during the second half of the 19th century, have been attributed to dramatic increases in the intake of sugar and refined carbohydrates. Sugar consumption increased to double or even more in almost all European countries and also the introduction of ceramic mills in North America in 1875 produced flours of better quality that favoured its massive consumption.

The worldwide tendency of caries increase remained constant during the second half of the 19th century and the first half of the 20th century. The preventive modalities against caries did not have considerable effects until the second half of the 20th century. France and England were major manufacturers of toothbrushes in the 19th century; however, tooth-brushing was not an accepted practice and was considered as luxury item.

Early 20th century was exciting for dentistry as a whole. In 1903, Charles Land developed jacket crowns covering the entire surface of the tooth. In 1905, German scientist, Alfred Einhron developed new local anesthetic called Procaine.

Ritter Dental Company introduced Dental X-ray in 1920, which later improved with flexible X-ray head. Mckay in 1930 did research on fluorides and verified effects of fluoridated drinking water on caries. Trendley Dean in 1940 established the ideal fluoride level needed in drinking water to reduce caries without mottling.

Since 1970s, a striking decline in caries experiences has been observed throughout industrialized countries. This might be related to introduction of fluorides (the fluoride contained in water has been recognized as a control factor of caries but high amounts may lead to fluorosis). Fluorosis has been reported in many archaeological studies related to consumption of such waters. Also, the decline in dental caries rate might also be due to improvements in general health. In developing countries the high caries rates were associated with malnutrition, poor quality of life and absence of health services. The hypothesis of an increase in the susceptibility/resistance by genetic reasons or available cariogenic flora have not been sufficiently documented.

In the Western world and in other regions of the globe approximately 50% of the nourishment comes from carbohydrates, precisely sucrose. Until recently, several populations living in isolated areas of the world adapted to their environments and diets. Bacteriologic analyses of their oral flora showed cariogenic species, but those individuals developed few or no caries. However, when those populations modified their diet they started developing progressively destructive caries patterns.

Luis Pezo has quoted interesting story of Tristan da Cunha, a volcanic island in the South Atlantic. Until the Second World War their diet was based on fish and potatoes. Despite their poor hygiene, the majority of them were free of caries. When the war started many factories and military stations were built on the island, which led to change in lifestyle of the population, facilitating the importation of other foodstuff. The deterioration of their oral conditions was evident in the beginning of the 1950s. In 1962, when the volcanic activity obliged inhabitants to evacuate towards England, more than 40% of their teeth were affected by caries or had been destroyed. The notable change in lifestyle of those individuals was diet, with a decrease in the consumption of potatoes and increase in consumption of sugar.

The role of sugar in the caries etiology seems to be confirmed; however, it is disputable if starches play a similar role. Starches may have a relative low cariogenicity; however, it is effective if taken with sucrose. The frequency of its consumption is also important. Thus, starch has been recognized as 'co-cariogenic', especially when it is gelatinized by thermal effect. The gelatinization of starch might be the determining factor of its cariogenicity (During the process of cooking food, the starch granules are disintegrated by heat and mechanical forces. The liberation of these molecules is called gelatinization. The temperature and water-starch proportion necessary to generalization may vary). In general, only gelatinized starches were susceptible to enzymatic breakage (through salivary or bacterial processes) to produce highly cariogenic molecules.

The use of pottery (Eastern Russia, 7000 BC) for storage and cooking is significant for the rise of caries. Until the introduction of pottery, other cooking methods such as roasting by direct contact with fire and roasting by wrapping in bamboo canes were employed around the world, but those methods would hardly result in gelatinization of starch. The cooking of carbohydrates produces an increase in their retentive and stick capacity leading to slower clearance times. For instance, bread starch shows higher clearance times than starches from potatoes or rice.

A few authors opined that cooking can eliminate some protective agents (against the caries) of certain foodstuff. African population showed an increase in caries frequency after the adoption of a colonial diet. The amount of cereals and sugar consumption was the same, however they were refined. The increase in caries was attributed to the absence of phytate, an organic phosphate contained in cereals that can be extracted easily by boiling. It is observed that the softer texture and the elimination of 'protective factors' through cooking increased cariogenicity.

On the other hand, there were some foods that inhibited the initiation/progression of caries. Diets rich in meat lead to low caries frequencies due to the fatty acids' antibacterial potential and their capacity to reduce the adherence of plaque on dental surfaces. The intake of dairy products and fish (foods rich in calcium and casein that can increase urea concentration) modified pH values and the quantity of salivary production, inhibiting the formation of dental plaque. And also, a food rich in polyphenols (such as cacao, coffee and tea) inhibited the bacterial metabolism and stimulates the salivary secretion, thereby preventing caries.

The type of carbohydrate; texture and technique employed in preparation of meals might not show different caries experiences. The effects of non-refined abrasive diet have been observed in Paleolithic and Mesolithic populations. In Neolithic populations the change to better processed diets leads to a low wear of masticatory surfaces, a factor

responsible for early development of caries. Such relation between dental wear and caries has been also observed in fishermen and sailors from the South American Pacific coast from 18th to 19th centuries.

A positive correlation between caries and dental wear, as observed in Mesolithic populations from Portugal and Sicily has also been reported where the consumption of carbohydrates could initiate caries even in attrition surfaces. This phenomenon has also been noticed for the Pecos from South-West USA during the Archaic Period (4000–1000 BC) with caries prevalence of 14%. Thus, the cariogenic potential of natural sugars contained in honey and sweet fruits have been confirmed in almost every part of the world. In general, excessive consumption of refined sucrose or gelatinized starches as etiological agents in caries activity has been established; however, there are many other socio-historical factors, specific for each population that should also be considered before generalizing the etiological evidence of caries.

MISCELLANEOUS FACTORS IN CARIES

The studies carried out in hunter-gatherers and farmers during different periods have documented that women show higher caries prevalence than men.

Studies in the recent past have revealed that physiological differences between sexes have an indirect impact on oral ecology. The saliva's chemical composition and flow are modified in various manners according to hormonal fluctuations associated with puberty, menstruation and pregnancy. These processes create cariogenic oral environment in females than in males. Estrogen levels are positively correlated with caries rates, whereas androgens do not affect them. Studies further revealed that pregnancy reduces the buffer capacity of saliva and produces xerostomia that promotes bacterial growth, increasing the susceptibility to caries.

It has been suggested that the increase of fertility had a significant effect on the increase in caries rates. It is established that pregnancy results in a deterioration of oral health along with a weakening in the tooth structure and subsequent caries development and tooth loss. The tooth loss due to pregnancy is controversial; however, repeated pregnancy might lead to poor development of teeth and also poor hygiene might predispose to caries.

The higher prevalence of caries in women might be attributed to the earlier eruption of the female dentition comparatively exposing the teeth for longer time. It is observed that if the reasons were strictly physiological, then differences between men and women should be universal, but it is not so. In general there are many archaeological studies that suggested the existence of other factors also.

In populations where caries prevalence is higher in women, there is possibility of difference in consumption of foods: men consuming more meat (rough diet) and women consuming more carbohydrates (soft diet). Furthermore, men consume big meals; whereas women consume several small meals leading to susceptibility to caries.

In South American population the carious lesions were much more frequent in males. This pattern has been observed in other samples also. In Andean and Amazonian populations, higher prevalence of caries was observed in women, who were responsible for chewing maize and manioc as a part of preparing fermentable beverages.

It is established that members from different social classes, consuming different foods, may have different patterns of caries. The burials in Copan (Honduras) and Lamanai (Baelize) showed significantly more caries in high-status individuals than in low status ones. It was observed that low-status individuals eat mainly carbohydrates; whereas elite individuals consumed much less carbohydrate preferring protein in their diet.

In Zalavar (Hungary), rich individuals showed significantly lower caries frequencies

(6.4%) than poor people (12.1%). In post-medieval Europe caries affected more the rich class than the poor class due to the regular consumption of sweet foods.

It has been documented that high caries frequencies were associated with poverty and a diet rich in carbohydrates. It is also documented that better economic conditions might also lead to intake of more cariogenic diet. Other socioeconomical factors should also be considered; such as the unfavourable dental development due to malnutrition and hypocalcification that turns tooth much more vulnerable to caries attack. Further, enamel defects may facilitate the development of carious lesions under the presence of cariogenic diets.

The relationship between caries and carbohydrates in the diet was based on the assumption that all these carbohydrates were cariogenic. This assumption inferred that the increase of caries was linked with agricultural produce of that era. However, the lower caries rates observed in Asiatic rice-eating farmers contradicted this assertion.

The clear association between age and caries experience was difficult to evaluate in archaeological populations. Caries progressed with the age and the proportion of teeth affected by coronal or root caries increased with age. In general, caries experience may vary among individuals and may obscure the perception of caries frequencies in whole populations.

Approximately 15% of teeth were lost during the process of human remains recovery. These sockets were difficult to be considered for caries indices because lost teeth could, or could not, have been affected by caries. The correct information could not be ascertained in various archaeological studies.

The new challenge of oral paleopathology is to determine the impact of different kinds of crops and diet on location and extent of caries. The ideal method for paleodietary reconstruction (The methods commonly used for paleodietary reconstructions are: (a) the identification of botanical and zoological macro-remains from excavations; (b) the physico-chemical analyses in bones and (c) the identification of botanical micro-remains from dental calculus, coprolites and artifacts.) is the characterization of specific paleopathological models depicting caries, periodontal disease and dental wear patterns. Caries extent and location along with other oral conditions need to be considered in the context of oral ecology. The observation comparing people living in the same place at different times or groups living in different sites at the same time is more significant than studying an isolated site/population. The knowledge of past definitely make us understand the future in a better way. Last but not the least, most of the archaeological studies have not been documented clearly; and also others do depend upon assumptions. However, as regard prevalence and distribution of caries, the archaeological studies have documented clearly.

Bibliography

1. Anderson T. Dental treatment in Medieval England. Br. Dent. J. 2004;197:419–25.
2. Asbell MB. Research in dental caries in the United States: 1820–1920. Compendium of Continuing Education in Dentistry: 1992;14:792–8.
3. Bailey SE. Dental morphological affinities among late pleistocane and recent humans. Dent. Anthropology: 2000;14:1–8.
4. Bartsiokas A and Day MH. Lead poisoning and dental caries in the Broken Hill hominid. Journal of Human Evolution: 1993;24:243–9.
5. Bernal V, Novellino P, Gonzalez P and Perez I. Role of wild plant foods among Late Holocene hunter-gatherers from central and north Patagonia (South America): An approach from dental evidence. American Journal of Physical Anthropology: 2007;33:1047–59.
6. Boydstun SB, Trinkaus E and Vandermeersch B. Dental caries in the Qafzeh 3 yearly modern human (abstract). American Journal of Physical Anthropology: 1988;75:188–9.
7. Carlos JP and Gittelsohn AM. Longitudinal studies of the natural history of caries II. A life-table study of caries incidence in the permanent teeth. Arch. Oral Biol.: 1965;10:739–51.
8. Caselitz P. Caries ancient plague of humankind. Dental Anthropology 1998;203–26.
9. Clement AJ. The antiquity of caries. British Dental Journal: 1958;104:115–22.
10. Costa RL. Age, sex and ante-mortem loss of teeth in prehistoric Eskimo skeletal samples from Point Hope and Kodiak Island, Alaska. American Journal of Physical Anthropology: 1980;53:579–87.
11. Crovella S and Ardito G. Frequencies of oral pathologies in a sample of 767 non-human primates. Primates: 1994;35:225–30.
12. Cucina A, Tiesler V and Sierra T. Sex Differences in oral pathologies at the Late Classic Maya Site of Xcambo, Yucatan1. Dental Anthropology: 2003;16:45–51.
13. Delgado-Darias T, Velasco-Vazquez J, Arnay-De La Rosa M and Gonzalez-Reimers E. Dental caries among the pre-Hispanic population from Gran Canaria. American Journal of Physical Anthropology: 2005;1289:560–8.
14. Duyar I and Erdal YS. A new approach for calibrating dental caries frequency of skeletal remains. Homo, Journal of Comparative Human Biology: 2003;54:57–70.
15. Eshed V, Gopher A and Hershkovitz I. Tooth wear and dental pathology at the advent of agriculture: new evidence from the Levant. American Journal of Physical Anthropology: 2006;130:145–59.
16. Grine FE, Gwinnett AJ and Oaks JH. Early hominid dental pathology: Interproximal caries in 1.5 million-year-old Paranthropus robustus from Swartkrans. Archives of Oral Biology: 1990;35:381–6.
17. Harris EF. Dental age: effects of estimating different events during mineralization. 2011;24, 59–63.
18. Hillson SW. Recording dental caries in archaeological human remains. International Journal of Osteoarchaeology: 2001;11:249–89.
19. Keene HJ. Dental caries prevalence in early Polynesians from the Hawaiian Islands. Journal of Dental Research: 1986;65:935–8.
20. Kerr NW, Bruce MF and Cross JF. Caries in Medieval Scots. American Journal of Physical Anthropology: 1990;83:69–76.
21. Langsjoen OM. Dental effects of diet and coca-leaf chewing on two pre-historical cultures of northern Chile. American Journal of Physical Anthropology: 1996;101:475–89.

22. Luckas JR and Largaespada L. Explaining sex differences in dental caries prevalence: saliva, hormones and 'life-history' aetiologies. American Journal of Human Biology: 2006;18:540–55.

23. Lukacs JR. Dental paleopathology and agricultural intensification in South Asia: New evidence from Bronze Age Harappa. American Journal of Physical Anthropology: 1992;87:133–50.

24. Lukacs JR. Sex differences in dental caries rates with the origin of Agriculture in South Asia. Current Anthropology 1996;37:147–53.

25. Lukacs JR. Fertility an agriculture accentuate sex differences in dental caries rate. Current Anthropology 2008;49:901–14.

26. Lukacs JR. Sex differences in dental caries experience: clinical evidence, complex etiology. Clinical Oral Investigations 2011;15:649–56.

27. Maat GJR and Van der Velde EA. The caries-attrition competition. International Journal of Anthropology: 1987;2:281–92.

28. Mandel ID. Caries through the ages: a worm's eye view. J. Dent. Res. 1983;62:926–9.

29. Matsumur H and Hudson MJ. Dental perspective on the population history of south east Asia. Am. J. Phys. Anthropology: 2005;32:97–104.

30. Moore WJ and Corbett ME. The distribution of dental caries in ancient British populations. II. Iron Age, Romano-British and Mediaeval periods. Caries Research: 1973;7:139–53.

31. Moore WJ and Corbett ME. Distribution of dental caries in ancient British populations. III. The 17th Century. Caries Research: 1975;9:163–75.

32. Moore WJ and Corbett ME. The distribution of dental caries in ancient British populations. I. Anglo-Saxon period. Caries Research: 1971;5:151–68.

33. Nelson GC and Luckas JR. Early ante-mortem tooth loss due to caries in a late Iron Age sample from the Sultanate of Oman. American Journal of Physical Anthropology: 1994;18:152.

34. Nelson GC, Luckas JR and Yule P. Dates, caries and early tooth loss during the Iron Age of Oman. American Journal of Physical Anthropology: 1999;108:333–43.

35. Pedersen PO. Some dental aspects of anthropology. Dental Record: 1952;72:170–8.

36. Pezo-Lanfranco L and Eggers S. The usefulness of caries frequency, depth and location in determining cariogenicity and past subsistence: a test on early and later agriculturalists from the Peruvian coast. American Journal of Physical Anthropology: 2010;143:75–91.

37. Puech PFF. Dentistry in ancient Egypt: Junkers' teeth. Dental anthropology newsletter, 1995;10:5–7.

38. Richards MP. A brief review of the archaeological evidence for Paleolithic and Neolithic susbsistence. Eur. J. Clin. Nutr. 2002;56:12–16.

39. Saunders S, De Vito C and Katzenberg A. Dental caries in nineteenth century Upper Canada. American Journal of Physical Anthropology: 1997;104:71–87.

40. Stuiver M, Reimer PJ and Braziunas TF. High precision radiocarbon age calibration for terrestrial and marine samples. Radiocarbon: 1998;40:1127–51.

41. Tayles N, Domett K and Halcrow S. Can dental caries be interpreted as evidence of farming? The Asian experience. Frontiers of Oral Biology 2009;13:162–6.

42. Tayles N, Dommet K and Nelsen K. Agriculture and dental caries? The case of rice in prehistoric Southeast Asia. World Archaeology 2000;32:678–83.

43. Temple DH. Variability in dental caries prevalence between male and female foragers from the Late/Final Jomon period: Implications for dietary behavior and reproductive ecology. Am. J. Hum. Biol. 2011;23:107–17.

44. Tompkins RL. Human population's variability in relative dental development. Am. J. Phys. Anthropology: 1996;99:79–102.

45. Trinkaus E, Smith R and Lebel S. Dental Caries in the Aubesier 5 Neanderthal Primary Molar. Journal of Archaeological Science: 2000;27:1017–21.

46. Turner CG II. Micro-revolutionary interpretations from the dentition. Am. J. Phys. Anthropology: 1969;30:421–6.

47. Ungar PS, Grine FE, Teaford M and Perez-Perez A. A review of interproximal wear grooves on fossil hominid teeth with new evidence from Olduvai Gorge. Archives of Oral Biology: 2001;46:285–92.

48. Varrela TM. Prevalence and distribution of dental caries in a late medieval population in Finland. Archives of Oral Biology: 1991;36:553–9.

49. Vodanovic M, Brkic H, Slaus M and Demo Z. The frequency and distribution of caries in the mediaeval population of Bijelo Brdo in Croatia (10th-11th century). Archives of Oral Biology: 2005;50:669–80.

50. Walker MJ, Zapata J, Lombradi AV and Trinkaus E. New Evidence of Dental Pathology in 40,000-

year-old Neanderthals. Journal of Dental Research: 2011;90:428–32.

51. Watt ME, Lunt DA and Gilmouv BH. Caries prevalence in the permanent dentition of a mediaeval population from the southwest of Scotland. Archives of Oral Biology: 1997;42:601–20.

52. Zandona AF, Santiago E, Eckert GJ, Katz BP, Pereira de Oliveira S, Capin OR, Mau M and Zero DT. The Natural History of Dental Caries Lesions: A 4-year Observational Study. J Dent. Res.: 2012; 91:841–6.

3

Epidemiology of Dental Caries

Epidemiology is the study of origin and cause of diseases in a community. The word epidemiology is of Greek origin, derived from 'Epi' means upon, 'Demos' means people and 'Logos' is the study; meaning by the study upon people. Epidemiology is the study of health and disease in a specific population for the purpose of (i) understanding disease dynamics (ii) controlling disease and (iii) promoting health. Epidemiology, a branch of public health, is concerned with human populations and seeks to understand and explain health related problems in a defined community. Clinical epidemiology, however, is patient oriented and is considered as a branch of medicine, which aids in decision making in clinical cases.

Definitions

Epidemiology has been defined by various authors. The accepted definition is *the study of the distribution and determinants of health states or events in specified populations and the application of this study to control the health problems.* Epidemiology is also defined as *the study of the frequency, distribution and determinants of morbidity and mortality in human population.*

Importance of Epidemiology

Epidemiology provides basis for describing disease occurrence in a community. It is also important to public health, because it provides basis for developing, prioritizing and evaluating public health programs. Epidemiology can be used to evaluate the success of the programs. Significant reduction in risk-taking behaviour and incidence of disease or mortality are the useful epidemiological measures for evaluating long term success of a program.

COMPONENTS OF EPIDEMIOLOGY

Three basic components of epidemiology are:
   i. Frequency of disease.
   ii. Distribution of disease.
   iii. Determinants of disease.

i. Frequency of Disease

The frequency implies rates and ratios (prevalence, incidence, etc.) of any disease process. Specifically, when new cases are to be studied, term 'incidence' is applied; and for total new and old cases, term 'prevalence' is used. The disease frequency in different populations or subgroups of the same population is an important step in the development of strategies for prevention and control.

ii. Distribution of Disease

Health and disease are never uniformly distributed in human population. The distribution is concerned with when (time), where (place) and whom (person) of health related events.

When (time): Concerned with behaviour of disease on the basis of hours, weeks, month and years, etc.

Where (place): Provides an idea about the geographical distribution of disease, viz. part of the world, country, state, village, mohalla, etc.

Whom (person): Presents magnitude of disease by age, sex, caste, socio-economic status, etc.

The epidemiologist examines the concentration of the particular disease in one subgroup and also increase/decrease of the same disease over the years. The variations so obtained are helpful in deciding the preventive regimes. This aspect of the epidemiology is known as *Descriptive Epidemiology.*

iii. Determinants of Disease

To determine the answer to 'why', the factors responsible for causation of the disease. The health related events in terms of agent, host and environment are studied. The study of etiology or the risk factors of the disease is known as *analytical epidemiology.* Analytical studies help in developing programs and policies for sound health.

MEASUREMENTS OF EPIDEMIOLOGY

The measurement tools used in epidemiology are rate, ratio, proportion, percentage, etc. along with numerator and denominator concepts.

Numerator: Numerator is the number of events, viz. disease, deaths, births, accidents, etc.

Denominator: The total population or the specific population going to be affected by that event. The purpose of denominator is to express the rate in a manner that the frequencies of disease/event being calculated should highlight the true picture of that particular situation. The denominator should be relevant as to highlight the magnitude of the problem properly. The population at the risk is to be considered, i.e. the population which is susceptible. For example, calculating fertility, denominator should be 15–50 years old women (less than 15 and more than 50 may not be counted in susceptible).

Rate: It is a measure of frequency of events or simply counting of cases in a given population. Rate provides scientific information which can be used for comparisons.

Ratio: Ratio relates to two different quantities, i.e. numerator and denominator are two different entities. For example, dentist-population ratio, male-female ratio, etc.

Proportion: Proportion expresses relationship between a part and the whole. The numerator is the part of denominator. For example:

One-tenth of population is geriatric, i.e.

$$\text{Proportion} = \frac{\text{Number of geriatric individuals}}{\text{Total number of population}}$$

Percentage: A proportion multiplied by 100 gives the value in percentage; for example, 10% of geriatric population.

Morbidity: Morbidity is the term used to describe the percentage of population suffering from any disease, say dental caries, at any given point of time. It provides information whether the individual has the disease or not. The severity, intensity or extent of the disease is not measured. These measurements are used for planning the strategies for prevention of the disease.

Incidence: Incidence measures the rate of appearance of new cases in a population.

It is the number of new cases of specific diseases occurring in a defined population during a specified period of time.

It is the average percentage of unaffected person who will develop that particular disease during a given period of time.

$$Incidence = \frac{\text{Number of new cases of a specific disease during a given time period}}{\text{Population at risk during that period}} \times 100$$

The incidence gives the frequency of new events on the first attacks. It should always include a dimension of time (day, month, year, etc.).

Prevalence: Prevalence refers to all current cases (old + new) existing at a given point of time or over a period of time in a given population.

The point prevalence rate of a disease is:

$$Point\ prevalence = \frac{\text{Number of persons who manifest the disease at the specific time in a given population}}{\text{Number of persons in that population at that time}} \times 1000$$

Sometimes, period prevalence is calculated.

$$Period\ prevalence = \frac{\text{Total number of persons having disease during a specific period (say, one year, six months, etc.)}}{\text{Total population or attribute midway through the period}} \times 1000$$

Prevalence rates are helpful in planning healthcare services. It identifies potentially high-risk population.

EPIDEMIOLOGY OF CARIES

The special considerations to dental caries as regard to epidemiological studies are as follows:

- Dental caries is age related. The prevalence may vary with different age groups.
- Dental caries exists in all populations; may vary in severity and prevalence.
- Caries is irreversible disease. The epidemiological information provides data not only on the current disease pattern, but also on previous disease experience.

- The profiles of caries vary for different population groups with different socio-economic levels and environmental conditions.

That is why the study of epidemiology of dental caries is necessary. The public health dentist needs epidemiological data, which facilitates his fight against caries. The data also help in developing a full understanding of the predisposing causes of the disease and also aid in planning the public programs for managing caries.

Factors Influencing Epidemiology of Caries

Following factors are important for epidemiological study on caries:

1. *Sex:* Girls usually have a higher rate of caries in younger age, chiefly because of the earlier eruption of their teeth and the consequent longer exposure time. Boys have higher caries rate than girls during adolescent (being less conscious for their oral hygiene).

2. *Race:* Racial characteristics affect caries; may get influenced by cultural characteristics and individual habits.

3. *Heredity:* In general, children of parents with low caries susceptibility have lesser carious lesions. Role of heredity has been established in various studies.

4. *Genetic effects:* The amelogenin gene is responsible for X-linked amelogenesis imperfecta. The decreased amount of amelogenin protein leads to disruption of enamel matrix formation, subsequently increased caries susceptibility.

5. *Pregnancy:* Pregnancy usually lead to hormonal fluctuations, salivary alterations, immune suppression and other physiological changes that may adversely affect the host resistance to caries.

6. *Diet:* Diet influences caries prevalence in different ways.

The Vipeholm study observed that the physical form of carbohydrates was more important than the total amount of sugar ingested.

The Hopewood House study observed that dental caries could be reduced by a particular diet, even in the presence of unfavourable oral hygiene.

Other forms of dietary nutrients might affect caries.

Deficiency of vitamins and minerals may indirectly influence caries.

7. *Systemic disturbances:* Systemic diseases may not directly influence the initiation of dental caries. Diseases of nutritional deficiencies and dominant gene transfers may produce alteration in the calcification of enamel and dentin, which may influence progress of dental caries.

CHANGING TRENDS IN DENTAL CARIES

Caries in Prehistoric Man (3000–750 BC)

Dental caries is considered a disease of advancing civilization. Consumption of refined carbohydrates and other processed foods in the more civilized populations might be the reason for correlating caries with advancing civilization.

The prevalence of the disease is proportionate to the stage of civilization for any specified rate.

The prehistoric crania kept in the museums of America when examined, indicated that the percentage of carious teeth ranged from 2 to 7% during that era (Table 3.1).

Caries in Ancient British Populations

In a survey of the prevalence of dental caries according to tooth type and period of history, Moore and Corbett (1971, 1973, 1976) studied dentitions of ancient populations in British Isles, spanning the period from iron age to the 19th century. In the periods from iron age to middle ages, the frequent sites of carious attack were at the cementoenamel junction. By the 17th century, the number of such cavities declined from the preceding periods. In the 19th century, the absolute number of junctional cavities was greater than in the earlier periods, especially in the adult age groups. These changes in the prevalence of caries coincided in their timing and rate with the increases in the consumption of sugar and other refined carbohydrates which probably began in the middle ages and were well established in the 17th century. By the beginning of the 19th century, these dietary trends had made only moderate progress and they became further intensified as a result of the removal of the port duty on sugar and repeal of the corn laws.

Caries in Contemporary Isolated Populations

Isolated populations that did not acquire the dietary habits of modern, industrialized man remained relatively free from dental caries.

In East Greenland, where native food prevailed except at trading posts where imported food was available; Pedersen (1938, 1967), reported that 4.3% of males living in isolated settlements had caries, as compared to 43.2% of a comparable Eskimo population living at a trading post.

The dental caries experience of the Canadian Inuit population (population of the

Table 3.1: Percentage of carious teeth found in prehistoric crania of man (Patrick, 1914)		
Race	Number of teeth examined	Percentage of carious teeth
Asians (Malays, Chinese, Burmese etc.)	2,180	2.0
Egyptians and Africans	3,306	3.4
Polynesians and Australians	2,738	4.3
Central Americans	930	4.8
North Americans	27,362	5.0
South Americans	6,719	5.8
Europeans	3,422	7.0

same culture) during 1969-1973 was increased by 66% in the 4-year period and was most significant in the younger age groups. This could be attributed to the fact that by 1973 there was a major shift from a natural diet to one consisting of refined carbohydrates including snacks, confectionery and canned soft drinks.

Caries in Contemporary Global Populations

The caries prevalence is ubiquitous in modern man living in highly industrialized societies; the caries experience may vary among countries, within countries or even within societies.

It is established that caries prevalence follows definite regional patterns. Caries prevalence is lowest (0.5–1.7 DMF) for Asian and African countries and highest (12–18 DMF) for the Americans and other western countries. Consistently low to moderate caries rates were found in populations of the Indo-Chinese peninsula, Malaysia, central and southern Thailand, India, Taiwan and New Guinea. Only those populations in the western hemisphere who live in areas where water supplies contain significant levels of fluoride have caries prevalence comparable to those living in Far East. The lowest caries prevalence in the USA was found in the populations living in Colorado Springs where water fluoride levels were found to be 1.5 ppm or even more.

WHO findings observed 60–90% prevalence of dental caries globally in schoolgoing children, with DMFT index among 2 years old being 2.5.

In Europe, variations in prevalence were observed with countries such as Spain recording 60% total prevalence with DMFT score 1.52 (Symth, et al 2007). In Italy, the total prevalence recorded was 45% with DMFT score 1.44 (Ferro, et al 2007).

In Saudi Arabia, prevalence of dental caries among 12-year-old was 68.9%, while in Thailand the prevalence was 70%.

In South Africa, the prevalence of caries among 12-year-old was 22% with DMFT of 0.7. In Zimbabwe and Uganda, the prevalence was 27.6% and 40% respectively. Tanzania showed prevalence of 42% with DMFT score 0.7 (Mwakotobe, 2007). In Kenya, the prevalence of schoolchildren (age 13–15 years) was higher at 50% with mean DMFT of 1.8 (Valderhang, 1992).

Decline in Caries Prevalence in the Later Part of 20th Century

The decline in caries prevalence, especially in the western world has been observed by various authors. National surveys conducted by these authors have suggested that the previously high DMF scores in high-income countries were diminishing (Fejerskov, et al 1982, Stookey, et al 1985).

In USA, the decline in caries prevalence was confirmed by results from the various National survey conducted on schoolchildren in early eighties. One such survey found that mean DMF scores among children aged 5–17 years were 32% lower than those in the similar survey conducted ten years ago.

De Paola, et al (1982) surveyed 9000 schoolchildren in Massachusetts (USA); the DMFT was compared to a similar survey performed in 1951. The results indicated 50% decline in the prevalence of caries. Many studies over the years indicated that the pattern of caries was reversing, resulting in fewer decayed teeth and more caries-free individuals.

The reduction in dental caries worldwide was achieved with the use of systemic and topical fluorides, toothpastes, sealants, improvements in diet, oral health education, etc. (International Conferences on Declining Caries, 1982 and 1984).

The reduction of caries has not occurred evenly as regard tooth surfaces; it is proportionately greater in smooth and proximal surfaces than in pit and fissure surfaces.

As caries prevalence falls, the least susceptible sites (proximal and smooth surfaces) reduce by the greatest proportion, while the most susceptible sites (occlusal) reduce by the smallest proportion (McDonald & Sheiham, 1992).

The factors contributed in decline of caries prevalence were improved oral health care regimes, sugar substitutes, better nutrition, use of fluoride dentifrices, dietary fluoride supplements and topical fluoride regimens, etc.

The Global Increase in Dental Caries

An exhaustive review of the epidemiological data from many countries indicated marked increase in the prevalence of dental caries in recent years (Bagramian 2009).

The disparities in prevalence and treatment of dental caries throughout the world remained a matter of concern for public health personnel. The social impact of differences in dental caries for specific groups of individuals is also an important fact. The increase in caries was observed in lower socioeconomic groups, new immigrants and children. The reasons which cause increase in caries are not clear; however, it is hypothesized that these group of individuals might not be able to undertake the preventive regimes (Table 3.2). The World Health Organization's 2003 report on oral health provides an overview of global caries epidemiology. Globally, the caries prevalence in school-age children was observed to be 60–90% and somewhat similar prevalence was observed among adults.

Table 3.2: Global prevalence of dental caries

Country (year)	Age (in years)	Sample size	Prevalence (%)
China (2001)	6	1587	84
China (2002)	5	140712	76
Philippines (2003)	2–6	993	59–92
UK (2003)	8	5580	50
USA (2004)	5–6	1598	50
USA (2004)	17	3249	78
Brazil (2004)	12	1151	53.6
Philippines (2005)	6–12	1200	92.3
Armenia (2005)	12	117	86
Philippines (2006)	6	4050	97.1
Taiwan (2006)	1–6	178	89.4
Taiwan (2006)	1–6	981	52.9
Argentina (2006)	7–9	121	78.5
Mexico (2006)	6–12	3048	90.2
Mexico (2006)	6–9	452	34.7
Norway (2006)	12	48168	59.8
China (2007)	3–5	2014	55
Brazil (2007)	0–5	1487	40
Brazil (2007)	1–2.5	186	20
China (2008)	5–74	350000	100
Turkey (2009)	5–6	542	76.8
Europe (2010)	Variable	2383	Max 62.4 Min 37.6
Russia (North-west) (2011)	15	352	91.8
Russia (2012)	6	532	93.4
Saudi Arabia (2015)	6–12	711	73.0
Norway (2015)	14–72	7519	10

Dental Caries among 12-year-old (Globally)

Most of the epidemiological studies, globally, focus on 12-year-old children, for the purposes of comparative epidemiology. WHO has divided the world into seven demographic regions to study caries epidemiology amongst 12-year-old children (Fig. 3.1). The data of prevalence of dental caries in Antarctica region is not available. Dental caries experience in children is relatively high in the American (DMFT = 3.5) and in the European Region (DMFT = 2.6), whereas the index is lower in most African countries (DMFT = 1.7).

Caries Distribution in 12-year-old (Country wise)

The maps (Figs 3.2–3.7) show a clear pattern of higher caries experience in North and South

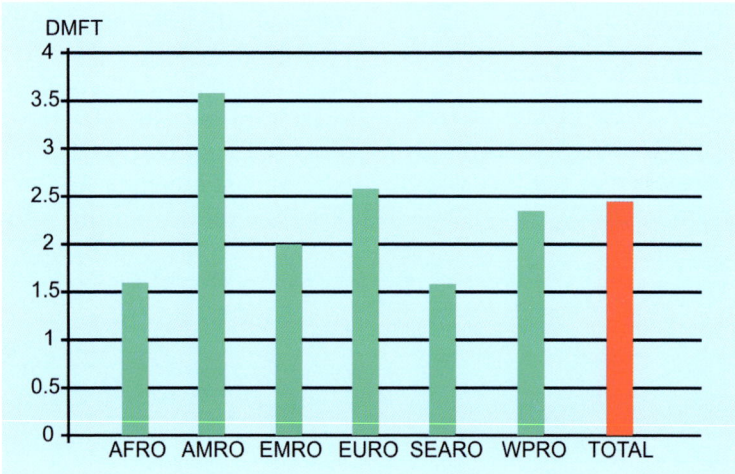

Fig. 3.1: Severity of dental caries (12-year-old children), in demographic regions of the world. AFRO: Africa; AMRO: America; EMRO: Eastern Mediterranean; EURO: Europe; SEARO: South-East Asia; WPRO: Western Pacific

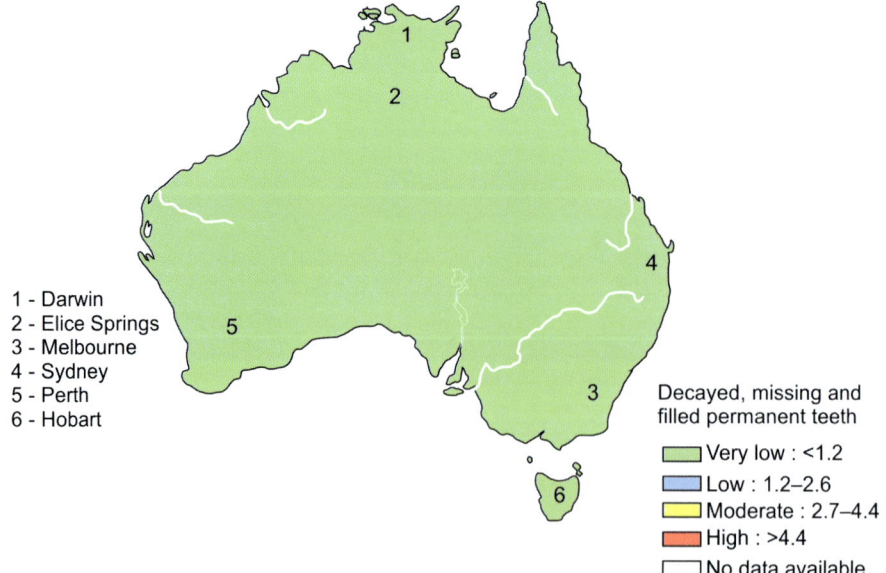

1 - Darwin
2 - Elice Springs
3 - Melbourne
4 - Sydney
5 - Perth
6 - Hobart

Decayed, missing and filled permanent teeth

Very low : <1.2
Low : 1.2–2.6
Moderate : 2.7–4.4
High : >4.4
No data available

Fig. 3.2: Caries distribution in Australian region (12-year-old)

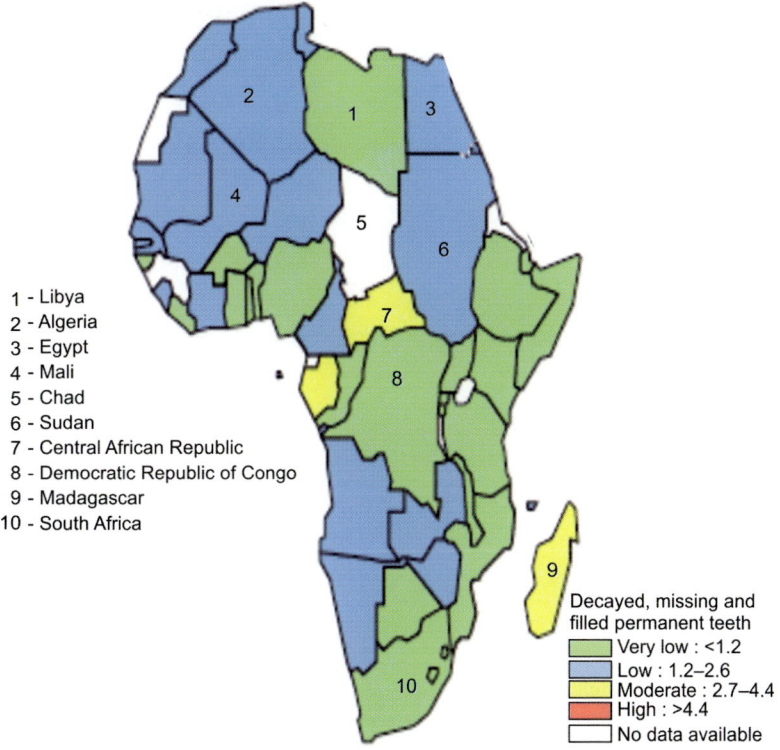

1 - Libya
2 - Algeria
3 - Egypt
4 - Mali
5 - Chad
6 - Sudan
7 - Central African Republic
8 - Democratic Republic of Congo
9 - Madagascar
10 - South Africa

Decayed, missing and
filled permanent teeth

Very low : <1.2
Low : 1.2–2.6
Moderate : 2.7–4.4
High : >4.4
No data available

Fig. 3.3: Caries distribution in African region (12-year-old)

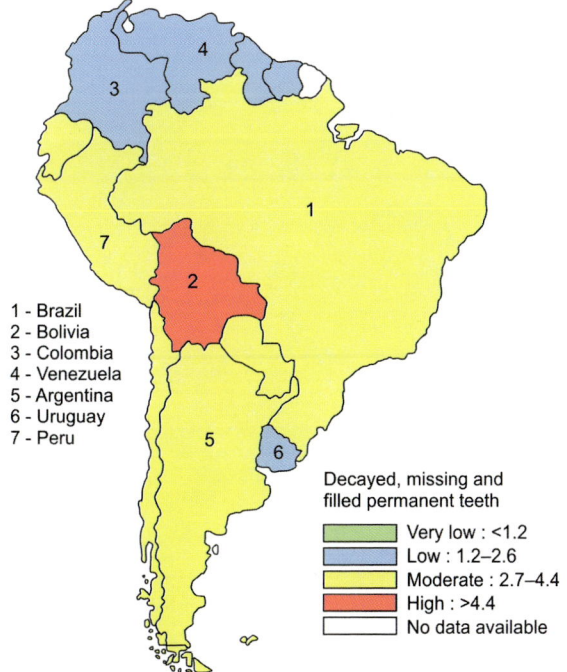

1 - Brazil
2 - Bolivia
3 - Colombia
4 - Venezuela
5 - Argentina
6 - Uruguay
7 - Peru

Decayed, missing and
filled permanent teeth

Very low : <1.2
Low : 1.2–2.6
Moderate : 2.7–4.4
High : >4.4
No data available

Fig. 3.4: Caries distribution in South American region (12-year-old)

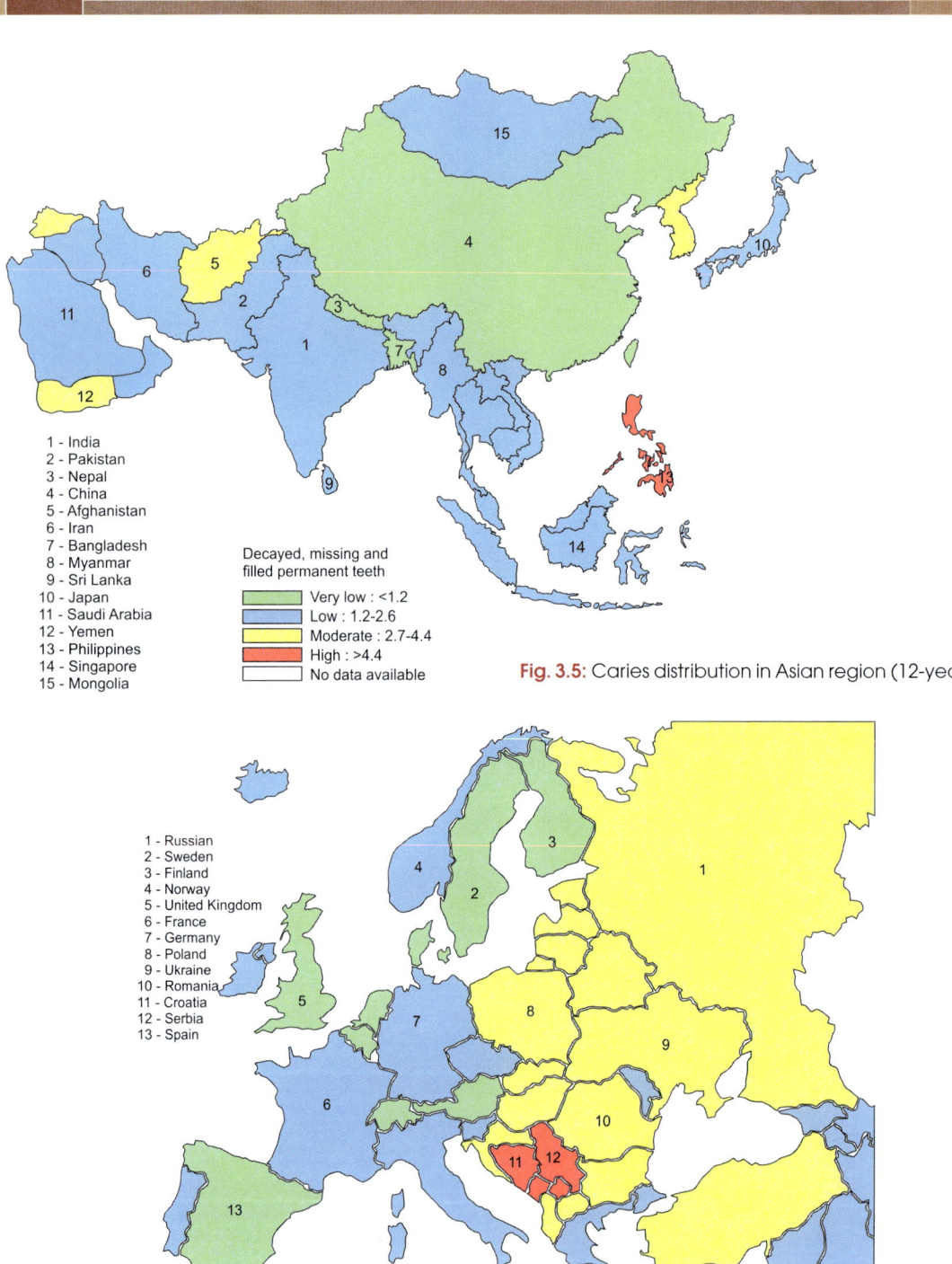

1 - India
2 - Pakistan
3 - Nepal
4 - China
5 - Afghanistan
6 - Iran
7 - Bangladesh
8 - Myanmar
9 - Sri Lanka
10 - Japan
11 - Saudi Arabia
12 - Yemen
13 - Philippines
14 - Singapore
15 - Mongolia

Decayed, missing and
filled permanent teeth

Very low : <1.2
Low : 1.2-2.6
Moderate : 2.7-4.4
High : >4.4
No data available

Fig. 3.5: Caries distribution in Asian region (12-year-old)

1 - Russian
2 - Sweden
3 - Finland
4 - Norway
5 - United Kingdom
6 - France
7 - Germany
8 - Poland
9 - Ukraine
10 - Romania
11 - Croatia
12 - Serbia
13 - Spain

Decayed, missing and
filled permanent teeth

Very low : <1.2
Low : 1.2-2.6
Moderate : 2.7-4.4
High : >4.4
No data available

Fig. 3.6: Caries distribution in European region (12-year-old)

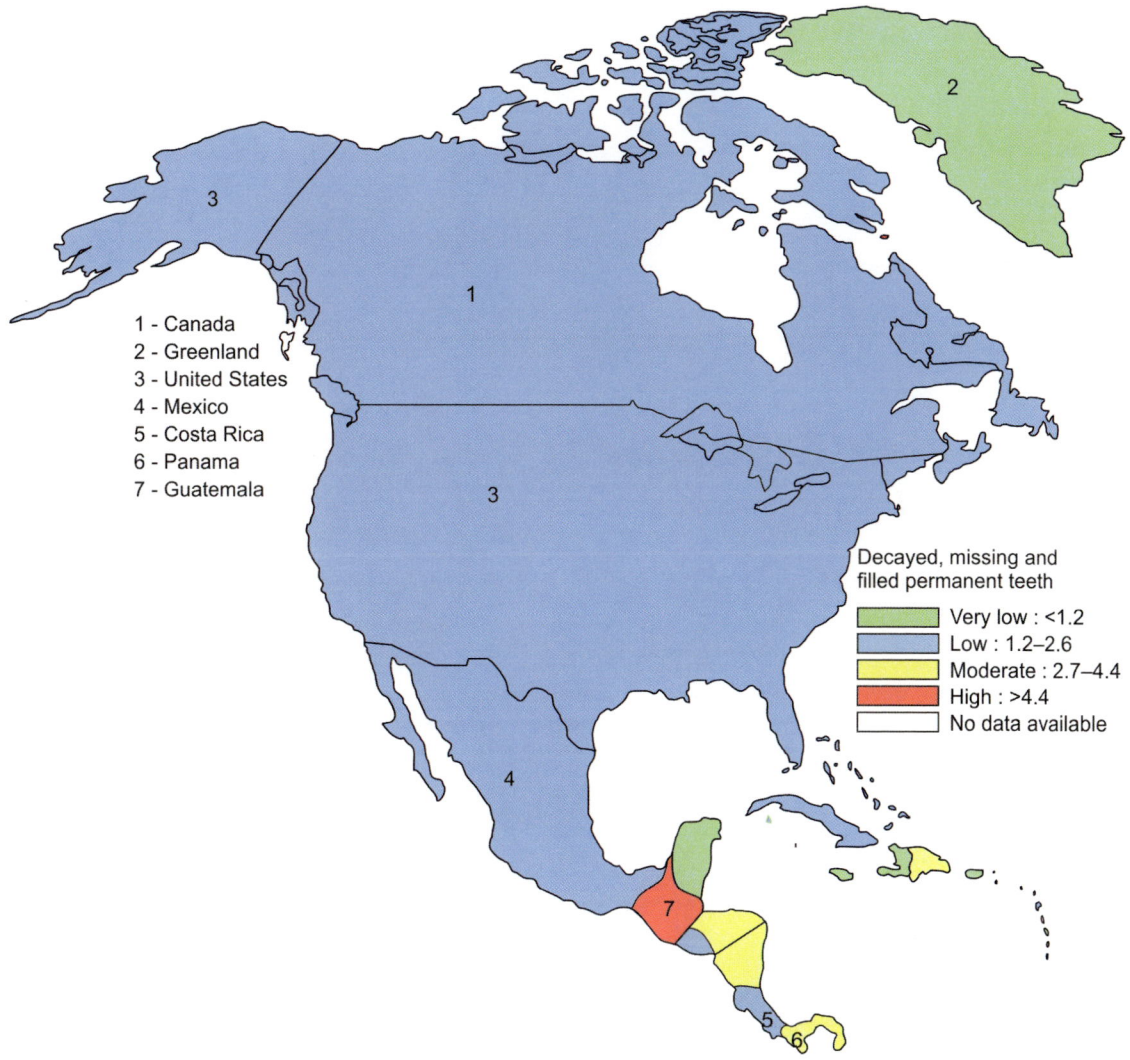

1 - Canada
2 - Greenland
3 - United States
4 - Mexico
5 - Costa Rica
6 - Panama
7 - Guatemala

Decayed, missing and filled permanent teeth

Very low : <1.2
Low : 1.2–2.6
Moderate : 2.7–4.4
High : >4.4
No data available

Fig. 3.7: Caries distribution in North American region (12-year-old)

America, Western Europe and much of Northern Africa; moderate caries experience in South America, Russia and the former Soviet Republics and low levels of caries in Eastern Africa, China, Australia and Greenland. WHO has also observed that developed countries have higher rates of caries experience, whereas developing countries have lower rates.

Dental Caries among 35–44-year-old

The prevalence of dental caries among 35–44 years old adults is high as the disease affects nearly 100% of the population in majority of the countries. The levels of dental caries (DMFT index) among 35–44 years old is illustrated in Figs 3.8–3.13.

Most industrialized countries and some countries of Latin Americas show high DMFT values. The dental caries experiences are much lower in the developing countries usually in several industrialized countries, older people have had their teeth extracted early in life.

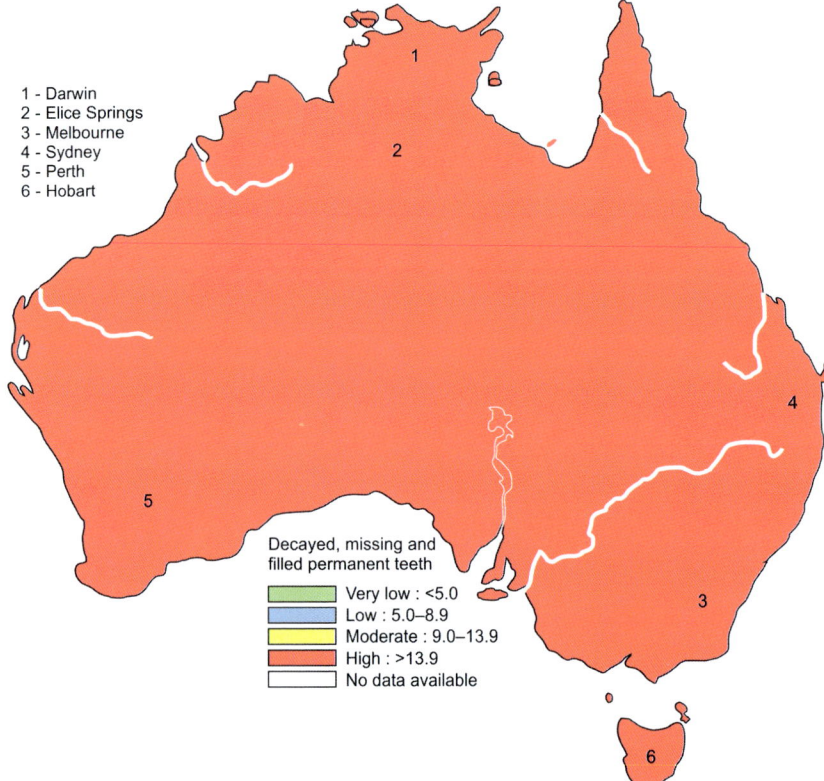

1 - Darwin
2 - Elice Springs
3 - Melbourne
4 - Sydney
5 - Perth
6 - Hobart

Decayed, missing and
filled permanent teeth

Very low : <5.0
Low : 5.0–8.9
Moderate : 9.0–13.9
High : >13.9
No data available

Fig. 3.8: Caries distribution in Australian region (35–44-year-old)

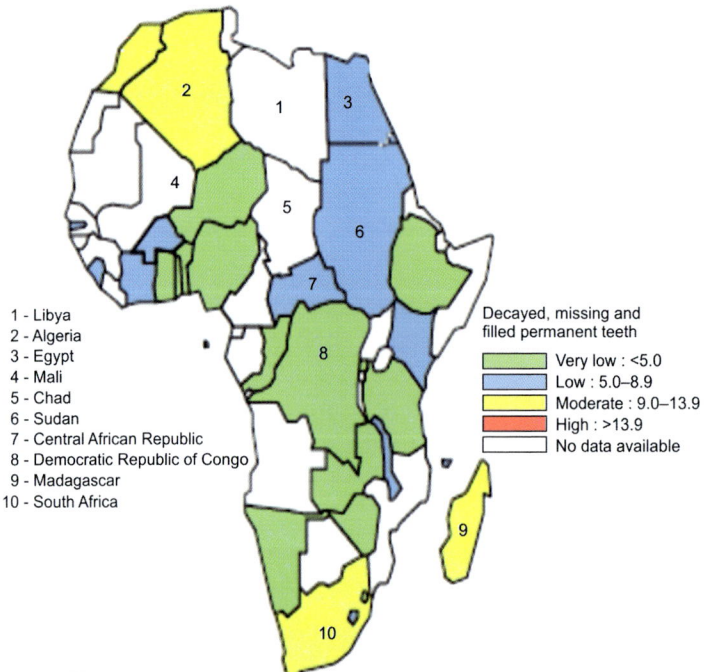

1 - Libya
2 - Algeria
3 - Egypt
4 - Mali
5 - Chad
6 - Sudan
7 - Central African Republic
8 - Democratic Republic of Congo
9 - Madagascar
10 - South Africa

Decayed, missing and
filled permanent teeth

Very low : <5.0
Low : 5.0–8.9
Moderate : 9.0–13.9
High : >13.9
No data available

Fig. 3.9: Caries distribution in African region (35–44-year-old)

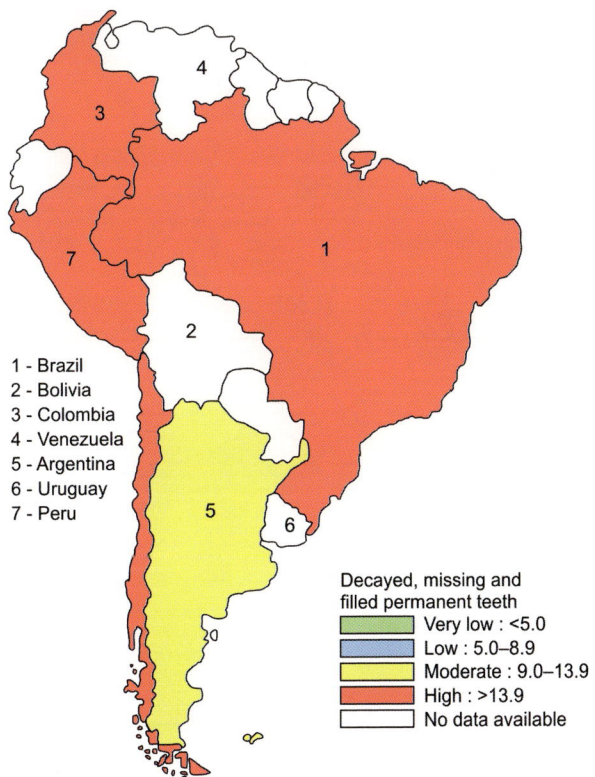

1 - Brazil
2 - Bolivia
3 - Colombia
4 - Venezuela
5 - Argentina
6 - Uruguay
7 - Peru

Decayed, missing and
filled permanent teeth

(green)	Very low : <5.0
(blue)	Low : 5.0–8.9
(yellow)	Moderate : 9.0–13.9
(red)	High : >13.9
(white)	No data available

Fig. 3.10: Caries distribution in South American region (35–44-year-old)

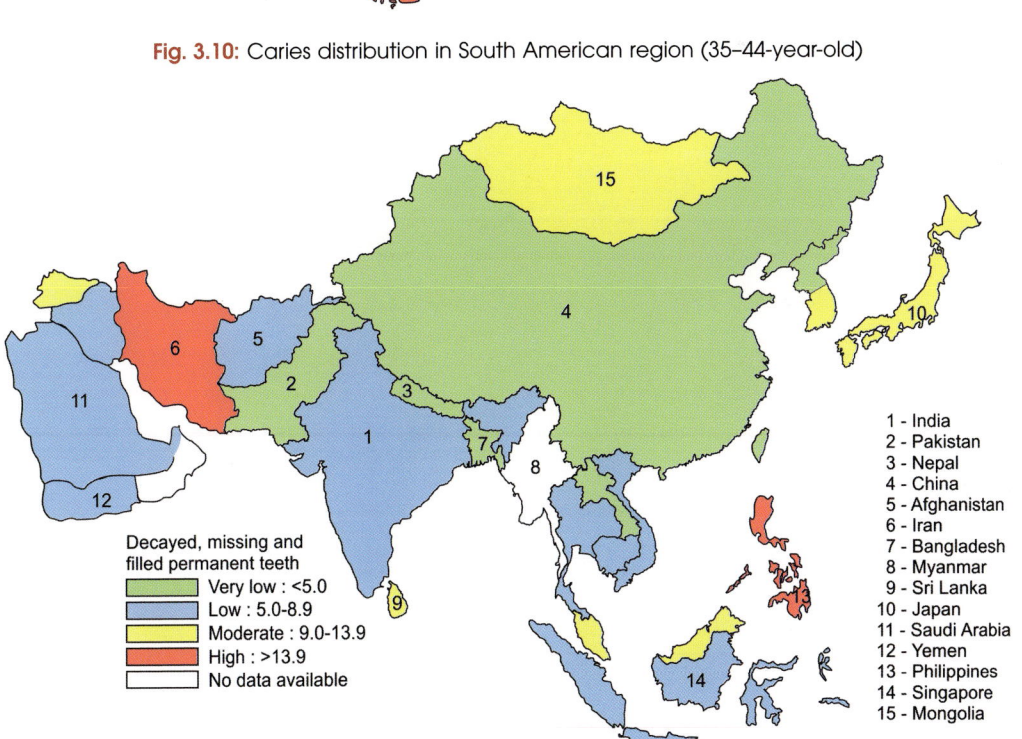

Decayed, missing and
filled permanent teeth

(green)	Very low : <5.0
(blue)	Low : 5.0-8.9
(yellow)	Moderate : 9.0-13.9
(red)	High : >13.9
(white)	No data available

1 - India
2 - Pakistan
3 - Nepal
4 - China
5 - Afghanistan
6 - Iran
7 - Bangladesh
8 - Myanmar
9 - Sri Lanka
10 - Japan
11 - Saudi Arabia
12 - Yemen
13 - Philippines
14 - Singapore
15 - Mongolia

Fig. 3.11: Caries distribution in Asian region (35–44-year-old)

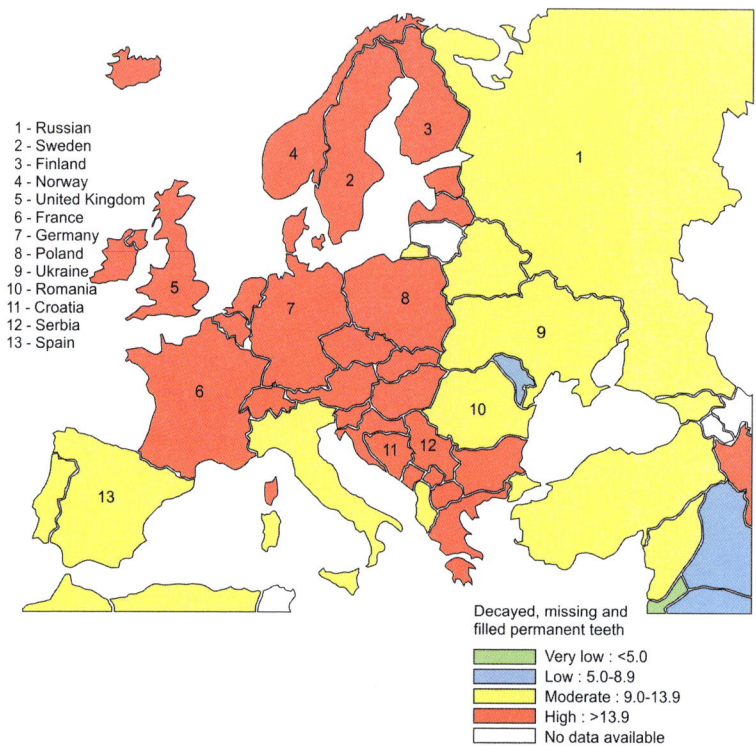

1 - Russian
2 - Sweden
3 - Finland
4 - Norway
5 - United Kingdom
6 - France
7 - Germany
8 - Poland
9 - Ukraine
10 - Romania
11 - Croatia
12 - Serbia
13 - Spain

Decayed, missing and
filled permanent teeth

Very low : <5.0
Low : 5.0-8.9
Moderate : 9.0-13.9
High : >13.9
No data available

Fig. 3.12: Caries distribution in European region (35–44-year-old)

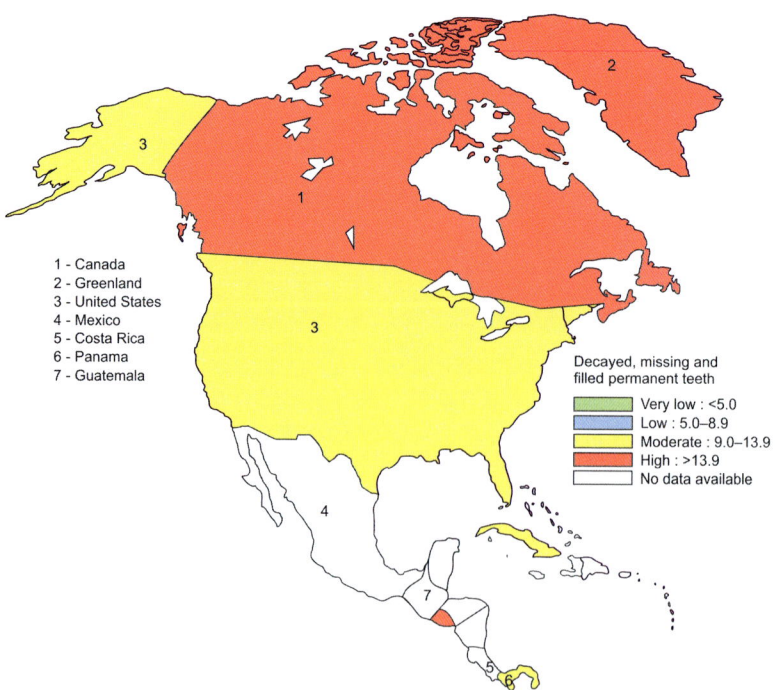

1 - Canada
2 - Greenland
3 - United States
4 - Mexico
5 - Costa Rica
6 - Panama
7 - Guatemala

Decayed, missing and
filled permanent teeth

Very low : <5.0
Low : 5.0–8.9
Moderate : 9.0–13.9
High : >13.9
No data available

Fig. 3.13: Caries distribution in North American region (35–44-year-old)

Distribution of Caries in European Population

The Global Oral Data Bank of WHO provides substantial information on caries experience worldwide. Data for Czechoslovakia and Sweden is not included in the global oral data bank (Tables 3.3–3.9) (Fig. 3.14).

Table 3.3: Changes in mean DMFT scores for 12-year-old in European Union member countries

Country	DMFT score in the 1980s	DMFT score in the 2000s
Austria	3.8 (1984)	1.04 (2002)
Cyprus	2.2 (1990)	0.65 (2003-2004)
Denmark	5 (1980)	0.7 (2008)
France	4.2 (1987)	1.23 (2006)
Germany	3.8 (1989)	0.7 (2005)
Ireland	2.6 (1984)	1.4 (2001-2002)
Italy	4.9 (1986)	1.1 (2004-2005)
Lithuania	4.5 (1983)	3.7 (2005)
Poland	4.4 (1985)	3.2 (2003)
Romania	3.1 (1986)	2.8 (2000)
Spain	4.2 (1984)	1.3 (2005)
England	3.1 (1983)	0.7 (2008-2009)

Table 3.4: DMFT at 12 years of age in Northern countries of Western Europe

Country (year)	DMFT
Austria (1983)	4.0
German Federal Republic (1983)	6.3
UK (1983)	3.1
Ireland (1984)	3.0
Norway (1984)	3.7
Switzerland (1985)	3.0
Denmark (1986)	3.0
Finland (1987)	1.7
Belgium (1988)	3.1
Netherland (1988)	2.5
Sweden (1988)	2.6

Table 3.5: DMFT score in Southern countries of Western Europe

Country (year)	DMFT
Portugal (1984)	3.8
Greece (1985)	4.4
Italy (1985)	3.0
Spain (1985)	4.2
Melta (1986)	1.6
France (1987)	4.2

It is seen that for these countries DMFT are higher than those for Northern Europe. The global oral data bank recorded a 2.7 DMFT for the Spanish province of Andalusia. The differences between the north and south areas might be because the use of fluoride dentifrice was less popular in Southern than in Northern Western Europe.

Table 3.6: Mean DMFT of 12-year-old children in Central and Eastern Europe

Country (year)	DMFT
Albania (2000)	3.0
Belarus (20000	2.7
Bosnia & Herzegovina (1997)	6.2
Bulgaria (2000)	4.4
Croatia (1999)	3.5
Czech Rep. (2002)	2.5
Estonia (1998)	2.7
Georgia (1990)	2.4
Hungary (1996)	3.8
Latvia (2002)	3.5
Lithuania (2001)	3.6
Macedonia (1999)	3.0
Moldova (1992)	2.3
Poland (2000)	3.8
Romania (1998)	7.3
Russia (1995)	3.7
Slovakia (1998)	4.3
Slovenia (1998)	1.8
Ukraine (1992)	4.4

Table 3.7: DMFT score at 12 years of age in different regions of UK

Region (year)	DMFT
England (1983)	2.9
Wales (2005)	3.3
	1.0
Scotland (2012)	4.5
	1.3
Northern Ireland (2002)	4.8
	3.6
United Kingdom (1999)	3.1
	1.5

Caries Prevalence in Netherlands

It is observed that mean DMFT levels remained around 3 in the Netherland regions. The highest value of 6.3 observed for the German

Federal Republic might be due to small sample from the city of Hamburg. The DMFT of 3.0 for Ireland was a mean value calculated from pooled data for fluoridated (dmft = 2.6) and non-fluoridated (dmft = 3.2) areas. It is noteworthy that Finland registered an exceptionally low DMFT of 1.7. No data were available for Luxemburg.

Caries Prevalence in Finland

Drinking water is not fluoridated in Finland and the level of fluoride in drinking water in most parts of the country varies between 0 and 0.3 mg/liter. The level is high (> 0.8 mg/liter) only in south eastern and south western regions. In urban areas, a significantly bigger proportion of conscripts (67.8%) had a mean DMFT ≤ 4 compared to rural areas (61.1%). The difference between urban (DMF = 0) and rural (DMF > 9) areas was most distinct. Of the conscripts from urban areas, 59.4% had no cariological treatment need, whereas the respective figure in the rural areas was almost 7% lower.

Table 3.8: DMFT score in Soviet Union

Country (year)	DMFT
Russia (1984)	4.04
Russia (2011)	4.9
Ukraine (1985)	4.7
Ukraine (2012)	2.7
Byelorussia (1986)	3.6
Byelorussia (2011)	2.1
Georgia (1986)	2.1
Moldavia (1986)	1.3
Latvia (1987)	6.7
Latvia (2003)	3.1

Caries Distribution in Urban Versus Rural Population

A prominent feature of urbanization is the increase in consumption of processed foods, particularly sugar. This accounts for the higher caries prevalence in urban than in rural areas in developing countries.

Variation in DMFT at 12 years of age in Urban and Rural areas of selected European countries and Soviet Republics is given in Table 3.9.

Table 3.9: DMFT of 12-year-old in Urban and Rural areas of European countries and Soviet Republic

Country (year)	Urban	Rural
Portugal (1984)	3.8	3.6
Portugal (1999)	2.4	2.2
Spain (1985)	4.7	4.5
Spain (2008)	2.6	2.8
Hungary (1985)	4.6	5.4
Hungary (2004)	2.9	3.0
Byelorussia (1986)	3.4	4.0
Byelorussia (2009)	1.9	2.2
Georgia (1986)	2.5	1.8
Moldavia (1986)	1.8	0.9
Latvia (1987)	7.0	6.5

Distribution of Caries in Canadian Population

The Canadian population is divided into 10 provinces; each province has complete control over all matters pertaining to public education and health. A national dental survey and comprehensive nation-wide dental statistics are not available in Canada. The provincial data is available, estimating dental health for selected Canadian population.

Caries Experience in 13–14-year-old Canadian Children

The data regarding caries experience in the provinces of British Columbia, Alberta and Ontario has DMFT scores of approximately 3 or less in 13-year-old children. In Saskatchewan, 13-year-old had a DMFT of 4.0. The other six provinces have mean DMFT scores between 5.0 and 6.0.

Dental caries in Canada has fallen substantially (studies during the period of 1958-87); but it increased (studies in the year 2004) due to significant changes in dietary pattern (Sabrina Peressini, 2004).

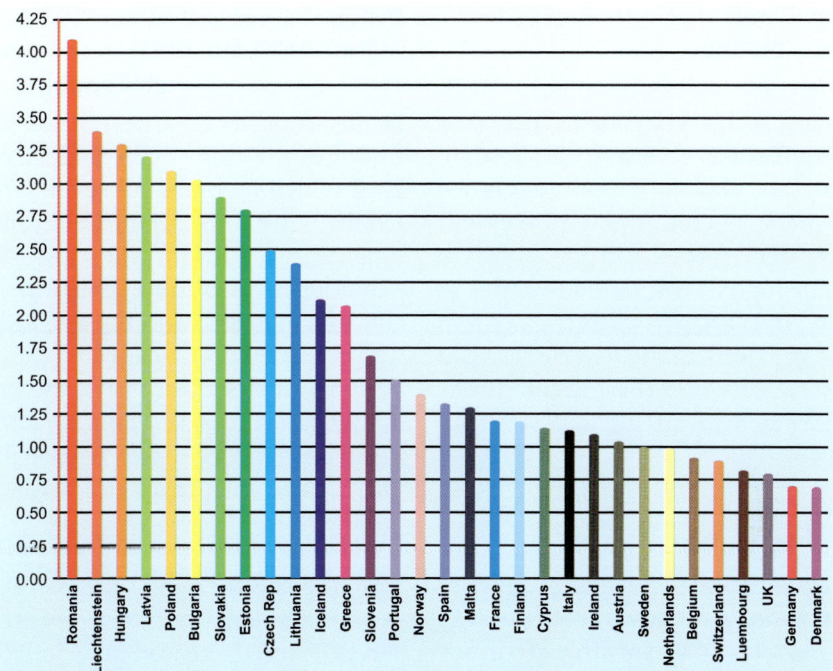

Fig. 3.14: Mean DMFT values in 12-year-old in EU/EEA (*Source:* European dentists manual of dental practice 2014 (5th edition))

Caries Distribution in United States of America

In the United States of America, during late eighteenth and early nineteenth century, mostly the population had defective or deficient teeth.

A study conducted in 1920 on more than 12,000 people revealed that those aged 20–24 years had more than half of their teeth affected by caries.

Table 3.10 reveals the enormous decrease in aggregate caries experience amongst US schoolchildren over the years. In every age group, the DMFS index is less than half of what was approximately 15 years before.

In 1960, white children aged 6–11 years had a significantly higher DMFT than non-whites. The difference between the two groups had shrunk by 1976 and in 1986, the difference was essentially non-existing.

Caries distributions by tooth surface among United States children according to various studies is tabulated in Table 3.11.

Table 3.10: Age-specific DMFS levels in USA

Age (years)	1971-76	1979-80	1986-87
5	0.15	0.11	0.07
6	0.41	0.20	0.13
7	0.69	0.58	0.41
8	1.86	1.25	0.71
9	3.59	1.90	1.14
10	4.14	2.60	1.69
11	4.58	3.00	2.33
12	6.36	4.18	2.66
13	8.67	5.41	3.76
14	9.60	6.53	4.68
15	11.67	8.07	5.71
16	15.12	9.58	6.68
17	16.90	11.04	8.04

Table 3.11: Caries distribution by tooth surface among Children of the United States of America

Study	Age	DMFS
NCHS 1971-74	5–17	7.1
NIDR 1979-80	5–17	4.8
NIDR 1986-87	5–17	3.1

Distribution of Caries in Arab League Countries

Countries in the Arab League are Algeria, Chad, Egypt, Ethiopia, Liberia, Mauritania, Morocco, Somalia, Sudan, Tunisia, Bahrain, Iraq, Jordan, Kuwait, Lebanon, Oman, Palestine, Qatar, Saudi Arabia, Syria, United Arab Emirates and Yemen. The incidence of caries in primary teeth was found to be high as compared to caries in permanent in Arab League countries (Khan 2014). The mean DMFT in the 6 to 20-year-old population was 2.4 while the prevalence of caries in primary teeth (dmft) in 2 to 12 years old children was 4.3.

Distribution of Caries in Saudi Arabia Population

The prevalence of dental caries and its severity in children in Saudi Arabia was estimated to be approximately 80% for the primary dentition with a mean DMFT 5.0 and approximately 70% for childrens' permanent dentition with a mean DMFT score 3.5. Khan, et al (2013) conducted study in Damman schoolchildren (2 to 12 years for primary teeth) and (6 to 18 years for permanent teeth). They observed mean dmft 5.38 and mean DMFT 3.34 in their study. The current estimates indicate that the World Health Organization 2000 goals are still unmet for Saudi Arabian children.

Distribution of Caries in United Arab Emirates

The first comprehensive national survey of oral health on schoolchildren in the United Arab Emirates was done by El-Nadeef, et al. in 2001-2002 which included all seven emirates (Abu Dhabi, Dubai, Sharjah, Umm al-Aaiwaibn, Fujairah, Ajman and Ra's al-Khaimah). The prevalence of dental caries in 5 years old children was 83% and the average dmft score was 5.1. In the 12-year-old group, where all permanent teeth were new, the prevalence of dental caries was 54% and the DMFT 1.6. The mean dmft in 5-year-old children in Abu Dhabi was 5.1 and the prevalence was 80–95%.

Distribution of Caries in Australia

The mean decayed, missing and filled deciduous teeth (dmft) for 6 years children was 3 in 1977 and decreased to 1.6 in 1996. Decayed, missing and filled permanent teeth (DMFT) for 12-year-old decreased from 4.8 in 1977 to 0.89 in 1998. However, since the mid to late 1990s, 6-year-old dmft increased by 24 percent and 12-year-old DMFT increased by almost 15 percent. Improvements in the oral health of Australian children halted during the mid 1990s after which caries experience had increased caries prevalence (DMFT and dmft) in permanent dentition of Australian Aboriginal children given in Table 3.12.

Table 3.12: Caries prevalence (DMFT and dmft) in permanent dentition of Australian Aboriginal children

State (Year)	Age (Years)	Location	Total number	DMFT	dmft
Western Australia (1963)	12	Rural-NF	15	2.13	1.50
Western Australia (1968)	12	Rural-NF	4	9.75	2.29
New South Wales (1983)	12	Rural - NF	62	2.20	4.60
Northern Territory (1992)	12	Overall	407	1.20	3.20
South Australia (2001)	12	Overall	nr	1.13	1.80
South Australia (2000)	12	Rural-F	125	0.90	3.20
New South Wales (2000)	12	Overall	206	0.87	2.09
Northern Territory (2002)	12	Overall	369	1.13	3.94
South Australia (2003)	12	Overall	169	1.28	3.95
Queensland (2004)	12	Rural-NF	38	3.50	6.63
Australia (2000-03)	12	Overall	752	1.25	3.68
New South Wales (2007)	11–12	Overall	147	1.17	3.04
Northern Territory (2009)	12	Overall	118	3.80	6.20

NF: non-fluoridated; F: fluoridated; nr: not reported

Distribution of Caries in Various Islands

Pacific Islands

Pacific islands region is difficult to define geographically. Islands lying south of the Tropic of Cancer (except Australia) are traditionally grouped into three divisions:

- Polynesia
- Melanesia
- Micronesia

Polynesia: Studies carried out in Polynesia in 1970s showed marked geographical differences in caries experience (Table 3.13). In the Cook Island, the mean dmft for 6 years old in Rarotonga was 0.31 compared to 0.27 in Mangaia; mean DMFT for 12-year-old were 6.13 and 3.12 respectively. Comparisons of two surveys conducted amongst the Tokelau community in 1963 and 1999 reveals that for children aged 5–10 years, the mean number of decayed and filled teeth had risen from approximately 3 in 1963 to 5 in 1999.

Table 3.13: DMFT score of 12-year-old children (WHO, 2008)

Region (year)	DMFT
Cook Islands (1995)	1.3
French Polynesia (1986-88)	3.2
French Polynesia (1994)	3.2
Nine (1984)	2.5
Nine (1995)	1.8
Samoa (1987)	2.5
Samoa (1994)	2.5
Tokelau (1999)	4.8
Tonga (1986)	1.0
Tonga (1998)	3.1
Tuvalu (1986)	2.4
Tuvalu (1994)	2.0

Melanesia: The urban areas of Vila and Santo had mean DMFT scores of 3.32 and 2.43 respectively for 12-year-old. The outer islands of Aoba and Ambryn reported mean DMFT scores for this age group as 0.88 and 0.17 respectively.

The regions of New Caledonia showed marked differences in dental health. Mean DMFT for 11–12-year-old was 5.13 in Noumea, 3.64 in the rural part of the main island and 2.18 in the outer lying Loyalty islands. A survey undertaken in 1995 gave an overall DMFT of 4.09 placing New Caledonia in the 'moderate' category on the WHO scale of caries severity.

The prevalence of dental caries in Fiji was recorded in 1979 as 0.5 and 1.4 for 8-year-old and 11-year-old respectively in an urban area and 0.6 and 21.8 for the same age groups in a rural area. A national oral health survey conducted in 1985/86 revealed a DMFT of 0.6 in 7–8-year-old and 1.1 in 11–12-year-old. This DMFT data puts Fiji ahead of the WHO goals for 12-year-old which aims for a DMFT of 3.0 or below.

An oral health survey carried out in the Solomon Islands in 1970 reported moderate to low levels of caries experience in the permanent dentition and a high caries prevalence in the deciduous dentition. Mean DMFT for 12-year-old was found to be 0.62.

Micronesia: A study carried out on the Gilbert Islands in 1971 (Table 3.14) revealed some of the lowest DMFT scores in the Pacific Islands. Mean DMFT for 11–12-year-old was 0.45 and mean DMFT for 7–8-year-old was reported as 0.

Table 3.14: DMFT score of 12-year-old children (South Pacific Commission, 1990)

	DMFT
Palau	3.7
Marshall Islands	4.0
Federated States of Micronesia	
• Kosrae (main island)	2.2
• Yap (outer island)	0.9
• Gram	1.6

Distribution of Dental Caries in Developing Countries

World Health Organization (WHO) recognizes India, Bhutan, Nepal, Bangladesh, Burma, Sri Lanka, Maldives, Thailand, Indonesia and Mongolia in Southeast Asia as developing and third world countries. Most of these countries are grappling with health problems such as tuberculosis and high infant mortality rates. Oral health is not yet regarded as a priority in these countries. Furthermore, data on dental caries are not available from most of these countries at the national level. However, a few area-wise studies have been conducted in these countries from which trends can be determined regarding prevalence of dental caries as related to time and age.

Distribution of Caries in African Populations

African population spread over 46 countries as recognized by WHO. Most of the studies observed DMFT on an average of 1.7 (+1.3). African region will achieve the goal of DMFT 3 by the year 2050. In this way, at least with respect to decay, the region does not present a precarious scenario. The index ranged from 0.3 to 5.5, half of the countries had an index of 1.3. It was found that Mozambique had a risk of 3.2 times higher than the average for the region. Tongo and Tanzania exhibited lower range than the regional average.

Distribution of Caries in Singapore

Singapore is unique in that it has 100% urban community with majority of the population living in a homogeneous environment. The mean d(123)t (incipient caries, enamel caries and dentinal caries tooth) and d(123)s (incipient caries, enamel caries and dentinal caries surfaces) scores were 2.2 + 3.3 and 3.0 + 5.6 respectively has been reported in the limited studies conducted in Singapore. There was no contributing 'f' or 'm' component because none of the children had any filled or extracted teeth. 10% of children displayed early childhood caries and 38.4% had severe early childhood caries. The mean DMFT scores for various age groups in Singapore [Chang and Tseng (2011)] are given in Table 3.15. Gao, et al (2009) in their study on 1782 children (3–6-year-old) observed that 40% children had caries. The mean deft and

Table 3.15: Mean DMFT scores for various age groups in Singapore

Age (Years)	Mean DMFT
5 (2005)	2.03
6 (1970)	0.41
6 (1979)	0.39
6 (1984)	0.15
6 (1989)	0.13
6(1994)	0.09
6–11 (1970)	2.6
6–11 (1979)	2.1
6–11 (1984)	1.9
6–11 (1989)	1.3
6–11 (1994)	1.1
12 (1970)	2.97
12 (1979)	2.84
12 (1984)	2.47
12 (1989)	1.39
12 (1994)	0.98
12 (2003)	0.54
12–18 (1970)	4.6
12–18 (1979)	3.8
12–18 (1984)	3.2
12–18 (1989)	2.5

defs were 1.54 and 3.30 respectively. They further observed that 16.5% children had rampant caries.

Distribution of Caries in Pakistan

Khan (1992) conducted survey on 12-year and 15-year-old schoolchildren of Lahore (Pakistan). He reported that DMFT score of 12-year-old children reduced from 2.1 in 1979 to 1.2 in 1988. Similarly, 15-year-old showed reduction from 3.2 in 1979 to 1.8 in 1988.

Charmia, et al (2011) conducted study on 419, 3–5-year-old pre-school children, of Karachi. The caries prevalence was observed as 29.1% with mean DMFT as 1.14 + 2.23. The study observed significant relationship of caries with income of the family.

Dawani, et al (2012) conducted study on 1000, 3.6-year-old pre-school children of Karachi. Caries prevalence was observed to be 51% with mean dmft score being 2.08 (males: 2.3, females: 1.90). The mean dmft for

3, 4, 5 and 6 years was 1.65, 2.0, 2.16 and 3.0 respectively.

Shamsher Ali (2012) investigated prevalence of dental caries among 5–14 years old children of Lahore (Pakistan) belonging to poor families. A total of 1673 children were examined. The overall caries prevalence observed was 71%. The mean DMFT score among 12–14 years age group was 3.70; whereas df score in 5–11 years group was 2.98. The study strongly emphasized the need for re-orientation of oral health programs in that locality.

Mirza, et al (2013) evaluated prevalence of dental caries amongst 3–8-year-old children of army school in Lahore. The study showed that only 39.06% students were caries free. The mean DMFT score was 2.69 (boys 3.02 and girls 2.37). 'F' component was very low; only 4.05% had fillings. Significant caries index, as evaluated, was 6.58, showing high caries distribution.

Siddiqui, et al (2013) conducted cross-sectional study comprising of 500 patients from deprived areas of Karachi. The age group examined was 18–35 years. Dental caries were observed in 221 individual from rural areas and 198 from urban locality.

Distribution of Caries in China

China is the second largest country in Asia according to geographical area. It has 56 ethnic groups. Han, the predominant ethnic group, constitutes approximately 92% of total population of 1.351 billion in 2012. The other 55 ethnic groups account for only 8% of total population in China.

According to second national health survey held in China, mean DMFT varied from 4.5 at age 5 (mean dmft), 1.0 in 12-year-old, 1.4 in 15-year-old, 1.6 in 18-year-old, 2.1 in 35–44-year-old to 12.4 in 65–74-year-old. Among adolescents and young adults, caries levels were high in urban areas while caries experience was high for old age people of rural areas. In adults, caries experience was higher in females than males.

A study carried out by MQ Du, et al (2009) on 1080 residents, 35–44 years old (group A) and 1080 residents, 65–74 years old (group B) in Hubei observed the root surface caries prevalence of 13.1% in group A (middle-age group) and 43.95% in group B (elderly group).

A community-based, cross-sectional study, carried out in north-east China on 2376 elderly subjects (age 65–74 years), observed that 67.5% of the subjects had dental caries and also the prevalence was higher in urban areas. Missing teeth accounted for 80.72% and filled teeth due to caries accounted for 2.08%.

An oral health survey was performed between 2011 and 2012 on 833 5-year-old children (Dai ethnic group). Dental caries experience was measured using "dmft" index and severe caries was assessed using "pa" index, modified from "pufa" index. Caries prevalence was 89% and 49% had carious teeth with pulpal involvement. The prevalence of carious teeth was in the order; lower second molars (52%), lower first molars (37%) and upper central incisors (31%).

A similar study was carried on 5-year-old Bulang children. It showed that caries prevalence was 85% and 38% out of them had pulpal involvement.

A cross-sectional survey was conducted on a representative sample of Chinese preschool children (2,014) aged 3–5 years in 2007. Results demonstrated a prevalence of 55% with regular dental caries and 14% with rampant dental caries. Another study in 2005 on 957 children aged 3–5-year-old in Guangxi province observed that 60% children had dental caries and 9–13% had rampant caries.

In 2008, Deyy Hu presented a report entitled *Dental Caries: Trends in China* from a review of 3 National Health Surveys which presented the results from oral health assessments conducted in over 70 provinces and cities. The total number of subjects in 3 surveys was over 350,000 and included all age groups from 5 to 74 years. The results of surveys reported as follows:

The number of untreated caries in the primary teeth of 5–6 years old showed no improvement over the past 10 years. The permanent teeth of adults aged 35–44 and 65–74 years have more caries and less restorations. Root surface caries in the older population has become more common.

Based on standards of National Oral Epidemiological Survey of China and WHO Oral Health Surveys, 1907 Tibetan students from 3 senior high schools were examined for caries, periodontitis, dental fluorosis and oral hygiene status. Dental caries prevalence was 39.96% and mean DMFT was 0.97. It was observed that students had poor oral health practices and unaware of their needs for oral health services.

A cross-sectional study of 2-year-old was carried out to explore the relationship between Early Childhood Caries (ECC) and socioeconomic status, behavioural and biological experiences of children. 394 children were examined with 109 having ECC. The mean dmft score of ECC group was 3.65 + 3.12 with decayed teeth making up 100% of the score. ECC was significantly associated with mother's schooling at child's birth, visual plaque index (VPI) score and *Streptococcus mutans*.

Distribution of Caries in Bhutan

The epidemiological data on dental caries in Bhutan are meagre; one study by Singh (1985) from the capital, Thimpu and nearby Paro has been reported, but no information is available for the rest of the country.

The urban and rural areas are almost equally affected and caries experience appears to be increasing with age.

Distribution of Caries in Nepal

This is a small country in the Himalayan region to the north of India, consisting of three geographical zones, viz. the relatively flat cultivated and forested Terai on the southern border, the central hilly terrain and the high Himalayan area to the North.

The quality of dentistry is poor in Nepal, so is the priority of epidemiological studies on oral health. A few studies have been conducted in major cities of Nepal.

Subedi (2011) conducted study on 5–6-year and 12–13-year-old children in different cities of Nepal. The level of caries was found in an increasing order from Bhaktapur, Lalitpur to Kathmandu and in the 5–6 years age groups, it was found significantly higher ($p>0.01$) among schoolchildren from Kathmandu, with a high significant caries index (SiC) value which may be due to the different pattern of lifestyle, urbanization and more use of sugary foods.

In both the age groups (5–6 years and 12–13 years), no significant difference in caries prevalence was observed in the government and private schools.

Distribution of Caries in Bangladesh

Bangladesh is situated east of India with a meager dentist: population ratio.

Limited epidemiological studies have been conducted both in urban and rural areas. In Dacca, the DMFT at 12 years in 1979 was 3.0 and in 1984,1.5; at 15 years of age in 1979, it was 2.0 and in 1984, it was 1.90. Thus, caries experience appears to be increasing with time in Dacca; Caries scores were higher in the Chittagong area with DMFT of 2.8 at 12 and 15 years, in 1982. Caries scores were lower in the Western rural areas of Jessore, the DMFT being 0.9 at 15 years old and 1.3 at 35–44 years old in 1984. In rural areas of Khulna, the DMFT at 12 years in 1984 was 1.7 and at 15 years, 2.8 which compared well with data from 15-year-old in Chittagong and 12-year-old in Dacca. Rahman, et al (2010) conducted study of 672 children evaluating prevalence of dental caries and observed 44.34% prevalence. The study further observed that prevalence of dental caries was high among children under five years of age.

Distribution of Caries in Burma (Myanmar)

Burma is a small country, situated in the east of India and Bangladesh. It has a tropical climate and an agricultural society, primarily rice eaters.

Ogawa, et al (2003) evaluated 739 individuals of Myanmar (Burma) as regard to prevalence of caries (DMFT score). The age group selected were 12 years, 35–44 years and 65–74 years. The DMFT score of total population was 4.53 + 6.68. The scores for 12-year-old was 0.65 + 1.02; for 35–44 years was 3.97 + 11.61 and for 65–74 years 11.78 + 10.08. The mean number of decayed teeth were higher in rural areas than in urban and mean number of filled teeth were higher in urban areas than rural.

Chu, et al (2012) conducted cross-sectional study of Myanmar (Burma) children evaluating prevalence of dental caries and oral health status. A total of 95 (5 years) and 82 (12 years) children were examined. The mean dmft score of 5-year-old was 0.9 while the mean DMFT score of 12-year-old was 0.2.

Distribution of Caries in Sri Lanka

Sri Lanka is an island situated east of the southern tip of India in the Indian Ocean. It is a tropical country with a population of about 15 million. Limited studies are available on caries prevalence of the province.

Prevalence of dental caries remained high throughout the country. Caries activity have been shown to increase over the years. The national data observed more than 90% of the population affected in the 35–44 years age group, with a mean DMFT of 9.2; the mean DMFT at the age of 12 years was 1.9 and at 6 years the mean dmft was 4.6. The average caries experience was found to be almost equal in urban and rural areas. The provincial data show that caries experience is highest in the central, southern and eastern of the country.

Dasnayke (2002) conducted study on Sri Lankan veddha children (2–9-year-old and 5–17-year-old) and observed 33% caries free primary dentition and 72% were caries free permanent dentition (Mean deft 2.7 and DMFT 0.9).

Perera, et al (2012) conducted cross-sectional study on 410 children between 2 and 5 years of age. The study observed gradual increase of caries prevalence with age (Table 3.16).

Table 3.16: Prevalence of dental caries (2–5 years) in Sri Lankan population

Age (months)	Prevalence (%)
24–29	08.9
30–35	21.3
36–41	29.7
42–47	46.09
48–53	55.2
54–59	68.8

The deft score of total children was 1.41 and significant caries index was 4.09. Girls were having significantly higher caries (43.6%) prevalence than boys (33.7%).

Distribution of Caries in Thailand

Thailand is bordered on the west and northwest by Burma and has a tropical climate.

On comparing the national data of 1963 with that of 1984 it is inferred that dental caries is increasing. (The DMFT was lowest in the north-east province in the year 1963.)

Caries experience in the central, southern and northern provinces was higher than in the north-east and highest in Bangkok province.

The data from the northern region over the years suggest that caries experience is much lower in the city, the DMFT at 12 years in the northern region being 1.4 and that in Chiang Mai 0.48. Two factors might explain this difference. The government of Thailand, in collaboration with WHO, has established an Inter-country centre for oral health in Chiang Mai and has launched a comprehensive preventive and restorative program in the region, whereby people might have opted for preventive regimes. The other contributing factor could be that this area has optimal natural fluoridation.

A national survey conducted in 1994 by Ministry of Health indicated that the level of dental caries was substantially higher in southern Thailand than for other regions and the mean caries experience was higher among urban children than rural children.

Petersen, et al (2001) conducted a cross-sectional study on Thai children (age 6–12 years) and observed that at the age 6, 93.3% children had caries with mean dmft 8%; whereas in 12-year-old children, 70% had caries in permanent teeth and the level of DMFT was 2.4%.

Distribution of Caries in Indonesia

Indonesia is a small tropical country consisting of 100 islands situated at the junction of the Indian and Pacific Oceans. Dental care has been designated by the government as an essential service in health centers and has been made a part of integrated primary health care.

Out of the limited studies, the caries experience was observed highest in Barnco island, whereas it was lowest in Bali Island. The data from Sumatra and Sulawesi islands revealed that the southern parts of both the islands had higher caries scores in 8–14-year-old in both urban and rural areas.

In Indonesia, caries increased with age, with urban areas having more caries than rural.

DISTRIBUTION OF CARIES IN INDIA

India has the vast geographical area with varying socioeconomic, cultural and dietary habits. Out of 25 million population, approximately one-third might not be suitably literate and financially sound. These features may have an inevitable effect upon the incidence and severity of dental caries.

A comprehensive National Oral Health Survey was conducted in 2002-2003 in order to ascertain the oral health status of individual of almost all age groups. The prevalence of dental caries for the various age groups for both coronal and root surface caries was observed as follows:

- 51.9% in 5-year-old children
- 53.8% in 12-year-old children
- 63.1% in 15-year-old teenagers
- 80.2% in adults aged 35–44 years old
- 85.0% in adults aged 65–74 years old

The report concluded and suggested that a preventive program, such as water fluoridation, should be initiated to address the problem of such a magnitude.

Another survey was conducted by Ministry of Health and Family Welfare, Government of India in collaboration with World Health Organization in 2007. The observations are depicted in Table 3.17.

Various studies suggest that oral health status of disabled population is poor. Data of a few studies is summarized in Tables 3.18–3.20.

Table 3.17: Caries prevalence (mean dmft/DMFT) in India (WHO 2007)

Age group (in years)	Percentage	Rural	Urban	Mean
5	40–45	2.0	1.9	1.9–2.2
12	45–50	1.8	1.8	2.3–2.6
15	50–55	2.3	2.4	2.7–3.1
35–44	60–75	5.5	5.0	5.1–5.5
65–74	75–85	14.9	14.7	5.8–6.2

Table 3.18: Prevalence of dental caries in 3–14-year-old handicapped children of Calcutta (DP Gupta, et al. 1993)

Handicap condition	Total children	Children with caries
Deaf and dumb	261	146
Physically handicapped	202	121
Mentally retarded	164	127
Blind	155	101
Cerebral palsy	74	72
Epilepsy	72	44
Down's syndrome	47	28
Cleft lip/palate	36	21
Microcephaly	17	14
Congenital heart disease	15	10

Table 3.19: Dental caries in 12–24-year-old handicapped children of Bombay (JP Bhavsar and Damle 1995)

Groups	Total children	DMFT
Orthopaedically handicapped	109	88
Deaf and dumb	134	78
Mentally subnormal	204	77
Cerebral palsy	77	90
Blind	69	64

Table 3.20: Dental caries in 6–12-year-old disabled children in Chennai (Gardens SJ et al 2014)

Groups	Total children	DMFT
Mental retardation (MR)	132	2.30
MR + cerebral palsy	97	2.01
MR + autism	55	1.27
Down's syndrome	54	2.44
MR + visual impairment	8	1.13
MR + speech and hearing disability	20	2.25
MR + attention deficit hyper-activity disorder (ADHD)	22	1.59
MR + dyslexia	14	2.07

Zonal Distribution

For convenience, the vast Indian population is divided into different zones, which represent population with different cultural and dietary habits.

In the North Zone, the prevalence of the dental caries was evaluated in two age groups: 15 years and 5–6 years. A very low prevalence was observed amongst both the age groups. It was also observed that the prevalence remained static in northern region over the past 15 years.

In an another study, (Grewal, et al 2009), 67.26% prevalence was observed in the age group of 7–9 years and 80.86% in 10–12 years with DMFT and deft of 1.97 and 2.61, respectively. It was further observed that there were greater treatment needs in older age group population.

Abdul Khan, et al (2008) conducted studies in Gwalior (India) and observed higher incidence of dental caries in females than males. The study further observed that vegetarian population were more affected, especially in the age group of 21–30 years (Tables 3.21–3.25).

In the West Zone, the prevalence of the dental caries was evaluated in the age group of 15 years and found to be in the moderate range (1.99). There has been gradual decline in the caries prevalence over the period of 15 years from the high value of 4.7 to 1.99 (Tables 3.21–3.25).

In the South Zone, the caries prevalence was evaluated in the age group of 15 years and 5 years with the prevalence rate in the range of very low to low and almost static over the period of 15 years in (Tables 3.21–3.25).

In the East Zone, the caries prevalence have declined over the period of 15 years and data from these states indicates the prevalence to be very low and low in the age group of 15 years and 5 years respectively (Tables 3.21–3.25).

Table 3.21: Prevalence of dental caries in children below 5 years from Indian cities

Author (Year) Place	Index used	Total number	Point prevalence (%)	Mean DMFT/DMFS
Virjee Aradhya (1987) Bangalore		673	66.3 (4–5 yr)	2.9
Sarkar and Chowdhary (1992) Dum Dum	WHO (1971)	40	0.0 (1 yr)	-
		40	13.2 (3 yr)	-
		50	25.5 (4 yr)	-
Mandal, et al (1994) West Bengal	WHO (1983)	-	52.42	1.86 (3.84)
Sethi and Tandon (1996) Udupi	William (1994)	404	65.5 (3–5 yr)	-
Goyal, et al (1997) Chandigarh	WHO (1983)	135	1.5 (1 yr)	0.04 (0.04)
		128	12.0 (2 yr)	0.3 (0.4)
		120	23.0 (3 yr)	0.6 (0.8)
		111	32.0 (4 yr)	0.9 (1.4)
		124	48.0 (5 yr)	1.5 (2.7)
Kuriakose & Joseph (1999) Thiruvananthapuram	WHO (1997)	600	57.0	2.28 (4.10)
Sharma, et al (2000) Chandigarh	Koch's modified (1967)	139	2.88 (16–18 months)	0.12 (0.29)
		139	13.67 (34–36 months)	0.76 (1.73)
Gautam, et al (2001) NCR-Delhi	WHO (1997)	-	35.12	1.18 (2.95)

Table 3.22: Prevalence of dental caries in 5–6 years old children of different regions of India

Author (Year) Place	Index used	Total number	Point prevalence (%)	Mean DMFT/DMFS
NORTHERN REGION				
Shourie (1941) Delhi	Day and Sedwik (1934)	69	50.8	2.83
Shourie (1947) Ajmer	Day and Sedwik (1934)	178	50	2.1
Gill and Prasad (1968) Lucknow	-	138	44.0	1.1
Tewari and Chawla (1977) Chandigarh	WHO (1971)	65	70.6	2.6
Damle, et al (1982) Narayangarh	Moller (1966)	123	74.0	3.3 (5.3)
Chopra, et al (1983) Amritsar	WHO (1962)	141	61.1	1.72

Contd...

Table 3.22: Prevalence of dental caries in 5–6 years old children of different regions of India (*Contd...*)

Author (Year) Place	Index used	Total number	Point prevalence (%)	Mean DMFT/DMFS
Khera N, et al (1984) Chandigarh	Moller's (1966)	-	90.02	3.26
Khera, et al (1984) Haryana	WHO (converted)	-	60.99	1.19
Tewari, et al (1985) Chandigarh	WHO (1983)	204	59.0	2.26
Tewari, et al (1985) Himachal Pradesh	WHO (1983)	227	53.0	2.0
Mehta, et al (1987) Dehradun	WHO (1983)	-	54.7	2.1 (3.9)
Thaper, et al (1989) Jaipur	Moller (1966)	-	68.6	2.1
Chopra, et al (1995) Delhi	WHO (1987)	381	34.1	1.14
Norboo, et al (1998) Leh	WHO (1987)	62	74.6	4.3 (11.6)
Tewari (1999) Rohtak	WHO (1987)	113	36.3	0.87
Chawla, et al (2000) Chandigarh	WHO (1983)	131	60.3	2.7 (6.10)
Pankaj, et al (2002-03) Delhi	WHO (1997)	113	29.9	1.1
Arora, et al (2012) Greater Noida	WHO (1997)	1031	30.06	1.68
Ramandeep K. (2012) Chandigarh	WHO (2007)	579	-	1.8
EASTERN REGION				
Dutta (1965) Calcutta	WHO (1962)	79	67.1	2.96
Tewari, et al (1985) Bihar	WHO (1983)	212	54.0	1.5
Sahoo, et al (1994) Orissa	WHO (1983)	170	58.82	2.52 (3.96)
Sharma, et al (1988) Shillong	WHO (1983)	180	88.33	6.36 (16.26)
Joyson Moses (2012) Chidambaram	WHO (1987)	-	63.83	-
WESTERN REGION				
Sehgal (1960) Mumbai	-	69	39.36	5.9 (6.14)

Contd...

Table 3.22: Prevalence of dental caries in 5–6 years old children of different regions of India (*Contd...*)

Author (Year) Place	Index used	Total number	Point prevalence (%)	Mean DMFT/DMFS
Tewari, et al (1985) Mumbai	WHO (1983)	220	89.0	5.30
Abhay, et al (2002-03) Bhandara	WHO (1997)	322	78.8	4.2
Madhuri, et al (2002-03) Nasik	WHO (1997)	208	39.6	1.6
Vaishali, et al (2002-03) Ahmednagar	WHO (1997)	316	51.7	2.1
Rahul, et al (2002-03) Amravati	WHO (1997)	285	56.3	2.1
Rawalani, et al (2002-03) Wardha	WHO (1997)	406	38.1	1.4
SOUTHERN REGION				
Gupta, et al (1987) Bangalore	WHO (1983)	100	70.0	1.66 (2.18)
Menon & Indushekhar (1999) Dharwad	WHO (1987)	624	2.56	0.03
Rao, et al (1999) Moodbidri	WHO (1987)	550	75.3	0.2
Gopinath, et al (1999) Tamil Nadu	WHO (1987)	97	36.0	(M)1.36 (F)1.17
Retnakumari (2000) Thiruvananthapuram	WHO (1997)	80	67.5	2.425
Goel, et al (2000) Putur	WHO (1987)	224 109(F) 115(M)	81.25 77.06 85.21	4.86 4.57 4.97
Mahesh, et al (2005) Chennai	WHO (1997)	600	83	3.51
Mahejabeen (2006) Dharwad	WHO (1997)	1500	54.1	2.70
Karunakaran, et al (2014) Namakkal	-	850	65.9	2.89

Table 3.23 Prevalence of dental caries in 12-year-old children of different regions of India

Author (Year) Place	Index used	Total number	Point prevalence%	Mean DMFT/DMFS
NORTHERN REGION				
Shourie (1941) Delhi	-	95	54.8	5.7
Chaudhary, et al (1957) Lucknow	Own criteria	368	32.0	1.15
Gill, et al (1968) Lucknow	WHO (1962)	99	43.3	0.8
Tewari, et al (1977) Chandigarh	WHO (1971)	216	78.2	3.4
Damle, et al (1982) Haryana	Moller (1966)	152	89.5	3.2 (4.9)
Gauba, et al (1983) Ludhiana	Moller (1966)	173	86.1	3.9 (4.6)
Chopra, et al (1983) Punjab	WHO (1962)	255	67.2	1.3
Thaper, et al (1989) Rajasthan	Moller	-	31.4	0.5
Chawla, et al (1993) Chandigarh	WHO (1983)	-	-	1.2
Hariprakash, et al (1993) New Delhi	WHO (1987)	-	87.0	0.86 (1.46)
Norboo, et al (1998) Leh	WHO (1987)	74	43.2	0.87 (1.54)
Singh, et al (1999) Faridabad	WHO (1987)	233	33.1	0.79
Chawla, et al (2000) Chandigarh	WHO (1983)	223	53	1.25 (2.0)
Pankaj, et al (2002-03) Delhi	WHO (1997)	107	44.8	1.14
Grewal, et al (2009) Nainital	WHO (1997)	722	77.7	1.97
Grewal, et al (2011) Delhi	WHO (1997)	520	52.3	0.53
Shweta, et al (2012) Noida	WHO (1997)	-	-	(2.92)
Ramandeep (2012) Chandigarh	WHO (1997)	534	-	0.5
EASTERN REGION				
Dutta (1965) Calcutta	-	116	74.1	2.4
Mishra & Shee (1985) Orissa	-	-	61.1	-
Tewari et al (1985) Orissa	WHO (1983)	174	63.8	2.1

Contd...

Table 3.23: Prevalence of dental caries in 12-year-old children of different regions of India *(Contd...)*

Author (Year) Place	Index used	Total number	Point prevalence (%)	Mean DMFT/DMFS
Sahoo et al (1986) Orissa	WHO (1983)	-	63.8	2.1
WESTERN REGION				
Sehgal (1960) Mumbai	-	144	89.9	5.6
Damle & Ghonmode (1993) Nagpur	WHO (1983)	-	83.3	4.1 (5.0)
Damle & Patel (1994) Mumbai	WHO (1983)	367	80.0	3.8 (5.1)
Rodrigues & Damle (1998) Mumbai	WHO (1997)	358	63.4	1.23
Rodrigues & Damle (1998) Bhiwandi	WHO (1997)	256	55.5	1.08
Abhay, et al (2002-03) Bhandara	WHO (1997)	348	91.4	5.0
Madhuri, et al (2002-03) Nasik	WHO (1997)	210	49.8	1.7
Vaishali, et al (2002-03) Ahmednagar	WHO (1997)	316	39.9	1.1
Rahul, et al (2002-03) Amravati	WHO (1997)	298	42.0	1.1
Rawalani, et al (2002-03) Wardha	WHO (1997)	416	59.3	1.8
Malvannia, et al (2014) Vadodara	WHO (1997)	1539	17.15	0.26
SOUTHERN REGION				
Shourie (1942) Tamil Nadu	Day & Sedwick (1934)	53	55.0	1.5
Rudrigues & Damle (1998) Mumbai	WHO (1997)	-	63.4	1.23
Menon & Indushekhar (1999) Dharwad	WHO (1987)	300	31.0	0.78
Rao, et al (1999) Moodbidri	WHO (1987)	771	67.1	1.29
Gopinath, et al (1999) Tamil Nadu	WHO (1987)	232	61.2	(M) 0.32 (F)0.37
Retnakumari N (2000) Varkala	WHO (1997)	119	67.2	2.067
Goel P, et al (2000) Puttur	WHO (1987)	203 116(M) 87(F)	59.6 62.06 59.3	1.87 2.93 3.13
Sogi & Bhaskar (2001) Davangere	Klein Palmer Knutson Index (1938)	936 107	- -	2.85 (3.76) 3.40 (4.56)
Kulkarni Deshpande (2002) Belgaum	WHO (1987)	2005	45.12	1.18
Mahesh, et al (2005) Chennai	WHO (1997)	600	80	3.94
Hegde, et al (2005) Belgaum	WHO (1997)	400	59.60	2.41

Table 3.24: Prevalence of dental caries in 15-year-old children of different regions of India

Author (Year) Place	Index used	Total number	Point prevalence (%)	Mean DMFT/DMFS
NORTHERN REGION				
Shourie (1941) Delhi	Day and Sedwick (1934)	19	52.7	1.20
Shourie (1947) Ajmer	Day and Sedwick (1934)	-	56.3	-
Chowdhury, et al (1957) Lucknow	Own criteria	107	32.7	-
Gill, et al (1968) Lucknow	WHO (1971)	23	62.0	1.1
Tiwari & Chawla (1977) Chandigarh	WHO (1971)	82	86.6	4.7
Damle, et al (1982) Naraingarh (Haryana)	Moller Index (1966)	230	77.2	2.4
Gauba, et al (1983) Ludhiana Chandigarh	Moller Index (1966) (1966)	101	88.1	5.0
Khera, et al (1984) Chandigarh	WHO	88.12	4.98	1.38
Tiwari, et al (1985) Chandigarh	WHO (1983)	217 205	51.1 47.5	1.38 1.30
Tiwari, et al (1985) Himachal Pradesh	WHO (1983)	178	50.0	1.3
Tiwari, et al (1985) Haryana	WHO (1983)	229	50.0	1.35
Mehta, Kavita (1987) Dehradun	WHO(1983)	202	45.0	1.0 (1.6)
Mehta, Kavita (1987) Dehradun	WHO(1983)	112	38.2	0.8 (1.3)
Thapar, et al (1989) Rajasthan	Moller (1966)	-	77.6	1.16
Thapar et al (1989) Rajasthan	Moller (1966)	-	41.33	1.16
Chopra, et al (1995) Jalandhar	WHO(1987)	150	42.0	0.9 (1.39)
Norboo, et al (1998) Leh	WHO(1987)	70	60.0	1.01 (4.6)
Singh, et al (1999) Faridabad	WHO 1987	207	42.5	1.29
Chawla, et al (2000) Chandigarh	WHO (1983)	155	56	1.12 (1.55)
Gautam, et al (2001) NCR-Delhi	WHO (1997)	2097	23.95	0.53 (0.81)
Pankaj, et al (2002-03) Delhi	WHO (1997)	105	50.5	1.5

Contd...

Table 3.24: Prevalence of dental caries in 15-year-old children of different regions of India (*Contd...*)

Author (Year) Place	Index used	Total number	Point prevalence (%)	Mean DMFT/DMFS
EASTERN REGION				
Tiwari, et al (1985) Bihar	WHO (1983)	160	42.5	1.2
Sahoo, et al (1986) Orissa	WHO(1983)	175	62.3	2.0 (2.9)
Sharma, et al (1988) Meghalaya	WHO(1983)	183	60.1	2.1 (4.2)
Mandal, et al (1994) Calcutta	WHO (1987)	119	21.0	0.35 (0.66)
WESTERN REGION				
Sehgal, U (1960) Mumbai	-	96	86.4	7.0
Damle, et al (1985) Mumbai	WHO(1983)	202	96.0	4.7
Tewari & Mandal (1985) Indore	WHO (1983)	162	68.0	2.8
Damle & Ghonomode (1993) Nagpur	WHO(1983)	-	82.6	4.0 (5.0)
Damle & Patel (1984) Mumbai	WHO (1983)		78.0	3.6 (5.9)
Rodrigues & Damle (1988) Mumbai	WHO (1997)	334	70.4	1.99
Abhay, et al (2002-03) Bhandara	WHO (1997)	244	86.0	4.7
Madhuri, et al (2002-03) Nasik	WHO (1997)	318	44.1	1.2
Vaishali, et al (2002-03) Ahmednagar	WHO (1997)	318	44.1	1.2
Rahul, et al (2002-03) Amravati	WHO (1997)	287	61.3	1.9
Rawalani, et al (2002-03) Wardha	WHO (1997)	417	71.5	2.8
Pratiti Datta (2013) Bhubaneshwar	DMFT (1997)	-	72	-
SOUTHERN REGION				
Shourie (1942) Tamil Nadu	Day and Sedwik (1934)	42	57.0	2.0
Gupta, et al (1987) Davangere	WHO (1983)	98	42.86	1.07 (1.45)
Menon & Indushekhar (1999) Dharwad	WHO (1987)	106	55.7	1.09
Menon & Indushekhar (1999) Calicut	WHO (1987)	-	45.65	0.91

Table 3.25: Prevalence of dental caries in 32–35-year-old individuals of different regions of India

Author (Year) Place	Index used	Total number	Point prevalence(%)	Mean DMFT/DMFS
NORTHERN REGION				
Damle, et al (1982) Haryana	Mollers (1966)	667	61	1.70
Tewari, et al (1985) Chandigarh	WHO (1983)	156	81.4	4.38
Chopra, et al (1985) Jalandhar	WHO(1987)	144	34.72	1.08 (1.97)
Chopra, et al (1995) Delhi	WHO 1987	388	24.5	0.5 (0.99)
Pankaj, et al (2002-03) Delhi	WHO (1997)	1213	78.0	3.9
EASTERN REGION				
Tiwari, et al (1995) Bihar	WHO (1983)	149	69.1	1.75
Sharma, et al (1985) Meghalaya	WHO (1983)	196	54.6	1.18 (3.05)
Mandal, et al (1994) Calcutta	WHO (1987)	118	19.49	0.47 (1.30)
WESTERN REGION				
Tewari and Mandal (1985) Indore	WHO(1983)	66	70.0	3.80
Abhay, et al (2002-03) Bhandara	WHO (1997)	391	88.3	4.9
Madhuri, et al (2002-03) Nasik	WHO (1997)	288	77.8	4.1
Vaishali, et al (2002-03) Ahmednagar	WHO (1997)	316	63.2	2.8
Rahul, et al (2002-03) Amravati	WHO (1997)	308	78.0	3.1
Rawalani, et al (2002-03) Wardha	WHO (1997)	413	83.2	5.2
SOUTHERN REGION				
Ramachandran, et al (1973) Tamil Nadu	WHO (1967)	-		2.88
Gupta, et al (1985) Thiruvananthapuram	WHO (1983)	103	79.61	2.21 (6.34)

Bibliography

1. Al Agili DE: A systematic review of population-based caries studies among children in Saudi Arabia. The Saudi Dental Journal, 2013;25:3–11.

2. Al-Bluwi GSM. Epidemiology of dental caries in children in the United Arab Emirates. Int. Dent. J. 2014;64:219–228.

3. Almeida CM, Petersen PE and Andre SJ, T. A changing oral health status of 6 and 2 years old schoolchildren in Portugal. Comm. Dent. Health: 2003;20:211–6.

4. Antunes JL, Narvai PC and Nugent ZJ. Measuring inequalities in the distribution of dental caries. Community Dent. Oral Epidemiol.: 2004;32:41–48.

5. Armfield JM and Spencer AJ. Quarter of a century of change: caries experience in Australian children, 1977–2002. Aust. Dent. J. 2008;53:151–159.

6. Arora SA, Setia S, Ahuja P, Singh D and Chandna, A. Prevalence of dental caries among pre-school children of Greater Noida City, UP (India). Ind. J. Dent. Sci.: 2012;4:4–6.

7. Bagramian AR, Godoy FG and Volpe AR. The global increase in dental caries. A pending public health crisis. Am. J. Dent. 2009;22:3–8.

8. Bailleul-Forestier I, Lopes K, Souames M, Azoguy-Levy S, Frelut ML and Boy-Lefevre ML. Caries experience in a severely obese adolescent population. Int. J. Paediatr. Dent.: 2007;17:358–363.

9. Bajoma AS and Rudolph MJ. Dental caries in 6, 12 and 15 years old venda children in South Africa. East Afr. Med. J.: 2004;81:236–43.

10. Baume LJ. Caries prevalence and caries intensity among 12,344 schoolchildren of French Polynesia. Archives of Oral Biology 1969;14: 181–205.

11. Bedos C, Brodeur JM, Arpin S and Nicolau B. Dental caries experience: a two-generation study. J. Dent. Res.:2005;84:931–936.

12. Bernabe E and Sheiham A. Extent of difference in dental caries in permanent teeth between childhood and adulthood in 26 countries. Int. Dent. J.: 2014;64:241–245.

13. Bhowate RR, Borle SR, Chinchkede DH and Gondhalekar RV. Dental health amongst 11–15 years old children in Sevagram, Maharashtra. Indian J. Dent. Res.: 1994;5:65–73.

14. Bratthall D. Introducing the significant caries index together with a proposal for a new global oral health goal for 12 years old. Int. Dent. J.: 2000;50:378–384.

15. Brian AB. Dietary patterns related to caries in a low-income adult population. Caries Res.: 2006;40:473–480.

16. Broadbent JM, Thomson WM and Poulton R. Trajectory patterns of dental caries experience in the permanent dentition to the fourth decade of life. J. Dent. Res.: 2008;87:69–72.

17. Campus G, Sacio G, Cagetli M and Abati S. Changing trends of caries from 1989 to 2004 among 12 years old Sardinin children. BMC Public Health: 2007;7:28.

18. Chandra S and Chawla TN. Incidence of dental caries in Lucknow schoolgoing children. J. Ind. Dent. Assoc.: 1979;51:109–10.

19. Chaturvedi TP, Singh RK, Vivek R, Singh A and Mishra CP. Prevalence of dental caries and treatment needs among schoolgoing children in urban and suburban areas of Varanasi District, UP (India). Nd. J. Prev. Soc. Med.: 2012;43:31–34.

20. Dash JK, Sahoo PK, Bhuyan SK and Sahoo SK. Prevalence of dental caries and treatment needs among children of Cuttack (Orissa). J. Indian Soc. Pedod. Prev. Dent.: 2002;20:139–43.

21. Datta P and Datta PP. Prevalence of dental caries among school children in Sundarban, India. Epidemiol.: 2013;3:135.

22. Dhar V, Jain A, Van Dyke TE and Kohli A. Prevalence of dental caries and treatment needs in the schoolgoing children of rural areas in Udaipur district. J. Indian Soc. Pedod. Prev. Dent.: 2007;25:119–121.

23. Dixit LP, Shakya A, Shrestha M and Shrestha A. Dental caries prevalence, oral health knowledge and practice among indigenous Chepang schoolchildren of Nepal. BMC Oral Health: 2013;13:20.

24. Dobloug A and Crytten J. A Ten-year longitudinal study of caries among patients aged 14–72 years in Norway. Caries Res. 2015;49:384–389.

25. Douglass JM, Tinanoff N, Tang JMQW and Altman DS. Dental caries patterns and dental health behaviors in Arizona infants and toddlers. Comm. Dent. Oral Epidemiol. 2001;29:14–22.

26. Downer MC. Changing trends in dental caries experience in Great Britain. Adv. Dent. Rest.: 1993;7:19.

27. Du MQ, Jiang H, Tai BJ, Zhou Y, Wu B and Bian Z. Root caries patterns and risk factors of middle-aged and elderly people in China. Community Dent and Oral Epidemiol (in press).

28. Dummer MH, Addy M, Hicks R and Kingdom, A. The effect of social class on the prevalence of caries, plaque, gingivitis and pocketing in 11–12 years old children in South Wales. J. Dent.: 1987;15: 185–90.

29. Farooqi FA, Khabeer A, Moheet IA, Khan SQ, Farooq I and ArRejaie AS. Prevalence of dental caries in primary and permanent teeth and its relation with tooth brushing habits among schoolchildren in Eastern Saudi Arabia. Saudi Med J. 2015, 36, 737–742.

30. Ferraro M and Vieira AR. Explaining gender differences in caries: a multifactorial approach to a multifactorial disease. Int. J. Dent.: 2010;1–5.

31. Gao XL, Hsu CY, Loh T, Koh D, Hwamg HB and Xu Y. Dental caries prevalence and distribution among preschoolers in Singapore. Community Dent Health 2009;26:12–17.

32. Gauba K, Tiwari A and Chawla HS. Frequency distribution of children according to dental caries status in rural areas of northern India (Punjab). J. Indian Dent. Assoc.: 1986;58:505–12.

33. Goyal A, Gauba K, Chawla HS, Kaur M and Kapur A. Epidemiology of dental caries in Chandigarh schoolchildren and trends over the last 25 years. J. Indian Soc. Pedod. Prev. Dent.: 2007;25:115–18.

34. Goyal A, Gauba K, Chawla HS, Kaur M and Kapur A. Epidemiology of dental caries in Chandigarh schoolchildren and trends over the last 25 years. J. Indian Soc. Pedod. Prev. Dent.: 2007; 115–118.

35. Grewal H, Kumar A and Verma M. Prevalence of dental caries and treatment needs in the rural child population of Nainital District, Uttaranchal. J. Indian Soc. Pedod. Prev. Dent.: 2009;27:224–226.

36. Hashim R, Thomson MW, Ayers KM, Lewsey JD and Awad M. Dental caries experience and use of dental service among preschool children in Ajman, UAE. Int. J. Pediatr. Dent.: 2006;16:257–62.

37. Heloe LA and Haugejorden O. "The rise and fall" of dental caries: some global aspects of dental caries epidemiology. Comm. Dent. Oral Epidemiol.: 1981;9:294–299.

38. Hugoson A, Hellqvist L, Rolandsson M and Birkhed D. Dental caries in relation to smoking and the use of Swedish snus: epidemiological studies covering 20 years (1983-2003). Acta. Odontol. Scand. : 2001;70:289–296.

39. Jones PC and Fatti P. Dental caries trends in Africa. Epidemiol.: 1999;27:316–20.

40. Joshi N and Rajesh R. Prevalence of dental caries among schoolchildren in Kulasekharam village: A correlated prevalence survey. J. Indian Soc. Pedod. Prev. Dent.: 2005;23:138–40.

41. Kallestal C and Wall S. Socio-economic effect on caries. Incidence data among Swedish 12–14 years old. Community Dent. Oral Epidemiol. 2002;30:108–14.

42. Kar S, Sarkar S, Kundu G, Zahir S and Mukherjee, A. Prevalence of dental caries in IVF children of West Bengal. J. Int. Acad. Res. for Multi-disciplinary: 2013;1:173–179.

43. Khan AA, Jain SK and Shrivastav A. Prevalence of dental caries among the population of Gwalior (India) in relation of different associated factors. Euro. Dent.: 2008;2:81–5.

44. Khan AA, Jain SK and Shrivastava A. Prevalence of dental caries among the population of Gwalior (India) in relation of different associated factors. Eur. J. Dent.: 2008;2:81–85.

45. Khan SQ, Khan NB and Arrejaie AS. Dental caries. A meta-analysis on a Saudi population. Saudi Med J. 2013;34:744–749

46. Khan SQ. Dental caries in Arab League countries: a systematic review and meta-analysis. Int. Dent. J.: 2014;64:173–180.

47. Khera N, Tewari A and Chawla HS. Inter-comparison of prevalence and severity of dental caries in urban and rural areas of Northern India. J. Indian Soc. Pedod. Prev. Dent.: 1984;2:19–25.

48. Kulkarni SS and Deshpande SD. Caries prevalence and treatment needs in 11–15 years old children of Belgaum city. J. Indian Soc. Pedod. Prev. Dent.: 2002;20:12–5.

49. Mahejabeen R, Sudha P, Kulkarni SS and Anegundi R. Dental caries prevalence among preschool children of Hubli: Dharwad city. J. Ind. Soc. Pedod. Prev. Dent.: 2006;19–22.

50. Mahesh KP, Joseph T, Varma RB and Jayanthi M. Oral health status of 5 years and 12 years schoolgoing children in Chennai city: An epidemiological study. J. Indian Soc. Pedod. Prev. Dent.: 2005;23:17–22.

51. Malvania EA, Ajithkrishnan CG, Thanveer K and Hongal S. Prevalence of dental caries and treatment needs among 12 years old schoolgoing children in Vadodara city, Gujarat, India: A cross-sectional study. Ind. J. Oral Sci. 2014;5:3–9.

52. Mandal KP, Tewari A, Chawla HS and Gauba K. Prevalence and severity of dental caries and treatment needs among population in the Eastern states of India. J. Indian Soc. Pedod. Prev. Dent.: 2001;19:85–91.

53. Marthaler TM, Brunelle J, Downer MC, Konig KG, Kunzel W and O'mullane DM. The prevalence of dental caries in Europe 1990–1995. ORCA Saturday afternoon symposium 1995. Caries Res.: 1996;30:237–55.

54. Marthaler TM, Menghini G and Steiner M. Trends in coronal caries prevalence in Southwestern Europe. Int. Dent. J.: 1996;46:193–7.

55. Marthaler TM, Menghini G and Steiner M. Use of the significant caries index in quantifying the changes in caries in Switzerland from 1964 to 2000. Comm. Dent. Oral Epidemiol.: 2005;33:159–66.

56. Marthaler TM, Menghini G, Steiner M and Bandi A. Caries prevalence in Switzerland. Int. Dent. J.: 1994;44:393–401.

57. Marthaler TM. Changes in dental caries 1953-2003. Caries Res.: 2004;38:173–181.

58. Meghashgyam B, Nagesh L and Ankola A. Dental caries status and treatment needs of children of

fisher folk communities, residing in the coastal areas of Karnataka region, South India. West Ind. Med. J.: 2007;56:96–98.

59. Mishra FM and Shee BK. Prevalence of dental caries in school going tribal children in Ganjam District, Orissa. J. Indian Dent. Assoc.: 1982;54: 375–77.

60. Mittal M, Chaudhary P, Chopra R and Khattar, V. Oral health status of 5 years and 12 years old school going children in rural Gurgaon, India: An epidemiological study. J. Indian Soc. Pedod. Prev. Dent.: 2014;32:3–8.

61. Morton LM, Cahill J and Hartge P. Reporting participation in epidemiologic studies: a survey of practice. Am. J. Epidemiol.: 2006;163:197–203.

62. Moses J, Rangeeth BN and Gurunathan D. Prevalence of dental caries, socio-economic status and treatment needs among 5 to 15 years old school going children of Chidambaram. J. Clin. Diag. Res.: 2011;5:146–151.

63. Munjal V, Gupta A, Kaur P and Garewal R. Dental caries prevalence and treatment needs in 12 and 15 years old schoolchildren of Ludhiana city. Indian J. Oral Sci.: 2013;4:27–30.

64. Naidu R, Prevatt I and Simeon D. The oral health and treatment needs of schoolchildren in Trinidad and Tobago: findings of a national survey. Int. J. Paediatr. Dent.: 2006;16:412–18.

65. Nishi M, Stjernswad J, Carlsson P and Bratthall D. Caries experience of some countries and areas expressed by the significant caries index. Comm. Dent. Oral Epidemiol.: 2002;30:296–301.

66. Nurelhuda NM, Trovik TA, Ali RW and Ahmed MA. Oral health status of 12 years old school-children in Khartoum state, the Sudan: a school-based survey. BMC Oral Health: 2009;15:15–23.

67. Patel S, Bay RC and Glick M. A systematic review of dental recall intervals and incidence of dental caries. J. Am. Dent. Assoc.: 2010;141:527–539.

68. Patro BK, Kuar RB, Goswami A, Mathur VP and Nongkynrih B. Prevalence of dental caries among adults and elderly in an urban resettlement colony of New Delhi. Ind. J. Dent. Res.: 2008;19: 95–98.

69. Peterson PE, Hoerup N, Poomviset N, Prommajan J and Watanapa H; Oral health status and oral health behavior of urban and rural schoolchildren in southern Thailand. Int. Dent. J. 2001;51:95–102.

70. Prakash H, Sidhu SS and Sundaram KR. Prevalence of dental caries among Delhi school children. J. Ind. Dent. Assoc.: 1997;760:12–6.

71. Psoter WJ, Saint Jean HL, Morse DE, Prophte SE, Joseph JR and Katz RV. Dental caries in twelve and fifteen year old: results from the basic oral health survey in Haiti. J. Public Health Dent.: 2005;65:209–14.

72. Rao A, Sequeira SP and Peter S. Prevalence of dental caries among schoolchildren of Moodbidri. J. Indian Soc. Pedod. Prev. Dent.: 1999; 17:45–53.

73. Rodrigues JS and Damle SG. Prevalence of dental caries and treatment need in 12–15 year old municipal school children of Mumbai. J. Indian Soc. Pedod. Prev. Dent.: 1998;16:31–6.

74. Saha S and Sarkar S. Prevalence and severity of dental caries and oral hygiene status in rural and urban areas of Calcutta. J. Indian Soc. Pedod. Prev. Dent.: 1996;14:17–20.

75. Saimbi CS, Mehrotra AK, Mehrotra KK and Kharbanda O. Incidence of dental caries in individual teeth. J. Indian Dent. Assoc.: 1993;55: 23–6.

76. Saravanan S, Anuradha KP and Bhaskar DJ. Prevalence of dental caries and treatment needs among schoolgoing children of Pondicherry, India. J. Indian Soc. Pedod. Prev. Dent.: 2003;21: 1–12.

77. Saravanan S, Kalyani V, Vijayarani MP, Jayakodi P, Felix JWA, Arunmozhi P, Krishnan V and Sampath KP. Caries prevalence and treatment needs of rural school children in Chidambaram Taluk, Tamil Nadu, South India. Indian J. Dent. Res.: 2008;19:186–90.

78. Schwendicke F, Dorfer CE, Schlattmann P, Foster Page L, Thompson WM and Paris S. Socioeconomic inequality and caries : A systematic review and meta-analysis. J. Dent Res 2015; 94: 10–18

79. Shailee F, Sogi GM, Sharma KR and Nidhi P. Dental caries prevalence and treatment needs among 12 and 15 years old schoolchildren in Shimla city, Himachal Pradesh, India. Indian J. Dent. Res.: 2012;23:579–84.

80. Shammery A and Guile EF. Prevalence of caries in primary schoolchildren in Saudi Arabia. Comm. Dent. Oral Epid.: 1990;18:320–21.

81. Shekar C, Cheluvaiah MB and Namile D. Prevalence of dental caries and dental fluorosis among 12 and 15 years old schoolchildren in relation to fluoride concentration in drinking water in an endemic fluoride belt of Andhra Pradesh. Ind. J. Public Health: 2012;56:122–128.

82. Singh AA, Singh B, Kharbanda OP, Shukla DK, Goswami K and Gupta S. A study of dental caries

in schoolchildren from rural Haryana. J. Indian Soc. Pedod. Prev. Dent.: 1999;17:24–8.

83. Singh S. Dental caries rates in South Africa: Implications for oral health planning. South Afr. J. Epidemiol. Infect.: 2011;26:259–261.

84. Sogi G and Bhaskar DJ. Dental caries and oral hygiene status of 13–14 year old schoolchildren of Davangere. J. Indian Soc. Pedod. Prev. Dent.: 2001;19:113–17.

85. Sonika R, Goel S, Vijaylakshmi S and Goel NK. Prevalence of dental caries and its association with Snyder test among preschool children in anganwadis of a North Indian city. Int. J. Public Health Dent.: 2012;3:1–10.

86. Srivastava R, Gupta SK, Mathur VP, Goswami A and Nongkynrih B. Prevalence of dental caries and periodontal diseases and their association with socio-demographic risk factors among older persons in Delhi, India : A Community based study. Southeast Asian J. Trop. Med. Pub. Health: 2013;44:523–533.

87. Subedi B, Shakya P, KCU, Jnawali M, Paudyal BD, Acharya A, Koirala S and Singh A. Prevalence of dental caries in 5–6 years and 12–13 years age group of schoolchildren of Kathmandu valley. J. Nepal Med. Assoc.: 2011;51:176–81.

88. Sudha P, Bhasin S and Anegundi RT. Prevalence of dental caries among 5–13 year old children of Mangalore city. J. Indian Soc. Pedod. Prev. Dent.: 2005;74–79.

89. Thomas, Raja RV, Kutty R, Strayer MS. Pattern of the caries experience among elderly population in South India. Int. Dent. J.: 1994;44:617–622.

90. Varenne B, Petersen PE and Ouattara S. Oral health status of children and adults in urban and rural areas of Burkina Faso, Africa. Int. Dent. J.: 2004;54:83–89.

91. Vargas CM, Crall JJ and Schneider DA. Socio-demographic distribution of pediatric dental caries. NHANES III, 1988-1994. JADA.: 1998;129: 1229–1238.

92. Vargas CM, Monajemy N, Khurana P and Tinanoff N. Oral health status of preschool children attending Head Start in Maryland, 2000. Pediatr. Dent.: 2002;24:257–263.

93. Walls AWG, Silver PT, Steele JG. Impact of treatment provision as the epidemiological recording of root caries. Eur. J. Oral Sci.:2000;108:3.

94. Whelton H. Overview of the impact of changing global patterns of dental caries experience on caries clinical trials. J. Dent. Res.: 2004;83:29–34.

95. Wright FAC, Deng H and Shi ST. The dental health status of 6 and 12 years old Beijing school-children in 1987. Comm. Dent. Health: 1989;6: 121–30.

96. Wyatt CC, Wang D, Aleksejuniene J. Incidence of dental caries among susceptible community-dwelling older adults using fluoride toothpaste: 2-year follow-up study. J. Can. Dent. Assoc.: 2014; 80:1–7.

4

Indices for Caries

An index is an expression of clinical observations of numerical values. It is usually used to describe the relative status of the individual or the group with respect to a particular condition being measured. Indices using various criteria have been developed to compare the extent and severity of any disease process. These measurements, individually and collectively, aid in assessing the overall status of the health of an individual.

Similarly, the dental indices, considered as the tools of epidemiological studies, are used to assess incidence, prevalence and severity of the dental diseases. The preventive programs are planned and implemented on the basis of such assessments.

The main objective of using dental indices in epidemiological studies is to increase understanding of the oral diseases along with measuring the prevalence and incidence of that particular disease. It also attempts to discover populations at high and low risk of a particular disease specifying problems of that region. The indices must assess the efficiency of remedial measures undertaken to overcome/prevent the disease. The reduction in the index means improved health status.

To understand epidemiological indices, it is important to understand the definitions of the following terms:

a. Prevalence

Prevalence is the measurement of all individuals affected by a disease at a specific point of time. Prevalence describes a proportion (expressed as percentage); For example, the prevalence of caries in Asian subcontinents is approximately 70%. Prevalence is further categorized as *point prevalence* (measure of proportion of people in a population who have a disease/condition at a particular time/date) and *period prevalence* (the proportion of the population with the given disease/condition over a specific period, say one year).

The *point prevalence* of a disease is:

$$\frac{\text{Number of persons in a defined population who manifest the disease (old and new cases) at a given point of time}}{\text{Number of persons in that population at that time}} \times 1000$$

The *period prevalence* (usually calculated for a year) is the proportion of the population manifesting the disease over the course of the year; those already showing at the beginning (point prevalence) plus the new cases and the relapses which might have occurred during that year. The denominator is the number of people in the population that has been studied during that year.

The *period prevalence* of the disease is:

$$\frac{\text{Number of cases that occurred in}}{\text{a given period (say one year)}}$$
$$\frac{}{\text{Number of people in the population}}$$
$$\text{during the period}$$

b. Incidence

Incidence is the measurement of the number of new individuals who manifest a disease in a population during a given interval of time. The incidence of a disease annually is expressed as:

$$\frac{\begin{array}{c}\text{Number of persons in a population}\\\text{who newly manifest the disease}\\\text{during a given year}\end{array}}{\begin{array}{c}\text{Number of persons in population}\\\text{in that year}\end{array}} \times 1000$$

Incidence, therefore, gives the frequency of new events or the first attacks. The more chronic the condition, the greater is the difference between incidence and prevalence.

c. Trend

Trend is the change or difference in the prevalence or incidence of disease with respect to time, location and socioeconomics.

Definitions of Index

An index is defined as 'an expression of clinical observation in numerical value which is used to describe the status of the individual or a group with respect to the condition being measured.'

An index is also defined as 'a numerical value describing the relative status of a population on a graduated scale with definite upper and lower limits, which is designed to permit and facilitate comparison with other populations classified by the same criteria and methods' (Russell AL).

The measurement scales for indices include, 'nominal' (simply name condition) or 'ordinal' (conditions in order of severity).

Characteristics of a Good Index

A good index should have the following characteristics:

- Easy to use.
- Permit examination of many people in a short period of time.
- Must define clinical conditions objectively.
- Should be highly reproducible in assessing a clinical condition when used by one or more examiner.
- Should be strongly numerically related to clinical stage of the specific disease under investigation.
- Be amenable to statistical analysis.

An ideal index is only valuable if the information it provides fulfills the following features:

i. Validity

The index must measure what it is intended to measure and should correspond with the clinical stages of the disease under study.

ii. Reliability

The index should measure consistently at different times and conditions. An index should be reproducible and repeatable, which means the index be interpreted in the same way by the same (intra-examiner) or different examiners (inter-examiner).

iii. Clarity, Simplicity and Objectivity

The examiner should be able to remember the rules of the index clearly; hence, the index should be simple and easy to apply. The criteria for the index should be objective and unambiguous, with mutually exclusive categories.

iv. Quantifiability

An index should be amenable to statistical analysis, so that the status of a group can be expressed by statistical measures.

v. *Sensitivity*

The index should be able to detect any shifts in either direction under the study conditions.

vi. *Acceptability*

The use of an index should not raise any objections by the subjects. It should not be time demanding or demeaning to the participants.

CLASSIFICATION OF INDICES

The indices are classified on the following basis:

a. Direction in which the Scores can Fluctuate on Subsequent Examinations

i. *Irreversible Indices*

An index that measures conditions which cannot return to normal (whose scores will not change on subsequent examinations). The typical feature of an irreversible index is that it assesses the damage caused by the disease rather than the disease itself.

The DMF index is an excellent example of an irreversible index as it only takes into consideration open cavities (D), filled cavities (F) and missing teeth (M), which are assumed to have been extracted due to caries. A carious lesion can never heal itself returning to normal stage, just like certain diseases like common cold, etc. where the conditions can be normal again. A carious (D) lesion can be filled (F) but this change does not lead to overall reversal of the DMF score.

X-ray indices for measuring alveolar bone loss may have many similarities with the DMF index. They all measure the irreversible damage caused by the disease process. The numerical values remain the same regardless of whether the bone loss was associated with inflammation or any other reason.

ii. *Reversible Indices*

The index that measures conditions which can return to normal. The reversible index score values can decrease or increase on subsequent examination. Mostly gingival indices are reversible.

iii. *Composite Indices*

The composite indices are the combination of reversible and irreversible aspects of the disease; for example, Periodontal Index by Russell. One class of morbidity indices is exclusively concerned with the clinical signs of active gingival inflammation; whereas another class takes into account the destructiveness of the condition (pocket deepening and bone resorption).

b. Extent to which Areas of Oral Cavity are Measured

i. *Full Mouth Index*

The index measures the patient's entire periodontium or dentition. For example, Dean's index, Russell's periodontal index, etc.

ii. *Simplified Index*

The index measures only a representative sample of teeth or tissues. For example, Simplified Oral Hygiene Index (OHI-S).

iii. *The Entity being Measured*

a. Disease index, measures the disease entity (e.g. decayed teeth).
b. Treatment index, measures the treated entity (e.g. filled teeth).
c. Symptom index, measures the symptoms (e.g. papilla bleeding index).

iv. *Miscellaneous*

a. Simple index, measures the presence/ absence of the condition (e.g. calculus surface index).
b. Cumulative index, measures all the past and present evidence of the condition (e.g. DMF index).

Uses of Dental Indices

The indices are used at individual level, community level and/or research purposes (Table 4.1).

Table 4.1: Uses of dental indices		
Individual level	*Research purpose*	*Community level*
• Individual assessment • Effectiveness of oral hygiene practices • Evaluate the success of professional treatment over a period of time • Self motivation	• Data determination before commencing any experimental study • Evaluate effectiveness of specific agents/devices in preventive/curative programs	• Measure prevalence and incidence of any dental condition • Assess needs of the community as regard to curative and preventive measures • Compare and evaluate the outcome of a community preventive program

INDICES FOR DENTAL CARIES

As early as 1931, Bodecker and Bodecker described a caries index, which was sensitive but too complex for use in epidemiological surveys.

Later, Bodecker (1939) modified the same index; where, in addition to counting the surfaces decayed, an extra count was allotted for those surfaces that could experience multiple carious attacks. But this was not used in major epidemiological studies.

The approach to measure caries by counting the numbers of teeth affected by caries was first used in a systematic manner by Dean and associates in their studies of dental caries in relation to fluorides.

Mellanby (1934) described the carious lesions as: (i) slight caries, (ii) moderate caries and (iii) advanced caries depending upon the degree of severity.

One major problem in studying the epidemiology of dental caries is the lack of standard method for recording the occurrence, progression and severity of the disease.

The need for having uniform standards for measuring dental caries has always been the matter of concern. Epidemiological studies of caries require the disease be accurately measured and quantified based on scientific principles. Such studies help investigating dental caries in a given population, planning and evaluating public health programs and evaluating outcome of the preventive initiative taken.

The prevalence of dental caries can be measured in terms of (i) Percentage of persons affected, (ii) Number of teeth/tooth surfaces affected, (iii) Number of discrete cavities, (iv) Progression of lesion, (v) Severity of each carious lesion and (vi) Consequences of caries.

The quantitative measurement of caries commonly relies on 'Index'.

Various indices used to quantify caries are as follows:

1. DMFT index.
2. DMFS index.
3. def index.
4. DMFI index.
5. Modified DMFT index.
6. CLR index.
7. ECSI index.
8. Moller's index.
9. Stone's index.
10. Czechoslovakian caries index.
11. Caries severity index for primary teeth.
12. Caries susceptibility index.
13. Oral health status index.
14. Function measure index.
15. Tissue health index.
16. Root caries index.
17. Specific caries index.
18. Nyvad criteria for caries assessment in primary teeth.
19. International caries detection and assessment system (ICDAS).
20. Lesion activity assessment (LAA) system.
21. The PUFA Index.

22. Caries assessment spectrum and treatment index (CAST).
23. Significant caries index.

1. DMFT (DECAYED-MISSING-FILLED TEETH) INDEX

DMFT (Decayed-Missing-Filled Teeth) Index was developed by Henry, et al in 1938 to determine the prevalence of coronal caries (Fig. 4.1). Initially DMF values were meant to describe the dental status and treatment need in elementary schoolchildren. Soon it was applied to determine caries experience in the given population. It is one of the simplest and most commonly used index of dental caries to be utilized in epidemiologic surveys. Its use in oral health surveys in describing caries experience in adults and the elderly has been endorsed by WHO.

This index is based on the fact that the caries do not heal and may leave some sort of scar. The tooth remains decayed or, if treated, either extracted or filled. The DMFT index is therefore an irreversible index measuring the lifetime caries experience.

The DMFT index is applied only to permanent teeth. It is composed of three components: 'D', denotes the decayed teeth; 'M', denotes the missing teeth due to caries and 'F', denotes the teeth that have been filled due to caries. Dental caries is recorded when:

- The lesion is clinically visible.
- There is discoloration or loss of translucency inferring undermined/demineralized enamel.
- The explorer tip in a pit or fissure catches/resists removal after moderate to firm pressure.
- The explorer tip may penetrate into dentin.

Principles in Recording DMFT

- All the 28 permanent teeth are examined, excluding all primary teeth and the third molars.
- A tooth is considered to be erupted when the occlusal surface or incisal edge is exposed or can be exposed by manually reflecting the overlying gingival tissue.
- A tooth is considered to be present even if the crown has been destroyed leaving only the roots.

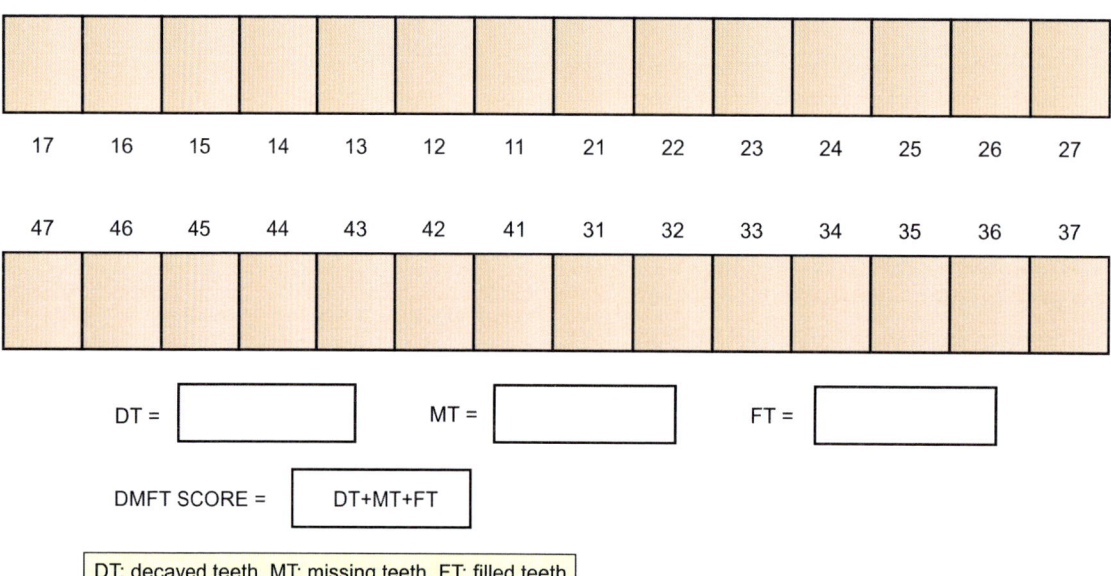

Fig. 4.1: Recording format for DMFT index

- No tooth be counted more than once. It is either decayed, missing, filled or sound.
- Decayed, missing and filled teeth should be recorded separately.
- Care must be taken to record as 'missing' only those teeth, which have been lost due to caries. (Also include those teeth which are badly decayed and are indicated for extraction).
- A tooth may have several restorations but it is counted as one.

Examination

A clean mouth mirror and a sharp explorer are used to carry out the examination.

DMFT is divided into three components, viz. component 'D', 'M' and 'F'. The description of individual components is as follows:

I. Component 'D'

It describes the decayed teeth, which include:
a. Carious tooth (the explorer should fall into the carious lesion and not just in a deep groove).
b. Filled tooth with recurrent decay.
c. Only the roots are left.
d. Defective filling with caries.
e. Temporary filling.
f. Filled tooth surface with caries on other surface.

II. Component 'M'

It indicates the number of missing permanent teeth due to decay. The teeth which are badly decayed and are indicated for extraction are counted as missing.

The teeth missing, not due to caries, are excluded. These are:
a. Teeth extracted due to reasons other than caries:
   - Orthodontic treatment.
   - Impaction.
   - Periodontal disease.
b. Un-erupted teeth.

c. Congenitally missing teeth.
d. Avulsed teeth due to trauma or accident.

III. Component 'F'

It indicates the number of carious permanent teeth that have been restored. Teeth are considered filled when one or more permanent restorations are present and there is no secondary (recurrent) caries or other area of the tooth with primary caries. A tooth may have several fillings but it is counted as one, i.e. a tooth may have restoration on one surface and caries on another, it is counted as decayed, i.e. D.

Teeth restored for reasons other than dental caries should be excluded, which include:
a. Restoration of fractured/traumatized teeth.
b. Hypoplastic teeth restored for esthetics.
c. Bridge abutments.
d. Fissure sealant.
e. Preventive infiltration.

Calculation of the Index

The maximum number for an individual DMFT score is 28 (32 if third molars are included).

A. For an Individual

D + M + F = DMF

For example; Decayed = 5, Missing = 2 and Filled = 3

D + M + F = 5 + 2 + 3 = 10, i.e. DMF score is 10. (The intact/sound teeth = 28 − 10 = 18)

B. For Population

Total the D, M, F values obtained for each individual. Then, divide the total 'DMF' by the number of individuals in the group.

$$\text{Mean DMF} = \frac{\text{Total DMF}}{\text{Total number of individuals examined in that group}}$$

C. Percentage of Decayed Teeth

It is calculated as ('D' component):

$$\text{Percentage of decayed teeth} = \frac{\text{Total number of decayed teeth}}{\text{Total number of teeth examined}} \times 100$$

D. *Percentage of Teeth Lost*

It is calculated as follows ('M' component):

$$\text{Percentage of teeth lost} = \frac{\text{Total number of missing teeth}}{\text{Total number of teeth examined}} \times 100$$

E. *Percent of Filled Teeth*

It is calculated as follows ('F' component):

$$\text{Percentage of teeth filled} = \frac{\text{Total number of filled teeth}}{\text{Total number of teeth examined}} \times 100$$

Advantages

- Simple and rapid to perform.
- Versatile.
- Universally accepted and applicable.
- Measurements have been used widely.

Shortcomings

Though DMFT has been universally accepted as an index, yet it has certain shortcomings, which are as follows.

1. The main drawback of DMF index is that it tends to equate a diseased state with a treated condition. While a carious tooth is given a score one, the filled tooth is also given a score one, thus making no differentiation in the filled and carious tooth. For example, a person with 4 teeth which need filling will be equated with the person who has already 4 filled teeth. The DMF index for both would be 4. Consequently the DMF index never changes even after the treatment. The DMF 4 of any individual will remain 4, even after getting the teeth filled.

2. Arrested caries is also a controversial component of the DMF index. Certain authors take these teeth as carious while others are of the view that these should be taken as sound.

3. In DMFT scoring, if both caries and a filling are present on the same tooth, only the caries will be scored, since each tooth is counted only once (priority to caries over fillings). The F component of the index does not reflect the true scope of restorative phase already provided to the population group. The authors who favour equating carious tooth with filled tooth, are of the view that the carious disease is irreversible and even after filling the tooth cannot be taken as normal. Other authors opine that even if the disease process is irreversible it is not irreparable. The tooth can be restored to function after restoration. Such teeth should be considered as 'treated' rather than diseased. Even missing tooth should be taken as treated, if replaced by appropriate prosthesis.

4. The index is not effective in analyzing the treatment outcome, which can be useful in controlling the disease.

5. The scoring system does not differentiate stages of progress of caries. A small restorable pit is equated to a grossly carious non-restorable tooth or a restorable tooth equated to a tooth missing due to caries. All the three are given a score of 1 which is not justifiable. (WHO has modified the scoring; D (Decayed) is split into D and I, i.e. restorable decayed teeth and non-restorable teeth indicated for extraction respectively. This is DIMF index).

6. The index provides information on carious and restored teeth; no information is provided on the clinical consequences of untreated dental caries, such as pulpal involvement, etc.

7. DMFT index fails to compensate for the prosthetic replacement of lost teeth. The index takes into consideration only the

tooth lost due to caries and ignores the prosthetic replacement.

8. The index is not an efficient tool for assessing the effects of preventive modalities undertaken by the individual or the population at large.

9. The index does not specify the number of teeth at risk.

10. The index may be invalid in older adults because missing teeth might be due to reasons other than caries. Similarly in children whose teeth have been extracted due to orthodontic reasons.

11. The index can overestimate caries experience, because teeth treated with preventive infiltrations are counted as filled.

WHO Modifications

WHO modified DMFT index in 1987. The modifications were:

a. All third molars are included.

b. Temporary restorations are considered as D.

c. Only carious cavities are considered as 'D', the initial lesions (Chalky spots, stained fissures, etc.) are not considered as D.

WHO further modified the index in 1997 as:
Until now, the teeth missing due to caries were included in 'M' component. WHO (1997) has stated that for individuals older than 30 years, the M component should comprise teeth missing due to caries or for any other reason; however, for subjects under 30 years of age, the M component will include teeth missing due to caries only.

The DMF index was further modified to DMC_sC_d index.

It is equivalent to DMF index, only the F component is divided into C_sC_d as follows:

D = Decayed

M = Missing

C_s = Conserved (filled) and sound

C_d = Conserved but with cavities present on same or any other surface.

2. DMFS (DECAYED, MISSING, FILLED SURFACES) INDEX

DMFS (Decayed, missing, filled surfaces) index was proposed by Klein, Palmer and Knutson in 1938. DMFS stands for: D—Decayed; M—Missing; F—Filled and S—Surfaces of tooth (The tooth surfaces recorded are Buccal, Lingual/Palatal, Mesial, Distal and Incisal/Occlusal).

A plain mirror and fine explorer are usually used to clinically evaluate the tooth surfaces. Initially, the DMFS index was designed for clinical evaluation only. Later, the clinical findings augmented by radiographs (revealing the proximal caries) were included as additional feature.

Third molars are not included in this index.

The maximum number of surface at risk is 128. If third molars are included, maximum number of surface at risk would be 148.

Anterior teeth surfaces

Total number of anterior teeth present (6 + 6 = 12) $\times$ Surface examined for a single anterior tooth (4)

$$= 48$$

Posterior teeth surfaces

Total number of posterior teeth present (8 + 8 = 16) $\times$ Surface examined for a single posterior tooth (5)

$$= 80$$

Difference in opinion exists as regard how many surface entities should be counted for molars and premolars which are crowned or lost due to caries. Crowned or extracted premolars and molars are counted as 3 to 5 F (filled) or 3 to 5 M (missing) surfaces respectively (consensus is to count '5' surfaces).

Procedure

The recording of D, M, F surfaces is done as (Fig. 4.2):

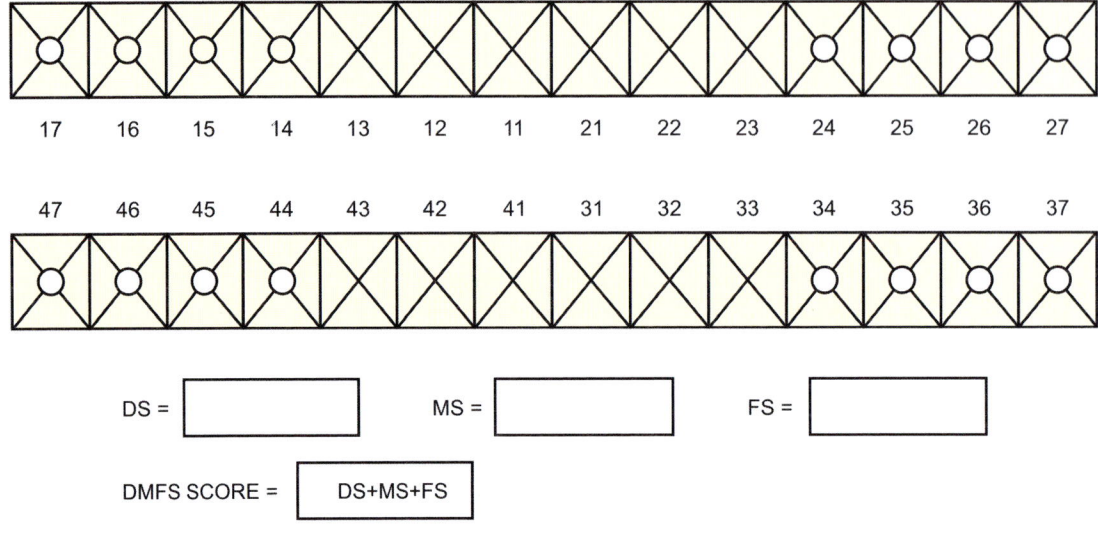

DS = [   ] MS = [   ] FS = [   ]

DMFS SCORE = [DS+MS+FS]

DS = Decayed surface, MS = Missing surface, FS = Filled surface

Fig. 4.2: Recording format for DMFS index

a. D (Decayed) (Codes: 1, 2, 3, 4)

Initial lesions (chalky spots) as well as frank lesions (carious defects) are counted. Cervical areas must be evaluated thoroughly for any initial white spot (lesion might be hidden under the gingiva).

Grading of lesion severity for pits and fissures
Grade 0: Healthy.
Grade 1: Thin light line, chalky margin.
Grade 2: Thin, brown to black line.
Grade 3: Frank defect less than 2.0 mm.
Grade 4: Frank defect more than 2.0 mm.

Grading of lesion severity for smooth surfaces (proximal surfaces)
Grade 0: Healthy.
Grade 1: Chalky spot less than 2.0 mm.
Grade 2: Chalky spot greater than 2.0 mm.
Grade 3: Frank defect less than 2.0 mm.
Grade 4: Frank defect greater than 2.0 mm.
- DMFS index in which initial lesions are also included is referred to as D_{1-4}MFS index.
- If both, a smooth surface lesion of grade 2 severity and a pit lesion of grade 3 severity,

are detected on the same surface, only the more severe of the two is counted.
- If no caries is detected clinically, the surface is scored as healthy even if the examiner is not certain (common finding with the proximal surfaces).

Radiographic grade of lesion severity (proximal surfaces)
Grade 1: Radiolucency in the outermost half of the enamel, initial lesion.
Grade 2: Radiolucency extended to inner half of the enamel, no dentinal involvement.
Grade 3: Radiolucency covering enamel with evident extension in peripheral dentin.
Grade 4: Obvious dentin radiolucency, close to the pulp.

When detectable radiolucency exists in pits and fissures/smooth surfaces, the clinical grade 4 carious defects, i.e. with large cavity is assigned.

b. F (Filled) (Code: 5)

If a filling with secondary caries is detected on a tooth surface, a separate category 'D+F' may be employed or taken as decayed 'D'.

If gold crown or post-crown is present, the counting is as follows:

On molars   Count all 5 surfaces
On bicuspids   Count all 5 surfaces
On anteriors   Count all 4 surfaces

c. M (Missing) (Code: 6)

For missing teeth, counting is carried out as:

Missing molars   count all 5 surfaces
Missing bicuspid   count all 5 surfaces
Missing anterior tooth   count all 4 surfaces

(Note: Initially bicuspid surfaces were counted as '3'; however, overcoming the controversy, the surfaces counted are '5').

d. Un-erupted (Code: 7)

Procedure of clinical recording: Clinical recording is initiated from the maxillary teeth followed by mandibular teeth. First right and then left quadrant is examined. Initially, the teeth are examined visually. The explorer is used only in case of doubt. Surfaces are examined in the following order: occlusal, facial, lingual, distal and mesial.

Procedure of radiographic recording: Proximal lesions are better analyzed by radiographic means. In case the proximal surfaces cannot be adequately examined because of the overlapping of X-ray projections or malaligned teeth, an "X" is scored for such surfaces. The final DMFS score is calculated from the clinical examination only.

3. def INDEX

The 'def' index was designed for measuring dental caries in primary dentition (Gruebbel 1944). The criteria for examining decayed teeth remain the same as for DMF index. 't' is added for teeth (deft) and 's' is added for surfaces (defs). def stands for:

'd'—Indicates primary teeth that are carious.

'e'—Indicates deciduous teeth which have been extracted due to caries, or which are indicated for extraction. Estimation of 'e'

becomes difficult as there can be wide variation in the time of exfoliation of deciduous teeth. A tooth missing, whether was normally exfoliated or was extracted because of advanced caries also creates problem in recording.

Differentiation between missing tooth due to caries and due to exfoliation:
- Age of the patient (whether near to exfoliation time or not).
- The shape of ridge (concave in carious missing tooth and straight in exfoliated one along with permanent successor).
- DMF/dmf index is higher in association with carious missing tooth especially in adjacent and contralateral teeth.
- Bad oral hygiene is mainly associated with carious teeth.

Differentiation between tooth missing due to caries and due to orthodontic treatment:
- Type of teeth (in orthodontic treatment, teeth to be extracted are 4, 5/c₍ d; while in carious missing teeth any tooth may be involved).
- Bilateral and/or opposing missing teeth are generally associated with orthodontic treatment (crowding can also be evident); while in carious missing teeth it is not necessary.
- DMF/def index is higher in association with carious missing tooth especially in adjacent and contralateral teeth.
- Appliance may be seen in orthodontic treatment.

'f'—Indicates number of carious deciduous teeth that have been restored without any recurrent decay. A tooth may have several fillings but it is counted as one tooth. A filled tooth showing evidence of recurrent decay, is counted as a decayed tooth.

In case of missing tooth, the coding is modified as:

'O'—Missing tooth (un-erupted or congenitally missing for any other reason).

'X'—Extracted deciduous teeth.

Calculation

Maximum deft score = 20 (Total number of deciduous teeth); Maximum defs score = 88 (Total number of tooth surfaces). The scoring is carried out as:

a. For one child

    def = d + e + f (Total of decayed, exfoliated and filled teeth)

b. For a group of children (say in population)

    Total the d, e and f for each child and divide the total def by the number of children examined.

$$\text{Mean def} = \frac{\text{Total def of each child}}{\text{Total number of the children examined}}$$

c. Percentage of decayed teeth

$$\text{Percentage of decayed teeth} = \frac{\text{Total number of decayed teeth}}{\text{Total number of children examined}} \times 100$$

Modifications of def Index

i. dmf Index

For children over 7 years and up to 11 or 12 years (before the age of exfoliation), the decayed, missing and filled primary teeth have been categorized as decayed-missing-filled teeth (dmft), when teeth are counted; or decayed-missing-filled surfaces (dmfs) when surfaces are counted.

ii. df Index

The exfoliated teeth are ignored; scored as dft for decayed, filled teeth and dfs for decayed-filled surfaces.

iii. Mixed Dentition

The caries indices for permanent as well as the deciduous teeth are to be carried out separately. Each child is given a separate index for permanent teeth and another for primary teeth. The index for the permanent teeth is determined first, followed by index for the primary teeth.

4. DMFI INDEX

The DMF index was modified by WHO in 1971 to DMFI index by subdividing decayed teeth into unfilled carious teeth (D), secondary decayed-filled teeth (DF) and decayed but indicated for extraction (I).

D—Unfilled teeth with caries.

DF—Filled teeth with secondary caries.

M—Missing teeth (extracted as a result of caries).

F—Filled teeth that show no signs of secondary caries.

I—Filled/unfilled teeth, indicated for extraction.

5. MODIFIED DMFT INDEX

Joseph Anaise (1983) modified the existing DMFT index, improving the recording criteria so as to provide an accurate description of the dental care status. The modified version also measures the severity of the carious attack, warranting the need for appropriate dental care.

Procedure

The modification involves division of the 'D' component into the following four categories:

    "C" = unfilled teeth that are carious.

    "CF" = restored teeth that are either carious around the margins of the restorations (secondary caries) or primarily on a tooth surface other than the 'restored one.'

    "IX" = carious teeth either filled or unfilled that are indicated for extraction.

    "IRC" = carious teeth either filled or unfilled that are indicated for root canal treatment (irreversible pulp involvement).

    In addition to these four categories of decayed teeth, the remaining two categories of the DMFT index (F – filled teeth, with no decay and 'M' – missing teeth) are recorded as usual.

    The DMF score is the sum of all six categories and the calculation of the individual component as well as the sum remain the same as the original DMFT index.

Condensed Criteria of Determining DMFT

The criteria of DMF recording are condensed for use in large surveys for determining the prevalence of caries. These are:

a. *Half mouth method:* WHO devised a criteria whereby half of the upper arch and the contralateral half of the lower arch is scored and the results are doubled. The objective was to obtain caries prevalence in a population which has not been previously scored (initial level surveys). This method is commonly used in epidemiological surveys for assessment of periodontal and gingival diseases.

b. *McLendon method:* He described a method where only first molar and upper central incisors are recorded.

c. *Viegas method:* Viegas has developed three methods for estimating average, whole-mouth scores for DMFT amongst 7 to 12-year-old children when only a part of oral cavity is examined. Method I (used in areas of low prevalence) requires only the examination of the right lower first molars. Method II (used in areas of moderate to high prevalence) requires an examination of the upper right and left central incisors in addition to lower molars. Method III is used by applying Method I for 7-year-old and Method II for 11-year-old. Then scores for 8-, 9-, 10- and 12-year-old are determined, without examining the children, but by constructing a graph based on the findings for the 7- and 11-year-old. The purpose is to determine how the estimates of prevalence of DMFT obtained from Viegas' Method II, correspond to the findings of DMFT made from examining the entire dentition of children.

d. *Grainger's method:* The method includes examination of both primary and permanent teeth. The buccal and lingual surfaces of posterior teeth (those without developmental pits) and the lingual surfaces of the anterior teeth are not included in the examination.

The examination proceeds as (Table 4.2):

1. The proximal surfaces between the mandibular anterior teeth are examined for decay or fillings; if one or more are found, the individual is assigned to Severity Zone 5 and the examination is terminated.

2. The labial surfaces of the maxillary and mandibular anterior teeth are examined for decay or fillings; if one or more are found, the individual is assigned to Severity Zone 4 and the examination is terminated.

3. The proximal surfaces between the maxillary anterior teeth are examined for decay or fillings; if one or more are found, the individual is assigned to Severity Zone 3 and the examination is terminated.

4. The proximal surfaces between the posterior teeth are examined for decay or fillings; if one or more are found, the individual is assigned to Severity Zone 2 and the examination is terminated.

5. The pit and fissures of posterior teeth are examined for decay of fillings; if one or more are found, the individual is assigned to Severity Zone 1 and the examination is terminated.

6. If the individual has not been assigned to any of the above severity zones, he is assigned to Severity Zone 0.

Table 4.2: Criteria for classification of individual according to severity zone of dental caries

Severity zone	Teeth/Surfaces involved
5	Proximal surfaces of mandibular anterior teeth (excluding distal surfaces of cuspids).
4	Labial surfaces of maxillary and mandibular incisors and cuspids.
3	Proximal surfaces of maxillary incisors and cuspids.
2	Proximal surfaces of molars and premolars (including distal surfaces of cuspids).
1	Pit and fissure surfaces of posterior teeth.
0	None of the above.

6. CLR INDEX

Karthikeyan (1997) suggested a new index simplifying the DMF index. This is named CLR index, i.e. Carious, Lost and Restored index. Restorations (R) can be of any type, viz. fillings, crowns, bridges, dentures, etc.

Carious 'C' can be further divided into two, i.e. (i) restorable carious teeth – 'C' and (ii) non-restorable carious teeth indicated for extraction, 'I'.

- C_1I_1L are given a score of 1.
- R is given ½ score.
- An arrested carious tooth without structural loss is given a score of ½ and is treated like a restored tooth.

Similarities between DMF and CLR index are:

- For permanent and deciduous teeth, capital letters and small letters are used respectively (i.e. CLR and clr).
- When a tooth has a filling and is also carious, it is counted only once (as a carious tooth).
- Tooth loss due to periodontal disease, trauma, congenitally missing teeth, teeth extracted for orthodontic purposes are excluded.
- In longitudinal studies, clr index like the dmf index is irrelevant as almost all deciduous teeth exfoliate.

Differences between DMF and CLR index are:

- Correctly restored tooth (filled tooth) is given a score of ½.
- Arrested caries with no structural loss is given a score of ½.
- Correctly placed prosthetic replacement is given a score of ½ when it replaces a lost tooth due to caries. In such situation for missing (due to caries) tooth, score 1 is not given.
- If the existing prosthesis is not satisfactory (need repetition), then ignoring the prosthesis, the missing tooth (due to caries) is scored as 1.
- In longitudinal studies comprising of young children with more permanent teeth

to erupt, the CLR index could be expressed as a fraction (i.e. numerator denoting the total carious, lost or restored teeth and the denominator representing the number of permanent teeth present in the child's oral cavity).

7. ECSI INDEX

ECSI (Extrapolated carious surface incremental index) evaluates caries progression intended to supplement rather than to replace existing indices (Wagg, et al 1974). It takes into account the enlargement of existing lesions as well as initiation of new ones. Degrees of caries are designated as follows:

0 = No carious attack.

1 = Carious attack confined to enamel.

2 = Carious attack involving enamel and dentin but not pulp.

3 = Carious attack involving the pulp.

The ECSI index is similar to DMFS index, having an additional component representing the extension of existing lesions.

8. MOLLER'S INDEX

Moller's index (1966) is quantitatively and qualitatively sensitive index as it records severity of carious lesions ranging from incipient to frank/obvious caries.

The characteristics of Moller's Index are:

S—Sound.

D_1–D_4—Carious (decayed) teeth (Table 4.3).

M—Missing (not erupted; extracted because of caries).

F—Filled.

FD—Filled and decayed (visible caries with loss of surface continuity in contact with a filling, i.e. secondary caries).

Arrested caries should be recorded as caries, because it is difficult to distinguish between acute and arrested caries.

9. STONE'S INDEX

It was developed by Stone, et al in 1949. The criteria of scoring are tabulated in Table 4.4.

Table 4.3: Coding of decayed teeth

	D_1	D_2	D_3	D_4
Smooth surface	White opaque area with loss of lustre	Slight discontinuity in enamel	Dentin involvement	Pulp involvement
Pit and fissures	Discoloration, all confined to a small narrow line; no definite sticking	Slight discontinuity in enamel, "sticky fissure" with or without discoloration (the probe requires a definite pull for removal)	Definite cavity with dentin involvement	Pulp involvement

Table 4.4: Criteria of scoring Stone's Index

Scoring	Criteria
1	One or more cavities in the same tooth where the lesion has not penetrated through the enamel to involve the dentin.
2	One or more cavities in the same tooth where the dentin is involved, where a total of less than a quarter of the crown is estimated to have been destroyed.
3	One or more cavities in the same tooth resulting in a destruction of more than a quarter of the crown.

10. CZECHOSLOVAKIAN CARIES INDEX

The Czechoslovakian Caries Index was introduced by Poncova, et al in 1956.

This index is mainly used to compare caries experience in one group with that of the other groups with a similar population density but living in different environments. In this index, the 'variables' seem to be controlled. During evaluation, the average number of teeth, tooth surfaces/areas and the condition of previously extracted or crowned teeth are considered. The following formula serves as the basis for this index (in adults):

$$\frac{1 - C - FC - 4/5E - 2/3AT}{Base}$$

C—Caries, FC—Fillings and Crowns, E—Extractions, AT—Anchorage teeth.

The proposed formula can be applied as a basis for an individual or a collective index. In individual examination, the "Base" is given by the amount of teeth in adult dentition (32) and in collective studies, the "Base" is the number of persons examined multiplied by 32 to establish the correct base figure. The average index value will then be between 0 and 1. More is the proximation of index value to 1, the higher the caries frequency.

11. CARIES SEVERITY INDEX FOR PRIMARY TEETH

Caries severity index, developed by Tank and Storvik in 1960 was initially utilized for permanent teeth to study the depth and extent of the carious surfaces and the extent of pulpal involvement. The criteria of scoring are tabulated in Table 4.5. Very few studies have utilized this scoring system.

Chosack (1986) however re-framed caries severity index to be used for primary teeth. The reframed criteria for scoring different surfaces and teeth are as follows:

A. Occlusal Surface Caries and Pit and Fissure Caries on Buccal or Palatal Surfaces of Molars

1. Early pit and fissure caries where the explorer catches or resists removal with moderate to firm pressure and is accompanied by either a softness at the base of the area or an opacity adjacent to the pit or fissure as evidence of undermining or demineralization; or softened enamel

Table 4.5: Criteria of scoring Caries Severity Index

Scoring	Criteria
1	Superficial (caries in enamel).
2	Moderate (caries in enamel and superficial dentin).
3	Moderately severe (enamel undermined).
4	Severe (approaching pulp).
5	Pulpitis (caused either by deep seated caries or by trauma without caries).
6	Death of pulp (caused either by deep seated caries or by trauma without caries).
7	Periapical infection (caused either by deep seated caries or by trauma without caries).

adjacent to the pit or fissure which may be scraped away with the explorer.

2. Cavitation of at least 1.0 mm across the smallest diameter at the tooth surface.
3. Cavitation with breakdown or undermining (seen by obvious discoloration) of at least half a cusp.

B. Buccal, Lingual and Palatal Smooth Surface Caries

1. A white lesion not extending to the embrasure areas, found to be soft and sticky by penetration with the explorer.
2. Cavitation of at least 1.0 mm but less than 2.0 mm across the smallest diameter, or a soft sticky white lesion extending into an embrasure.
3. Cavitation of at least 2.0 mm in the smallest diameter, or a soft sticky white lesion extending into both embrasures.

C. Proximal Surfaces of Molars

1. A discontinuity of the enamel (an explorer will 'catch' and there is softening).
2. Cavitation with early breakdown or obvious discoloration indicating undermining of the ridge.
3. Breakdown of the marginal ridge with cavitation extending to the mesial or distal extensions of the occlusal fissures.

In case of proximal caries "3", this will not be counted as occlusal caries unless the caries extends past the distal or mesial extensions of the fissures; in such cases occlusal caries will be scored as in section A.

D. Proximal Surfaces of Incisors and Canines

1. A discontinuity of the enamel (an explorer will 'catch' and there is softening).
2. Cavitation with breakdown or obvious discoloration, indicating undermining for at least 1.0 mm on the buccal or lingual surfaces.
3. Cavitation with breakdown of the incisal edge or undermining of the edge as indicated by obvious discoloration.

Caries seen on buccal, lingual and palatal surfaces in all teeth continuous with occlusal or proximal caries is only scored for those surfaces when normal pits or fissures of these surfaces are affected or included, or when the caries extends along at least half the gingival third of these surfaces.

Only the largest caries involvement is scored for any one surface. Scores of two or more lesions on one surface are not combined.

A filled surface is given a score of 1. Secondary caries at the margin of a restoration is given a score of 2. A full crown restoration gives a total score of 5 for that tooth. A tooth extracted because of caries is given a total score of 6.

The caries severity index for the given population is the mean of the scores of the carious teeth. Teeth free of caries are not included in this calculation.

12. CARIES SUSCEPTIBILITY INDEX

The caries susceptibility index was developed by Richardson in 1961. This index is based on

Bodecker and Mellanby Caries indices. Two factors are important in measuring caries susceptibility, namely:

a. Amount of tooth surface at risk.

b. Amount of caries developing during the period of observation.

Measure of susceptibility can be calculated by dividing 'b' with 'a'.

Procedure

Each tooth is divided into various surfaces and one carious tooth surface is measured as one unit. Susceptible surfaces are scored as follows:

Incisors – Mesial, Distal, Lingual, Labial = Total 4 surfaces.

Canine – Mesial, Distal, Lingual, Labial = Total 4 surfaces.

Premolar – Mesial, Distal, Lingual, Buccal, Occlusal = Total 5 surfaces.

Molar – Mesial, Distal, Lingual, Buccal, Occlusal = Total 5 surfaces.

Permanent dentition would have a total of 148 susceptible surfaces, whereas deciduous dentition would have a total of 88 susceptible surfaces.

Each individual is examined initially for tooth surfaces with caries and restored surfaces.

The individual is re-examined after an observation period of 6 months or 12 months and the caries developed in each surface is noted.

From the initial examination the number of susceptible surfaces is calculated for each individual. Each tooth surface which is caries-free and had not been restored is considered susceptible.

The caries score is calculated in the second inspection (i.e. 6 months or 12 months after the initial inspection). The caries score is divided by the number of susceptible surfaces to give a ratio. This ratio is designated as *susceptibility ratio* (SR).

$$\text{Susceptibility ratio (SR)} = \frac{\substack{\text{Number of carious surfaces} \\ \text{developed during the} \\ \text{period of observation}}}{\substack{\text{Number of susceptible} \\ \text{surfaces determined during} \\ \text{initial examination}}}$$

$$\substack{\text{Susceptibility} \\ \text{index (SI)}} = \substack{\text{Susceptibility} \\ \text{ratio (SR)}} \times 100$$

13. ORAL HEALTH STATUS INDEX (OHSI)

Marcus, et al (1980) developed the Oral Health Status Index (OHSI).

This index include components of the DMFT (Decayed, Missing and Filled teeth) and 15 other variables such as temporomandibular dysfunction, degree of periodontal disease and tumors, etc. A prior planning is required to develop an examination protocol, including all measurements to evaluate given population.

The Oral Health Index is modified adding emphasis to decayed, fractured and replaced teeth. It is considered as more efficient in revealing the behavioural factors associated with dental health status. This modified index is easier to use in epidemiological studies.

14. FUNCTIONAL MEASURE INDEX (FMI)

The Functional Measure Index (FMI) was proposed by Sheiham, et al in 1987. This index is the first comprehensive index to measure dental health and functional status rather than disease.

In FMI, the 'Filled' and the 'Sound' teeth are weighed equally, while, the 'Decayed' and 'Missing' teeth are given 'zero' weight. FMI considered the functional measure or the number of functioning teeth, defined as the aggregate or healthy restored (i.e. filled) teeth (otherwise sound) and sound teeth with no decay. The argument being that sound and restored teeth have equivalent function.

The FMI is calculated by adding the filled and sound teeth and then dividing by total number of teeth present, i.e. 28 (excluding third molar).

$$FMI = \frac{Filled + Sound}{28}$$

The FMI scores range from 0 to 1.

Very less number of studies have utilized this index.

15. TISSUE HEALTH INDEX (THI)

The Tissue Health Index measures the number of sound teeth that represents the total amount of sound tooth tissue at a given point of time.

It infers average weight of decayed teeth, filled (otherwise sound) teeth and sound teeth. In principle, the weights represent the relative amount of sound tissue surrounding these three categories of teeth. In other words, a sound tooth contains more sound tissue on average, than a filled tooth, while a filled tooth contains more sound tissue than a decayed tooth. On this basis, missing teeth are considered as having zero sound tissue.

In the THI, selective weightage is given for Decayed, Filled and Sound teeth (i.e. '1' – Decayed, '2' – Filled and '4' – Sound).

The THI is calculated using the formula,

$$THI = \frac{\frac{1}{4} \, (1 \times Decayed + 2 \times Filled + 4 \times Sound)}{28}$$

The total number of teeth present is taken as 28, as third molars are excluded. The THI scores range from 0 to 1.

As in the case of functional measure index, less studies have utilized this index. This is also considered as a reliable indicator of dental health status and more efficient at revealing behavioral factors associated with dental health status.

16. ROOT CARIES INDEX

Katz (1984) proposed an index for measuring root caries. This index is commonly utilized in epidemiological surveys. The caries are recorded along with the gingival recession without the help of radiographs. The root caries index take into account the peculiar nature of root surface caries (caries appears only on teeth with exposed cementum). The clinical criteria are as follows:

- Presence of a discrete, well defined and discolored soft area.
- The explorer entered easily and displayed some resistance to withdrawal.
- The lesion was located either at the cemento-enamel junction or wholly on cementum.

The root caries index (RCI) is calculated as follows:

$$RCI = \frac{RD + RF}{RD + RF + RN} \times 100$$

where,

RD = total number of decayed root surfaces.

RF = total number of filled root surfaces.

RN = total number of exposed root surfaces.

RCI is expressed as percentage.

Restored lesion was counted as root caries only if it was obvious that the lesion originated at cemento-enamel junction or was completely confined to root surfaces.

17. SPECIFIC CARIES INDEX

Specific caries index provides qualitative and quantitative information about untreated dental caries in an individual based on clinical examination. Along with DMFS index, this index can be helpful in planning oral health care for a given population. The scoring criteria are tabulated in Table 4.6.

SCI scores for both 6 and 6A remain the same, i.e. 6.

Calculation

The SCI score is calculated by adding the individual tooth scores. The SCI scores for an individual can range from 0 to 192 (for 32 teeth).

18. NYVAD CRITERIA FOR CARIES ASSESSMENT IN PRIMARY TEETH

The Nyvad caries assessment criteria (Nyvad, et al 1999) classify the activities of both non-cavitated and cavitated lesions. The coding criteria are tabulated in Table 4.7.

Table 4.6: Scoring criteria for Specific Caries Index

Scoring	Criteria
0	No carious lesion.
1	Carious lesion on the occlusal, buccal pits and fissures of molars and premolars and the lingual pits of the anterior teeth.
2	Proximal caries affecting the molars and premolars.
3	Carious lesion on the proximal surface of the anteriors, not involving the incisal angle.
4	Carious lesion on the proximal surface of the anteriors, involving the incisal angle.
5	Carious lesion on the cervical region of the tooth.
6	• Carious lesion on the occlusal cusp tips of molars and premolars and on the incisal edges of incisors.
6A	• Grossly decayed tooth/root stumps indicated for extraction.

Table 4.7: Coding criteria for Nyvad's caries assessment

Score	Category	Criteria
0	Sound	Normal enamel translucency and texture (slight staining allowed in otherwise sound fissure).
1	Active caries (intact surface)	Surface of enamel is whitish/yellowish opaque with loss of luster; feels rough when the tip of the probe is moved gently across the surface; generally covered with plaque. No clinically detectable loss of substance. Intact fissure morphology; lesion extending along the walls of the fissure.
2	Active caries (surface discontinuity)	Same criteria as score 1. Localized surface defect (microcavity) in enamel only. No undermined enamel or softened floor detectable with the explorer.
3	Active caries (cavity)	Enamel/dentin cavity easily visible with the naked eye; surface of the cavity feels soft or leathery on gentle probing. There may or may not be pulpal involvement.
4	Inactive caries (intact surface)	Surface of enamel is whitish, brownish or black. Enamel may be shiny and feels hard and smooth when the tip of the probe is moved gently across the surface. No clinically detectable loss of substance. Intact fissure morphology; lesion extending along the walls of the fissure.
5	Inactive caries (surface discontinuity)	Same criteria as score 4. Localized surface defect (microcavity) in enamel only. No undermined enamel or softened floor detectable with the explorer.
6	Inactive caries (cavity)	Enamel/dentin cavity easily visible with the naked eye; surface of the cavity feels shiny and feels hard on gentle probing. No pulpal involvement.
7		Filling (sound surface): same as score 0.
8		Filling with an active caries: (lesion may be cavitated or non-cavitated).
9		Filling with an inactive caries: (lesion may be cavitated or non-cavitated).

Advantages

• Assesses the progress and activity of the lesions simultaneously.

• Differentiates between enamel discontinuity and the dentin caries; provides information for monitoring the progress of caries.

- Suggest possible treatment option depending upon the diagnosis.

Procedure

The tooth surface must be dried and visualized under good illumination for detecting non-cavitated lesions. The compressed air and artificial light is a pre-requisite for Nyvad caries assessment system. Visual examination and a sharp probe is used to classify activity of the carious lesions.

The tip of probe is placed at an angle of about 30° to the tooth surface (enamel) and moved gently, so that the difference between the smooth texture of sound surface (inactive lesion) and the rough texture of caries-demineralized surface (active lesion) can be felt. For dentin lesions, tactile examination using slight pressure, differentiates hard tissue from soft tissue (leathery consistency). The surface texture is considered to be a better indicator of activity than color. That is why the activity assessment should not be based only on the color of lesion, especially for dentin lesion. The dark brown dentin lesion having leathery consistency may indicate that they are still active. As the transition between active and inactive stages may not be instant, mixed lesions are considered as active.

Shortcomings

This index is restricted to scoring conse-quences of infection in teeth and surrounding tissues as a result of the carious process.

19. THE INTERNATIONAL CARIES DETECTION AND ASSESSMENT SYSTEM (ICDAS)

The ICDAS criteria were developed by an international team of researchers integrating several criteria into one standard system for caries detection and assessment (Ismail, et al 2007). The ICDAS provides flexibility for clinician and researchers to choose the stage of caries process as per their research requirements. It detects six stages of carious process, ranging from the early clinically visible changes in enamel to extensive distinct cavity.

The stages of caries process are given codes as under:

Code	Description
0	Sound
1	First visual change in enamel
2	Distinct visual change in enamel
3	Localized enamel break down (without clinical signs of dentin involvement)
4	Involvement of dentin (underlying dark shadow of dentin)
5	Distinct cavity with visible dentin
6	Extensive distinct cavity with visible dentin (involving more than half of the surfaces)

The initial ICDAS criteria included detection of coronal caries; the assessment of lesion activity and root caries were not included. ICDAS coordination committee in 2009 modified the assessment criteria, which include coronal caries, caries associated with sealants and root caries (ICDAS II).

The detection 'D' and assessment 'A' assumes importance in International Caries Detection and Assessment system. The detection is carried out following the stages as:

    i. Stage of caries process.

    ii. Topography (pits and fissures or smooth surfaces).

    iii. Anatomy (crowns versus roots).

    iv. Restoration or sealant status.

The assessment implies caries process by 'stage' (non-cavitated or cavitated) and 'activity' (active or arrested). The present version of ICDAS does not yet include an assessment of lesion activity (being in the process of development).

A. Caries Detection Criteria for Coronal Tooth Surfaces

a. Pit and Fissure Caries/Smooth Surface Caries

Code 0: *Sound tooth surface*

There should be no evidence of caries (either no or questionable change in enamel translucency after prolonged air drying (accepted drying time is 5 seconds). Surfaces with developmental defects such as enamel hypoplasia, fluorosis, tooth wear (attrition, abrasion and erosion) and extrinsic/intrinsic strains will be recorded as sound. The examiner should score as sound a surface with multiple stained fissures if such a condition is seen in other pits and fissures; a condition consistent with certain habits (e.g. staining due to frequent tea drinking, smoking, etc.).

The differential diagnostic criteria between dental fluorosis (mild form) and other opacities of enamel are given in Table 4.8.

Code 1: *First visual change in enamel*

There is no evidence of any change in color indicating carious activity, when seen wet; however, after prolonged air drying (5 seconds is considered adequate to dehydrate a carious lesion in enamel) an opacity or discoloration (white or brown) is visible that is not consistent with the clinical appearance of sound enamel. OR

When there is change of color because of caries which is not consistent with the clinical appearance of sound enamel and is limited to the confines of the pit and fissure area (whether seen dry or wet). The stained pits and fissures are designated in code 0.

Code 2: *Distinct visual change in enamel*

The tooth must be viewed wet. When wet, there is a (i) clear opacity (white spot lesion) and/or (ii) brown carious discoloration which is wider than the natural fissure/fossa that is not consistent with the clinical appearance of

Table 4.8: Differential diagnosis between dental fluorosis (mild form) and other opacities of enamel (Conceived from Russel-1961)

Lesion characteristics	Dental fluorosis (mild form)	Other enamel opacities
Area affected	Usually seen on or near tips of cusps or incisal edges	Usually centered in smooth surface; may affect entire crown
Shape of lesion	Resembles line shading; lines follow incremental lines in cuspal enamel	Often round or oval
Demarcation	Shades off demarcation not imperceptible; merges into normal enamel	Clearly differentiated from adjacent enamel
Color	Slightly more opaque than normal enamel; paper white incisal edges; tips of cusps may have frosted appearance; No staining at time of eruption	Usually pigmented at time of eruption (creamy-yellow to dark reddish orange)
Teeth affected	Most frequent on teeth that calcify slowly (cuspids, bicuspids; second and third molars); rare on lower incisors; extremely rare in deciduous teeth	Any tooth may be affected. Frequent on labial surfaces of lower incisors; usually one to three teeth get affected; common in deciduous teeth
Gross hypoplasia	None. Pitting of enamel does not occur in the mild form. Enamel surface has glazed appearance and feels smooth to explorer	None to severe. Enamel surface may seem etched and feels rough to explorer
Detection	Often invisible under strong light; can be detected by line of light tangential to tooth crown	Seen easily under strong light or light perpendicular to tooth surface

sound enamel. The lesion should also be visible when dry.

Code 3: *Localized enamel breakdown (without clinical signs of dentin involvement)*

The tooth viewed wet may have a clear opacity (white spot lesion) and/or brown discoloration which is wider than the natural fissure/fossa that is not consistent with the clinical appearance of sound enamel. Once dried for approximately five seconds, there is loss of tooth structure at the entrance, or within the pit or fissure/fossa. This will be seen visually as evidence of demineralization [opaque (white), brown or dark brown walls] at the entrance or within the fissure or pit and although the pit or fissure may appear substantially and unnaturally wider than normal, the dentin is not visible along the walls or base of the cavity/discontinuity.

If in doubt, or to confirm visual assessment, the WHO/CPI/PSR probe can be used gently across the tooth surface to confirm the presence of a cavity confined to the enamel. This is achieved by sliding the ball-end of the probe along the suspected pit or fissure and a limited discontinuity is detected if the ball drops into the surface of the suspected enamel cavity/discontinuity.

Code 4: *Without localized enamel breakdown*

This lesion appears as a shadow or discolored dentin visible through the intact enamel surface which may or may not show signs of localized breakdown (loss of continuity of the surface, not showing the dentin). The appearance of shadow or discoloration is seen easily when the tooth is wet. The darkened area is an intrinsic shadow which may appear as grey, blue or brown in color. The shadow must clearly represent caries that initiated on the tooth surface being evaluated. If in the opinion of the examiner, the carious lesion has initiated on an adjacent surface and there is no evidence of any caries on the surface being scored then the surface should be coded '0'.

Code 5: *Cavity with visible dentin*

Cavity is visible in opaque/discolored enamel exposing the dentin. The tooth if viewed wet may have darkening of the dentin. Once dried, there is visual evidence of loss of tooth structure at the entrance or within the pit or fissure, i.e. frank cavitation. In the recording, the dentin is regarded as *exposed*.

The WHO/CPI/PSR probe can be used to confirm the presence of a cavity in dentin. This is achieved by sliding the ball-end of the probe along the suspected pit or fissure and a dentin cavity is detected if the ball enters the opening of the cavity and the examiner confirms the ball touching the dentin (avoid probing deep dentin; caries approaching pulp).

Code 6: *Extensive distinct cavity with visible dentin*

The cavity is deep and wide and the dentin is clearly visible on the walls and at the base. An extensive cavity involves at least half the tooth surface or approaching the pulp (obvious loss of tooth structure).

b. Free Smooth Surface (buccal and lingual) and examination of mesial and distal surfaces with no adjacent teeth

Code 0: *Sound tooth surface*

There should be no evidence of caries, either no or questionable change in enamel translucency after prolonged air drying (approximately 5 seconds). Surfaces with developmental defects such as enamel hypoplasias, fluorosis, tooth wear (attrition, abrasion and erosion) and extrinsic/intrinsic stains will be recorded as sound.

Code 1: *First visual change in enamel*

There is no evidence of any change in color indicating carious activity; however, after prolonged air drying an opacity is visible that is not consistent with the clinical appearance of sound enamel.

Code 2: *Distinct visual change in enamel when viewed wet*

There is opacity or discoloration that is not consistent with the clinical appearance of sound enamel. The lesion should also be visible when dry. The lesion is located in close proximity (touching or within 1.0 mm) of the gingival margin.

Code 3: *Localized enamel breakdown due to caries with no visible dentin*

Once dried, there is loss of surface integrity without visible dentin.

   If in doubt or to confirm the visual assessment, the CPI probe can be used without pressure to confirm the loss of surface integrity.

Code 4: *Underlying dark shadow from dentin with or without localized enamel breakdown*

The lesion appears as a shadow of discolored dentin visible through the enamel surface beyond the white or brown spot lesion, which may or may not show signs of localized breakdown. This appearance is often seen more easily when the tooth is wet and is a darkening and intrinsic shadow which may be grey, blue or brown in color.

Code 5: *Distinct cavity with visible dentin cavitation in opaque or discolored enamel exposing the dentin beneath*

Cavitation in opaque or discolored enamel exploring the dentin beneath involving less than half of the tooth surface.

Code 6: *Extensive distinct cavity with visible dentin*

Obvious loss of tooth structure; the cavity is deep and wide and the dentin is clearly visible on the walls and at the base.

c. Caries associated with Restorations and Sealants

Code 0: *Sound tooth surface with restoration or sealant*

There should be no evidence of caries; either no or questionable change in enamel translucency after air drying for 5 seconds; surfaces with marginal defects less than 0.5 mm in width (i.e. will not admit the ball-end of the CPI probe).

Code 1: *First visual change in enamel*

Same as described earlier.

Code 2: *Distinct visual change in enamel/ dentin adjacent to a restoration/sealant margin*

- If the restoration margin is placed on enamel, the tooth must be viewed wet. When wet there is opacity consistent with demineralization or discoloration that is not consistent with the clinical appearance of sound enamel.
- If the restoration margin is placed on dentin, code 2 applies to discoloration that is not consistent with the clinical appearance of sound dentin or cementum.

Code 3: *Carious defects of less than 0.5 mm with the signs of code 2*

Carious defect at the margin of the restoration/sealant less than 0.5 mm, in addition to either an opacity or discoloration consistent with demineralization that is not consistent with the clinical appearance of sound enamel or with a shadow of discolored dentin.

Code 4: *Marginal caries in enamel/dentin/ cementum adjacent to restoration/sealant with underlying dark shadow from dentin*

The tooth surface may have characteristics of code 2 and has a shadow of discolored dentin which is visible through an intact enamel surface with a localized breakdown in enamel but no visible dentin. This appearance is seen easily when the tooth is wet and the darkening/intrinsic shadow may be grey, blue, orange or brown.

Code 5: *Distinct cavity adjacent to restoration/sealant*

Distinct cavity adjacent to restoration/sealant with visible dentin in the interfacial space with signs of caries as described in codes 4, in addition to a gap of less than 0.5 mm in width or in case margins are not visible, there is evidence of discontinuity at the margin of restoration/sealant and the underlying dentin detected by moving 0.5 mm ball-end probe along the restoration/sealant margin.

Code 6: *Extensive distinct cavity with visible dentin*

Obvious loss of tooth structure; the cavity may be deep or wide and the dentin is clearly visible on both the walls at the base.

The scoring criteria for ICDAS II are summarized in Table 4.9.

ICDAS Two-digit Coding Method

A two-number coding system is suggested to identify restorations/sealants with the first digit, followed by the appropriate caries code. For example, a tooth restored with amalgam which also exhibited an extensive distinct cavity with visible dentin would be coded 4 (for an amalgam restoration), 6 (distinct cavity), an unrestored tooth with a distinct cavity would be 06. The suggested restoration/ sealant coding system is as follows:

0 = Sound: i.e. surface not restored or sealed (use with the codes for primary caries).

1 = Sealant, partial.

2 = Sealant, full.

3 = Tooth colored restoration.

4 = Amalgam restoration.

5 = Stainless steel crown.

6 = Porcelain or gold or PFM (porcelain fused to metal crown) crown or veneer or inlay or onlay or other restorative material.

7 = Lost or broken restoration.

8 = Temporary restoration.

9 = Used for the following conditions.

9.0 = Implant for other non-carious related reasons.

9.1 = Implant placed due to caries.

9.2 = Pontic placed for reasons other than caries.

9.3 = Pontic placed for carious reasons.

9.6 = Tooth surface cannot be examined: surface excluded.

Table 4.9: Scoring criteria for ICDAS-II

Scoring	Criteria
0	Sound tooth surface: no evidence of caries after prolonged air drying (5 s).
1	First visual change in enamel: opacity or discoloration (white or brown) is visible at the entrance of the pit or fissure after prolonged air drying, which is not or hardly seen on a wet surface.
2	Distinct visual change in enamel: opacity or discoloration distinctly visible at the entrance of the pit and fissure when wet, lesion must still be visible when dry.
3	Localized enamel breakdown due to caries with no visible dentin or underlying shadow: opacity or discoloration wider than the natural fissure/fossa when wet and after prolonged air drying.
4	Underlying dark shadow from dentin +/– localized enamel breakdown.
5	Distinct cavity with visible dentin: visual evidence of demineralization and dentin exposed.
6	Extensive distinct cavity with visible dentin and more than half of the surface involved.
	Caries associated with restoration and sealants
0	Sound tooth surface with restoration and sealant.
1	First visual change in enamel.
2	Distinct visual change in enamel/dentin adjacent to restoration/sealant margin.
3	Carious defect of >0.5 mm, with signs of code-2.
4	Marginal caries in enamel/dentin/cementum adjacent to restoration/sealant, with underlying dark shadow from dentin.
5	Distinct cavity adjacent to enamel/dentin.
6	Extensive distinct cavity with visible dentin.

9.7 = Tooth missing because of caries (tooth surfaces will be coded 9.7).

9.8 = Tooth missing for reasons other than caries (all tooth surfaces will be coded 9.8).

9.9 = Unerupted (tooth surfaces coded 9.9).

B. Caries Detection Criteria for Root Surface Caries

One score will be assigned per root surface. The facial, mesial, distal and lingual root surfaces of each tooth should be coded as follows:

Code E: If the root surface cannot be visualized directly (as a result of gingival recession or by gentle air drying), then it is excluded. The calculus should be removed prior to determining the status of the root surface.

Code O: The root surface does not exhibit any unusual discoloration that distinguishes it from the surrounding or adjacent root areas nor does it exhibit a surface defect either at the cemento-enamel junction or wholly on the root surface. The root surface has a natural anatomical contour; OR

The root surface may exhibit a definite loss of surface continuity or anatomical contour that is not consistent with the dental caries process.

The loss of surface integrity is usually associated with dietary habits or lesions such as abrasion or erosion. Abrasion is characterized by a clearly defined outline with a sharp border; whereas erosion has a more diffuse border. Neither condition shows discoloration.

Code 1: There is a clear demarcated area on the root surface or at the cemento-enamel junction (CEJ) that is discolored; however, there is no cavitation present.

Code 2: There is clear demarcated area on the root surface or at the cemento-enamel junction (CEJ) that is discolored and there is cavitation present.

Caries associated with Root Restorations

When a root surface is filled and there is caries adjacent to the restoration, the surface is scored as caries. The criteria for caries associated with restorations on the roots of teeth are the same as those for caries on non-restored root surfaces.

Special Considerations

Whenever both coronal and root surface are affected by a single carious lesion that extends at least 1.0 mm past the CEJ in both the incisal and apical directions, both surfaces should be scored as caries. However, for a lesion affecting both crown and root surface that does not meet the 1.0 mm or greater extent of involvement, only the coronal or root surface that involves the greater portion (more than 50%) of the lesion should be scored as caries. When it is impossible to invoke the 50% rule (i.e., when both coronal and root surfaces appear equally affected), both surfaces should be scored as caries.

When a carious lesion on a root surface extends beyond the line angle of the root to involve at least 1/3rd of the distance across the adjacent surface, that adjacent surface also should be scored as caries.

If more than one lesion is present on the same root surface, the most severe one is scored.

Non-vital teeth are scored in the same way as vital teeth.

Shortcomings of ICDAS-II Index

- It does not correlate well with the detection and assessment of the condition of sealants and various types of restorations.
- Incorporating non-primary carious lesion related condition makes the use of the ICDAS-II index complicated.
- It may lead to an overestimation of the seriousness of dental caries experience.
- When using ICDAS-II in epidemiological surveys, the chance that every person in the

world is affected by dental caries becomes very high, showing the low discriminating power of the index.

International Caries Classification and Management System (ICCMS)

The International Caries Classification and Management System (ICCMS) incorporates a range of options designed to accommodate the needs of different users across the ICDAS domains of clinical practice, dental education, research and public health.

There are four ICCMS elements, which depicts that caries management pathway is cyclical as each element follows in turn (Fig. 4.3). The cycle restarts after each risk based recall interval.

20. LESION ACTIVITY ASSESSMENT (LAA) SYSTEM

The lesion activity assessment (LAA) Criteria, developed by Ekstrand, et al 2007-2009, for use in association with the ICDAS scoring system based on using three clinical parameters: Parameter 1 (visual appearance), Parameter 2 (plaque stagnation), Parameter 3

(surface texture), evaluated by drawing the probe across the surface (Table 4.10). The scores so obtained are added and the total score is used to determine if the lesion is to be designated as 'active' or 'arrested'. The total score of 4 to 7 indicate an inactive lesion; whereas a total score more than 7 indicate an active lesion.

The total numbers of individuals are examined by two examiners in order to assess intra- and inter-examiner agreement. In case the examiners do not agree in their examination, a consensus is to be reached on the basis of re-examination by both the examiners.

The association on LAA and ICDAS codes involves lesion detection and coding, thereby estimating its depth or severity and assessing its activity. Most of the *in-vitro* studies could not observe any major difference between the Nyvad System and the ICDAS-LAA system in assessing caries activity in primary teeth; however, in clinical studies ICDAS-LAA system may overestimate the caries activity assessment of the occlusal lesions in primary teeth compared to the Nyvad System.

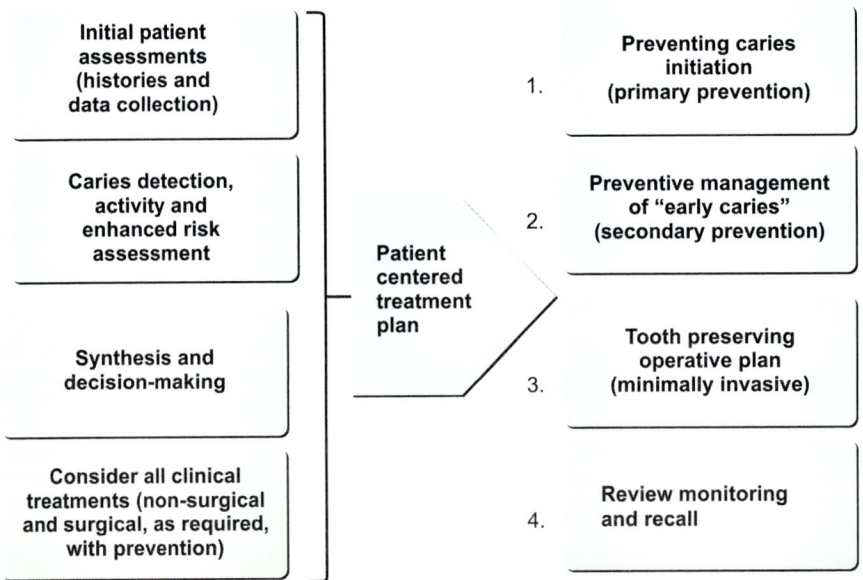

Fig. 4.3: International caries classification and management system (ICCMS)

Table 4.10: Assessment of activity by the LAA system

Criterion	Activity score
Clinical parameter 1 (visual appearance)	
ICDAS score 1, 2 (brown lesions)	1
ICDAS score 1, 2 (white lesions)	3
ICDAS score 3, 4, 5 or 6	4
Clinical parameter 2 (plaque stagnation)	
Plaque stagnation area	3
Non-plaque stagnation area	1
Clinical parameter 3 (surface texture)	
Rough or soft surface on gentle probing	4
Smooth or hard surface on gentle probing	2

21. THE PUFA INDEX

The PUFA index measures/quantifies the prevalence and severity of oral conditions resulting from untreated dental caries. The PUFA index is recorded separately, which complements classical caries indices with relevant information, subsequently helpful for planning oral health strategies.

Rules

1. The index is recorded separately from the DMFT/dmft and shows the presence of either a visible pulp, ulceration of the oral mucosa due to root fragments or a fistula/an abscess in the surrounding tissues. Any lesion not related to a tooth with visible pulpal involvement as a result of caries, is not included.

2. The assessment is made visually without the use of an instrument.

3. Only one score is assigned per tooth.

4. In case of doubt concerning the extent of odontogenic infection, the basic score (P/p for pulp involvement) is given.

5. If the primary tooth and its permanent successor tooth are present depicting stages of odontogenic infection, both teeth will be scored.

6. Upper case letters are used for the permanent dentition and lower case letters used for the primary dentition.

Criteria and Codes

The capital letters (P, U, F, A) refer to permanent teeth, whereas small letters (p, u, f, a) denotes primary teeth.

P/p: Pulpal involvement is recorded when the opening of the pulp chamber is visible or when the coronal tooth structures have been destroyed by the carious process and only roots or root fragments are left. Probing is not used to diagnose pulpal involvement.

U/u: Ulceration due to trauma (sharp pieces of tooth) is recorded when sharp edges of a dislocated tooth with pulpal involvement or root fragments that have caused traumatic ulceration of the surrounding soft tissues, i.e. tongue or buccal mucosa.

F/f: Fistula is recorded when a pus releasing sinus tract related to a tooth with pulpal involvement is present.

A/a: Abscess is scored when a pus containing swelling related to a tooth with pulpal involvement is present.

Calculation

The PUFA/pufa score per person is calculated in the same way as for the DMFT/dmft and represents the number of teeth that meet the PUFA/pufa criteria.

The PUFA for permanent teeth and pufa for primary teeth are reported separately.

Thus, for an individual, the score can range from 0 to 20 pufa for the primary dentition and 0–32 PUFA for the permanent dentition.

The prevalence of PUFA/pufa is calculated as percentage of the population with a PUFA/pufa score of one or more. The PUFA/pufa experience for a population is computed as a mean figure and can therefore have decimal values.

The 'untreated caries, PUFA ratio' is calculated as:

$$\frac{PUFA + pufa}{D + d} \times 100$$

22. CARIES ASSESSMENT SPECTRUM AND TREATMENT INDEX (CAST)

Caries assessment spectrum and a treatment index (CAST) was developed by Frencken in 2011. The index is based upon the combined strength of ICDAS II, PUFA and the DMF indices. CAST index is proposed on a spectrum (means a complete range of situations, from one extreme to its opposite), since it not only provides information regarding the number of non-cavitated and cavitated lesions, but also inform the consequences of the untreated ones by recording pulpal involvement due to carious process. The CAST index is considered useful in assessing the stages of carious lesion progression.

It describes the stages of progression of carious lesions from no carious lesion, through caries protection (sealant), restoring carious tooth, differentiating caries in enamel and dentin, the advanced stages of caries (pulpal involvement, fistula/sinus etc.), subsequently tooth loss. The codes and description of CAST index is tabulated in Table 4.11.

Advantages
- Used only for epidemiological surveys.
- It is built on strength of ICDAS, DMF and PUFA indices.
- Visual/tactile hierarchical one digit coding system.
- A DMF score can be easily calculated from the CAST score.

Limitations
- It does not record active and inactive carious lesions.
- It has not been validated, nor has its reliability been tested.
- It is not suggested for use in clinical trials.
- It does not provide data on treatment or preventive measures required for each code.

Table 4.11: Codes and descriptions of the CAST index

Characteristic	Code	Description
Sound	0	No visible evidence of a distinct carious lesion.
Sealed	1	Pits and fissures sealed with a sealant material, may be partially.
Restored	2	A cavity restored with an indirect restorative material.
Enamel	3	Distinct visual change in enamel. A clear discoloration (white or brown in color) simulating carious discoloration, including localized enamel breakdown without clinical signs of dentin involvement.
Dentin	4	Internal discoloration in dentin (carious effect). The lesion appears as shadows of discolored dentin visible through enamel which may or may not exhibit a visible localized breakdown.
Dentin	5	Distinct cavitation into dentin without pulpal involvement.
Pulp	6	Involvement of pulp. Distinct cavitation reaching the pulp.
Abscess/fistula	7	A swelling containing pus or a pus releasing sinus tract related to that tooth with pulpal involvement.
Lost	8	The tooth extracted because of dental caries.
Other	9	Does not match with any of the above categories.

23. SIGNIFICANT CARIES INDEX (SiC)

Significant caries index (SiC) was proposed by Bratthall in 2000 in order to highlight those individuals who have higher caries score in a given population. The SiC index is the mean DMFT of one-third of the group with highest caries score. This index is mainly used as a complement to the mean DMFT value. DMF and SiC indices when used together help in highlighting the oral health inequalities more accurately among different population groups within the community.

The index tries to overcome limitation of the mean DMFT value in accurately assessing the distribution of dental caries in a given population.

Calculating SiC Index

To calculate SiC index, the DMFT score of the group in a given population is presented first. For example, to simplify, only 15 individuals are taken (in original surveys, the numbers are much more). The mean DMFT score is calculated as described in Table 4.12.

Table 4.12: Calculating mean DMFT

Serial number	DMFT score	
1	1	
2	2	
3	1	
4	1	
5	0	
6	0	Calculate the sum of
7	1	all DMFT values. Then
*8	5	divide the sum by the
*9	4	total number of
*10	6	individuals to get mean
*11	7	DMFT.
12	0	39/15 = 2.6
*13	7	
14	2	
15	2	

Total (15)	39

Mean DMFT = 2.6

*Serial number with highest scores

Table 4.13: Calculating SiC index

Serial number with highest score	DMFT score	
13	7	The sum of DMFT (in the
11	7	selected one-third with highest
10	6	score) is 27. Divide this sum by
8	5	the total number of individuals
9	4	in the sub-group to get the
Total (5)	**27**	SiC Index. The SiC value
(one-third of 15)		would be 27/5 = 5.4

Now re-examine the individuals' scores and analyze how many are in the 'one-third' group. One-third of 15 is 5 (in case of odd numbers, round-off the fraction).

The five individuals with highest DMFT scores are separated. SiC value is calculated as described in Table 4.13.

Limitations

Being extension of DMF index, it follows same criteria for assessing dental caries; since having same limitations as DMF index.

Bibliography

1. Acharya AB and Mainali S. Are dental indexes useful in sex assessment? J. Forensic Odonto-stomatol: 2008;26:53–9.
2. Acharya S. Specific Caries Index: A new system for describing untreated dental caries experience in developing countries. J. Public Health Dent.: 2006;66:285–7.
3. Agbaje JO, Lesaffre E and Declerck D. Assessment of caries experience in epidemio-logical surveys: a review. Comm. Dent. Health: 2012;29:14–9.
4. Aherne CA, O' Mullane D and Barrett BE. Indices of root surface caries. J. Dent. Res.: 1990;69:1222–6.
5. Anaise JZ: Measurement of dental caries experience–modification of the DMFT index. Comm. Dent. Oral Epidemiol.: 1984;12:43–6.
6. Assaf AV, Meneghim Mde C, Zanin L, Mialhe FL, Pereira AC and Ambrosano GM. Assessment of different methods for diagnosing dental caries in epidemiological surveys. Comm. Dent. Oral Epidemiol.: 2004;32:418–25.

7. Bernabe E, Suominen-Taipale AL, Vehkalahti MM, Nordblad A and Sheiham A. The T-Health index: a composite indicator of dental health. Eur J Oral Sci. 2009;117:385–9.

8. Bodecker CF. The modified dental caries index. J. Am. Dent. Assoc.: 1939;26:1453–60.

9. Bodecker CF and Bodecker HWC. A practical index of the varying susceptibility to dental caries in man. Dent. Cosmos.: 1931;77:707–16.

10. Braga MM, Mendes FM, Martignon S, Ricketts DN and Ekstrand KR. *In vitro* comparison of Nyvad's system and ICDAS-II with lesion activity assessment for evaluation of severity and activity of occlusal caries lesions in primary teeth. Caries Res.: 2009;43:405–12.

11. Braga MM, Oliveira LB, Bonini GA, Bonecker M and Mendes FM. Feasibility of the international caries detection and assessment system (ICDAS-II) in epidemiological surveys and comparability with standard World Health Organization criteria. Caries Res.: 2009;43:245–9.

12. Bratthall D. Introducing the significant caries index together with a proposal for a new global oral health goal for 12 years old. Int. Dent. J.: 2000; 50:378–84.

13. Broadbent JM and Thomson WM. For debate: problems with the DMF index pertinent to dental caries data analysis. Comm. Dent. Oral Epidemiol.: 2005;33:400–9.

14. Chosack A. A dental caries severity index for primary teeth. Comm. Dent. Oral Epidemiol.: 1986;14:86–9.

15. Clara J, Bourgeois D and Muller-Bolla M. DMF from WHO basic methods to ICDAS II advanced methods: a systematic review of literature. Odontostomatol. Trop.: 2012;35:5–11.

16. Cypriano S, Sousa Mda L and Wada RS. The current applicability of viegas simplified indices to dental caries in epidemiological surveys. Cad. Saude Publica: 2004;20:1495–1502.

17. de Souza AL, Sanden WJM, Leal SC and Frencken E. The caries assessment spectrum and treatment (CAST) index: face and content validation. Int. Dent. J.: 2012;62:270–6.

18. Diniz MB, Rodrigues JA, Hug I, Cordeiro Rde C and Lussi A. Reproducibility and accuracy of the ICDAS-II for occlusal caries detection. Comm. Dent. Oral Epidemiol.: 2009;37:399–404.

19. Ditmyer M, Dounis G, Mobley C and Schwartz E. Inequalities of caries experience in Nevada youth expressed by DMFT index vs. significant caries index (SiC) over time. BMC Oral Health: 2011;11:12–21.

20. Downer MC. Do we really need another system for recording caries? Thoughts on ICDAS. Comm. Dent. Health: 2012;29:258–9.

21. Ekstrand KR, Martignon S, Ricketts DJ and Qvist V. Detection and activity assessment of primary coronal caries lesions: a methodologic study. Operative Dentistry 2007;32: 225–5.

22. Ekstrand KR, Zero DT, Martignon S and Pitts NB. Lesion activity assessment. Monographs of Oral Science 2009;21:63–90.

23. Frencken JE, Amorim RG, Faber J and Leal SC. The caries assessment spectrum and treatment (CAST) index: rational and development. Int. Dent. J.: 2011;61:117–23.

24. Frencken JE, de Souza AL, vander Sanden WJ, Bronkhorst EM and Leal SC. The caries assessment and treatment (CAST) instrument. Comm. Dent. Oral Epidemiol.: 2013;41:e71–7.

25. Iranzo-Cortes JE, Montiel-Company JM and Almerich-Silla JM. Caries diagnosis: agreement between WHO and ICDAS II criteria in epidemiological surveys. Comm. Dent. Health: 2013;30:108–11.

26. Ismail AI, Sohn W, Amaya A, Sen A, Hassan H and Pitts NB. The International Caries Detection and Assessment System (ICDAS): an integrated system for measuring dental caries. Comm. Dent. Oral Epidemiol. 2007;35:170–8.

27. Jablonski-Momeni A, Stachniss V, Ricketts DN, Heinzel-Gutenbrunner M and Pieper KJ. Reproducibility and accuracy of the ICDAS-II for detection of occlusal caries *in vitro*. Caries Res.: 2008;42:79–87.

28. Karthikeyan KS. DMF Index: its shortcomings and suggested rectification. JIDA: 2008;68:19–24.

29. Katz RV. Development of an index for the prevalence of root caries. JDR: 1984;63:814–9.

30. Knutson JW. An index of the prevalence of dental caries in schoolchildren. Public Health Rep.: 1944;59:253–63.

31. Koroluk L, Hoover JN and Komiyama K. The sensitivity and specificity of a colorimetric microbiological caries activity test (Cariostat) in preschool children. Pediatric Dent.: 1994;16:276–81.

32. Lang WP, Borgnakke WS, Taylor GW, Woolfolk MW, Ronis DL and Nyquist LV. Evaluation and use of an index of oral health status. J. Public Health Dent.: 1997;57:233–42.

33. Larmas M. Has dental caries prevalence some connection with caries index values in adults? Caries Research: 2010;44:81–4.

34. Mehta A. Comprehensive review of caries assessment systems developed over the last decade. RSBO: 2012;9:316–21.

35. Mendes FM, Braga MM, Oliveira LB, Antunes JL, Ardenghi TM and Bonecker M. Discriminant validity of the international caries detection and assessment system (ICDAS) and comparability with World Health Organization criteria in a cross-sectional study. Comm. Dent. Oral Epidemiol.: 2010;38:398–407.

36. Milgram P and Tanzer JM. Perspectives on PACS: Where is caries prevention clinical research going? J. Dent. Res.: 20129;1:122–4.

37. Moller IJ and Paulsen S. A standardized system for diagnosing, recording and analyzing dental caries data. Scand. J. Dent. Res.: 1973;81:1–11.

38. Monre B, Heinrich WR, Benzian H and Holmgren C. PUFA – An index of clinical consequences of untreated dental caries. Comm. Dent. Oral Epidemiol.: 2010;38:77–82.

39. Peterson PE. World Oral Health Report-2003. Comm. Dent. Oral Epidemiol.: 2003;31:3–24.

40. Pitts NB, Ekstrand KR. International caries detection and assessment system (ICDAS) and its international caries classification and management system (ICCMS) – methods for staging of the caries process and enabling dentists to manage caries. Comm Dent Oral Epid 2013;41:e41–e52.

41. Poulsen S and Horowitz HS. An evaluation of a hierarchical method of describing the pattern of dental caries attack. Community Dent. Oral Epidemiol. 1974, 2, 7–11.

42. Powell LV. Caries prediction: a review of the literature. Comm. Dent. Oral Epidemiol.: 1998;26: 361–71.

43. Schuller AA, Holst D. Oral status indicators DMFT and FS-I: Reflection on index selection. Eur. J. Oral Sci.: 2001;109:155–9.

44. Sellos MC and Soviero VM. Reliability of the Nyvad criteria for caries assessment in primary teeth. Eur. J. Oral Sci.: 2011;119:225.

45. Shivakumar K, Prasad S and Chandu G. International caries detection and assessment system: A new paradigm in detection of dental caries. J. Conserv. Dent.: 2009;12:10–16.

46. Shoaib L, Deery C, Ricketts DN and Nugent ZJ. Validity and reproducibility of ICDAS II in primary teeth. Caries Res.: 2009;43:442–8.

47. Slade GD and Caplan DJ. Methodological issues in longitudinal epidemiologic studies of dental caries. Comm. Dent. Oral Epidemiol.: 1999;27: 236–48.

48. Viegas AR. Simplified indices for estimating the prevalence of dental caries-experience in children seven to twelve years of age. J. Public Health Dent.: 1969;29:76–91.

5

Etiology of Dental Caries

The etiology of dental caries is undoubtedly a complex problem complicated by many direct and indirect factors. The universally accepted opinion as regard to etiology of dental caries could not be established till date. Numerous references of dental caries including early theories attempting to explain its etiology, have been recorded in history. Caries occurs in different individuals at different ages, at different sites and at different rates of progress. Evidence for caries was observed in Homosapiens since Paleolithic times. The disease occurs at sites with a pre-existing quantum of diverse microflora, while even more complex micro-organisms might not be implicated with pathology. The etiology is particularly challenging because it depends on determining which species are implicated directly in active lesions and which are merely present causing no harm.

The traditional model of caries is that decay is a one-way process of acidic demineralization of the hard tissues of tooth. The process is initiated by frequent intake of refined sugars coupled with plaque deposition onto the tooth surfaces. However, the newer concepts, over the years, compelled the researchers re-analyze the traditional model. A few authors have reported decline in caries for the last couple of decades. The declining trend continued even when sugar consumption and plaque control measures changed a little. Appropriate fluoride consumption was considered to be the cause of declining caries. Fluoride in its many forms could provide buffer against caries. It was established that high rate of caries was associated with deficiency of fluoride intake, reduced salivary protection or with excessive frequency of carbohydrate consumption. Later, it was concluded that decline and increase in caries activity are time specific and population specific. At one place with specific individuals, there might be decline; whereas at some other place the scenario be opposite. To understand more, let us explain the existing old and new theories of etiology of caries.

Many theories have evolved over the years; however, no single theory could explain the definite etiology.

Various theories hypothesized from time to time are as follows:

1. Humoral theory.
2. Worm theory.
3. Vital theory.
4. Putrefaction theory.
5. Parasitic theory.
6. Sulfatase theory.
7. Theory of inflammation.
8. Chemical theory.
9. Septic theory.

10. Acidogenic theory.
11. Diet detergent theory.
12. Environment and nutritional theory.
13. Osmotic theory.
14. Chelation theory.
15. Proteolytic theory.
16. Proteolysis-chelation theory.
17. Genetic theory.
18. Autoimmune theory.
19. Sucrose chelation theory.
20. Bioelectric phenomena.
21. Levine's theory.
22. Bandlish theory.
23. Caries balance concept.
24. Systemic theory.

1. Humoral Theory

Hippocrates (400 BC) and Galen (130 AD) were of the view that caries was due to humoral pathology and opined that a state of health or a specific disease was determined by the relative amount of humor, viz. blood, phlegm, yellow bile and black bile. They further suggested that dental decay was due to accumulation of certain juices in the tooth. Galen once stated that "when the head becomes disordered in nature, it produces many excrements from which lesions of lower organs occurs." Therefore, the excrement readily passes to mouth. Dental decay, mouth ulcers, pyorrhea are due to catarrhal idioms descending to them from head.

According to him, dental caries is produced by internal action of acid and corroding humors. The imbalance in these humors results in the disease process. Hippocrates and couple of other authors favored this concept and also added that accumulated debris around the teeth helped in corroding action.

2. Worm Theory (the Legend of the Worm)

Guy de Chauliac (1300-1368) was the first to report worms causing dental diseases. The early history of India, Egypt and Homer writings have also referred 'worm' as the cause of toothache. Therefore, it was hypothesized that caries could be recognized as a worm over tooth surface.

Van Leeuwenhoek, the father of microscopy, observed three different worms from the extracted teeth that act as demons and substituted foods as likely source. Early researchers were of the view that the tooth cavity, which they referred as 'hole', was the result of worm boring into a tooth. It has the appearance similarly to the worm hole evident in wood. Perhaps the Guinea worm, Dracunculus medinensis, a worm of drinking water was the tooth worm. The common treatment for worms at that time was to place a few drops of oil of vitriol (sulphuric acid) onto the tooth.

3. Vital Theory

Earlier authors postulated that tooth decay originated from within the tooth itself like 'gangrene'. They observed wider area beneath and smaller pin-point area on the top of the tooth histologically.

4. Putrefaction Theory

A few authors suggested putrefaction as the cause of dental decay. But the availability of skeletal remains and the evidence that putrefaction did not advance the dental lesion quickly dispelled the idea.

5. Parasitic Theory

Erdl (1843) described filamentous parasites in the membrane of tooth surfaces. Dental caries was thought to develop as a result of infiltration and decomposition of enamel cuticle (a surface protein membrane on the teeth).

The filamentous parasites in the membrane of tooth surfaces were considered as the causative agent for dental caries.

He suggested that it was not the tooth worm but filamentous organisms on the tooth surface, which might have infiltrated into the tooth and produced dental caries.

6. Sulfatase Theory

Bacterial toxins hydrolyze the 'Mucoitin sulfate' of enamel and 'chondroitin sulfate' of dentin producing sulphuric acid that in turn causes decalcification of dental tissues. Since the concentration of sulfated polysaccharides in enamel is very less and also not readily accessible, the hypothesis was not accepted.

7. Theory of Inflammation

John Hunter (1778) and Thomas Bell (1831) opined that dental decay was because of internal inflammation. It continued to be advocated by prominent physicians of that era. However, W.D. Miller demonstrated that it was not possible to produce an inflammatory process in the hard structures of teeth. He pointed out that filling gold foil might produce an acute inflammatory process in bone or other tissues, but it would not affect the tooth. The inflammatory process as the cause of dental decay could not be substantiated and was discarded.

8. Chemical (Acid) Theory

A few authors in early 19th century (Parmly, 1819) suggested that the teeth were destroyed by unidentified chemical agent (acid) formed in the oral cavity. Various hypothesis as how the acid is produced were put forward. Robertson (1835) proposed that the acid was formed by fermentation of food particles around teeth. Another suggestion was that the putrefaction of protein produced ammonia, which was subsequently oxidized to nitric acid. Till then, the activity of bacteria was not recognized.

Ficnus (1847) attributed dental caries to 'denticolae', the generic term for decay related micro-organisms. Leber and Rotenstein (1867) reported presence of micro-organisms in caries affected teeth. A couple of other authors, Clark (1871), Tomes (1873) and Magitot (1878) opined that bacteria were essential for initiation of caries, although they suggested an exogenous source of acids. They

further observed that caries was due to the solvent action of acids generated by fermentation of food present around the teeth. The tooth worm disappeared from the prevailing view and investigators recognized fungi and long leptirichia-type organisms on the tooth surface and within the carious lesion. Conceptually, they substituted bacteria for the tooth worm.

9. Septic Theory

Underwood and Milles (1880) hypothesized that acid capable of causing decalcification was actually produced by bacteria. They reported micrococci as well as other forms of organisms in sections of decayed teeth.

10. Acidogenic Theory/ Chemicoparasitic Theory

The acidogenic/chemicoparasitic theory is a blend of chemical and septic theories. WD Miller (1882) working at the University of Berlin, the pioneer investigator on dental caries, hypothesized this concept. According to this theory caries is caused by acids produced by micro-organisms of the oral cavity. The results of his studies were extensively discussed, documented and were widely accepted.

He opined that the dental decay is a chemicoparasitic process, whereby enamel is decalcified by chemical process and the dentin dissolution consists of two stages; the decalcification of dentin followed by dissolution of softened residue. The acid which affects the primary decalcification is derived from fermentation of starches and sugar lodged in the retaining areas of the teeth. Miller found that bread, meat and sugar, incubated *in vitro* with saliva at body temperature produced enough acid capable of decalcifying enamel and dentin. Subsequently, he isolated numerous micro-organisms from the oral cavity, many of which were acidogenic and some were proteolytic. Most of these bacterial forms were capable of forming lactic acid. After extensive research, Miller believed that caries was not caused by any single organism, but rather by a variety of micro-organisms.

Two main factors were recognized in the caries process:

a. Quantity and quality of carbohydrates.
b. Acid producing oral micro-organisms.

a. Quantity and Quality of Carbohydrates

It has been referred earlier that members of isolated primitive societies who have relatively low caries index manifest a remarkable increase in caries incidence after exposure to refined diets (mostly carbohydrate). The readily available fermentable carbohydrates were presumed to be responsible for increase in caries incidence. Numerous studies endorsed this belief.

Miller in his early studies observed decalcification when teeth were incubated in mixtures of saliva and bread/sugar. There was no effect on the teeth when meat/fat was used in place of the carbohydrate. Both cane sugar and cooked starches produced acid; however, a little acid was formed when food was substituted with raw starches. A few authors disagreed and reported the production of similar quantities of acid from mixtures of either sucrose or starch incubated with saliva with no difference in acid production between raw and refined sugarcane.

The uncontaminated human saliva contains small amounts of carbohydrates. Salivary carbohydrates are bound to proteins and other compounds and are not readily available for microbial degradation. The cariogenic carbohydrates are dietary in origin. The cariogenicity of these carbohydrates varies with the frequency of ingestion, physical form, chemical composition, route of administration and presence of other food constituents.

Sticky, solid carbohydrates are more cariogenic than those consumed as liquids. Carbohydrates in detergent foods are less damaging to the teeth than the same in soft retentive foods. Carbohydrates, which are rapidly cleared from the oral cavity, are less conducive to caries than those which are slowly cleared. Polysaccharides are less easily fermented by plaque bacteria than mono-saccharides and disaccharides. Plaque organisms produce a little acid from sugar alcohols, sorbitol and mannitol. Glucose or sucrose, fed by stomach tube or IV does not contribute to decay as they are unavailable for microbial breakdown. Meals high in fat, protein or salts reduce the oral retentiveness of carbohydrates. Refined pure carbohydrates are more cariogenic than crude carbohydrates. The dental caries results subsequent to interaction between oral bacteria and local carbohydrates producing acids and affecting the dissolution of hard tooth tissues.

b. Acid Producing Oral Micro-organisms

Miller confirming the role of acids in caries production demonstrated the presence of micro-organism within tubules of decayed teeth, mainly cocci and leptothrix.

Earlier authors emphasized more on gram-positive bacillus (*B. nacrodentin*) from carious dentin; however, subsequent authors agreed on certain streptococci to be the causative agents.

Clarke (1924) isolated *Streptococcus mutans* from carious lesions and described the same as the main culprit agent. Bunting (1928) suggested a definite correlation between *Lactobacillus acidophilus* and dental caries.

Considerable emphasis has been placed on diet-bacteria interactions, which are involved in caries initiation on different tooth surfaces. Specific micro-organisms as well as combination of organisms including *Lactobacilli*, Streptococci, Actinomyces species and others have been studied. The studies confirmed that a number of organisms, including streptococci and lactobacilli, are associated with dental caries. The possibility exists that one or more organisms are implicated in the initiation of caries while different organisms may influence the progress of disease.

Keyes (1960) demonstrated that under certain laboratory conditions, caries could be considered as an infectious and transmissible disease, which fulfills the biologic principles governing any infectious process.

It has been established that the streptococcal organisms studied by Keyes and Fitzgerald were actually rodent strains of *Streptococcus mutans*, an efficient cariogenic micro-organisms. The epidemiologic studies over the years have confirmed that *Streptococcus mutans* is pandemic in its geographic distribution and is particularly prevalent in societies where sucrose consumption is high.

Miller's acidogenic/chemicoparasitic theory is the backbone of current knowledge and understanding of the etiology of dental caries. However, Miller's work could not explain predilection of specific sites on a tooth to dental caries, the initiation of smooth surface caries and phenomenon of arrested and recurrent caries. Also, this theory does not clarify why some population is caries free in spite of having same diet and other environmental features.

A few authors argued that Miller's theory could not explain the quantitative and reproducible feature of age distribution. Acid production may be necessary, but it is certainly not a sufficient condition for dental caries.

11. Diet Detergent Theory

Wallace (1910) hypothesized that the fibrous part of diet acts as detergent, which leads to physical removal of substrate required for initiation of caries. He classified food into two categories; one which tends to leave viscous and fermentable carbohydrates and second which tends to brush tooth surface during mastication. The fibrous food is subjected to crushing and disintegration between the teeth many times. A lack of fibrous matter reduced the need for mastication and, as a consequence,

food debris was removed from the teeth less effectively. It was observed that refined carbohydrates, because of their shorter time spent during chewing, accumulated in the film that naturally covered the teeth. These carbohydrates along with micro-organisms form acids that initiated the first phase of caries. If no carbohydrate is lodged in the oral cavity, the bacteria which are best adapted for the medium would either be starved out or if present will not be active. The author opined that an irregular dentition might be an important predisposing cause of caries. The irregular dentition and malocclusion do not allow easy cleaning, thereby predisposing to the accumulation of food debris and subsequently leading to caries.

12. Environmental and Nutritional Theory

It is established that the vitamins and minerals available in nutrition play an important role in development of teeth. The continuous availability of these vitamins and minerals also affects disintegration and dissolution of enamel. A few authors were of the view that only environmental factors play role in initiation and progress of caries, whereas vitamins/minerals affect only during development of tooth tissues. The altered tooth tissues might become susceptible to caries.

13. Osmotic Theory

Eckerman (1920) hypothesized two kinds of caries: Primary (physio-pathological process within the tooth) and Secondary (breaking down of tissues by micro-organisms). Primary caries commences from within, beginning at the tooth pulp and spreading outwards to the surface of the enamel. This outward spread simulates osmotic flow of blood plasma and red blood cells, brought about by an excess of common salt or sugar in the saliva. The interchange takes place via dentinal tubules and certain spindle-like spaces in the enamel communicating with the peripheral ends of the dentinal tubules. Occasionally the interchange follows under the Nasmyth's membrane, which forms the osmotic membrane. The channel so formed was designated as 'caries canals'. Caries canal is a cone-shaped area in dentin exhibiting different color, having its apex towards the pulp and its base under the carious enamel. Color of this area (carious dentin) is due to blood plasma. Primary caries is limited to the crown of the tooth; that might be because of the fact that owing to early eruption or malnutrition, the enamel not matured properly allows osmotic force to effectively create disturbances. The consequence of this outpouring of plasma into the dentin is an excess of organic matter in that tissue. The micro-organisms become effective and the "primary" merges into "secondary" caries, which is a bacterial process. Secondary caries was limited to areas such as exposed roots of teeth or where food debris can be held for sufficient time. Various authors later disagreed with Eckerman's concept since it could not explain lateral extension of caries; also it was established that 'caries canals' appeared at the later stage of decay.

14. Chelation Theory

Earlier authors established that chelation was the most important mechanism for the dissolution, transportation and utilization of minerals. The alkaline blood maintains calcium in solution by means of chelation. The normal turnover/replacement, and pathologic demolition of bone also involves chelation. This might be true for dissolution of primary tooth roots. The two most important pigments in the plant and animal kingdoms are chelate complexes. Hemoglobin is an iron chelate and chlorophyll is a magnesium chelate. According to this concept, tooth decay results from demineralization by chelating agents which dissolve enamel minerals by forming complexes. The chelation theory recognizes a wide variety of agents, which include acids and alkaline compounds that form calcium chelates under acidic and non-acidic conditions.

15. Proteolytic Theory

According to this theory (Gottleib, 1944 and others), the proteolytic enzymes liberated by oral bacteria destroy the organic matrix of enamel (enamel lamellae and enamel rod sheaths), resulting in loosening of apatite crystals with eventual loss of minerals. This theory differs in that the initial attack on enamel is proteolytic rather than acidic. The gram-negative bacilli produce sulphuric acid during their invasion of organic pathway, subsequently destroying the inorganic minerals. Once enamel is collapsed forming cavity, the micro-organisms can enter deeper dentinal tissues.

They further opined that a radiopaque layer as seen in caries progression is the result of maturation process in the tooth surface following exposure to the oral environment. Minor variations in the organic and inorganic components of the tooth are seen as determining features in the initiation and progress of caries. It implies that the caries may penetrate either through enamel rods or extend along the course of a number of rods or involve segments of numerous rods. Although the proteolysis of organic matrix of dentin may occur after demineralization, it could not be established that the initial attack on enamel was proteolytic.

Later Pincus (1949) also maintained that the initial process in caries was the proteolytic breakdown of the dental cuticle. The organic membrane was found on all the teeth followed by destruction of the prism sheaths. The loosened prisms then fell out mechanically. He proposed that the Nasmyths membrane and enamel proteins, which are acted upon by the sulfatase enzyme of the bacilli yield sulphuric acid.

Limitations

- Areas of enamel with relatively high organic content such as lamellae and tufts do not show susceptibility to caries.
- Studies have shown the occurrence of caries even in the absence of proteolytic micro-organisms.
- Not possible to simulate caries with proteolytic agents.
- Though enamel contains 1.0–1.5% organic matrix, out of which 0.6% is protein; initiation of caries with the breakdown of small percentage of protein is debatable.
- The sulfatase of gram-negative Bacilli which are considered to dissolve by enamel proteins have not been found in abundance in experimental studies.

16. The Proteolysis-chelation Theory

The proteolysis-chelation theory, proposed by Schatz, et al (1956), implies a simultaneous microbial degradation of organic components (proteolysis), and the dissolution of minerals of the tooth by a process known as 'chelation'. The hypothesis was based on the chemical aspects of chelation, with a little direct evidence of proteolysis-chelation as a mechanism in the caries process.

Chelation is a process involving the complexing of a metallic ion to a complex substance through a coordinate covalent bond which results in a highly stable, poorly dissociated or weakly ionized compound.

The widely accepted examples are the chlorophyll molecule of green plants linked to magnesium and hemoglobin linked to iron mechanism of chelation.

The proteolysis-chelation theory considers dental caries to be a bacterial destruction of teeth where the initial attack is on the organic components of enamel. The breakdown products of this organic matter have chelating properties, thereby dissolve the enamel minerals. This results in formation of substances which may form soluble chelates with the mineralized component of the tooth and thereby decalcify the enamel at a neutral

or even alkaline pH. Enamel also contains other organic components besides keratins, such as mucopolysaccharides, lipids and citrate, which may be susceptible to bacterial attack and act as chelators. The proteolysis-chelation theory clarifies the argument as to whether the initial attack of dental caries is on the organic or inorganic portion of enamel by stating that both may be attacked simultaneously.

However, proteolysis-chelation theory do not fulfill the following observations:

Increased caries incidence with increased sugar consumption.

Increased lactobacillus count with high caries activity.

Decreased caries incidence following topical/systemic administration of fluoride.

Researchers favoring the theory explained that the increased caries incidence concomitant with increased carbohydrate consumption might be because carbohydrates facilitate proteolysis; producing conditions whereby keratinous proteins are less stable. And also the increased caries incidence along with increased lactobacillus counts might be the result of caries process, rather than its cause. Proteolysis may provide ammonia which prevents a 'Hydrogen drop' that would tend to inhibit growth of the lactobacilli. The release of calcium from hydroxyapatite by chelation might also encourage the growth of lactobacilli.

Calcium exerts a vitamin-sparing action on some bacilli. Reduced caries incidence following administration of fluoride might be because of formation of fluorapatite, which strengthen the linkages between the organic and inorganic phases of the enamel. Although these explanations seem authentic, yet the exact mechanism of caries etiology could not be explained.

The analysis of evidence supporting the three main theories of dental caries, i.e. acidogenic theory, proteolysis theory and proteolysis-chelation theory is summarized in Table 5.1.

Table 5.1: Summary analysis of evidence supporting three main theories of dental caries

Factors studied	Acidogenic	Proteolysis	Chelation
A. Clinical			
i. Site of cavities (caries occurs at places where fermentable carbohydrate food is retained on tooth surfaces)	+ The localization of cavities is confirmed by various authors supported by our clinical experience	− No evidence only proteolysis would account for localization and since carbohydrates are used for bacterial energy in preference to protein, proteolysis will be delayed in areas where carbohydrates are retained	− No evidence why chelation account for localization
ii. Diet and caries High incidence of caries found in persons using high carbohydrate diet	+ Clinical studies have established the relationship of caries and carbohydrates. Elimination of diet, which forms acids in mouth has been shown to reduce caries Fluorides increase the resistance of enamel to decalcification to acids and hence reduce caries	− No similar association exists in relation to attack by proteolysis. No such studies reported Increased resistance by adding zinc chloride was not approved	− No similar association exists in relation to chelation. No such studies reported effect of fluoride on keratinase lacks scientific support
iii. Animal studies Caries detected in animals when fed on carbohydrate diets and prevented by agents which inhibit fermentation	+ Agents such as iodoacetic acid and dicalcium phosphate reduce caries in animals	− Doubtful questionable evidence given	− No studies
B. Mechanism of destruction			
i. Destruction of inorganic part has been shown both *in vivo* and *in vitro*	+ Decalcification by acid production has been proved	± (doubtful) No mechanism has been established to show how proteolysis will destroy the calcified tissues	± (doubtful) The keratin in enamel is dissolved by mouth organisms, thereby forming chelating agents which dissolve enamel. Evidence reported that the total keratin changed into chelating compounds can dissolve only 1% of calcium in enamel so not convincing evidence to produce detectable caries
ii. Destruction of organic part has doubtful evidence	± Since organic portion is fragile, it disintegrates	± Proteolytic agents destroy human enamel protein	± It was only presumed that oxygen uptake

(Contd.)

Table 5.1: Summary analysis of evidence supporting three main theories of dental caries (*Contd...*)

Factors studied	Acidogenic	Proteolysis	Chelation
in all the three theories	as decalcification takes place	is partially supported by scientific evidence	was observed when proteolytic bacterium culture grew in human enamel. But actual organisms were not isolated from enamel. The uptake of oxygen by enamel was as good as auto-respiration
C. Histology of caries			
i. Destruction of enamel is accompanied by loss of calcific material and the organic portion persists	+ Different zones found in caries in enamel can be explained by acid theory	Doubtful Bacteria penetrate along the organic tracts in enamel but proteolysis does not explain different zones	– No evidence
ii. Appearance of radiolucent area in X-rays	+ Radiolucency seen in radiographs because of loss of calcium	– No support	– No support
iii. Increase of nitrogen and loss of specific gravity and hardness	+ Loss of inorganic material and persistence of organic material occurs in initial stage which accounts for increase of nitrogen and loss of specific gravity and hardness	– No evidence reported	– No evidence
D. Bacteriology			
i. Isolation of appropriate bacteria from enamel caries	+ Bacteria producing acid from fermentable carbohydrates is isolated from caries sites	– No evidence	Doubtful Doubtful keratolytic organisms have not been isolated from initial enamel caries but found in deeper cavities
ii. Presence of necessary bacteria in oral cavity	+ Bacterial flora capable of producing decalcifying acids always present in the oral cavity and on the tooth surface	+ Proteolytic types such as *Actinomyces bovis, Streptococcus mitis* are generally present in the oral cavity	Doubtful
iii. Bacterial antagonists reduce caries	+ Certain bacterial antagonists such as iodoacetic acid, penicillin, etc. reduce caries in animals and man	No evidence	No evidence

17. Genetic Theory

Caries has been established as a multifactorial disease, affected by the action and interaction of genetic, environmental, and behavioral factors. Horowitz, et al (1958) investigating 'caries experience rate' observed definite correlation of hereditary to caries susceptibility. The genetic aspect of the host influences factors such as host immune response, effect of salivary components and dietary habits that affect the nature of the available substrate upon which the cariogenic organisms grow and multiply. Various authors have confirmed the role of genetics in caries susceptibility. Book and Grahnen (1953) in their study on parents and siblings concluded that environmental factors play no role in caries susceptibility; however, genetics play a vital role in individuals' resistance against caries. Many studies provided evidence of genetic contributions, salivary gland functions, structural modification of enamel and varied immune response to cariogenic micro-organisms. Only specific genes have been associated with caries risk, such as genes involved in enamel formation (amelogenin, ameloblastin, tuffelin). The role of proline-rich proteins (PRP—proteins coded by chromosomes) in saliva and other forms of glycoproteins have been evaluated.

The genetic/hereditary involvement of preferences of carbohydrate intake vis-à-vis taste of individuals have also been studied. Studies examining genetically determined taste sensitivity to 6-n-propylthiouracil showed that individuals with low sensitivity experience a low caries risk than those with high testing sensitivity. Evaluating genes TAS2R38, TAS1R2 and GNAT3, it was established that taste plays a vital role in caries initiation.

Heritability is the ratio of the genetic component of variance to the total variance of the trait, expressed as a proportion or percentage. Heritability may vary among populations with different patterns of environmental factors, and may even change with age within a given population. Recently genetic factors such as DNA methylation, which is modified by environmental factors and nutrition have been observed to play vital role in the genetic determinant of caries (Chmurzynstea, 2010).

18. Autoimmune Theory

Burnet (1959) hypothesized 'forbidden clone'concept, describing caries as the 'auto-immune' disease. He proposed that the normal state of immunological self tolerance might be induced by gene mutations in mesenchymal stem cells. A mutant cell propagates formation of 'forbidden clone'. These mutant cells synthesize cellular or humoral autoantibodies, which circulate through the body fluid and attack target cells (odontoblasts cells in caries). The theory enables us to understand, how somatic mutations affect large number of target cells at various parts of the body.

Burch and Jackson (1966) later analyzed caries epidemiologic data and suggested that partially mutational genes determine whether a site on a tooth is at risk or not.

Since most of the data was based on epidemiologic studies, its authenticity could not be established.

19. The Sucrose Chelation Theory

Egglers-Lura (1967) proposed that sucrose itself, and not the acid so produced can cause dissolution of enamel. The calcium forms an ionized calcium saccharate with sucrose. The calcium saccharates require inorganic phosphate, which is subsequently removed from the enamel by phosphorylating enzymes. However, different researchers disagreed and observed that soluble complex can be formed between sucrose and calcium even at alkaline pH values.

20. Bioelectric Phenomena

The electric forces might be the causative agents in dental decay; a new concept hypothesized by Parker (1969). It has been recognized that certain living objects have the potential to produce an electrical voltage. The mechanism of producing such electrical voltage can be: (a) The piezoelectric effect and the related semiconductor mechanism, (b) The ion pump and membrane potential involved in nerve activity, (c) A difference in electron concentrations where high- and low-redox potentials exist in some proximity to one another and have electrical continuity between them. The tooth surfaces and the surroundings may develop electrical voltages since the enamel surface because of its crystalline structure may act as an ion-permeable membrane and also the bacterial colonies in plaque.

Earlier authors have established that enamel because of its permeability function as an ion-selective membrane. They further opined that non-uniform distribution of potassium ions across membranes of sound human teeth resulted in significant electrical potentials. The passage of this current through enamel surfaces along with change in reflectance of light was correlated with demineralization of enamel. When dental plaque covered the surfaces of teeth, reflectance again changes leading to lowering of the electrical resistance. When the tooth surface was made positive by passage of electrical current, demineralization was observed. Remineralization occurred when an external electrical voltage of negative potential was applied to the tooth surface.

21. Levine's Theory

Miller's acidogenic concept was accepted widely till nineteenth century. Almost all studies favoured 'acid' as the main causative agent. However, two different postulates were also flouted simultaneously.

The first was proteolysis theory which suggested that the initial stage of caries initiation was the enzymatic destruction of organic matrix of enamel, which facilitates colonization and growth of bacteria which produced acid for removal/dissolution of inorganic contents of enamel. The process subsequently invades dentin.

The second was proteolysis-chelation theory, which suggested that after an initial proteolytic attack on enamel, chemicals were released which removed the calcium of the mineral phase (getting chelated). The chelated contents help dissolution of the tooth tissues.

The factors associated with caries initiation and progression are divided in two groups: first the factors which govern the resistance of tooth surface to acid attack and second the factors which determine the source and potential of acid generation.

a. Factors governing resistance of tooth surfaces.
   - Tooth morphology.
   - Enamel microstructure and composition.
   - Aberration in enamel anatomy.
b. Factors governing acid production.
   - Oral flora producing plaque and acids.
   - Diet having potential to invite cariogenic micro-organisms.
   - Flow, viscosity and buffering capacity of saliva.

Levine hypothesized that caries may be considered as a demineralizing process with the passage of mineral ions from enamel modified by the presence of plaque which acts as diffusion barriers. He and his colleagues illustrated this fact by putting acid on enamel surface *in vitro*. The enamel was removed layer by layer; whereas when enamel was covered by a barrier which partially restricts the movement of ions from the surface, such as gelatin then the characteristic subsurface demineralization pattern was observed. It implies that 'acid' alone may not show the potential to initiate caries process.

If more ions leave the enamel than enter in a given time interval, then there is net demineralization and the start of the carious process. The focus of interest is on those factors which affect this delicate ionic balance

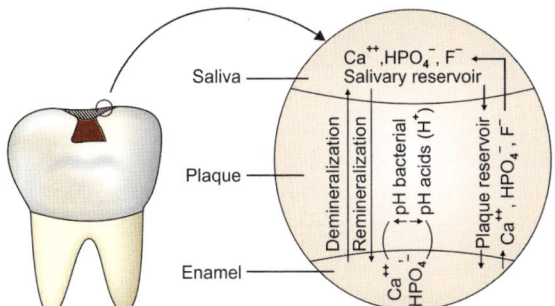

Fig. 5.1: Levine's ionic see-saw theory of dental caries

and also the factors which favor remineralization of enamel surface (Fig. 5.1).

The factors which influence ionic exchange between enamel and plaque are:

- pH.
- Calcium and phosphate ion concentration.
- Fluoride in different forms.

Fluorides help precipitation of calcium and phosphate ions from the solution, especially at low concentration. Free mineral ions in the plaque-enamel interface are to be deposited as hydroxyapatite on enamel crystals. However, at higher concentration, calcium fluoride is deposited initially. The fluoride concentrations as low as 5 ppm can reverse the net movement of ions from solid to solution. The fluorides have the potential to tilt the 'see-saw' in enamel's favor.

22. Bandlish's Theory

Signifying role of attrition in caries etiology, Bandlish (1982) hypothesized that oral fluids protect the enamel by providing a protecting covering on the enamel surface. Attrition makes the fissures wider and removes the superficial layer of the enamel along with the initial carious lesion, if present. The new layer of enamel becomes protective again with the help of oral fluids. In areas where the oral fluid cannot reach (e.g. contact areas) enamel cannot be made protective against the carious attack.

Organic acids produced by bacterial fermentation of the carbohydrate cause surface demineralization of the enamel. At this stage, the bacteria do not penetrate the intact enamel surface. The demineralized products are redeposited into the enamel during the process of remineralization. Caries occur only if there is more demineralization and less remineralization.

Caries starts at the contact area where the protective action of oral fluid is lacking, i.e. the perimeter of the contact area. Smaller the area, more is the perimeter/unit area; as the area becomes large, the perimeter/unit area falls. Similarly smaller the contact area, more the perimeter per unit area, as the contact area becomes more (may be physiologic or with attrition), the perimeter/unit area falls. The effect of acid attack depends upon the perimeter/unit area. Greater the perimeter, stronger the attack. As the length of perimeter/unit area increase with decrease in size of the contact area, the carious lesion progress faster in a smaller contact area, if other conditions are kept constant.

The convexity of the adjoining surfaces affects the intensity of caries. The more the convex surface, the smaller is the contact area; the less the convex surface, the larger is the contact area. When there is contact between two surfaces of varying convexities, the contact on the more convex surface is smaller. Accordingly, the caries incidence is higher in more convex surfaces (Figs 5.2A and B). The above mentioned concept of convexities when applied to caries incidence of different adjacent surfaces seems to be correct except in the case of contact between the permanent first molar and second molar. Mesial surface of first permanent molar is less convex still this surface is more prone to caries. The reason could be that some caries might have been initiated during the period the first molar remained in contact with second deciduous molar.

Bandlish was of the view that meticulous contact through brushing and cleaning reduces caries not by removing plaque but by removing some part of enamel.

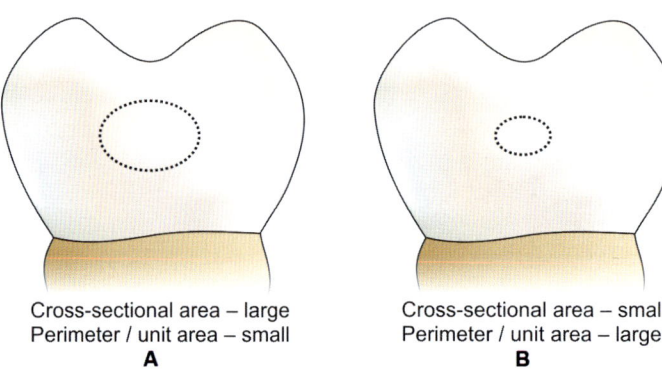

Cross-sectional area – large
Perimeter / unit area – small
A

Cross-sectional area – small
Perimeter / unit area – large
B

Figs 5.2A and B: Progression of caries is faster in tooth B as compared to tooth A

It is suggested that gradual recession of active enamel lesion to a larger extent is a result of surface wear. Plaque acts as a reservoir of minerals and with its buffering capabilities helps in maturation of enamel surface, thereby reducing caries.

The approximal surface gains the beneficial effect of oral fluids during functional movement of teeth. During the buccolingual movement of teeth, there is more movement at occlusal border of the contact area and less at the cervical border (less movement near the fulcrum). Where there is more movement there is less incidence of caries. Accordingly, the cervical border of contact area is more prone to caries.

In case of occlusal caries, caries starts at places where there is least attrition and least plaque, i.e. where contact of two or more enamel surface occurs like in fissures and at cusp tips. He opined that pits and fissures are not usually full of plaque as the general belief is, but there may be little plaque in the functioning pits and fissures. It is not the depth of a fissure, which is important but the narrowness of the fissure, which makes it more caries prone. Maximum enamel caries occurs in a fissure where the two walls of a fissure either meet or come close to each other. The plunging action of masticatory forces helps to pump the oral secretions into the region of contact area. Food consumption habits are changing with modernization; less

fibrous and softer food being consumed more, the masticatory forces are reduced. The reduced masticatory forces do not force oral secretions into the unprotected areas, thereby making these areas more prone to caries.

23. Caries Balance Concept

Featherstone (1999) proposed 'caries balance concept' and hypothesized that the caries is the outcome of disturbance in balance between pathological and protective factors. The caries progress if the pathological factors overweigh the protective factors.

The pathological factors are:
• Cariogenic/acidogenic micro-organisms.
• Quality of fermentable carbohydrates.
• Frequency of intake of carbohydrates and their clearance.
• Inadequate mineral content and flow of saliva.

The protective factors are:
• Adequate mineral contents and flow of saliva.
• Supply of fluorides from extrinsic sources (fluoride, along with salivary calcium and phosphates provide ingredients for remineralization).
• Effective use of antiplaque.

This balance between pathologic factors on one side and protective factors on the other side dynamically changes throughout the day.

According to the caries balance concept, caries does not result from a single factor; rather, it is the outcome of the complex interaction of pathologic and protective factors. The risk factors, the potential of these may vary with time, must be assessed regularly. The basic concept can be used to treat or arrest/reverse caries in individuals and also at community levels. By checking the pathological factors and increasing the protective factors, one can dream of caries-free dentition.

24. Systemic Theory

The body organs constantly move between states of health and disease based on oxidative stresses and the inflammatory responses. Such reactions continuously take place in the body, including the teeth and supporting structures. The body has sensing and control mechanisms to regulate hormones and fluid flows. Dentinal fluid flow is regulated by the endocrine portion of the parotid gland, which receives signals from the hypothalamus. Free radicals, produced in the hypothalamus increases with the elevated blood glucose, which in turn affects the parotid hormones, subsequently resulting in caries. Minimizing the effect of free radicals on hypothalamus with antioxidant can avoid negative effect on the parotid hormone, maintaining the proper dentinal fluid flow. The process effectively controls the inflammation inside the tooth by replenishing antioxidant stores.

A high sucrose diet affects the tooth externally by enabling the bacteria to produce acid and internally by reducing the dentinal fluid flow, which controls the inflammatory process in the dentin. Antioxidants can protect teeth by minimizing the effect of free radicals, thereby decreasing acid erosion and subsequently the caries.

Bibliography

1. Abott F. Caries of human teeth. Dental Cosmos.: 1879;21:57–184.
2. Bandlish LK. Attrition and plaque defense mechanism of teeth. The Probe 1981;23:67.
3. Bibby BG, Gustafson G, and Davies GN. A critique of three theories of caries attack. 1958;8:685.
4. Bradshaw DJ and Lynch RJM. Diet and the microbial aetiology of dental caries: new paradigms. Int. Dent. J.: 2013;63:64–72.
5. Bubby GB, et al. A Critique of Three Theories of Caries Attack. Int. Dent. J: 1958;8:685–94.
6. Burch PRJ and Jackson D. Periodontal disease and dental caries. Some new aetiological considera-tion. Brit. Dent. J.: 1966;120:127–34.
7. Carvalho JC. Caries process on occlusal surfaces: evolving evidence and understanding. Caries Res.: 2014;48:339–46.
8. Chaussain-Miller C, Fioretti F, Glodberg M Menashi S. The role of matrix metalloproteinases (MMPs) in human cavities. J. Dent. Res.: 2006;85:22–32.
9. Clarke JK. On the bacterial factor in the aetiology of dental caries. Br. J. Exp. Pathol.: 1924;5:141–7.
10. Cochrane NJ, Cai F, Huq NL, Burrow MF and Reynolds EC. New approaches to enhanced remineralization of tooth enamel. J. Dent. Res.: 2010;89:1187–97.
11. Curtis EK. Meth mouth: A review of metham-phetamine abuse and its oral manifestations. Gen. Dent.: 2006;54:125–9.
12. Dawes C. What is the critical pH and why does a tooth dissolve in acid? J. Can. Dent. Assoc.: 2003;69:722–4.
13. De Soet JJ, Nyvad B and Kilian M. Strain-related acid production by oral streptococci. Caries Res.: 2000;34:486–90.
14. Featherstone JDB. The caries balance: Contributing factors and early detection. CDA Jounral: 2003;31:257–69.
15. Featherstone JDB. Caries prevention and reversal based on the caries balance. Pediat. Dent.: 2006;28:128–32.
16. Ferraro M and Vieira AR. Explaining gender differences in caries: a multifactorial approach to a multifactorial disease. Int. J. Dent.: 2010.
17. Gonalez-Cabezas C. The chemistry of caries: remineralization and demineralization events with direct clinical relevance. Dent. Clin. North Am.: 2010;54:469–78.
18. Gracia-Godoy F. Familial caries distribution in human permanent teeth: buccal and lingual pits of first molars. J. Pedod.: 1983;7:318–23.
19. J Houte V. Role of Micro-organisms in Caries Etiology. J. Dent. Res.: 1994;73:672–81.

20. Jackson D.Genes and dental caries Proc. Roy. Soc. Med.: 1968;61:265–9.

21. Jackson D and Burch PRJ Dental caries as a degenerative disease. Gerontologia: 1969;1:203–16.

22. Kidd EAM and Fejerskov O. What constitutes dental caries? Histopathology of carious enamel and dentin related to the action of cariogenic biofilms. Journal of Dental Research: 2004;83:35–8.

23. Levine RS. The Aetiology of Dental Caries—An Outline of Current Thought. Int. Dent. J.: 1977;27:344–48.

24. Lukacs JR and Largesepada LL. Explaining sex differences in dental caries prevalence: saliva, hormones, and "life history" etiologies. Am. J. Human Biol.: 2006;18:540–55.

25. Parker RB. Bioelectrical phenomenon in dental decay. J.Dent. Res.: 1969;48–795.

26. Patir A, Seymen F and Yildirim M. Deeley K, Cooper ME, Maragita ML, Vieiro AR. Enamel formation genes are associated with high caries experience in Turkish children. Caries Res.: 2008;42:394–400.

27. Pearce E. Plaque minerals and dental caries. Nz. Dent. J.: 1998;94:12–15.

28. Reynolds EC. Calcium phosphate-based re-mineralization systems: scientific evidence? Aust. Dent. J.: 2008;53:268–73.

29. Schatz A and Martin JJ. The Proteolysis-Chelation Theory of Dental Caries. JADA: 1962;65:386–75.

30. Schatz A, Martin JJ and Schatz V. The Chelation and Proteolysis Chelation Theories of Dental Caries—Their Origin, Evolution and Physiology l. NY state DJ: 1972;38:285–95.

31. Shaw L and Muyrray JJ. A family history study of caries-resistance and caries-susceptibility. Br. Dent. J.: 1980;148:231–5.

32. Shuler CF. Inherited risks for susceptibility to dental caries. J. Dent. Ed.: 2001;65:1038–45.

33. Silverstone LM. Remineralization phenomena. Caries Res.: 1974;11:59.

34. Simon-Soro A and Mira A. Solving the etiology of dental caries. Trends in Microbiology 2015;23:76–82.

35. Slayton RL, Cooper ME and Marazita ML. Tuftrelin, mutans streptococci, and dental caries susceptibility. J. Dent. Res.: 2005;84:711–4.

36. Soafer JA. Genetics and site attack in dental caries. Comments on Jackson's theory. Br. Dent. J.: 1982;152:267–73.

37. Soderling EM. Xylitol, mutans streptococci, and dental plaque. Adv. Dent. Res.: 2009;21:74–8.

38. Southward K. The systemic theory of dental caries. General Dentistry: 2011;367–73.

39. Tanzer JM. Dental caries is a transmissible infectious disease: the Keyes and Fitzgerald revolution. Journal of Dental Research: 1995;74:1536–42.

40. ten Cate JM. Remineralization of caries lesions extending into dentin. J. Dent. Res.: 2001;80:1407–11.

41. Thylstrup A, Bruun C and Holmen L. In vivo caries models: mechanisms of caries initiation and arrestment. Adv. Dent. Res.: 1994;8:144–57.

42. Tomita Y, et al. Lipids in Human Parotid Saliva with regard to Caries Experience. Joleo Sci.: 2008;57:115–21.

43. Vieira AR, Marazita ML and Goldstein-McHenry, T. Genome-wide scan finds suggestive caries loci. J. Dent. Res.: 2008;87:435–9.

44. Wallace JS. The effects of foodstuffs in the causation and prevention of dental caries. Br. Med. J.: 1910;617.

45. Wojcik M, Burzynska-Fedzwiatr I and Wozniak IA. A review of natural and synthetic antitoxidants important for health and longevity. Curre. Med. Chem.: 2010;17:3262–88.

46. Wright JT. Defining the contribution of genetics in the etiology of dental caries. J. Dent.Res.: 2010;89:1173–4.

47. Zero DT. Dental caries process. Dental Clinics of North America: 1999;43:635–64.

6

Saliva and Caries

Saliva is a blend of exocrine secretions secreted mainly by three major salivary glands, i.e. parotid, submandibular and sublingual glands along with slight contribution from many minor glands in the oral cavity. Salivary secretion usually involves two stages; first, the acinar end pieces of glands secrete sodium chloride rich isotonic plasma-like primary saliva and second, this sodium chloride rich fluid when passes through ductal epithelium most of the sodium chloride is reabsorbed, while potassium and bicarbonates are secreted, making the final saliva hypotonic. Saliva is a biological material utilized for diagnostic, screening and epidemiological studies.

Saliva is composed of more than 99% water and less than 1% solids, mostly electrolytes (sodium, potassium, calcium, magnesium, bicarbonate, chloride, phosphate, etc.) and proteins (immunoglobulins, glycoproteins, traces of albumin and polypeptides) which are responsible for its characteristic viscosity. Daily production of saliva ranges from 0.5 to 1 liters. The whole saliva is contributed by parotid (20%), submandibular (65–70%) and sublingual glands (7–8%). Rest is from minor glands. In contrast to glandular saliva whole saliva has cloudy appearance and contains gingival crevicular fluid, vast amount of epithelial cells from oral mucosa and millions of bacteria. The salivary flow index classifies salivary flow as normal, low and very low. In adults, normal total stimulated salivary flow ranges from 1.0 to 3.0 mL/minute (unstimulated being 0.25 to 0.35 mL/minute) and very low stimulated salivary flow is less than 0.7 mL/minute (unstimulated being 0.1 mL/minute).

The organic and inorganic elements of saliva have made it a subject of interest in the past and current studies. It is observed that salivary composition depends on the changes taking place in oral cavity coupled with the series of processes occurring in the body.

The mechanisms by which saliva protects the teeth relates to both its fluid characteristics and the inherent components. Saliva forms a seromucosal covering (mucin-protein with high carbohydrate content) that lubricates and protect the oral tissues. Saliva also protects oral tissues against proteolytic attacks by micro-organisms. Mastication, deglutition and speech are aided by the lubricating effect of mucin-proteins. Saliva contributes to oral health performing various functions such as rinsing effect, clearance of materia alba, dilution of detritus, lubrication of tooth surfaces, protection of teeth by neutralization of acid by buffering actions, reinforcing hydroxyapatite and enamel pellicle formation and also the antimicrobial defence mechanism.

All these functions, mediated by inorganic and organic components should be considered in assessing the effects of saliva on dental caries. It has been established that the multifactorial caries disease may get influenced by inherited salivary factors. The salivary components are genetically regulated and have effect on colonization and clearance of oral bacteria.

Current research seeks to identify risk factors for caries and also identify inherent oral defences that may prevent caries development. These defences include factors which inhibit or reverse demineralization such as buffering action, antimicrobial activities including micro-organism adherence/clearance from the oral cavity and the secretion of antimicrobial peptides (immune surveillance). It is accepted that saliva plays an important role in caries etiopathogenesis. Saliva provides basic protection for hard dental tissues, periodontium and oral mucosa. A few authors recognize saliva as necessary for dental enamel as blood is for body cells and as the cellular activity is dependent on blood-stream providing it with nutrients and removing the catabolites, the enamel depends on saliva playing the similar role.

FACTORS INFLUENCING COMPOSITION AND FLOW OF SALIVA

The composition and flow of saliva vary greatly among individuals and also in the same individual during different times. The factors which may influence composition and salivary flow are:

    i. *Water intake:* It is established that when water content of the body is reduced to 8%, salivary flow virtually decreases to zero. Similarly hyperhydration causes an increase in salivary flow rate. During dehydration, salivary glands cease secretions to conserve water.

    ii. *Visual and mental stimulation:* A few studies have observed that by thinking of good food (food of choice) or viewing the same increases the salivary flow. However, it has been contradicted by other authors.

    iii. *Salivary flow index:* As the salivary flow increases, the concentration of proteins, sodium chloride, bicarbonate, etc. increases; whereas concentration of phosphates and magnesium decreases. Salivary flow index varies with the type, intensity and duration of the mechanical/chemical stimulus. There are definite evidence of increase in stimulated salivary flow with chewing gum; however, whether such stimulation increases unstimulated salivary flow has not been documented. Chewing acidic objects, being considered potent gustatory stimuli, enhances salivary flow.

    iv. *Age, sex and physical activity:* The effect of aging on salivary flow has not been confirmed. A few histological studies observed decrease in volume of acini of salivary glands in elderly individuals; however, functional studies observed no effect of aging on glandular capacity to produce saliva. Many studies observing low saliva production in elderly have related this to systemic diseases and the continuous use of medications, than aging.

It has been established that females, because of small glands, produce less saliva; and also the hormonal pattern contributes to diminished salivary secretions.

During physical exercises sympathetic stimulation may diminish or even inhibit salivary secretions. Exercise may also increase the electrolyte levels in saliva.

    v. *The circadian/circannual rhythms:* Salivary composition is related to circadian cycle and the flow is affected by circannual rhythms. It is established that the concentration of total proteins attains its peak at the end of afternoon, while the peak production of sodium and chloride occur in the morning. As regard to flow, it is established that less saliva flows from parotids in summer, while in winter the volumes are high.

vi. *Body postures and light:* Individuals in standing position secrete more saliva than sitting and lying. Light also affects the secretion; 30–40% decrease in salivary secretion occurs in the dark (blind people, however, have normal secretion).

vii. *Smoking and medication:* Individuals those who smoke have higher flow than non-smokers. It is established that the vitiating effect of tobacco increases glandular secretions.

Certain medications, such as antidepressants, antihistamines, etc. (drugs having anti-cholinergic action) cause reduction in salivary flow.

There are various features within saliva that protect the tooth surface or influence the caries development. The features are:

a. Salivary Flow Rate

Plenty of food items are being consumed daily by an individual. Many among those, especially fermentable carbohydrates, have a direct influence on caries process. One of the function of saliva is to dilute and eliminate all sticky components of food, which stick to oral tissues. This is a physiological process usually referred to as 'Oral clearance'. It is established that 0.8 to 1.2 ml total volume of saliva spreads as a thin film on oral tissues. Sucrose accumulation in that salivary film depends upon various factors, such as quality and frequency of sucrose intake along with salivary capacity of oral clearance. This is important for patients with low salivary flow rate. Salivary glands will be stimulated after intake of sugar by taste or chewing to increase the flow rate resulting in swallow which eliminates some of the sugar from oral cavity. The clearance rate depends upon several factors, most important being salivary flow rate. It has been demonstrated that sugar

accumulation differs between two individuals with different salivary flow rates.

Saliva influences caries process mainly by its rate of flow and by its content of fluoride. Stookey demonstrated that stimulating salivary flow through chewing of sugar-free gum after meals has been shown to reduce the incidence of dental caries. It is established that individuals with impaired saliva flow rate often show high caries incidence.

Salivary gland hypofunction is a common term used to cover both subjective symptoms and objective signs of dry mouth. Xerostomia or dry mouth is subjective oral dryness which impairs oral functions. Hyposalivation (low flow of saliva) leads to dry mouth. The decreased secretion of saliva may be because of systemic conditions, medications and/or head and neck radiography, influence diseases of oral cavity, subsequently affecting the overall health of an individual.

b. Salivary Minerals

Saliva provides protective and reparative environment by continuously supplying minerals to the oral tissues. The formation of organic acids as by-products of glucose metabolism is influenced by the presence of inorganic ions in the oral environment. Under physiological conditions the calcium and phosphate ions help maintain pH at near neutral level. Saturation of these ions accounts for buffering capacity of saliva.

Two main minerals, calcium and phosphates, play an important role as salivary electrolyte.

i. Salivary Calcium

Total calcium concentration (sum of protein bound, ionized and non-ionized) is in the range of 1.0 to 2.0 mmol/l. One fifth of whole saliva is bound to proteins and the rest is bound to phosphate and bicarbonate ions. When saliva pH and ionic strength increases at high flow rates, more calcium will be in un-ionized form. Calcium with two positive charges, can be bound to ions with two negative charges forming a chelate ring. After exposure to foodstuff, such as soft drinks and fruits that are rich in citric acid, it forms chelate ring; thereby the concentration of calcium in saliva is substantially reduced, subsequently accelerating demineralization of teeth.

ii. Salivary Phosphate

Salivary phosphate includes phosphoric acid (H_3PO_4), dihydrogen phosphate (H_2PO_4) and hydrogen phosphate (HPO_4). The lower the pH, the lower the concentration of phosphate; and higher the concentration of phosphoric acid and vice versa. Total phosphate concentration is determined by the salivary flow rate, i.e. the concentration of total phosphate decreases dramatically with increasing saliva flow rate. Low saliva pH values are more harmful for the teeth than low total phosphate concentration in saliva.

Calcium and phosphate in ionized forms are part of hydroxyapatite unit ($Ca_{10} (PO_4)_6 (OH)_2$). When the calcium, phosphate and hydroxyl ion activities are known, the ion activity product for hydroxyapatite (IAP_{HAP}) in saliva can be calculated by the formula:

$$IAP_{HAP} = (Ca^{2+})^{10} (PO_4^{3-})^6 (OH^-)^2$$

Both calcium and phosphate concentration of saliva influence the ion activity, the most important being saliva pH. A drop in pH of one unit (say pH 6 to pH 5), will reduce the hydroxyl ion activity ten fold and phosphate ion activity hundred fold, thereby reducing the overall ion activity for hydroxyapatite many times. If the ion activity product is larger than the solubility product, the saliva is supersaturated and remineralization may occur; if vice-versa, then demineralization follows. However, these activities are influenced by specific salivary proteins having inhibitory effects on these processes. These proteins are multifunctional; partly responsible for the remineralization capability of saliva.

CRITICAL pH

The critical pH in saliva is not constant, but a dynamic variable. The critical pH value, commonly fixed at 5.5, is the value when the ion activity product is equal to solubility product of hydroxyapatite. At this value, the process of demineralization and remineralization does not occur. The salivary critical pH may vary by up to one pH unit from the mean critical pH with different flow rates.

The salivary factors which prevent teeth from dissolving at pH above the critical pH level involve two processes. One is based on solubility of tooth enamel in saliva; involves salivary calcium and phosphate ions repressing tooth mineral dissolution by mass action and if the pH is sufficiently elevated, replacing lost tooth mineral by remineralization. Second is deposition of a salivary aggregate, consisting of calcium phosphate-carbonate-protein complex (salivary precipitin) into and onto plaque and teeth. It is usually present in amorphous or poorly crystalline form and is acid soluble, much more than the calcium phosphate of tooth substance. This means that when acid is produced by the plaque bacteria from fermentable carbohydrate and the pH drops, the calcium phosphate (saliva precipitin) in plaque, would dissolve before the hydroxyapatite of the tooth. Its role is one of a surrogate source of calcium and phosphate ions, which makes it possible to maintain calcium phosphate saturation of plaque fluid. Solubilization of salivary precipitin calcium phosphate may occur as the pH declines following exposure to fermentable carbohydrates and ceases, when pH rises. The pH at which solubilization ceases should be a point of saturation and the pH between the lowest pH reached during the pH fall and the critical pH should be zone of undersaturation.

Figure 6.1 shows role of saliva in the various calcium phosphate reactions that occur at the tooth-plaque-saliva interface.

However, these activities are directly influenced by saliva containing specific

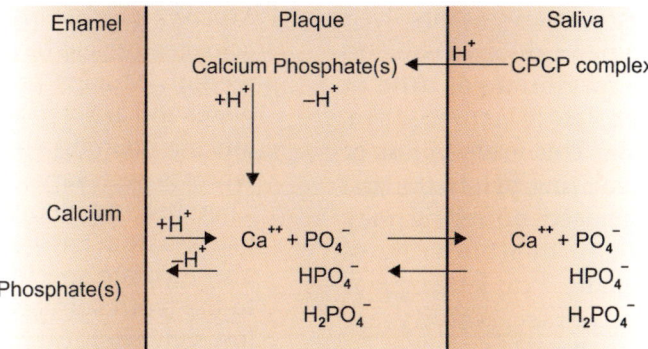

Fig. 6.1: Role of saliva at tooth-plaque-saliva interface, maintaining calcium phosphate interactions. CPCP = Calcium phosphate carbohydrate protein complex

proteins with inhibitory effects on these processes. These proteins are multifunctional in that they are partly responsible for the remineralization capacity of saliva, but they interact with some micro-organisms.

BUFFERING CAPACITY OF SALIVA

Buffering capacity of saliva protects the oral cavity by preventing colonization of pathogenic organisms, denying them the favorable environment. It also neutralizes and cleans the acid produced by acidogenic micro-organisms, thus preventing enamel demineralization.

Buffering capacity mainly depends upon the chemical nature (organic and inorganic components) of saliva. The thickness of biofilm and the number of bacteria present also determines the efficacy of buffering capacity.

After consuming sugary foodstuffs, the pH in plaque drops and remain lowered until the sugar is cleared from the oral cavity and also the acid produced is buffered. When pH drops below critical pH, tooth demineralization initiates; so, it is essential to reduce the time the pH remains below critical pH. An inverse relationship between buffering capacity and caries experience is well established. It has also been emphasized that the buffer capacity of unstimulated saliva varies so much that single measurement is not reliable for predicting caries development. Physical and chemical changes in saliva composition and particularly changes in its buffering capability play an important role in development and progression of caries.

The buffer effect is affected by altered general health, hormonal and metabolic changes. In women, buffer effect decreases gradually, independent of flow rate, during late pregnancy time and recovers after delivery.

The common chemical definition of buffer capacity is determined by following formula: $\beta = \Delta C_A / \Delta pH$ where β is buffer capacity, ΔC_A is increase in saliva acid concentration and ΔpH is change in salivary pH.

The addition of large amounts of acid if results in minor pH change, the buffer capacity is high and vice versa. Phosphate, bicarbonate and protein buffer systems are mainly responsible for maintaining the pH. Digestive enzymes and urea also play their role.

a. *Phosphate buffer:* As the total phosphate (hydrogen and dihydrogen phosphate forms) concentration in saliva decreases with increasing flow rate, buffer capacity decreases from around half in resting saliva to almost 10% in highly stimulated saliva.

b. *Bicarbonate buffer:* Bicarbonates are in dynamic relation with carbonic acid in saliva. The hydration of CO_2 to carbonic acid and vice versa is catalyzed by the enzyme carbonic anhydrase, present in saliva. CO_2 is present primarily as dissolved gas with a pCO_2 in parotid saliva equal to that of blood. The magnitude of drop in pCO_2 varies with the flow of air over saliva, i.e. during breathing. This leads to loss of CO_2 from saliva increasing pH. In the oral cavity extensive phased buffering may occur, allowing for further buffering of remaining bicarbonate. Two isoenzymes with carbonic anhydrase activity are involved in salivary physiology.

CA II is a high activity isoenzyme. It produces bicarbonate in the saliva. CAVI is the serous acinar cell isoenzyme secreted by parotid and submandibular glands. The low salivary concentration of CAVI appears to be associated with increased prevalence of caries. Since there is a positive correlation between CAVI concentration and salivary flow rate and a negative correlation with the DMFT index, it has been hypothesized that salivary CAVI plays a vital role in protecting the teeth from caries. CAVI has the ability to bind to the enamel pellicle and retain its enzymatic activity on the tooth surface. In the enamel pellicle, CAVI may catalyse the conversion of salivary bicarbonate and hydrogen ions to carbon dioxide and water.

The carbonic acid-bicarbonate buffer is important in stimulated saliva; while in unstimulated saliva, the phosphate buffer system is effective.

c. *Protein buffer:* Saliva contains many proteins (mainly glycoproteins), which can act as buffers when the pH is above or below their bioelectric point. Proteins accept protons when the pH is below and release protons when the pH is above bioelectric point. The buffering effect of proteins is far less than bicarbonate and phosphate in human saliva. In addition to their chemical buffering, some of the salivary proteins increase the viscosity of saliva when the pH becomes acidic and thereby physically protect the teeth against acidic attack by forming a diffusion barrier.

i. *Mucous glycoproteins:* Mucins are of acinar cell origin having a high molecular weight. Mucins are hydrophilic, hold water and are responsible for lubricating and maintaining a moist mucosal surface which is necessary for healthy oral cavity. They help accelerating the clearance of bacteria from the oral cavity. Mucins may also mediate specific bacterial adhesion to the tooth surface. In individuals with low saliva flow (dry mouth), the secretion of these proteins is reduced compromising the adhesion properties.

ii. *Serous glycoproteins:* The glycoproteins are a group of carbohydrate-linked proteins. Most salivary proteins such as secretory immunoglobulin A (IgA), lactoferrin, peroxidases and agglutinins, belong to this group.

iii. *Calcium binding proteins:* These are statherin and proline rich proteins frequently present in saliva. Supersaturation state of saliva with respect to calcium salts constitutes a protective and reparative environment, which is necessary for integrity of teeth. Proteases of oral mucosa are able to degrade statherin, but due to its high concentration it is effective only in the presence of saliva in the mouth. It also promotes adhesion of *Actinomyces viscosus* to tooth surfaces. Acidic proline rich proteins form a complex with a large number of genetic variants. These proteins are readily adsorbed from saliva to hydroxyapatite surfaces in the form of initial acquired pellicle and regulate hydroxyapatite crystal structure.

Negatively loaded residues on the salivary proteins also act as buffers. Sialin, a salivary peptide, plays an important role in increasing the biofilm pH after exposure to fermentable carbohydrates.

d. *Digestive enzymes:* α amylase constitutes 40–50% of total salivary gland produced protein. Function of amylase is to split starch into maltose, maltotriose and dextrins. Amylase in saliva clears food debris (mainly starch) from the oral cavity; however, during this process bacteria may produce sufficient acid.

e. *Urea:* Urea is another buffer present in total salivary fluid. It causes rapid increase in biofilm pH by releasing ammonia and carbon dioxide when hydrolyzed by bacterial ureases. Children with chronic renal insufficiency present with less caries than healthy children, due to increased level of salivary urea.

Antimicrobial Proteins in Saliva

Inert Defence Factors

Many salivary antimicrobial proteins interact with each other *in vitro* and result in additive, synergistic or inhibitory effects on mutans streptococci, lactobacilli and fungi. Most of the antimicrobial proteins inhibit the metabolism and adherence; however, their exact mode of action is not clearly documented. These proteins are known to limit bacterial or fungal growth, interfere with bacterial glucose metabolism and promote elimination of bacteria. Defensive proteins eliminate hydrogen peroxide, which is considered toxic for mammalian cells.

Lysozyme in whole saliva is contributed from major and minor salivary glands, gingival crevicular fluid and salivary leukocytes. It is present in newborn babies, exerting protection before tooth emergence. In addition to its muramidase activity, lysozyme a strongly cationic protein, can activate bacterial autolysins, which can destroy the cell walls.

Lactoferrin is an iron binding glycoprotein and its function is to expropriate iron from pathogenic micro-organisms.

Peroxidase systems in human saliva comprises two enzymes; salivary gland derived peroxidase and leukocyte myeloperoxidase, together with thiocyanate ions and hydrogen peroxide. They have two major functions; the antimicrobial activity and protection of host cells from toxicity of hydrogen peroxide. Antimetabolic activity may be of importance, since the more hypothiocyanite in saliva, the less acid production in dental plaque.

Cystatins are protective by inhibiting unwanted proteolysis, also effect calcium phosphate precipitation and have some antiviral activity. They play a minor role in calcium homeostasis in saliva. Histatins have a broad antimicrobial spectrum against bacteria as well as oral yeasts.

Agglutinins are glycoproteins which interact with unattached bacteria, resulting in clumping of bacteria into large aggregates. These aggregate of bacteria can easily be flushed away by saliva.

Specific Defense Factors

The immunoglobulins IgG, IgM, IgA and secretory IgA form the basis of the specific salivary defense against oral microbial flora. Two IgA subclasses, IgA1 and IgA2 are present in saliva. IgA1 forms the major component; however, the relative amount of IgA2 is higher in saliva than in other secretions. In human beings, maternally originated IgG is only immunoglobulin present in neonates. It decreases to non-detectable levels after some months and reappear as the tooth erupts. It mainly enters the saliva through gingival crevicular fluid. IgGs are also capable of opsonizing bacteria for phagocytes, which are reported to remain active in dental plaque and saliva. Salivary IgA is absent at birth but reappears at the age of one. The formation of specific IgAs in saliva correlates with the colonization of bacteria in oral cavity. Salivary Igs can bind to salivary pellicle and dental plaque. In the oral cavity, Igs act by neutralizing various microbial virulence factors, limiting microbial adherence and agglutinating the bacteria. These also prevent penetration of foreign antigens into the mucosa. Anti-streptococcal IgGs, mainly from maternal serum against caries and colonization of bacteria may have protective role; however, contradictory results also exist.

It must be noted that presence of active caries lesions may induce the formation of specific IgGs and they remain at higher levels for longer period till the eradication of lesions.

Other Caries Related Components in Saliva

Saliva contains certain elements, other than those of pure salivary origin, which may influence caries process.

An elevation of saliva-urea level in the oral cavity will lead to binding of hydrogen ions and more alkaline salivary pH. Therefore, these individuals experience less caries in spite of high plaque scores.

Diabetic patients usually present high glucose level in saliva with poor metabolic control. Such patients develop more caries.

A few elements from foodstuff and/or drinking water may influence salivary concentration, subsequently the caries. One such element, namely 'fluoride' has an important role against caries. The fluoride concentration in the saliva depends strongly on the fluoride present in the drinking water. With increasing fluoride concentration in the drinking water the risk of systemic fluorosis of the enamel increases, while the prevalence of caries decreases. The caries control protocol stresses the importance of presence of salivary fluorides close to the sites of action, i.e. where the dissolution of hard tissues is to take place. Therefore, most strategies to control caries involve measures to increase the fluoride concentration in oral fluids. Fluoride diffuses from saliva into plaque in short time, elevating the fluoride concentration in plaque. Fluoride in the form of mineral calcium fluoride is available both in saliva and in plaque. The calcium fluoride functions as a slow releaser of fluoride. When fluoride ions are present in plaque fluid along with dissolved hydroxyapatite and the pH is higher than 4.5, a fluorapatite like remineralized layer is formed over the remaining surface of the enamel. This layer is much more acid-resistant than the original hydroxyapatite and is formed more quickly than ordinarily remineralized enamel. The cavity-prevention effect of fluoride is partly due to these surface effects, which occur during and after tooth eruption. Fluoride also forms a complex ion with magnesium. Fluoride diffusing into micro-organisms prevents the enzyme enolase from taking part in glycolytic pathway by binding magnesium, which is needed for optimum enzymatic activities.

Maintaining Integrity of Enamel

Saliva modulates demineralization and remineralization activity, thereby playing a vital role in maintaining physico-chemical integrity of enamel. The features which control the stability of enamel are the salivary pH and the concentration of calcium, phosphate and fluoride in saliva. Higher concentration of calcium and phosphate may result in remineralization of already initiated carious process. The concentration of calcium is not affected by diet; however, salivary flow may affect calcium concentration. Intake of medicine, such as pilocarpine may increase calcium level in saliva. Certain diseases, such as cystic fibrosis may also be effective in increasing calcium levels.

The concentration of phosphates depends on salivary pH and varies with salivary flow. As the flow increases, the total concentration of inorganic phosphate decreases. The main function of phosphate is to maintain integrity of tooth tissues.

The concentration of fluoride in saliva depends upon its consumption, which is mostly from drinking water. The presence of fluoride ions in the liquid phase reduces mineral loss during drop in pH of biofilm, as these ions decrease the solubility of enamel hydroxyapatite making it resistant to demineralization. Fluoride also reduces production of acids in biofilms.

The concentration of hydrogen ions influences the equilibrium of calcium phosphate in the enamel. The higher the concentration of hydrogen ions, the lower is the pH and vice versa.

Bibliography

1. Aaltonen AS, Tenovuo J and Lehtonen OP. Increased dental caries activity of pre-school children with low baseline levels of serum IgG antibodies against the bacterium *Streptococcus mutans*. Arch. Oral Biol.: 1987;32:55–60.

2. Ahmadi-Motamayel F, Goodarzi MT, Hendi SS, Abdolsamadi H and Rafieian N. Evaluation of salivary flow rate, pH, buffering capacity, calcium and total protein levels in caries free and caries active adolescence. 2013;5:35–9.

3. Atkinson JC and Wu AJ. Salivary gland dysfunction: causes, symptoms, treatment. J. Am. Dent. Assoc.: 1994;125:409–16.

4. Azevedo LR, Damante JH, Lara VS and Lauris JR. Age-related changes in human sublingual glands: a post mortem study. Arch. Oral Biol.: 2005;50:565–74.

5. Badet C, Richard B, Castaing-Debat M and de Flaujae PM and Dorignac G. Adaptation of salivary lactobacillus strains to xylitol. Arch. Oral Biol.: 2004;49:161–4.

6. Bashir E and Lagerlof F. Effect of citric acid clearance on the saturation with respect to hydroxyapitite in saliva. Caries Res.: 1996;30:213–7.

7. Battino M, Ferreiro MS, Gallardo I, Newman HN and Bullon P. The antioxidant capacity of saliva. J. Clin. Periodontol.: 2002;29:189–94.

8. Bowen WH, Qhivey RG Jr and Smith AV. Glucosyltransferase inactivation reduces dental caries. J. Dent. Res.: 2001;80:1505–6.

9. Camling E, Gahnberg L, Krasse B and Wallman C. Crevicular IgG antibodies and *Streptococcus mutans* on erupting human first permanent molars. Arch. Oral Biol.: 1991;36:703–8.

10. Catalan MA, Nakamoto T and Melvin JE. The salivary gland fluid secretion mechanism. J. Med. Investig.: 2009;56:192–6.

11. Challacombe SJ. Serum and salivary antibodies to *Streptococcus mutans* in relation to development and treatment of human dental caries. Arch. Oral Biol.: 1980;25:495–502.

12. Chiappin S, Antonelli G, Gatti R and De Palo EF. Saliva specimen: A new laboratory tool for diagnostic and basic investigation. Clin. Chim. Acta.: 2007;383:30–40.

13. Dawes C. Effects of diet on salivary secretion and composition. J. Dent. Res.: 1970;49:1263–73.

14. Dawes C. Circadian rhythms in human salivary flow rate and composition. J. Physiol.: 1972;220:529–45.

15. Dawes C. A mathematical model of salivary clearance of sugar from the oral cavity. Caries Res.: 1983;17:321–34.

16. Dawes C. What is the critical pH and why does a tooth dissolve in acid? J. Can. Dent. Assoc.: 2003;69:722–4.

17. Dawes C. The unstimulated salivary flow rate after prolonged gum chewing. Arch. Oral Biol.: 2005;50:561–3.

18. de Almedia Pdel V, Gregio AM, Machado MA, de Lima AA and Azevedo LR. Saliva composition and functions: a comprehensive review. J. Contemp. Dent. Pract.: 2008;9:72–80.

19. Denny PC, et al. A novel saliva test for caries risk assessment. J. Calif. Dent. Assoc.: 2006;34:287.

20. Dreizen S and Mann AW. The buffer capacity of saliva as a measure of dental caries activity. J. Ala. Acad. Sci.: 1946;18:68–9.

21. Edgar WM. Saliva: its secretion, composition and functions. Br. Dent. J.: 1992;172:305–12.

22. Ericssion Y. Clinical investigations of the salivary buffering action. Acta. Odontol. Scand.: 1959;17:131–65.

23. Gopinath VK and Arzreanne AR. Saliva as a diagnostic tool for assessment of dental caries. Arch. Orofac. Sci.: 2006;1:57–9.

24. Grahn E, Tenovuo J, Lehtonen OP, Eerol E and Vilja P. Antimicrobial systems of human whole saliva in relation to dental caries, cariogenic bacteria and gingival inflammation in young adults. Acta. Odontol. Scand.: 1988;46:67–71.

25. Guggenheimer J and Moore PA. Xerostomia: etiology, recognition and treatment. J. Am. Dent. Assoc.: 2003;134:61–9.

26. Hedenbjork-Lager A, Bjorndal L, Gustafsson A, Sorsa T, Tjaderhana L, Akerman S and Ericson D. Caries correlates Strongly with salivary levels of Matrix Metalloproteinase-8. Caries Res. 2015, 49, 1–8.

27. Hegde MN, Hegde ND, Ashok A and Shetty S. Biochemical indicators of dental caries in saliva: an in vivo study. Caries Res.: 2014;48:170–3.

28. Heintze U. Secretion rate, buffer effect and number of lactobacilli and *Streptococcus mutans* of whole saliva of cigarette smokers and non-smokers. Scand. J. Dent. Res. 1984;92:294–301.

29. Heintze U, Birktied D and Bjorn H. Secretion rate and buffer effect of resting and stimulated whole saliva as a function of age and sex. Swed. Dent. J: 1983;7:227–38.

30. Humphrey SP and Williamson RT. A review of saliva: normal composition, flow and function. J. Prosthet. Dent.: 2001;85:162–9.

31. Inoue H, Ono K, Masuda W, Morimoto Y, Tanaka T, Yokota M and Inenaga K. Gender difference in unstimulated whole saliva flow rate and salivary gland sizes. Arch. Oral Biol.: 2006;51: 1055–60.

32. Jensdottir T, Nauntofte B, Buchwald C and Bardow A. Effects of sucking acitic acid candy on whole mouth saliva composition. Caries Res.: 2005;39;468–74.

33. Johnsson M, Richardson CF, Bergey EJ, Levine MJ and Nancollas GH. The effect of human salivary cystatins and statherin on hydroxyapatite crystallization. Arch. Oral Biol.: 1991;36:631–6.

34. Kadoya Y, Kuwahara H, Shimazaki M, Ogawa Y, Yagi T. Isolation of a novel carbonic anhydrase from human saliva and immunohistochemical demonstration of its related isoenzymes in salivary gland. Osaka City Med. J.: 1987;33:99–109.

35. Kivela J, Parkkila S, Parkkila A-K. and Rajaniemi, H. A low concentration of carbonic anhydrase isoenzyme VI in whole saliva is associated with caries prevalence. Caries Res.: 1999;33:178–84.

36. Kivela J, Parkkila S, Parkkila A-K, Leinonen J and Rajaniemi, H. Salivary carbonic anhydrase isoenzyme VI. J. Physiol.: 1999;520:315–20.

37. Lagerlof F. Effects of flow rate and pH on calcium phosphate saturation in human parotid saliva. Caries Res.: 1983;17:403–11.

38. Lagerlof F and Dawes C. The volume of saliva in the mouth before and after swallowing. J. Dent. Res.: 1984;63:18–21.

39. Lagerlof F and Lindqvist L. A method for determining concentrations of calcium complexes in human parotid saliva by gel filtration. Arch. Oral Biol.: 1982;27:735–8.

40. Lagerlof F and Olibeby A. Caries-protective factors in saliva. Adv. Dent. Res.: 1994;8:229–38.

41. Lagerlof F and Olliveby A. Caries protective factors in saliva. Adv. Dent. Res.: 1994;8:229–38.

42. Laine M, Tenovuo J, Lehtonen OP, Ojanotko-Harri A, Vilja P and Tuohimaa P. Pregnancy related changes in human whole saliva. Arch. Oral Biol.: 1988;33:913–7.

43. Lamkin MS. Oppenheim FG. Structural features of salivary function. Crit. Rev. Oral Biol. Med.: 1993;4:251–9.

44. Larmas M. Saliva and dental caries: diagnostic tests for normal dental practice. Int. Dent. J.: 1992;42:199–208.

45. Larsen MJ, Jensen AF, Madsen DM and Pearce EI. Individual variations of pH, buffer capacity and concentrations of calcium and phosphate in unstimulated whole saliva. Arch. Oral Biol.: 1999;44:111–7.

46. Lehner T, Murray JJ, Winter GB and Caldwell J. Antibodies to Streptococcus mutans serotypes in saliva for children ages 3 to 7 years. Arch. Oral Bio1.: 1978;23:1061–7.

47. Lehtonen OP, Grahn EM, Stahlberg TH and Laitinen LA. Amount and avidity of salivary and serum antibodies against Streptococcus mutans in two groups of human subjects with different caries susceptibility. Infect. Immun.: 1984;43:308–13.

48. Leinonen J, Kivela J, Parkkila S, Parkkila A-K and Rajaniemi H. Salivary carbonic anhydrase isoenzyme VI is located in the human enamel pellicle. Caries Res.: 1999;33:185–90.

49. Leone CW and Oppenheim FG. Physical and chemical aspects of saliva as indicators of risk for dental caries in humans. J. Dent. Educ.: 2001;65: 1054–62.

50. Lima DP, Diniz DG, Moimaz SA, Sumida DH and Okamoto AC. Saliva: Reflection of the body. Int. J. Infect. Dis.: 2010;14:184–8.

51. Lindfors B and Lagerlof F. Effect of sucrose concentration in saliva after a sucrose rinse on the hydronium ion concentration in dental plaque. Caries Res.: 1988;22:7–10.

52. Loesche WJ, Schork Terpenning MS, Chen YM and Stoll J. Factors which influence levels of selected organisms in saliva of older individuals. J. Clin. Microbiol.: 1995;33:2550–7.

53. Lukacs JR and Largaespada LL. Explaining sex differences in dental caries prevalence: saliva, hormones and "life-history" etiologies. Am. J. Hum. Biol.: 2006;18:540–55.

54. Lumikari LM, Loimaranta V. Saliva and dental caries. Adv. Dent. Res.: 2000;14:40–7.

55. McDevitt JT. Saliva as the next best diagnostic tool. J. Biochem.: 2006;456:23–5.

56. Melvin JE, Yule D, Shuttleworth T and Begenisich T. Regulation of fluid and electrolyte secretion in salivary gland acinar cells. Annu. Rev. Physiol.: 2005;67:445–69.

57. Mundorff SA, Eisenberg AD, Leverett DH, Espeland MA and Proskin HM. Correlations between numbers of microflora in plaque and saliva. Caries Res.: 1990;24:312–7.

58. Nagler RM, Klein L, Zaryhevsky N, Drgues N, Reynuk AZ. Characterization of differentiated antioxidant profile of human saliva. Free Rad. Biol. Med.: 2002;32:268.

59. Nagler RM. Salivary glands and the aging process: mechanistic aspects, health-status and medicinal-efficacy monitoring. Biogerontology: 2004;5:223–33.

60. Navazeshg M and Kumar SK. Measuring salivary flow: challenges and opportunities. J. Am. Dent. Assoc.: 2008;139:35–40.

61. Nederfors T. Xerostomia and hyposalivation. Adv. Dent. Res.: 2000;14:48–56.

62. Ou-Yang LW, Chang PC, Tsai AI, Jaing TH and Lin SY. Salivary microbial counts and buffer capacity in children with acute lymphoblastic leukemia. Pediatr. Dent.: 2010;32:218–22.

63. Papas AS, Joshi A, Mac Donald SL, Maravelis-Splagounias L, Pretara-Spanedda P and Curro FA. Caries prevalence in xerostomic individuals. J. Can. Dent. Assoc.: 1993;59:171–9.

64. Park YD, Jang JH, Oh YJ and Kwon HJ. Analyses of organic acids and inorganic anions and their relationship in human saliva before and after glucose intake. Archives Oral Biol.: 2014;59:1–11.

65. Petti S, Tarsitani G and DÁrca AS. A randomized clinical trial of the effect of yoghurt on the human salivary microflora. Arch. Oral Biol.: 2001;46:705–12.

66. Sakabe R, Tanaka H, Sakabe J, Nakajima I and Akasaka M. Adhesion of Lactobacillus salivarius to salivary pellicle on HA. J. Dent. Res.: 2004;83:3611.

67. Sawair FA, Ryalat S, Shayyab M and Saku T. The unstimulated salivary flow rate in a Jordonian healthy adult population. J. Clin. Med. Res.: 2009;1:219–25.

68. Scully C. Sjogrens syndrome: clinical and laboratory features, immunopathogenesis and management. Oral Surg., Oral Med., Oral Pathol.: 1986;62:10–23.

69. Shern RJ, Fox PC and Li SH. Influence of age on the secretory rates of the human minor salivary glands and whole saliva. Arch. Oral Biol.: 1993;38:755–61.

70. Ship JA, Pillemer SR and Baum BJ. Xerostomia and the geriatric patient. J. Am. Geriatr. Soc.: 2002;50:535–43.

71. Smith SI, Aweh AJ, Coker AO, Savage KO, Abosede DA and Oyedeji KS. Lactobacilli in human dental caries and saliva. Microbios.: 2001;105:77–85.

72. Spak CJ, Johnson G and Ekstrand J. Caries incidence, salivary flow rate and efficacy of fluoride gel treatment in irradiated patients. Caries Res.: 1994;28:388–93.

73. Stack KM and Papas AS. Xerostomia: etiology and clinical management. Nutr. Clin. Care: 2001;4:15–21.

74. Stookey GK. The effect of saliva on dental caries. J. Am. Dent. Assoc.: 2008;139:11–17.

75. Tappuni AR and Challacombe SJ. A comparison of salivary immunoglobulin A and IgA subclass concentrations in predentate and dentate children and adults. Oral Microbiol. Immunol.: 1994;9:142–5.

76. Tenovuo J. Antimicrobial function of human saliva—how important is it for oral health? Acta. Odontol. Scand.: 1998;56:250–56.

77. Tenovuo J, Grahn E, Lehtonen OP, Hyyppa T, Karhuvaara L and Vilja P. Antimicrobial factors in saliva: ontogeny and relation to oral health. J. Dent. Res.: 1987;66:475–9.

78. Tenovuo J, Lumikari M and Soukka T. Salivary lysozyme, lactoferrin and peroxidases: antibacterial effects against cariogenic bacteria and potential clinical applications in preventive dentistry. Proc. Finn. Dent. Soc.: 1991;87:197–208.

79. Thomson WM, Chalmers JM, Spencer AJ and Slade GD. Medication and dry mouth: findings from a cohort study of older people. J. Public Health Dent.: 2000;60:12–20.

80. Tulunoglu O, Demirtas S and Tulunoglu I. Total antioxidant levels of saliva in children related to caries, age and gender. Int. J. Paediatr. Dent.: 2006;16:186–91.

81. van Nieuw AA, Bolscher JG and Veerman EC. Salivary proteins: protective and diagnostic value in cariology. Caries Res.: 2004;38:247–53.

7

Diet and Caries

Dental caries has been established as a multifactorial disease. Nutritional factors and general health affect oral tissues as the nutrients in diet play an important role in maintaining the oral health. Diet along with environmental factors which encourage growth of cariogenic microflora are considered as the main causative agents in the development of caries. The microflora proliferate with fermentable diet modifying the tooth tissue substrate, subsequently leading to caries.

The importance of diet in production of caries has been recognized since ancient times. The frequency and quality of sugar intake along with local contribution of some minerals contributes to caries development. The dissolution and deposition of minerals is a continuous process. Fluoride as a mineral is important, since it inhibits proliferation of oral pathogens and also form acid resistant fluoroapatite in the enamel surface, which protect the surface from caries initiation. Sucrose provides substrate for lactic acid and also help in biofilm formation. Modification of dietary regimes has always been emphasized in caries prevention.

DIET VERSUS NUTRITION

Intake of food, water, etc. affects our systemic health and also the local environment as well. In simple terms, 'diet' constitutes whatever we eat or drink and the 'nutrition' means the components of diet which are absorbed and assimilated.

'Diet' is the sum total of food and drink consumed by any person from day to day; whereas 'Nutrition' is the absorption and assimilation of that consumed food (involves metabolic process wherein nutrients of food get absorbed).

Earlier malnutrition was considered to be the main cause of caries susceptibility; however, over the years the effects of nutritional status on caries have been varied. The population with the best nutrition presented with high caries prevalence; whereas lowest caries prevalence was observed in poor people. Relationship of nutritional deficiencies and caries has not been documented properly. It has also been observed that patients with eating disorders, such as anorexia nervosa might have high caries prevalence.

Various studies have suggested that prenatal deficiencies of proteins, minerals and vitamins predispose the off-spring to subsequent development of caries. A few animal studies have also demonstrated high caries in rats fed on protein deficient diet.

The nutritional deficiencies during the developmental stages may influence caries susceptibility by affecting enamel formation, salivary composition/function and also the immunological responses. There is no definite evidence that nutrition in the post development period has any influence on development of caries. It is postulated that the food consumed by an individual throughout his life and the nutrients thereof, could directly or indirectly affect the susceptibility of the teeth to decay through the following channels: (i) by alteration in the differentiation, development and maturation of teeth and their supporting structures (ii) by changes in the metabolic processes in the dental tissues and (iii) by alteration in the composition of saliva and also the food constituents.

The dietary interactions with environmental factors, viz. flow and quality of saliva, individual's systemic health, ethnic geographical and psychological factors are extremely important and complex. Dietary factors coupled with local environment affect the adherence and multiplication of microbes over the hard tissues. These factors may place the host at a higher risk of caries susceptibility.

Pre-eruptive Nutrition and Caries

The formation of organic matrix, mineralization and maturation start as early as 6th week of intrauterine life. Nutritional deficiencies, such as those of calcium, phosphate, vitamins A, C, D and proteins affect formation/development of tooth tissues. They may impair enamel and dentin quality and increase caries susceptibility. It is observed that hypoplastic teeth, may be the result of vitamin D deficiency, are more caries susceptible than the non-hypoplastic teeth.

The adverse effects of carbohydrates on erupted teeth are well known. A few authors have observed the effects of carbohydrates on pre-erupting teeth, making them caries susceptible after eruption. Animal experiments have shown that diet rich in sugar produce high enamel carbonate levels and low calcium: phosphate ratio resulting in caries.

NUTRITION AND ORAL MICROFLORA

The nutrients available in oral cavity coupled with the environmental conditions determine the kind and the quality of microflora. These further influence the metabolic and pathogenic potential of the organisms.

It is established that most of the microflora are fastidious, i.e. they need plenty of nutrients. Oral microbes exhibit great diversity in nutrient requirements. A few organisms use carbohydrates as their energy source while others use nitrogen. Some may need water soluble vitamins and even proteins.

The source of nutrition for oral microflora is usually Endogenous, viz. saliva, crevicular fluid, epithelial cells, blood, etc. and Exogenous, viz. diet and its constituents.

The food intake provides nutrition for bacteria. The organisms may gain access to the food during the ingestion and mastication or even after the food is modified with salivary ingredients.

Dietary Constituents affecting Bacterial Nutrition

The influence of dietary carbohydrate on oral flora has been studied exhaustively. A large group of oral micro-organisms utilize carbohydrates as their principal energy source. The organisms have the potential to adapt to the time of non-availability of carbohydrates since the availability of dietary carbohydrates may be intermittent in the oral environment. The enzyme systems of these organisms help converting sugar to storage material, which can be utilized later.

The cariogenic bacteria have the characteristic acidurance, i.e. capacity to ferment sugar to grow and survive in acidic environment. Bacteria which grow best at pH 4 or less are called 'Acidophilic', which grow at neutral pH are 'Neutrophilic' and at alkaline pH are 'Alkaliphilic'.

The cellular mechanism by which sugar is fermented and converted to other forms is explained in subsequent pages.

When lactobacilli and *Streptococcus mutans* grow in an environment with limited supply of sugar, they form formate, acetate and ethanol. They do not form any lactic acid because enzyme lactate dehydrogenase is dependent on fructose-1, 6-biphosphate for this activity. At low extracellular levels of sugar, the intracellular level of fructose 1, 6-biphosphate is low, thereby less lactic acid formation. High sugar concentration favors formation of lactic acid. The bacteria with lactic acid as fermentation product have the potential to produce acid at pH lower than bacteria having carboxylic acid as the fermentation products.

The effects of dietary proteins are limited on oral flora. The slow rate of dissolution and liberation of proteins from ingested food coupled with short exposure time to salivary proteolytic enzyme activity suggests that amino acids from dietary sources are relatively unavailable to oral micro-organisms.

The fat containing foodstuffs are less likely to adhere to the teeth and the fatty coating on carbohydrates render them less soluble, subsequently less availability to oral flora.

The physical consistency of food influences the retention of food at various sites in the oral cavity, affecting the growth of microflora at those sites. Diet consistency and taste have a selective influence on salivary gland function. Sticky food will adhere to both surface and fibrous foods may get lodged in interproximal spaces or periodontal pockets.

CARBOHYDRATES AND CARIES

Carbohydrates are important component of food worldwide. They are principally a source of energy and also help in synthesis of fatty acids and amino acids. They are also a part of structure of biologically important materials such as glycolipids, glycoproteins, nucleic acids and heparin.

Structurally, the carbohydrates contain carbon, hydrogen and oxygen.

Classification

a. *Monosaccharides:* Carbohydrates which cannot be broken down to simple sugars by acid hydrolysis, e.g. glucose, fructose, galactose.

b. *Disaccharides:* Formed by condensation of 2 monosaccharides, e.g. sucrose (glucose + fructose), maltose (glucose + glucose), lactose (glucose + galactose).

c. *Polysaccharides:* Polymers of many monosaccharides, e.g. starch, cellulose, glycogen (formed from glucose).

The nomenclature, examples and availability of carbohydrates are given in Table 7.1.

The nutritionally important carbohydrates are:

• Glucose (occurs mostly in combined form and is found in nearly all foods).

• Sucrose (most familiar and prominent sugar in domestic use).

• Lactose (unique to mammals and found in milk).

• Starch (energy stored in most plants and seeds).

• Glycogen (animal equivalent of starch).

The word 'sugar' has been derived from arabic word 'Sukkar'. It was introduced in western countries around 11th–15th century AD. One of the earliest use of sugar was to disguise acidic taste of medicines. 60% of sugar is derived from sugarcane and the rest 40% from sugar beet.

Various authors in early times have documented the role of sugar and sugar containing food items in the development of caries.

Arabian Mesu pointed to dates as the cause of caries, whereas Aristotle named figs as being cause of caries. Pierre Fauchard (1746) observed 'All sugary foods contribute not a little to destruction of teeth' and that 'those who like sucrose and use it frequently rarely have a good teeth'. Thomas Bardmore (1768) opined about sweets as "eat them seldom and always wash the teeth after that". William

Table 7.1: Carbohydrates: Form, examples and availability

Form of carbohydrates	Examples	Availability
Monosaccharides (Single sugar unit)	• Glucose • Fructose • Galactose	• Rarely found naturally in foods (except for fructose) • Fructose (apple, honey, etc.)
Disaccharides (Double sugar unit)	• Sucrose (50% glucose, 50% fructose) • Lactose (50% galactose, 50% glucose) • Maltose (100% glucose-glucose bond) • High fructose corn syrup (42–55% fructose)	• Occurs naturally in foods (sucrose, lactose) • Produced by starch digestion (maltose) • Sucrose/lactose (fruit, milk and sweet potatoes)
Oligosaccharides (Multiple sugar unit: 3–10) Polysaccharides (multiple glucose/sugar units)	• Raffinose • Stachyose • Starch • Glycogen (animal starch) (absorbed as glucose) • Resistant starch (do not get absorbed)	• Raffinose (dry beans and peas, onions, breast milk) • Available in starchy vegetables • Grains • Dry beans/seeds • Nuts • Dry beans • Pasta • Cooked potatoes
Polysaccharides/Lignin (multiple sugar/glucose units)	• Dietary fiber (non-digestible carbohydrate) mostly in plants • Functional fiber (isolated non-digestible carbohydrate) (may have beneficial effects)	• Dietary fibers pass intact through digestive track, whereas functional fibers may be fermented by colon microflora • Whole grains • Dry beans and peas • Nuts and seeds • Fruits • Vegetables

Robertosn (1845) was the pioneer researcher who concluded that caries was caused by "acids formed from lodgements of food". Motegazza (1864) showed that teeth could be decalcified by being placed into a mixture of saliva and sugar. He suggested that the formation of lactic acid and acetic acid was responsible for this decalcification. Later, Miller (1889) hypothesized that carbohydrates and micro-organisms produce acid, subsequently leading to caries process. Even the children consuming syrup containing sugar over the regular basis had a significantly higher caries experience than children who took medicines in tablet form. A couple of studies have confirmed these findings.

The long chain of starch molecules prevent them from being metabolized easily in oral cavity; therefore relatively little acid is secreted from their metabolism. However, during processing, starch undergoes partial denaturation and degradation increasing their potential of adhesion and subsequently the caries.

Epidemiologic Evidences

The evidences linking sucrose consumption and prevalence of caries can be found in several epidemiologic studies.

Kite, et al (1950) studied the importance of local effect of diet on caries. When intact or desalivated rats were fed on cariogenic diet by stomach tube, caries did not develop. In contrast, caries occurred in normally fed rats, the severity being much higher in desalivated animals.

A device was used to control feeding of rats. The device consisted of a circular tray with 18 feeding cups. A plastic tube led from each cage to the tray, one cup at a time being accessible. The machine imposed eating patterns of widely different frequency to rats. A highly positive correlation was found between frequency of eating and caries incidence.

Orland, et al (1954) compared the occurrence of caries in rats fed on a cariogenic diet kept in a germ-free environment and in normal flora. The experiment clearly showed that micro-organisms are essential for caries development.

Marthales (1978) compared the caries experience of 11–12 years old children in 19 countries with annual sugar consumption data and showed a positive correlation between caries and sugar consumption.

Sreenky (1982) observed positive correlation in caries experience in the primary dentition of 5–6 years old with sugar availability in 23 countries and of 12 years old with sugar availability in 47 countries.

Studies Correlating Increase/Decrease Consumption of Sugar

Many authors have correlated caries experience with sugar consumption in various studies. The population having habit of consuming excess sugar in routine food, tea, coffee, candy, etc. experience more caries.

Mac Gregor (1963) examined caries prevalence in 12 years old Ghana children between 1950 and 1960. Caries prevalence was highest (59%) in people with good living (sugar being a luxury item), 46% in people with fair living standard and 28% in people with poor living standards, correlating caries with increase in sugar consumption.

Anaise (1978) observed 71% higher caries experience in Israeli confectionary workers

than workers in textile factories. Kotayama (1979) in his study observed 17.2 DMFT in confectionary workers as compared to other workers with 11.4 DMFT.

Zitzon (1979) observed that Eskimos living on their natural diet have low caries experience; however, the caries increased rapidly after exposure to sugar rich diet.

The inhabitants of an island in South Atlantic (Island of Tristan da Cunha) lived remote from the rest of the world for many years consuming simple, less sugary diet. The prevalence of caries was negligible. But as the islanders developed contacts with the rest of the world and started consuming sugar products, the caries prevalence was much higher.

A study was conducted on a group of children of low socio-economic background at Hopewood House, in the Australian state of New South Wales. Children were examined from birth till they attain 12 years of age. Dental examination was conducted annually. Sugar and refined carbohydrates (e.g. white bread) were excluded from children's diet. They were fed with a vegetarian diet rich in proteins, fats, minerals and vitamins. The study began with 81 children. At the age of 4–9, 78% were caries free. At age 13, only 53% were caries free. Over the years, some of the dietary restrictions in the institution were relaxed, but at the conclusion of the study 35% of the 13 years old were still caries free.

The Vipeholm Study

The study was conducted on 436 adult inmates in a mental institution at the Vipeholm Hospital near Lund, Sweden in 1945. A mental institution was chosen because the patients on account of their mental illness were expected to remain there for sufficient time required for the study.

The first year was a preliminary (preparatory) period. The effect of vitamins and minerals on caries was studied in initial 18 months. This was Vitamin Study Period.

The caries activity was found to be low and without any significant differences between the groups.

Later, a relationship between carbohydrate intake and caries was evaluated during 1947-1949. It was referred to as Carbohydrate Study I.

During 1949-1951, the carbohydrate menu was selected as is for common Swedish household. This second study was referred to as Carbohydrate Study II.

Four different types of groups were selected for both these studies (I & II):

a. Control group (basic diet without additional carbohydrates but with supplementary fat to bring up the caloric level).
b. Sucrose group (basic diet with additional sugar in solution (not sticky form). The amount of sucrose was more than in any other groups).
c. Bread group (basic diet plus addition of sugar in bread (sticky form) consumed at meals).
d. Chocolate, caramel, 8-toffee, 24-toffee group (Basic diet plus addition of sugar in form of sweets (sticky form) consumed between meals).

a. Control Group

A group of 60 males with an average age of 34.9 years received a carbohydrate—poor, high fat diet practically free from refined sugar. Caries activity was observed to be negligible.

After 2 years the diet was replaced by ordinary diet, with refined sugar given at meal time. This change of diet resulted in statistically significant change in caries activity.

b. Sucrose Group

A group of 57 male patients with an average age of 34.7 years were fed on 300 gram sucrose in solution at mealtime for one and a half years. After 2 years, an extra 75 gram of sugar dissolved in beverages was given at meal time. These changes in intake of carbohydrates produced no statistically significant changes in caries activity.

c. Bread Group

A group of patients consisting of 41 males and 42 females received sweet bread at one meal every day for 2 years (345 gram sweet bread containing 50 gram refined sugar). It did not increase the caries activity.

During further 2 years, same sweet bread was served at all meals. During 2nd year of this 2 years period, an increase was observed in caries activity which was significant for males than females. It was because females had better oral hygiene and they might have consumed less.

d. Chocolate Group

A group of 47 males who received 300 gram refined sugar in solution at meals during first 2 years, which was later reduced to 110 gm. For next 2 years, they received 30 gram sugar between meals as 65 gram chocolate. It was served as four portions between meals.

This change was accompanied by significant increase in caries activity.

e. Caramel Group

A group of 62 males received 345 gram of sugar rich bread at one meal a day. After 2 years, they received 22 caramels daily in 2 portions between meals during 3rd year. In 4th year 22 caramels were given in 4 portions between meals. There was significant increase in caries activity which was followed by withdrawal of caramel and was replaced by an isocaloric quantity of fat. This withdrawal of caramels resulted in fall of caries increment.

f. 8-toffee Group

This group consisted of 40 males who received low carbohydrate, high-fat diet for one year. 8 toffees were added which was served in between meals for next 3 years. There was a marked increase in caries activity.

g. 24-toffee Group

This group consisted of 48 males and 39 females who received ordinary Swedish diet for first two years. During next two years, they received 160 grams of carbohydrates as 24 toffees in between meals which was withdrawn thereafter. There was marked increase in caries activity during the time patients were offered toffees followed by marked fall to original level on withdrawal.

Conclusions

- The consumption of sugar can increase caries activity.
- The risk of caries is greater if the sugar is consumed in a form that will be retained on the surfaces of the teeth.
- The risk of sugar increasing caries activity is greatest if sugar is consumed between meals.
- Upon withdrawal of sugar rich foods, the increased caries activity rapidly disappears.
- Caries lesion may continue to appear despite the avoidance of refined sugar and maximum restrictions of natural sugars and dietary carbohydrates.
- The increase in caries activity varies widely from one person to another.
- The increase in clearance time of the sugar increases the caries activity.

The study showed that the physical form of carbohydrates was much more important in cariogenicity than was the total amount of sugar ingested.

Cariogenicity of Carbohydrates

Dietary sucrose mostly is refined from sugarcane and sugar beets. Apart from the natural occurrence of sucrose in fruits, it is the most common sweetening agent in candies, baked goods (cookies, cakes and pastries), desserts, soft drinks, cereals, milk drink products, condiments (e.g. ketchup, jams, jellies, etc.). Sucrose is termed an 'arch criminal' in the process of caries development.

Sucrose is the source of energy for the most cariogenic plaque bacteria. Caries mainly depends on growth of dental plaque. Mutans streptococci have the ability to produce both intracellular and extracellular polysaccharides that favour adherence and colonization of micro-organisms. Plaque contains extracellular polysaccharides—glucans and levans. These are produced by the enzymes glucosyl transferase and fructosyl transferase which have been isolated from *Streptococcus mutans* and *Streptococcus sanguis*. The properties of these enzymes are:

- They are highly specific for sucrose and fructose respectively and will not utilize sugars such as glucose, maltose and lactose.
- They have a pH range, i.e. 5.2–7.0.
- In the presence of adequate nutrients, the enzymes can be made by organisms and sucrose is not required as an inducer.
- The equilibrium of reaction is:

$$nC_{12}H_{22}O_{11} \rightarrow (C_6H_{10}O_5)n + nC_6H_{12}O_6$$
$$\text{sucrose} \qquad \text{glucan} \qquad \text{fructose}$$

As long as sucrose is present in plaque, glucosyl transferase enzyme will continue to utilize it to form plaque matrix material and fructose. The relatively high energy bond between C-1 of glucose and C-2 of fructose in sucrose causes it to have a high free energy of hydrolysis so that it can serve directly as a glucosyl donor. Other disaccharides such as maltose and lactose have low free energy of hydrolysis and cannot serve directly as glucosyl donor.

Sugar is taken up by oral streptococci using the phosphoenol pyruvate dependent phosphotransferase system where sugar is modified to a phosphate ester before it appears inside the cell. The intracellular product sucrose is then allowed by sucrose hydrolase to yield glucose phosphate and fructose. The sugar phosphate is subsequently integrated into catabolic pathway. When the sugar is abundant, lactate is the major end product; when availability of sugar is limited, the major end products are ethanol, formate and acetate. The ability to ferment sucrose is increased in bacteria previously exposed to sucrose.

Mundroff, et al (1990) studied cariogenic potential of 22 different food items relative to sucrose. Cariogenic potential indices (CPI) were calculated based on number and severity of buccal/lingual caries. Foods with lowest CPI were peanuts, gelatin desserts, corn chips, yoghurt and bologna. Foods with highest CPI were sucrose, granola cereal, french fries, bananas, etc. Increased cariogenic potential was associated with foods containing approximately 1% or more hydrolysable starch in combination with sucrose or other sugars.

Naria, et al (1969) compared a caries promoting diet MIT-200 (ingredients: pulverized sucrose 67%, lactalbumin 20%, salt mixture 3%, vitamin 1%, cottonseed oil 3%, cellulose 6%) with a previous formulation MIT-10 (composed of natural food items). He observed that MIT-200 is more cariogenic than MIT-10 but caries did not penetrate up to dentin. They further opined that MIT-200 composition is reproducible and is adequate nutritionally; and can also be used for assay of cariostatic agents.

Factors Affecting Cariogenicity

The decalcification potential of a food is equivalent to retention of food product coupled with their potential of acid production.

The factors affecting cariogenicity of carbohydrates are divided into two groups:
a. Factors related to food products.
   i. Types of carbohydrates.
   ii. Quantity/concentration of carbo-hydrates.
   iii. Stickiness.
   iv. Chewing/swallowing.
b. Factors related to acid production.
   i. Frequency of intake.
   ii. Oral clearance.

   iii. Timings of intake.
   iv. Behavioural characteristic.

a. Factors related to food products

i. Types of carbohydrates

The major dietary source of carbohydrate is starch because it is the most common storage product of plants. Starch granules from plants are slowly fermented in oral cavity by salivary amylase. Cooking the starch causes degrada-tion and a change in form and allows amylase to provide metabolic substrate effectively as maltose, maltotriose, dextrins and small amounts of glucose.

Starch products when combined with sucrose for sweetness have been found to be more cariogenic than sucrose alone. Most of these products such as cookies, breads, etc. are consumed as between meal snacks, increasing their cariogenic contribution. In some food items such as soft drinks, starch hydrolysate (glucose group) is included, which may have even higher caries potential than processed and heated starch.

ii. Quantity/concentration of carbohydrates

The quantity and concentration of carbo-hydrates is important for development of caries; however, no linear relationship has been observed. The sucrose content of commonly ingested foods is tabulated in Table 7.2.

Sucrose solutions in the range of 0.05– 50% have been tested by Frostell (1969) and between 0.025 and 25% by Imfeld (1972). Their results were different. Frostell found that plaque pH was lower after rinsing with 50% concentration than with 5%; whereas Imfeld reported deep and similar curves after rinses containing 2.5%, 5.0% or 10% sucrose.

iii. Stickiness

The stickiness of food items enhances the retention time of sugars, resulting in a prolonged fall in pH, subsequently increased incidence of dental caries. High retention rates have been observed for products such as sweet biscuits, potato chips, etc.

Table 7.2: Sucrose content of commonly ingested food items

Food items	Mean percentage of sucrose content
Diet soft drinks	0.0
Conventional soft drinks	4.3
Cheese	0.0
Breads	0.1
Fresh fruits	2.0
Canned juice	2.5
Wafers	4.2
Ice-creams	15.1
Candies	38.9
Chocolate plain	56
Chocolate milk	45
Cough syrups, etc.	50

iv. Chewing/swallowing

Chewing results in increased contact of food items with the tooth surfaces, subsequently increased incidence of dental caries as compared to swallowing. However, acid in fruits juices and soft drinks may decrease the oral pH. The fall in pH may enhance fermentation of carbohydrates, leading to demineralization and caries.

b. Factors related to acid production

i. Frequency of intake

The frequency of intake of sugar may have a significant effect as regard cariogenicity of the diet. However, a few authors have observed that frequency of intake might not be related to the development of caries, but the time the sugars remain available to micro-organisms in the oral cavity is significant. The frequency of intake gains importance as caries is regarded as the outcome of balance of demineralization and remineralization. Higher frequency means more demineralization and less remineralization. The duration of the decrease in pH after intake of a cariogenic food is important.

ii. Oral clearance

Oral clearance implies clearance of carbohydrates from the oral cavity. It depends on metabolism by micro-organisms, degradation of carbohydrates by plaque and salivary enzymes and the flow of saliva. Most carbohydrates are cleared by these mechanisms. Retentiveness of foods is not the same as stickiness. A caramel or jellybean may be sticky, but its retentive properties are comparatively lower than foods such as cookies, etc. A short clearance time reduces the length of time the sugar remain available for acid production by the bacteria. During hyposalivation, may be due to Sjögren's syndrome, surgery or medication, or in older age groups with poor health, an increased caries rate is usually observed. The clearance rate is of great importance for elderly population, where medically induced low salivary secretion may lead to root caries. In all age groups, medical conditions, such as depression, eating disorders, malnutrition, etc. may influence salivary functions resulting in increased caries rate.

iii. Timing of intake

The timings of sugar intake, especially sleep time consumption of sugars is important feature for caries development. The low salivary flow during sleep decreases oral clearance of the sugars and increases the contact time, subsequently increasing the cariogenic potential of sugar and other food items.

iv. Behavioral characteristics

The food habits vary from individual to individual. A variety of factors such as availability, cost, traditions, taste, emotions and even advertisements, etc. govern our choice of food. The factors are summarized as:

- Ladies, especially working ladies, prefer snacks and avoid whole meal.
- Kids, especially girls, are influenced by advertisements.
- The taste of food is important (youngsters may like sweets).
- A few people may develop habit of taking off and on snacks because of their stressful occupations, sport activities, etc.

pH changes in plaque from food items: The most widely accepted theory of caries etiology is acidogenic theory. Thus measurement of plaque pH before, during and after a food is consumed should be a guide to cariogenic potential of that food.

There are four methods of measuring plaque pH:

a. Metal (Ir, Pd) probes can be inserted into plaque.

b. *Glass probes:* Glass probes are inserted into the plaque. Both these methods allow direct reading of pH on plaque surface. The drawback of these methods is that it may disrupt plaque structure and the accumulation of plaque over the probe may not provide exact information.

c. A miniature glass electrode is filled into a partial denture that stays in the oral cavity for several days. The plaque accumulates over the electrode and evaluated. Originally, glass electrodes were used; however, now a H^+ sensitive transistor electrode are being used. Bimetallic (Pt/Pd oxide) wire electrodes have also been used.

d. *Sampling method:* Plaque is removed from teeth and pH is measured outside the oral cavity. The disadvantage of this method is that plaque is disturbed each time the sample is taken. Secondly, the sample may represent pooling of plaque from different areas, providing intermittent information.

If a food or beverage does not cause plaque, pH to fall below 5.7 in three minutes after ingestion, it is safe for teeth. The relationship between dietary sucrose and caries is proportional. It is established that raising sucrose content of diet beyond certain level may not increase caries development.

Acidogenicity of Food Items

The acidogenicity of mid-meal snacks has been widely studied; however, acidogenicity of various other food items has not been documented properly.

Rugg-Gunn, et al (1975) reported that eating cheese after a sugary food prevented plaque pH to fall. Sugared coffee leads to drop in plaque pH.

He (1981) further investigated the effect of a three course breakfast—sugared coffee, boiled egg, bread and butter. When sugared coffee was taken at last, curve was deeper; however, shallowed when it was taken first or second. The most favorable curve was obtained when all three were taken together, implying that one food can influence the cariogenicity of another.

Geddes, et al (1977) observed that peanuts and sugarless chewing gum after sugary food prevented fall in plaque pH. Apples had a little beneficial effect when compared with peanuts.

Edgar (1981) studied the effect of cheese immediately after eating pears in preventing fall of plaque pH. He opined that if sugar containing food is followed by non-acidogenic food, pH drop is small as compared to meal which ends with acidogenic sugar foods. If meals began with sweets followed by savory food, the pH drop can be greatly reduced.

ROLE OF FATS

It has been established that dietary fats have limiting effect on dental caries. A study on Eskimos showed that as long as they lived a primitive life (fat content 65%), they had a little or no tooth decay; however, when they adopted civilized diet (fat content 25% or less), dental caries resulted.

Gustaffson (1955) observed that experimental dental caries decrease in rats by increasing the amounts of corn oil in diet. Medium chain fatty acids and their salts have antibacterial property at low pH; however, their mechanism is not well defined. Various studies carried out in institutionalized subjects, showed that inclusion of cod liver oil in diet reduced caries.

Potassium nanonate when added to diet being fed to rats reduces caries. Various studies have observed reduction in acidogenic organisms after daily rinsing with mouth-washes containing potassium nanonate. It has been shown that when nanonate is applied to a tooth prior to its exposure to acid-saliva mixture, it provides protection against decalcification of the tissues.

Certain fatty acids have exhibited antimicrobial effects and have been shown to inhibit carbohydrate metabolism in plaque.

The anticariogenic effects of dietary fats are attributed to:

- Dietary fats may alter the effect of diet by replacing carbohydrate in snacks.
- Dietary fat may form a physical barrier on tooth surface and prevent demineraliza-tion.
- Dietary fats enhance clearance of carbohydrates from the oral cavity.

ROLE OF PROTEINS

It has been established that protein deficiency during dental development leads to smaller teeth, delayed eruption and a greater susceptibility to caries. The mechanism by which protein deprivation induces caries susceptibility is not established; however, following factors may contribute:

- Reduction in salivary flow, subsequently the buffering capacity.
- Reduction in remineralization and antibacterial capacity.
- Tooth morphology may get modified/altered.
- Decrease in immune response (salivary IgA level falls).

It has been reported that dental caries in rats were accelerated when experimental diets were heat treated (heat leads to destruction of amino acids/lysine in diet). This effect has also been noted in experimental diet containing milk powder. Autoclaving of dry milk powder destroys the lysine and increases its caries producing capacity. The lysine probably reduces the rate of enamel decalcification by forming a complex with enamel.

Arginine rich peptides and vitamin B_6 (pyridoxine) may have protective effect against caries. Metabolism of these amino acids by plaque bacteria may inhibit/offset the production of demineralizing acids, resulting in increase in pH level within the plaque.

VITAMINS AND CARIES

Vitamin A

Vitamin A is essential for normal development of teeth and bones. This may be related to its potential in the synthesis of glucoproteins and maintenance of stability of cellular membranes. Vitamin A is concerned primarily with the process of differentiation of epithelial cells. Odontogenic epithelium fails to undergo normal histodifferentiation and morpho-differentiation in vitamin A deficiency and results in an increased rate of cell proliferation. The ameloblasts also fail to differentiate properly. Consequently their organizing influence on the adjacent mesenchymal cell is disturbed and atypical dentin, 'osteodentin' is formed. The epithelial invasion of pulpal tissue is characteristic feature in vitamin A deficiency.

The association of dental caries with vitamin A deficiency has not been documented exhaustively. In a few studies posteruptive vitamin A deficiency has been reported to result in higher dental caries score. This may be due to changes in salivary gland functions rather than changes in dental tissues. A few authors observed that cod liver oil (rich source of vitamin A) supplements were found to decrease the dental caries susceptibility.

Vitamin B Complex

Vitamin B complex is essential as growth factor for oral bacteria including *Streptococcus mutans*. These vitamins serve as components in coenzyme involved in glycolysis process of bacterial metabolism. In animal studies, vitamin B complex deficiencies have lead to disturbances in maintenance of tooth supporting tissues; however, their role in caries initiation is not documented.

Vitamin B₃ (Niacin)

There is strikingly low incidence of dental caries in dental patients with nicotinic acid deficiency because it acts both as essential nutrient for oral acidogenic flora and part of enzyme system concerned with the degradation of fermentable carbohydrates to organic acid in amount sufficient to alter tooth structure. Niacin appears to promote dental caries via stimulation of cariogenic oral flora.

Vitamin B₆ (pyridoxine) has shown some anti-cariogenic action as it promotes growth of non-cariogenic microflora in oral cavity, thereby hampering growth of cariogenic micro-organisms.

Vitamin B₇ (Biotin)

It is essential nutrient for all acid producing micro-organisms tested and as such may play a role in microbiology of caries.

Vitamin C

It is established that vitamin C is more involved in maintenance of gingival health than caries. Animal studies have also showed less concurrent results in this regard. Hanke (1932) claimed that vitamin C levels are inversely related to dental caries but this has not been confirmed by surveys and clinical trials.

Vitamin D

Enamel is the most mineralized tissue in the human body; inorganic contents being more than 99%. Calcium and phosphate are the main inorganic constituents. Vitamin D enhances absorption of calcium and phosphate from the food. The inorganic component increases the strength of teeth and their ability to fight demineralization.

Deficiency of vitamin D, especially during developmental stage, results in delayed eruption of teeth; and also the teeth may be smaller in size.

The beneficial effects of vitamin D are:

- Vitamin D affects calcium metabolism.
- Vitamin D, which is produced in response to light exposure, induces cathelicidin, an antimicrobial peptide, which has the potential to attack oral bacteria causing dental caries.

Schroth, et al (2010) studied the effects of vitamin D in pregnant Canadian women and whether or not their children developed early childhood caries (ECC). The observations were:

- Mothers of children who developed ECC had lower vitamin D levels.
- The early childhood caries were more severe if their mothers had low vitamin D levels during pregnancy.

The authors concluded that the vitamin D levels of a mother during pregnancy definitely related to their children's risk of developing ECC.

Schroth, et al (2013) further evaluated role of vitamin D in developing childhood caries (ECC) in their study on pre-school children. The authors measured the children's vitamin D levels and the parents answered questions on their child's nutritional habits, oral health and family information. The observations were:

- Children with severe ECC had lower vitamin D levels than the healthy children.
- Winter season was also related to low vitamin D levels in children with severe ECC.

Reviewing other studies, it was observed as follows:

- Taking vitamin D supplements result in substantial reduction of dental caries in children.
- Taking vitamin D supplements had no effect on caries, especially in older age.

It has also been established that geographic location and sun exposure are related to dental caries. People living closer to the equator with greater amounts of sun exposure are less likely to develop dental caries.

In early 1920s and 1930s, many studies were conducted evaluating role of vitamin D on dental caries.

The initial animal studies observed that vitamin D stimulated the calcification of teeth. Subsequently, the beneficial effect of vitamin D on dental caries was established.

A few studies were conducted on children in New York regarding dental caries with respect of season, artificial ultraviolet-B irradiance and oral intake of vitamin D. The authors observed that intake of vitamin D, prevent caries effectively.

Use of vitamin D appears to be a better option for reducing dental caries than fluoridation of community water supplies, as there are many additional health benefits of vitamin D and a number of adverse effects of water fluoridation such as fluorosis (mottling) of teeth and bones.

Vitamin K

Vitamin K may be effective in reducing caries, since it is known to reduce enzymatic activity in carbohydrate degradation cycle; however, studies observed that deficiency of vitamin K did not produce any increase in dental caries incidence.

MINERALS AND CARIES

Calcium and Phosphorus

Calcium (Ca) and phosphorus (P) are essential components of saliva and are required for remineralizing the demineralized tooth structure.

A significant cariostatic action has been demonstrated by inorganic phosphates when added to cariogenic diets of rats or hamsters. The exact mechanism of action of phosphate in caries reduction is unclear but evidence points to a local effect in mouth rather than a systemic influence through ingestion.

a. The ability of phosphate to reduce the rate of dissolution of hydroxyapatite of enamel.

b. Supersaturated solutions of phosphates can redeposit calcium phosphate particularly in areas of enamel that have been particularly demineralized.

c. Phosphates act to buffer organic acids formed by fermentation of plaque microorganisms.

d. Phosphate act to desorb proteins from the enamel surfaces, thereby modifying acquired pellicle.

Mechanism of Action of Calcium and Phosphorus

Concentration of calcium and phosphates in saliva is raised and critical pH for decalcification is lowered, i.e. teeth can tolerate lower pH without decalcification.

The insoluble salts of calcium and phosphates have better direct effect in raising ionic concentration. Since salts are present in fine powder form so they enter plaque along with food debris. If plaque becomes acidic, these salts dissolve more readily than enamel and by buffering the acid, raise local concentration of calcium and phosphates so tooth substance will not dissolve.

Calcium Lactate

A couple of demineralization/remineralization studies have shown calcium lactate having caries protective effects. It may keep plaque fluid saturated with calcium, subsequently not allowing sucrose induced plaque pH to fall.

Lynch RJM (2004) studied the anticaries effects of calcium glycerophosphate. The Calcium glycerophosphates may act in the following manner affecting caries process:

    i. Effects on enamel.

   ii. Buffering of plaque pH.

  iii. Modification in plaque metabolism.

  iv. Elevation of calcium and phosphorus levels in plaque.

i. Effects on Enamel

Monofluorophosphate (MFP) and calcium glycerophosphate (CaGP) in a definite ratio can effect the acid solubility of hydroxyapatite. The ratio ranging between 10:1 and 20:1 was significantly more effective than mono-fluorophosphate alone. The combined effect was attributed to increased uptake of fluoride in non-alkali soluble form at the expense of an alkali soluble fraction containing calcium fluoride. Other calcium compounds like acetate and chloride were studied for synergistic anticaries effect but no significant effect on monofluorophosphate activity was seen.

Various studies have suggested that calcium glycol phosphate interacted directly with outer layer of hydroxyapatite. This interaction is independent to the presence of fluoride.

ii. Buffering of Plaque pH

Presence of calcium glycerophosphate (CaGP) acts as buffer in plaque. It is established that inclusion of 0.25–1% calcium glycerophosphate into diet can effectively reduce the subsequent drop in plaque pH compared to the control.

iii. Modification in Plaque Metabolism

A few studies observed reduction in mean plaque scores after rinsing with glycero-phosphate solutions. This is because organic phosphates might have high affinity for tooth surface.

iv. Evaluation of Calcium and Phosphorus Levels in Plaque

The toothpastes containing calcium glycol phosphate lead to significant increase of calcium and phosphorus levels in plaque. This increase is responsible for anticaries efficiency.

Hydrolysis of starch from crackers by measurement of maltose was shown to be reduced by 70% after rinsing with tea. Removal of tannins from tea with gelatin resulted in negation of enzymatic inhibition.

Components of tea may therefore possibly reduce the cariogenic effect of starches retained in the oral cavity that act as slow release substrate reservoir for plaque.

Various studies have established cheese to have cariostatic properties. Grenby and Bull (1975) studied the effects of supplementing diet with glycerophosphates and calcium salts on dental caries. Calcium glycerophosphate showed more caries inhibitory effect than sodium glycerophosphate. It is also reported that activity of sodium glycerophosphate is augmented with calcium nitrate. It is established that calcium exhibited anticaries activity.

Silva, et al (1986) observed that chewing cheddar cheese prevents demineralization via two different mechanisms, i.e. stimulating salivary flow and by increasing calcium and phosphorus concentrations in dental plaque thus favoring remineralization.

Saroglu Sonmez and S. Aras (2007) observed white cheese and sugarless yoghurt did not lower plaque pH below 5.7. Plaque pH with any of these two did not reach 5.5, i.e. critical pH at which remineralization can occur.

Phosphates

Various studies have been conducted to evaluate the cariostatic effects of phosphates. Most of the studies reported phosphates to be effective anti-caries agents.

- 100 gm of diet of any individual should have 0.4 gm of phosphorus.
- The anti-caries activity of phosphates depend on type of anion, in the order:
  Cyclic $\rightarrow$ trimeta $\rightarrow$ tripoly $\rightarrow$ hexameta $\rightarrow$ ortho $\rightarrow$ pyro
- Phosphates of same series differ in cariostatic activity depending upon type of cation, in the order:
  $H^+ \rightarrow Na^+ \rightarrow K^+ \rightarrow Ca^{+2} \rightarrow Mg^{+2}$
- Phosphates have shown significant cariostatic activity when administered to rodents as freely mixed in diet or when baked in bread and mixed into diet.

- Phosphates with nearly neutral pH do not appear to be cariostatic when applied in concentrated solutions directly to tooth surface. Cariostatic action of phosphates appear to be largely due to a local action on tooth as these phosphates pass through mouth and then return to mouth through saliva.
- No correlation between cariostatic activity of phosphates and its water solubility/buffering capacity/chelating ability have been observed.
- Cariostatic activity of some phosphates appears to be exerted on structure of enamel, possibly by an initial demineralization and subsequent remineralization process.
- Adhesiveness or retentiveness of phosphate is important. The compounds which are themselves retentive on surfaces or pits and fissures and permit slow release of phosphate appear to be most effective.
- Phosphates combined with fluoride have an additive effect on control of dental caries; however, mechanism of action of both is different.
- Phosphates because of their detergent properties can interfere with adherence of plaque bacteria to enamel surface and can also reduce bacterial growth.
- Phosphate in oral environment minimizes its loss from tooth enamel.

Shannon Ira L (1964) studied parotid fluid flow rate, parotid fluid and serum inorganic phosphate concentration as related to dental caries. Inorganic phosphate determination was carried out on blood serum and parotid fluid was obtained from patients having dental caries. Parotid fluid and inorganic phosphate are inversely related to dental caries experience.

Collan, et al (1971) studied the effects of replacement of 4.0% sucrose with anticariogenic diet (alkaliphosphate salt combination). They observed nephrocalcinosis in every animal fed with this diet. The appearance of nephrocalcinosis is synchronous with caries protecting effect.

Sodium and Potassium

Salts of sodium (Na) and potassium (K) are extensively used in combination with fluoride for both topical and systemic application. Potassium is found in quite high concentration in enamel. Their individual effect on caries is not established; however, potassium intake showed statistically significant correlation between caries prone individuals and caries.

Trace Elements

Trace elements are a part of food as good as any other nutrient. Their availability is through soil or water, directly or indirectly.

Soil: Various studies have shown correlation of caries prevalence with mineral content of soil; low mineral content of soil and high caries prevalence. A few earlier studies correlated different caries levels to underlying differences in rock strata in addition to soils. Water running through these strata was also significant factor in carrying trace elements to human nutrition.

Water: Intake or consumption of water is either from ground or surface water. Ground water varies in hardness as compared to surface water. Hewat and Eastcott (1955) have shown a significant decrease in caries after consuming moderately hard water as compared to less hard water. This is largely due to calcium and fluoride; and also partially due to other trace elements like the alkaline ions. Commonly significant trace elements are:

1. Fluorine

Fluorine (F) is one of the most reactive elements and therefore is never found naturally in its elemental form. The fluoride ion, however, is abundant in nature and occurs almost universally in soils and water in varying concentrations. The concentration of fluorine in outer enamel surface is 421–573 ppm, whereas 122–205 ppm is in inner surface.

Mechanism of action of fluoride in preventing caries is based on two models pre-eruptive and post-eruptive. It has been hypothesized that pre-eruptive exposure to fluoride inhibits caries. It is hypothesized that fluoride is said to act by getting incorporated into the developing enamel hydroxyapatite crystal and thus reducing enamel solubility. It has been argued that pre-eruptive benefits are especially important for reducing pit-and-fissure lesions. Any pre-eruptive effect on caries inhibition is likely to be minor; the evidence for posteruptive action is much stronger. Three major mechanisms of action have been identified (one pre-eruptive and two post-eruptive), these are:

Pre-eruptive: Some reduction in enamel solubility in acid by pre-eruptive incorporation of fluoride into the hydroxyapatite crystals.

Post-eruptive:

- Promotion of remineralization and inhibition of demineralization of early caries.
- Inhibition of glycolysis, the process by which cariogenic bacteria metabolize fermentable carbohydrate.

Fluoride works best to prevent caries when a constant, low level of fluoride is maintained in the oral cavity. Its most important caries-inhibitory action is post-eruptive and takes place at the plaque-enamel interface. The action of fluoride in preventing caries is multifactorial; its effect comes from a combination of several mechanisms.

Fluoride introduced into the oral cavity is mainly taken up by dental plaque, where 95% is held in bound form rather than as ionic form. The bound fluoride can be released in response to lower pH and F is taken up by demineralized enamel than sound enamel. The availability of plaque fluoride to respond to the acid challenge leads to the gradual establishment of a well crystallized and more acid resistant apatite in the enamel surface during demineralization-remineralization cycle. Therefore, plaque acts as a major reservoir of fluoride in oral cavity and slow release of it helps in reducing caries.

Fluoride in plaque inhibits glycolysis, the process through which fermentable carbohydrate is metabolized by cariogenic bacteria to produce acid. There is also some evidence that plaque fluoride can inhibit the production of extracellular polysaccharide by cariogenic bacteria, a necessary process for plaque adherence to smooth enamel surfaces.

Fluoride can be delivered for human benefit in two ways—systemic and topical fluoride. Systemic fluoride is based on pre-eruptive model but it has topical effect also. Various vehicles for delivering systemic fluoride are, water, milk, salt, tablet and dietary supplements. All of them are for regular consumption in order to provide low concentration of fluoride. Most of the epidemiological studies on water, milk, salt fluoridation have shown to achieve around 50% reduction in dental caries in population. Caries reductions were greatest for the free smooth surfaces and proximal surfaces of teeth and were less pronounced for pit-and-fissure surfaces.

Topical fluoride provides large concentrations of fluoride to the erupted tooth surface. Their action is post-eruptive. Vehicles used are solution, gel, foam, varnish, prophylactic paste for professional use, fluoride dentifrices and mouthrinses for home use. These agents provide 30–40% reduction in caries incidence.

2. Zinc

Zinc (Zn) is second most abundant trace element in human enamel, next only to iron. Role of zinc in dental caries could not be authenticated. Various studies have shown zinc as cariogenic and also as cariostatic. Most animal studies have shown an increase in caries due to zinc deficiency. Different concentrations of zinc could control growth of *Streptococcus mutans*, initial plaque formation and inhibition of acid production. Effect of zinc supplementation in reducing dental caries has not been established.

Increased dental caries is seen with a decrease in plasma zinc level in contraceptive steroid-treated rats. A few authors observed higher saliva zinc concentration in caries-free individuals when compared with individuals having caries experience.

3. Copper

Many studies have established that Copper (Cu) reduces the acidogenicity of the dental plaque. Copper inhibits the H-ATP synthase, inhibits various metabolic enzymes through the oxidation of key trial group and forms the insoluble copper-potassium salts on tooth surface, thereby increasing its acid resistance. Its topical application to the teeth inhibited acid production by plaque, significantly reduced caries scores and produced lower *Streptococcus mutans* count. A few authors confirmed significant decrease in salivary copper level in individuals with caries as compared to those with no caries.

Copper is considered as a mild cariostatic agent but it is not established. Problem with research in studying effect of copper on human health is the difficulty of separating its effect from other inorganic elements freely available in food/water.

Copper is found in high level in carious lesions suggesting a caries arresting/prohibitive role of the element. Three distinct mechanisms for the increased levels of copper in the carious lesions have been proposed (i) the caries affected hydroxyapatite in the dentin has a higher affinity for binding aqueous oral copper than healthy dentin (ii) the bacteria responsible for cariogenesis may actively accumulate copper and (iii) the increased copper is secreted into tubules as an antibacterial defensive mechanism.

A few studies have observed that individuals with caries presented with decreased serum copper level as compared to healthy controls.

4. Molybdenum

Molybdenum (Mo) has been studied exhaustively for its relation with caries. Earlier studies have suggested a decrease in caries prevalence with high intake of molybdenum.

A few authors have suggested that lower caries prevalence in some communities was due to high molybdenum concentration (0.1 ppm) in water in those areas; however, another few could not find any beneficial effect of molybdenum in water when supplied to different population. Most of the animal studies could establish caries reduction phenomenon of molybdenum.

5. Selenium

Many studies conducted in different part of the world showed that an increased consumption of dietary selenium (Se) during tooth development phase leads to increased caries prevalence. A few authors have showed that high selenium concentration is bad for teeth and also provided evidence that selenium reduced cariostatic effect of fluoride as well.

Most of the animal studies observed that selenium has damaging effect on teeth as far as caries experience is concerned; however, it could not be established in human studies.

6. Vanadium

Many studies have reported an inverse relationship between vanadium (V) concentration in water and dental caries. It was also suggested that this relationship was unrelated to fluoride concentration in water. (Vanadium replaces the part of phosphorus in hydroxyapatite crystal and helps in caries inhibiting mechanisms.) Most of animal studies have suggested beneficial effect of vanadium; however, it could not be established in human studies.

7. Magnesium

Earlier studies associated low caries prevalence with high magnesium (Mg) concentration in diet or water supplies. However, presence of increased level of calcium and hardness in water (known for their caries reducing action) were not studied along with effects of magnesium. High magnesium is usually present with high calcium and it is difficult to prove any effect of magnesium on teeth without excluding calcium.

A few studies showed magnesium having protective effect on enamel in a population where dietary calcium was kept low, adding additional magnesium phosphate in the diet.

Animal studies have found either no effect of magnesium or an increase in caries incidence. Magnesium do occur in enamel as a constituent along with calcium and phosphorus. Summarily, animal studies observed increase of caries by magnesium; while epidemiologic studies suggested the opposite.

8. Manganese

A few studies observed positive correlation between manganese (Mn) and dental caries. It is hypothesized that high levels of Mn in both saliva and plaque cause increase in caries incidence. It was also observed that Mn concentration in the enamel of high caries group was greater than the low caries ones.

A few animal studies has also observed inhibiting effect of manganese on caries.

9. Sulfur

Sulfur (S) is primarily ingested in the form of various amino acids. Epidemiological studies fail to provide any direct correlation between sulfur and caries. Protein (amino acids) deficiency can effect tooth development; however, deficiencies of sulfur can have deleterious effect on tooth development or caries in humans could not be established. A few animal studies inferred that sulfites rich diet has cariostatic action.

10. Chromium

Since chromium (Cr) helps in sugar metabolism, its relationship with dental caries was of interest to researchers. Earlier it was documented that chromium content of soil was significantly higher in low caries areas; however, other studies could not authentisize the concept.

Although role of chromium in caries inhibition is not clear but lower level of chromium in oral environment might affect growth and metabolism of bacteria.

11. Cobalt

Cobalt (Co) may interfere with calcification of tooth by inhibiting apatite crystal formation and mineralization. However, its role in caries initiation/progression could not be established.

12. Iodine

Anti-bacterial effect of iodine (I) has long been established; however, no study has observed direct relation of iodine and caries. Most evidence on anticaries effect of iodine is documented in animal studies. A few authors have observed that iodine has an additive effect on reducing caries when used with fluoride. Potassium iodine has been used as preventive agent and produced significant reduction in caries. Effect of iodine as topical application is being studied for further reference.

13. Iron

Iron (Fe) is consistently present in tooth enamel. It has an antibacterial effect especially on *Streptococcus mutans* and it also interferes with biofilm formation. Caries inhibiting effect of iron might be due to its ability to inhibit the H-ATPase of *Streptococcus mutans*, affecting its acidogenicity and aciduricity. Iron also interferes with sucrose metabolism, leading to reduction in extracellular polysaccharides production. Iron reduces demineralization by forming acid resistant coating on enamel surface and has no role in the remineralization. Its definite role in caries has not been established. Miguel et al (1997) compared the effect of iron salts in sucrose (ferrous sulphate and ferric glycerophosphate) on the incidence of dental caries. They concluded that acidogenic activity of plaque in animals receiving either of iron-sucrose formulation tended to be lower than that of control groups. Further, the combination of iron-sugar may be effective in tackling anemia.

14. Nickel

Nickel (Ni) has been observed to have minor effect on caries reduction. No epidemiological study has evaluated correlation between caries and Nickel only; however, its effect in combination with copper, zinc, manganese, etc. has been documented.

15. Silicon

Silicon (Si) is an abundant element in earth crust and soil. It has been established that silicon is an essential element for bone formation particularly during mineralization. Topical application of silicon on animals produced no caries inhibiting effect. Silicon might incorporate into apatite crystals of enamel leading to increase in their solubility.

16. Lithium

Many studies have observed that lithium (Li) has anti-caries effect. Most of these studies evaluated other trace elements also. No clear conclusion can be drawn regarding anticariogenic effect of lithium but studies observed reduction in caries. Further experimental studies are required to authentisize the hypothesis of lithium reducing dental caries.

17. Titanium

A few authors reported reduction in caries in experimental animals after topical application of titanium nitrate. Topical application of titanium fluoride has also given similar effect.

Reed and Bibby observed titanium fluoride to have better caries resistance than acidulated fluoride.

It has also been hypothesized that titanium (Ti) may enhance the cariostatic effect of fluoride on systemic administration. Titanium is considered an effective cariostatic agent both topically and systemically.

18. Lead

It has been shown that lead (Pb) in excess is caries promoting; however, no correlation was observed with concentration of lead in enamel and caries. The studies on lead were not encouraged mainly because of its toxic nature.

19. Cadmium

Cadmium (Cd) toxicity commonly affects teeth, causes staining and active caries lesions. Most of the animal studies were conflicting observing cadmium as caries promoting and cariostatic agent.

20. Strontium

The concentration of strontium (Sr) in outer surface of enamel is 443–471 ppm and inner surface of enamel is 246–331 ppm. Various epidemiological studies have suggested that strontium exhibited cariostatic properties, predominantly in the presence of fluoride. Strontium concentration of 5–10 ppm in drinking water has been effective in inhibiting caries. It causes mottling of enamel; however, its definite role in caries prevention could not be established.

There is a need for further research, especially on the availability of strontium in the dental hard tissues, plaque and saliva and its association with caries.

Minerals and their effects on caries are summarized in Table 7.3.

DIET AND ROOT CARIES

It has been established that diet has definite role in the production of root caries. Various studies on diet and root caries have

Table 7.3: Minerals and their effects on caries	
Minerals	*Effect*
F, P	Cariostatic
Mo, V, Cu, Li, Fe, S, Cr, Sr	Mildly cariostatic
Co, Mn, Zn, I	Doubtful
Al, Ni, Ti	Caries inert
Se, Mg, Cd, Pb, Si	Caries promoting

recognized the effects of carbohydrates and other dietary items on root caries.

Root surfaces differ anatomically from enamel and have different physical and chemical compositions that make this tissue more sensitive to demineralization and caries.

Hecht and Friedman (1949) observed much higher cervical decay rate in institutionalized drug users than in control group; the main reasons were increased sugar intake and poor oral hygiene. A few authors were of the view that craving for sugar was the main cause of root caries in drug addicts. These addicts usually suffer from xerostomia also.

Revald (1994) has observed that frequent exposure to fermentable carbohydrates and higher intake of daily sugar were related to higher root caries in older adults. The stickiness of carbohydrates may be more detrimental to root caries. The association of root caries and periodontal diseases has also been observed.

Papas, et al (1995) in their study using food diaries observed 4.2% root caries related to sugar, 2.8% with plaque, 3.8% by total number of teeth and 5.6% with recession. Their data suggested that root caries has similar dietary etiology to coronal caries.

A few authors have reported negative association of root caries with cheese consumption. The dietary factors which affect enamel caries do affect root caries also. All cariogenic food items affect exposed roots leading to caries.

Dietary Counseling

A vast number of studies have established relation of diet and nutrition to dental caries.

Dietary counseling as regard to modifying dietary habits can control the initiation and progression of dental caries, especially in caries susceptible populations. A group of individuals in a given population can be selected for dietary counseling. The selected individuals are categorized as caries susceptible or normal by evaluating their saliva, determining the retained soluble carbohydrates. The important features are:

a. The individual's resistance should be assessed thoroughly evaluating dental and medical history. The level of education and motivation should also be evaluated as regard to need and other habits.

b. The individual's normal daily diet is examined as regard to need and other habits. Craving for sweets or any other food item should also be recorded. In case changes are required, the individual should be motivated and encouraged to follow the changed protocol of daily diet.

c. The forms of dietary modifications can be:
   i. Modifying the texture of food items.
   ii. Changing the components of routine diet.
   iii. Elimination/addition of specific food items.
   iv. The caries susceptible individuals are advised as follows:
   • Encouraged to have firm and detergent food instead of soft and sticky one.
   • Use of food items rich in proteins, fats, vitamins and minerals.
   • Minimizing intake of refined sugary food.
   • Differentiate between good and bad foods as regard to their cariogenicity.
   • The caloric values of different food items and also their effect on teeth should also be explained.

Food Components and their Anticariogenic Activity

A variety of foods and food components have the potential to act as anti-caries agents.

Characterization of their effectiveness has been confirmed through *in vitro* and *in vivo* studies using both animal and human subjects.

Minimum inhibitory concentration (MIC) is the lowest concentration of an antimicrobial that will inhibit the visible growth of a microorganism after overnight incubation.

Apple

Apple contains polyphenols (condensed tannins), which have inhibitory effects on the synthesis of water insoluble glucans by glycosyltransferase and adherence of bacterial cells to the tooth surface.

Nutmeg

Extract of nutmeg, a widely used spice, possess strong inhibitory activity against *Streptococcus mutans*. The compound has been identified as macelignan with a minimum inhibitory concentration of 3.9 µg/ml. It is also active against lactobacilli at the 2–31 µg/ml MIC range.

The specific activity and fast effectiveness of macelignan ascribes it as a potent natural anti-biofilm agent.

Coffee

Coffee is the dried seed of the fruit originated from a tree of the Coffea genus. Green coffee is composed of caffeine, chlorogenic acids, trigonelline, etc. The interactions between polyphenols and other organic compounds seem to inhibit the demineralization process. The interaction involves covalent, ionic, hydrogen bonding or hydrophobic processes, which induces the metamorphism of enamel organic matrix. The metamorphic organic matrix is precipitated in the enamel, resulting in a slowdown of the speed of mineral loss, subsequently inhibiting enamel demineralization. Roasted coffee, but not green coffee, showed antibacterial activity against *Streptococcus mutans* owing to its β-dicarbonyl compounds content. Roasted and green coffee

extracts interfere with *Streptococcus mutans* adsorption to hydroxyapatite. Low molecular weight trigonelline and nicotinic acid may prove active as antiadhesive.

Wine

Wine contains proanthocyanins which exert antibacterial activity against mutans streptococci. It interferes with the adhesion of streptococci to hydroxyapatite and inhibit the biofilms formation.

Tea

Tea, made from the leaves of *Camellia sinensis* (family Theaceae), is one of the most popular beverages worldwide.

Green tea is prepared from fresh tea leaves that are pan-fried or steamed and dried to inactivate enzymes. It contains polyphenolic catechins. Black tea is prepared by crushing tea leaves and allowing fermentation to occur, leading to the formation of flavins and arubigins. Oolong tea is partially fermented and contains catechins.

The catechin in green tea strongly inhibits glucosyltransferase activity reducing the caries activity. Minimum inhibitory concentration of epigallocatechin against streptococci is 31.25 g/ml. Polyphenols also exert the anticariogenic activity.

Propolis

It is a resinous substance produced by honey bees; the secretions are mixed with resins collected from different plants.

Propolis has the potential to reduce the streptococci count in saliva and plaque. It also interferes with the adhesion capacity of streptococci and reduces the production of insoluble polysaccharide.

Flavonoid propolis decreases the count of *Streptococcus mutans,* whereas non-flavonoid propolis lacked the killing activity against streptococcus; however, it inhibits the acid production.

Cocoa

Cocoa products rich in polyphenols, significantly reduced the caries incidence. Cocoa reduces the plaque pH, biofilms formation and also inhibits the glucosyltransferase activity. Cocoa products contain inhibitors of enzyme dextransucrase, responsible for the formation of the plaque extracellular polysaccharides from sucrose.

Ajowan/Ajwain/Carom

It is an aromatic spice, resembling thyme in flavor. It consists of naphthalene derivative (minimum inhibitory concentration of 156.25 µg/ml), which possesses anticariogenic potential. It reduces bacterial adherence and biofilm formation.

Barley Coffee

It is made from roasted barley. It has the potential to inhibit adherence of mutans streptococci to hydroxyapatite crystals and also restricts biofilm formation.

Cranberry

Cranberry inhibited *Streptococcus sobrinus* adhesion to hydroxyapatite. Cranberry polyphenols reduces acidogenicity of streptococci.

Mushroom

Mushrooms inhibit *Streptococcus mutans* adherence to hydroxyapatite and restrict the biofilms formation.

Tobacco

Tobacco has a strong anti-cariogenic effect. The active component present in plant extracts are tannins and other polyphenols. They interfere with the *Streptococcus mutans* ability to colonize teeth surfaces. The inhibition of glycosyltransferases and sucrose-dependent *Streptococcus mutans* colonization has also been reported.

Eugenol

Eugenol is an aromatic molecule found in essential oils and various plants, including cloves, bay leaves and cinnamon leaves.

Eugenol has been widely used in dentistry to treat toothache and pulpitis. Eugenol inhibits the growth and prevents the insoluble and soluble glucans synthesis of *Streptococcus sobrinus*. Eugenol significantly inhibited the reduction of pH induced by *Streptococcus mutans*.

Neem

Neem contains trimethylamine, chlorides, nimbidin, azadirachtin, lectin, fluorides in large amounts and silica, sulfur, vitamin C, tannins, saponins, flavonoids and sterols in small quantities. Maximum antimicrobial activity was observed on *Streptococcus mutans*. This may be due to the presence of fluoride, which is known to exert an anticariogenic action and silica acting as an abrasive and preventing accumulation of plaque. Tannins exert an astringent effect and form a coat over the enamel, thus protecting against tooth decay. Prior to exposure of bacteria to neem stick extract, may result in significant reduction in bacterial adhesion.

Mango (Mangifera indica)

Mango contains tannins, bitter gum and resins. Tannins and resins have an astringent effect on the mucous membrane and form a layer over enamel. The astringent layer provides protection against acid attack.

Tulsi

Tulsi (*Ocimum sanctum*), is a time-tested medicinal herb. Eugenol, the active constituent present in Tulsi, is responsible for its therapeutic potential. The other important constituents include ursolic acid and carvacrol. The antimicrobial activity of Tulsi can be attributed to these constituents. It has the antimicrobial potential against *Streptococcus mutans*.

Garlic (Allium sativum)

Garlic is effective in relieving tooth pain due to the allicin—a compound with a powerful antibiotic effect. It is possible that this may slow down bacterial activity; however, it is unlikely that garlic alone can be effective in inhibiting caries process.

Eucalyptus (Eucalyptus globulus)

Ethanol extracts from *Eucalyptus globulus* leaves reportedly possess antibacterial activity against various oral bacteria. The extracts exhibit potent antibacterial activity against *Streptococcus mutans* and *Streptococcus sobrinus*. Macrocarpals, which are polyphenols are major components of 60% ethanol extracts of eucalyptus leaves.

Myrtus Communis

Myrtus ethanolic extract is used in Mediterranean regions to prepare an alcoholic drink. The extract having a MIC value of 106.6 mg/ml is found to be potential anticariogenic.

Herbs

Certain herbs like Glycyrrhiza root extracts, Withania, etc. have anticariogenic effect. They inhibit the growth of *Streptococcus mutans* and *Streptococcus sobrinus*, the bacteria responsible for caries initiation.

Anticariogenic Potential of Milk and Milk Products

Dairy products are perceived to be important for one's overall and dental health. Milk and milk products contain nutrients that have anticariogenic properties: calcium (11%), potassium and sodium (3%), proteins (3%) and lipids (up to 3.8%). Milk also contains 4–5% disaccharide lactose, which can be fermented by oral biofilms' bacteria. Normally sucrose lowers the plaque pH to <5, while lactose lowers pH to approximately 6.0. Therefore, under normal conditions, the carbohydrate content of milk conferred to low cariogenic potential. The caries protective agents of milk are given as follows:

Milk Proteins

Milk contains two major protein groups; distinguished by their solubility in unheated milk at pH 4.6 and 20°C: caseins (insoluble) and whey proteins (soluble). Caseins account for 80% of the total protein in bovine milk and exist primarily as calcium phosphate stabilized micellar complexes. Caseins are a heterogeneous family of proteins predominated by αs1-, αs2-, κ- and β caseins.

Whey proteins (20% of total milk protein) are also a heterogeneous, polymorphic group of proteins composed of α-lactalbumin (α-LA, 20%), β-lactoglobulin (β-LG, 50%), serum albumin (BSA, 10%), immunoglobulins (10%) and proteose peptones (<10%). Glycomacropeptide (GMP) is a major component of cheese whey protein as it is 15–20% of the total protein. Glycomacropeptide is a glycophosphopeptide with no aromatic amino acids.

Prevention of dental caries by milk-derived bioactive peptides is a complex physical and chemical sequence of cascading events. In general, bioactive peptides with anticariogenic activity have multiple functions to prevent dental lesions including bacterial inhibition, competitive exclusion to enamel binding sites, improved buffering capacity in the pellicle surrounding teeth, reduced enamel demineralization and increased enamel remineralization.

Non-phosphorylated casein peptides had no anticariogenic effects. CPP-ACP increases the level of amorphous calcium phosphate in plaque depressing enamel demineralization and enhancing remineralization. CPP-ACP would compete with calcium for plaque Ca binding sites. This will reduce the amount of calcium bridging between the pellicle and adhering cells and between cells themselves.

Milk components casein phosphopeptide (CPP) and glycomacropeptide (GMP) incorporated into the salivary pellicle and reduced adherence of *Streptococcus sobrinus* and *Streptococcus mutans*.

Glycomacropeptide (GMP) reduces dental caries by changing the microbial population of dental plaque predominated by *Streptococcus mutans* and *Streptococcus sanguis* to a less cariogenic population predominated by *Actinomyces viscosus*.

Minor Milk Proteins

Lactoferrin is an iron-binding protein found in milk of many species including bovine and human. Lactoferrin has antibacterial activity towards Gram-negative bacteria including the dental cariogen *Streptococcus mutans*.

Lysozyme is an effective antibacterial enzyme isolated from milk, tears and saliva. Human milk is a better source of lysozymes. The mechanism of action for lysozyme is to hydrolyze $\alpha(1\text{-}4)$-glucosidic linkages in bacterial cell wall peptidoglycan.

Lactoferricin B is an induced bioactive peptide encrypted within lactoferrin and can be liberated by the digestive enzyme pepsin. Lactoferricin is active against both Gram-positive and Gram-negative bacteria. The effect of Lactoferricin B against oral odontopathogenic bacteria has not been investigated.

Milk Products

Yogurt

Yogurt consumption led to a rapid drop in the plaque pH. The initial fall in plaque pH was due to the acidic nature of the yogurt (4.0–4.5 pH). The increase in pH after 20 and 30 minutes may be due to the buffering capacity of stimulated saliva and the reduced lactose content of the yogurt due to fermentation. The increase in pH may also be due to the fact that the natural CPP content present in yogurt is higher than that of milk, due to the proteolytic activity of micro-organisms contained in the yogurt and the peptides and amino acids produced by the hydrolysis of casein.

Grenby, et al (2001) identified the anticaries component that existed in milk and milk products. They were of the view that removal of lactose, fat and other proteins from milk had a little influence on its protective ability. Main anti-caries agents in milk are calcium and phosphorus. These are sufficient to reduce demineralization of enamel.

Somnmez I. Saroghi and Aras SW (2007) studied the effect of white cheese and sugarless yoghurt on dental plaque acidogenicity and observed that none of them lowered the plaque pH under 5.7.

Cheese

Various studies have established cheese to have cariostatic properties. It showed an anticariogenic effect on subsequent sucrose challenges by using interproximal pH electrodes.

Rugg-Gunn, et al (1975) in their plaque pH study observed that the consumption of cheese along with other food items offering cariogenic challenge can obliterate any cariostatic effect of that item. A few authors have found that cheese extracts reduce acid demineralization *in vivo*.

Silva, et al (1986) observed that chewing cheddar cheese prevents demineralization via two different mechanisms, i.e. stimulating salivary flow and by increasing calcium and phosphorus concentrations in dental plaque thus favouring remineralization.

Saroglu Sonmez and S. Aras (2007) observed white cheese and sugarless yoghurt did not lower plaque pH below 5.7. Plaque pH with any of these two did not reach 5.5, i.e. critical pH at which remineralization can occur.

Grenby and Bull (1975) studied the effects of supplementing diet with glycerophosphates and calcium salts on the dental caries. Calcium glycerophosphate showed more caries inhibitory effect than sodium-glycerophosphate. It is also reported that activity of sodium glycerophosphate is augmented with calcium nitrate. It is concluded that calcium exhibited anticaries activity.

SUGAR SUBSTITUTES

All food items containing fermentable carbohydrates are potentially cariogenic. A non-profit organization called Tooth-friendly Sweets International (TFSI) is continuously working to promote healthy snacks, which can be consumed in between meals. The organization also help motivating population as regard importance of healthy food in dentistry and also the effects of oral hygiene on dental health.

The US Food and Drug Administration (FDA) prefers food items which do not promote tooth decay or reduce risk of dental caries. Such food items which are not or less fermented by plaque are selected and are labeled as Happy tooth food. The food items which does not drop pH to 5.7 within 3 minutes, is considered 'safe' and labeled as 'Happy tooth food'. The plaque pH model (pH 5.7) does not take into account other factors in caries process and remained controversial. It has been established that demineralization of root surfaces may occur at a much higher pH level (6.7–6.8), which is not conducive with parameter of good food.

To reduce cariogenicity, fermentable carbo-hydrates are usually replaced by non-fermentable food items. Certain sugar substitutes (artificial sweetener) are also used which have negligible effect as sugar.

Chemically, sugar substitute (sugar alcohols) differ from sugars in that the complex OH grouping is substituted by an alcohol (-OH) group. Sugar alcohols have a similar level of sweetness and caloric value as the sugar and are termed nutritive sweeteners. The most commonly used sugar-alcohols are sorbitols, mannitols, xylitol, maltitol, lactitol, hydrogenated starch and hydrolysates glucosyl.

These polyols or polyalcohols, formed by hydrogenating the sugar, are used as sugar substitute and the food items are termed 'sugarless' or 'sugarfree'.

Sugar substitutes, their form and commercial preparations, are tabulated in Table 7.4.

Mechanism of Action

Sugar substitutes produce a minimal fall in plaque pH; a few of them even do not get fermented. The reasons for weak fermenta-bility or non-fermentability are:

i. Very few plaque bacteria are capable of fermenting the sugar alcohols, especially the Xylitol. *Streptococcus mutans*, having

Table 7.4: Sugar substitutes, their form and commercial preparations			
Artificial sweeteners	*Sugar alcohols*	*Novel sweeteners*	*Natural sweeteners*
Acesulfame potassium (Sunett, Sweet One)	Erythritol	Stevia extracts (Pure via, Truvia)	Agave nectar
Aspartame (Equal, NutraSweet)	Hydrogenated starch hydrolysate	Tagatose (Naturlose)	Date sugar
Neotame	Isomalt	Trehalose	Fruit juice concentrate
Saccharin (SugarTwin, Sweet'N Low)	Lactitol		Honey
Sucralose (Splenda)	Maltitol		Maple syrup
Stevia	Mannitol		Molasses
Cyclamate	Sorbitol		
	Xylitol		
Advantame			

certain enzymes, can ferment mannitol and sorbitol. The glucose present in plaque environment, prevents net synthesis of enzymes involved in fermentation of sorbitol or mannitol. If the exposure time of plaque to these alcohols is short, the necessary enzymes could not be formed leading to minimal fermentation of sorbitol or mannitol or both.

ii. The nature of end products formed after fermentation from these alcohols may also relate to less fermentation. The fermentation reaction requires proper balancing of C, O and H atoms in the end products. For sucrose, glucose and fructose, this balance can be achieved by formation of lactic acid. However, sorbitol, mannitol and xylitol have two extra hydrogen atoms that need be deposited in end products. The microbes capable of fermenting these alcohols usually re-route the carbon atoms from an acid producing pathways to one in which alcohols are formed. Thus, sugar alcohols cannot be fermented to as low pH as sucrose or glucose. The extra H-atoms in these alcohols make these sucrose substitutes highly desirable in snack foods. The commonly used sugar substitutes are:

a. Xylitol

Xylitol is considered as the best choice because it has sweetness comparable to sucrose. Further, it is not fermented by cariogenic bacteria such as *Streptococcus mutans* and *Lactobacillus casei* and is metabolically inert within the plaque flora.

Xylitol is usually found in a variety of fruits and vegetables. The absorption of xylitol is slow but better than sorbitol. Xylitol was developed in Finland and remained as a part of Finnish culture, for several generations. The normal 'sugar' acts as:

- It is used by bacteria for energy.
- Bacteria produce lactic acid as waste product.

- Acid so produced decreases the pH of oral cavity, leading to demineralization of enamel.
- Usually the salivary components restore back the pH to neutral within 30 minutes; however, sugar should be avoided during this period.

Xylitol on the other hand:

- Cannot be used by bacteria as energy source.
- It also inhibits bacterial growth (bacteria get starved in the presence of xylitol).
- It is used as chewing gum (the chewing process promote salivary secretions neutralizing the acidic pH).

A two years study was conducted to evaluate the uses of xylitol instead of sugar. The study was divided into three adult groups. One group consumed xylitol sweetened food, second group consumed fructose-sweetened food and a third group consumed the normal sucrose containing diet. The study observed practically no new lesions in Xylitol group, four lesions per person in fructose group and seven in sucrose group.

Another study was conducted in Turku. The participants chewed a daily average of 4 sticks of gum containing xylitol, in addition to a normal diet. Control group individuals chewed same amount of gum containing sucrose, in addition to a normal diet. After one year observation, 0.3 new DMF surfaces appeared in experimental individuals as compared to nearly four surfaces in the control group.

Schienen, et al (1985) carried out a study in Hungary in 11 children homes. Children in 5 homes were fed xylitol confectionary, 3 institutions were given fluorinated milk/water and rest constituted the control group. The study observed 43% caries reduction in children fed on xylitol and 26% in fluoride group.

The effects of xylitol can be summarized as:

- Various clinical trials have shown marked reduction in caries with xylitol.

- Animal studies have also shown anti-cariogenicity; however, this is debated because of increase in salivary flow, decreased plaque accumulation and other factors related with xylitol chewing.
- Xylitol stimulates salivation, thereby increasing plaque pH and promoting remineralization (can be described as non-cariogenic but not anticariogenic). A few authors have observed specific anticariogenic activity with use of xylitol.
- The high expense of xylitol may be inhibitory as regard to its common use.

b. Sorbitol

Sorbitol has been used as a hypoacidogenic food item considered 'safe for teeth'. This sugar alcohol is found naturally in many fruits, berries, seaweed and algae. It is usually prepared from glucose by electrolytical hydrogenation. The daily intake is recommended as 150 mg/kg/day.

It is hypothesized that mutans streptococci are capable of fermenting sorbitol to pH below 5.0; however, clinical trials have demonstrated that pH lowers to only non-cariogenic level.

Sorbitol is non-cariogenic and may reduce the caries incidence about 10–20%. Various studies have established that when diet containing sorbitol was fed to rats and monkeys, little caries developed in comparison with glucose and sucrose diets.

c. Hydrogenated Starch

The hydrogenation process is used to treat partially hydrolyzed starch from corn, wheat or potato starch to form hydrogenated starch hydrolysates. They serve as bulk sweeteners, crystallization modifiers, humectants and cryoprecipitates.

d. Non-caloric Sweeteners approved by FDA

The FDA has approved only five non-caloric sweeteners, viz. saccharin, aspartame, acesulfame K, sucralose and neotame.

i. Aspartame is extensively used in puddings, beverages and snack foods used for in-between meal. It is 180 times sweeter than sugar.
ii. Saccharin is used as a tabletop sweetener in liquid and tablet forms. It is 300 times sweeter than sugar.
iii. Acesulfame-K has also been used in different food items. It is 200 times sweeter than sugar.
iv. Sucralose (1, 4, 6, trideoxy trichloro-galacto-sucrose) has been studied for use as sweetener in beverages such as tea and coffee and showed non-cariogenic properties. It is established that sucralose is not fermentable and does not serve as a substrate for glucosyltransferase and fructosyltransferase. It is 600 times sweeter than sugar.
v. *Neotame:* It is 7000–13000 times sweeter than sugar.
vi. *Cyclamate:* Not used today because of its carcinogenic effect. In 2013 cyclamate was banned by Philippine Food and Drug Administration.
vii. *Stevia:* Low calorie sweetener, has not yet been evaluated by FDA. Manufactured from leaves of shrubs that grow in South and Central America. It is 300 times sweeter than sugar.
viii. *Advantame:* Advantame is new non-caloric sweetener from Japan's Ajinomoto Cooperation. The US Food and Drug Administration has approved for general use. The natural resources defense council object FDA's decision claiming that it significantly affect the proper function of hypothalamus.

e. Hydrogenated Glucose Syrup (lycasin)

It is fermented slowly as compared to sucrose and causes minimum decrease in plaque pH. Its cariogenicity is much less than sucrose when fed to rats.

f. Glucosylsucrose (coupling sugar)

This is used in a variety of foods, viz. candies, chocolate, cookies, jam and jelly. It is fermented by various micro-organisms; however, the acidogenicity is much less than glucose or sucrose. Thus its cariogenic potential is less.

g. *Isomaltose*

It is a mixture of two sugar alcohols. Various studies have suggested that it resulted in lower plaque accumulation than sucrose. Further, use of isomaltulose in between meals resulted in decrease in *Streptococcus mutans* in saliva.

h. *Maltitol*

It has been observed that substituting maltitol for sucrose resulted in decrease in caries. Further, streptococci do not use maltitol for acid production.

i. *Erythritol*

Erythritol is 70–80% as sweet as sucrose. A few authors have reported a lower incidence of caries in specific pathogen-free rats when fed with erythritol diet as compared to sucrose diet.

The cariogenicity of sugar components and other sweeteners is tabulated in Table 7.5.

Table 7.5: Cariogenicity of sugar components and other sweeteners

Sugar component/Sweetener	Cariogenicity
Sucrose	Very high
Glucose	High
Fructose	High
Lactose	Slight to moderate
Maltose	High
Sarbose	Slight
Xylitol	Nil
Sorbitol	Nil
Mannitol	Nil
Leucoisose	Slight to nil
Isomaltose	Slight to nil
Lacital	Slight to nil
Nystose	Slight to nil
Isomaltitol	Slight to nil
Hydrogenated starch	Slight to nil
Hydrolysate glucosyl	Slight to nil
Na saccharins	Slight inhibitory
Acesulfame K	Slight inhibitory
Aspartame	Nil
Stevia	Nil
Neotame	Nil
Advantame	Nil
Cyclamate	Nil
Sucralose	Nil

CHEWING GUM

It has been established that Sugar-free gums are non-cariogenic and when used after meals or snacks, may have anti-caries effect. However, sucrose containing gums are cariogenic.

Macpherson and Daves (1993) observed that after the plaque became acidic following exposure to sucrose solution, rate at which pH returned to normal was faster than when sugar-free gum was chewed. Lee and Schachtile (1992) showed that if plaque pH was decreased by exposure to retentive food rather than sucrose solution, then chewing gum was not effective in bringing down the plaque pH to normal level.

Schirrmeister JF, et al (2007) studied the effects of various forms of calcium when added to chewing gum on carious lesions. They concluded that use of chewing gum offered no additional benefit, even if chewing gum contained calcium compounds.

SOFT DRINKS

Soft drinks are popular beverages consumed in routine, especially by youngsters. It is a matter of concern that over-consumption of soft drinks may result in caries and even erosion. Sugar-containing soft drinks can be cariogenic and their low pH can cause erosion in teeth. pH of soft drinks and other beverages is given in Table 7.6. One glass of soft drink may contain 30–40 gm of sugar (602 bottle of soft drink is equal of 16 gm of sugar). Soft drinks contain phosphoric acid,

Table 7.6: pH of soft drinks and other popular beverages

Beverage	pH
Coca -Cola	
Classic	2.53
Diet	3.39
Cherry	2.53
Sprite	3.42
7-Up	
Regular	3.19
Diet	3.67
Pepsi	
Regular	2.49
Diet	3.05
Mountain Dew	
Regular	3.22
Diet	3.34
Orange Slice	3.12
Tea	
Iced tea	3.86
Lemon iced-tea	2.90
Diet lemon iced-tea	2.55
Raspberry iced tea	2.95

citric acid, etc. which can lower the pH to 2.4 or less. Acid enters the pits and rough surface of enamel and cause subsurface structure loss. However, the oral clearance is rapid and the pH change is transitory. National Health and Nutrition Examination has suggested an association between sugared beverages and caries. Non-nutritive sweeteners found in diet soft drinks may not be directly cariogenic because cariogenic bacteria cannot ferment aspartame, saccharine, acesulfame-K and sucralose to produce acids.

Jandt Klause D. (2006) observed that use of soft drinks and confectionary products, especially in younger people, are the main cause of caries. Author suggested new functional soft drink, which may exhibit substantially lower erosion effects than conventional cold drinks.

Bibliography

1. Aires CP, Del Bel Cury AA, Tenuta LM, Klein MI, Koo H, Duarte S and Cury JA. Effect of starch and sucrose on dental biofilm formation and on root dentin demineralization. Caries Res.: 2008;42:380–6.
2. Aires CP, Tabchoury CP, Del Bel Cury AA, Koo H and Cury JA. Effect of sucrose concentration on dental biofilm formed in situ and on enamel demineralization. Caries Res.: 2006;40:28–32.
3. Ali MS, Batley H and Ahmed F. Bodybuilding supplementation and tooth decay. Br Dent J. 2015, 219: 35–39.
4. Allison LM, Walker LA, Sanders BJ, Yang Z, Eckert G and Gregory RL. Effect of human milk and its components on *Streptococcus mutans* Biofilm Formation. J. ClinPediatr. Dent. 2015;39:255–61.
5. Alvarez JO and Navia JM. Nutritional status, tooth eruption and dental caries: a review. Am. J. Clin. Nutr.: 1989;49:417–26.
6. Amit A and Robin WE. Is the consumption of fruit cariogenic? J. Investig. Clin. Dent.: 2012;3:17–22.
7. Anderson CA, Curzon ME and van Loveren C. Sucrose and dental caries: a review of the evidence. Obes. Rev.: 2009;10:41–54.
8. Anderson RJ. Dental caries prevalence in relation to trace elements. Br. Dent. J.: 1966;120:271–5.
9. Bergel E, Gibbons L, Rasines MG, Luetich A and Belizan JM. Maternal calcium supplementation during pregnancy and dental caries of children at 12 years of age: follow-up of a randomized controlled trial. Acta. Obstet. Gynecol. Scand.: 2010;89:1396–1402.
10. Birkhed D. Sugar substitutes - one consequence of the Vipeholm study? Scand. J. Dent. Res.: 1989;976:126–9.
11. Bona AD and Nedel F. Evaluation of Melia azedarach Extracts against *Streptococcus mutans*. J. Med.Food. 2015;18:259–63.
12. Bowen H. The Stephan Curve revisited. Odontology: 2013;101:2–8.
13. Bowen WH and Lawrence RA. Comparison of the cariogenicity of cola, honey, cow milk, human milk and sucrose. Pediatrics: 2005; 116:921–6.
14. Bowen WH and Pearson SK. Effects of milk on cariogenesis. Caries Res.: 1993;27:461–6.
15. Bowen WH, Amsbaugh SM, Monell-Torrens S, Brunelle J, Kuzmiak-Jones H and Cle MF. A

method to assess cariogenic potential of foodstuffs. J. Am. Dent. Assoc.: 1980;100:677–81.

16. Bowen WH. Food components and caries. Advances in Dental Research 1994;8:215–20.

17. Bradshaw DJ and Lynch RJM. Diet and the microbial aetiology of dental caries: new paradigms. Int. Dent. J.: 2013;63:64–72.

18. Brighenti FL, Gaetti-Jardim E Jr, Danelon M, Evangelista GV and Delbem AC. Effect of Psidium cattleianum leaf extract on enamel demineralization and dental biofilm composition in situ. Arch. Oral Biol.: 2012;57:1034–40.

19. Burt BA, Eklund SA, Morgan KJ, Larkin FE, Guire KE and Brown LO. The effects of sugars intake and frequency of ingestion on dental caries increment in a three-year longitudinal study. J. Dent. Res.: 1988;67:1422–29.

20. Burt BA, Kolker JL, Sandretto AM, Yuan Y, Sohn W and Ismail AI. Dietary patterns related to caries in a low-income adult population. Caries Res.: 2006;40:478–80.

21. Burt BA, Satishchandra P. Sugar consumption and caries risk: A systematic review. J. Dent. Edu.: 2001;65:1017–23.

22. Burtter W. Trace elements and dental caries in experiments on animals. Caries Res.: 1969;3:1–13.

23. Chou KH and Bell LN. Caffeine content of prepackaged national-brand and private-label carbonated beverages. J. Food Sci.: 2007; 72:C337–42.

24. Cochrane NJ and Reynolds EC. Calcium Phospopeptides-Mechanism of Action and Evidence for Clinical Efficacy. Adv. Dent. Res.: 2012;24:41–47.

25. Coss KJ, Huq NL and Reynolds EC. Casein phosphopeptides in oral health-Chemistry and clinical applications. Curr. Pharm. Des.: 2007;13:793–800.

26. Crossner CG, Hase JC and Birkhed D. Oral sugar clearance in children compared with adults. Caries Res.: 1991;25:201–6.

27. Curzon NEJ and Crocker DC. Relationships of trace elements in human tooth enamel to dental caries. Arch. Oral Biol.: 1978;23:647–53.

28. Dennison BA. Fruit juice consumption by infants and children: a review. J. Am. Coll. Nutr.: 1996;15: 4–11.

29. Durso SC, Vieira LM, Cruz JN, Azevedo CS, Rodrigues PH and Simionato MR. Sucrose substitutes affect the cariogenic potential of Streptococcus mutans biofilms. Caries Res.: 2014; 48:214–22.

30. Edgar WM and Geddes DAM. Chewing gum and dental health: a review. Br. Dent. J.: 1990;168:173.

31. Fang MM, Lei KY and Kilgore LT. Effect of zinc deficiency on dental caries in rats. J. Nutr.: 1980;110:1032–36.

32. Fontana M and Gonzalez-Cabezas C. Are we ready for definitive clinical guidelines on Xylitol/polyol use? Adv. Dent. Res.: 2012; 24:123–128.

33. Gazzani G, Daglia M and Papetti A. Food components with anticaries activity. Current Opinion in Biotechnology: 2011;23:1–7.

34. Geddes DA. Diet patterns and caries. Adv. Dent. Res.: 1994;8:221–4.

35. Giacaman RA and Munoz-Sandoval C. Cariogenicity of different commercially available bovine milk types in a biofilm caries model. Pediatr. Dent.: 2014;36:1–6.

36. Giacaman RA, Campos P, Munoz-Sandoval C and Castrol RJ. Cariogenic potential of commercial sweeteners in an experimental biofilm caries model on enamel. Arch. Oral Biol.: 2013;58:1116–22.

37. Giacaman RA, Munoz MJ, Ccahuana-Vasquez RA, Munoz-Sandoval C and Cury JA. Effect of fluoridated milk on enamel and root dentin demineralization evaluated by a biofilm caries model. Caries Res.: 2012;46:460–6.

38. Graf H. Potential cariogenicity of low and high sucrose dietary patterns. J. Clin. Periodontol.: 1983;10:636–42.

39. Grant WB and Holick MF. Benefits and requirements of vitamin D for optimal health: a review. Altern. Med. Rev.: 2005;10:94–111.

40. Grenby TH. Summary of the dental effects of starch. International Journal of Food Sciences and Nutrition: 1997;48:411–6.

41. Gupta P, Gupta N, Pawar AP, Birajdar SS, Natt AS and Singh HP. Role of sugar and sugar substitutes in dental caries: a review. ISRN Dent.: 2013;1–5.

42. Gustafsson BE, Quensel CE, Swenander Lanke L, Lundqvist C, Grahnen H, Bonow BE and Krasse B. The Vipeholm Dental Caries Study. The effects of different levels of carbohydrate intake in 436 individuals observed for five years. Acta Odontol. Scand.: 1954;11:232–364.

43. Gustafsson BE. The Vipeholm Dental Caries Study. Survey on the literature on carbo-

hydrates and dental caries. Acta Odontol. Scand.: 1954;11: 207–31.

44. Harel-Raviv M, Laskaris M and Chu KS. Dental caries and sugar consumption into the 21st century. Am. J. Dent.: 1996;9:184–90.

45. Harris HH, Vogt S, Eastgate H and Lay PA. A link between copper and dental caries in human teeth identified by X-ray fluorescence elemental mapping. J. Biol. Inorg. Chem.: 2008;13:303–6.

46. Hartles RL and Leach SA). Effect of diet on dental caries. Br. Med Bull.: 1975;31:137–41.

47. Hecht S and Fridman J. High incidence of cervical dental caries among drug addicts. O. Med, O. Patholog. 1949;2:1428–42.

48. Herod EL: The effect of cheese on dental caries: a review of literature. Aust. Dent. J. 1991;36:120.

49. Holick MF. Vitamin D deficiency. N. Engl. J. Med.: 2007;357:266–81.

50. Holloway PJ, James PMC and Slack GL. Dental disease in Tristan da Cunha. Br. Dent. J.: 1963;115:19.

51. Ikeda T. Sugar substitutes: reasons and indications for their use. Int. Dent. J.: 1982;32:33–43.

52. Jenkins GN and Tatevossian A. Sucrose and the role of saccharates in enamel caries. Caries Res.: 1971;5:28.

53. Kashket S and DePaola DP. Cheese consumption and the development and progression of dental caries. Nutrition Reviews: 2002;60:97–103.

54. Kleinberg I. Oral effects of sugars and sweeteners. Int. Dent. J.: 1985;35:180–9.

55. Krasse B. The Vipeholm Dental Caries Study: Recollections and Reflections of 509 years later. J. Dent. Res.: 2001;80:1785.

56. Larsson B, Johansson I and Ericson T. Prevalence of caries in adolescents in relation to diet. Comm. Dent. Oral Epidemiol.: 1992;20:133–7.

57. Lee JG and Messer LB. Intake of sweet drinks and sweet treats versus reported and observed caries experience. Eur. Arch. Paediatr. Dent.: 2010;11:5–17.

58. Leitao TJ, Tenuta LM, Ishi G and Cury JA. Calcium binding to *Streptococcus mutans* grown in the presence or absence of sucrose. Braz. Oral Res.: 2012;26:100–5.

59. Lingstrom P, van Houte J and Kashket S. Food starches and dental caries. Crit. Rev. Oral Biol. Med.: 2000;11:366–80.

60. Lippert F and Hara AT. Strontium and Caries: A Long and Complicated Relationship. Caries Res.: 2013;47:34–49.

61. Lodi CS, Manarelli MM, Sassaki KT, Fraiz FC, Delbem AC and Martinhon CC. Evaluation of fermented milk containing probiotic on dental enamel and biofilm: in situ study. Arch. Oral Biol.: 2010;55:29–33.

62. Luoma H. Fluoride in sugar. Int. Dent. J.: 1985;35:43–9.

63. Maniken KK. The rocky road of xylitol to its clinical application. J. Dent. Res.: 2000;79:1352–5.

64. Marshall Day CD, Sedwick HJ. The fat-soluble vitamins and dental caries in children. The Journal of Nutrition 1934;309–28.

65. Marthaller TM. Changes in the prevalence of dental caries: how much can be attributed to changes in diet? Caries Res.: 1990;24:3–15.

66. Milgrom P, Soderling EM and Nelson S. Clinical evidence for polyol efficacy. Adv. Dent. Res.: 2012;24:112–6.

67. Mobley C, Marshall TA, Milgrom P and Coldwell SE. The contribution of dietary factors to dental caries and disparities in caries. Academic Pediatrics: 2009;9:410–4.

68. Moynihan PJ and Kelly SAM. Effect on caries of restricting sugars intake. J. Dent. Res.: 2013;93:8–18.

69. Munoz-Sandoval C, Munoz-Cifuentes MJ, Giacaman RA, Ccahuana-Vasquez RA and Cury JA. Effect of bovine milk on *Streptococcus mutans* biofilm cariogenic properties and enamel and dentin demineralization. Pediatr. Dent.: 2012; 34:197–201.

70. Newburn E. Sucrose in the dynamics of the carious process. Int. Dent. J.: 1982;32:13–23.

71. Paes Leme AF, Koo H, Bellato CM, Bedi G and Cury JA. The role of sucrose in cariogenic dentin biofilm formation-new insight. J. Dent. Res.: 2006;85:878–87.

72. Papas AS, Joshi A, Palmer CA, Giunta JL and Dwyer JT. Relationship of diet to root caries. Am. J. Clin. Nutr.: 1995;61:423–9.

73. Pearce E. Plaque minerals and dental caries. Nz. Dent. J.: 1998;94:12–15.

74. Pecharki GD, Cury JA, Paes Leme AF, Tabchoury CP, Del Bel Cury AA, Rosalen PL and Bowen WH. Effect of sucrose containing iron (II) on dental biofilm and enamel demineralization in situ. Caries Res.: 2005;39:123–9.

75. Petti S and Scully C Polyphenols, oral health and disease: a review. J. Dent.: 2009;37:413–23.

76. Psoter WJ, Reid BC and Katz RV. Malnutrition and Dental Caries: A Review of the Literature. Caries Res.: 2005;39:441–7.

77. Ribeiro CC, Ccahuana-Vasquez RA, Carmo CD, Alves CM, Leitao TJ, Vidotti LR and Cury JA. The effect of iron on *Streptococcus mutans* biofilm and on enamel demineralization. Braz. Oral Res.: 2012;26:300–5.

78. Ribeiro CC, Tabchoury CP, Del Bel Cury AA, Tenuta LM, Rosalen PL and Cury JA. Effect of starch on the cariogenic potential of sucrose. Br. J. Nutr.: 2005;94:44–50.

79. Sandhu KS, Gupta N, Gupta P, Arora V and Mehta N. Caries protective foods: A futurist perspective. Int. J. Adv. Health Sci.: 2014;1:21–25.

80. Scheinin A, Makinen KK and Ylitalo K. Turku sugar studies. V final report on the effect of sucrose, fructose and Xylitol diets on the caries incidence in man. Acta Odontol. Scand.: 1975;33: 1.

81. Scheinin A. Xylitol in relation to oral and general health. Int. Dent. J.: 1979;29:237.

82. Schroth RJ, Lavelle C, Tate R, Bruce S, Billings RJ and Moffatt ME. Prenatal vitamin D and dental caries in infants. Pediatrics, 2014, 133, e1277–e1284.

83. Schroth RJ, Levi JA, Sellers EA, Friel J, Kliewer E and Moffatt MEK. Vitamin D status of children with severe early childhood caries: a case-control study. BMC Pediatrics. 2013;13:174.

84. Sheiham A and James WPT). A reappraisal of the quantitative relationship between sugar intake and dental caries: the need for new criteria for developing goals for sugar intake. BMC Pub. Health: 2014;14:863–70.

85. Sheiham A. Sucrose and dental caries. Nutr. Health: 1987;5:25–9.

86. Shenkin JD, Heller KE, Warren JJ and Marshall TA. Soft drink consumption and caries risk in children and adolescents. Gen. Dent.: 2003;51:30–6.

87. Shetty P and Kumara S. Serum copper level in dental caries patients: a case control study. Asian J. Med. Cli. Sci.: 2012;1:142–3.

88. Southward K. A hypothetical role of vitamin K2 in the endocrine and exocrine aspects of dental caries. Medical Hypotheses. 2015;84:276–80.

89. Sreebny LM. The sugar-caries axis. Int. Dent. J.: 1982;32:1–12.

90. Steele JL, Martinez-Mier EA, Sanders BJ, Jones JE, Jackson RD, Soto-Rojas AE, Tomlin AM and Eckert GJ). Fluoride content of infant foods. Gen. Dent.: 2014;72–5.

91. Tank G and Storvick CA. Effect of Naturally Occurring Selenium and Vanadium on Dental Caries. J. Dent. Res.: 1960;39:473–88.

92. Tenuta LM, Del Bel Cury AA, Bortolin MC, Vogel GL and Cury JA. Ca, P and F in the fluid of biofilm formed under sucrose. J. Dent. Res.: 2006;85:834–8.

93. Thurnheer T, Giertsen E, Gmur R and Guggenheim B. Cariogenicity of soluble starch in oral *in vitro* biofilm and experimental rat caries studies: a comparison. J. Appl. Microbiol.: 2008; 105:829–36.

94. Trahan L. Xylitol: a review of its action on mutans streptococci and dental plaque—its clinical significance. Int. Dent. J.: 1995;45:77–92.

95. Urvi GJ, Acharya BS, Velasquez GM, Vance BJ, Tate RH and Quock RL. Survey of fluoride levels in vended water stations. Gen. Dent.: 2014;47–50.

96. van Palenstein W, Matee M, van der Hoeven J and Mikx F. Cariogenicity depends more on diet than the prevailing mutans Streptococcal Specie. Journal of Dental Research: 1996;75:535–45.

97. Wei SHY. Diet and dental caries. Asia Pacific J. Clin. Nutr.: 1995;4:45–50.

98. Weiss ME and Bibby BG. Effects of milk on enamel solubility. Arch. Oral Biol.: 1966;11:49–57.

99. Yabao RN, Duante CA, Velandria FV, Lucas M, Kassu A and Nakamori M. Prevalence of dental caries and sugar consumption among 6–12-year-old schoolchildren in La Trinidad, Benguet, Philippines. Eur. J. Clin. Nutr.: 2005;59:1429–38.

100. Yem CJ, Lin CL, Hu CC, Jang ML, Chen WK and Chou MY. Effect of trace elements on dental caries in human tooth. Chung Shan Med. J.: 1991;2:72–81.

101. Yem CJ, Lin CL, Hu CC, Jang ML, Chen WK and Chou MY. Effects of trace elements on dental caries in human tooth. Chung Shan Med. J.: 1991;2:72–81.

102. Zero DT. Sugars—The arch criminal? Caries Res.: 2004;38:277–85.

103. Zita AC, McDonald RE and Andrews AL. Dietary habits and the dental caries experience in 200 children. J. Dent. Res.: 1959; 38:860.

104. Zheng X, Cheng X, Wang L, Qiu W, Wang S, Zhou Y, Li M, Li Y, Cheng L, Li J, Zhou X and Xu X. Combinatorial effects of arginine and fluoride on oral bacteria. J Dent Res 2015; 94: 344–53.

8

Microbiology of Caries

The earlier theories of dental caries along with results of various research studies have established that the micro-organisms play a vital role in initiation and progression of caries. Human oral cavity is a factory-store of micro-organisms. Over 700 species of bacteria, amounting to a total of more than 10 lac crore, are usual inhabitants of oral cavity.

It is accepted that the tooth can develop caries only when it comes in contact with micro-organisms. Infective pericoronitis and deep periodontal pockets may induce micro-organisms onto un-erupted teeth leading to caries. One certain parameter to develop caries is infection (bacteria). Gnotobiotic animals with no oral microbiota did not develop caries even when fed cariogenic diet; however, the same produce extensive caries with a normal oral microbiota.

The essentiality of the microbial flora to the pathogenesis of caries is confirmed; however, the role of microbial agent(s) and/or their toxins are to be analyzed. The search for specific microbial agent for dental caries has initiated ever since chemico-parasitic theory of dental caries came into existence. Under normal conditions, the microbial flora in the oral cavity remain in equilibrium, wherein the chemical by-products of some microbes are utilized by other microbes for their growth. Furthermore, the metabolic activities of some bacteria can utilize oxygen, creating conditions that are favorable for the growth of those bacteria that require oxygen-free conditions.

This equilibrium may break in certain circumstances, especially after sugar intake that is readily used by bacteria. The pH in the adherent community is lowered, which favors predominance of acid-loving bacteria; mainly Streptococci and Lactobacilli species. These species can further reinforce acidic environment leading to dissolution of hard tissues, thereby caries.

Virulence (the ability of a bacterium to cause infection) is significant in the development of caries. The virulence should be effective so as to invade the host tissues and encourage bacterial colonization; subsequently damaging the tissues.

Koch's postulates regulate the virulence of micro-organisms which are effective to change the host tissues to pathological state. The postulates are:

1. The individuals should harbour the bacteria required for the particular disease.

2. The bacteria should be isolated from the diseased tissue of the infected person.

3. Pure culture, when inoculated into a susceptible individual/animal should produce the same disease.

4. Same bacteria should be re-isolated from intentionally infected individual/animals.

However, Koch's postulates do not depict the exact virulence because of inherent limitations such as:

- Virulence is within the bacterium.
- Culture may not be feasible in certain bacteria.
- The virulence factor may vary with members of the same family.
- Bacteria may affect humans and may not cause the same effect in animals and vice-versa.

Following guidelines were formulated as a guide for investigators to specify the bacterial species which is/are the chief causative agent in caries.

- The causative micro-organism should favor acidogenic environment.
- The organisms should be able to endure the acidity that it produced in the carious lesion.
- The organism must be isolated from all stages of the carious lesion and grown in pure cultures.
- The micro-organisms after culture must be able to produce caries when inoculated into the oral cavity.
- The causative organism should be absent from the saliva of caries-free individuals.
- The micro-organisms that produce sufficient acids to decalcify enamel and dentin must not be present during the carious process. If they are present, it must be proved that the acid so produced cannot initiate/propagate a carious lesion.

Researchers over the years kept identifying possible pathogens of human dental caries. Miller (1880) explaining dental caries could not specify definite micro-organisms causing caries. However, later, he emphasized that streptococci could be the causative agent. Oral streptococci were implicated in dental caries because of their abundance in oral cavity and selective presence in and around carious lesions.

Streptococci are approximately 1000 times more numerous than lactobacilli. They were equally abundant in the oral cavities of children and adults. Streptococci have been isolated in abundance from precarious/carious plaque on enamel than any other bacterial species.

ROLE OF PLAQUE IN DENTAL CARIES

- Plaque is an adhesive layer comprising colonies of bacteria which deposits on the surface of the tooth.
- Plaque tends to stick to the surface of the teeth, facilitating bacteria to have cariogenic effect.
- The quantity and quality of plaque is also responsible for the carious process.

The chief micro-organisms associated with dental caries are:

i. Streptococcus.
   - *Streptococcus mutans.*
   - *Streptococcus sobrinus.*
ii. Lactobacillus.
   - *L. casei.*
   - *L. fermentum.*
   - *L. plantarium.*
iii. Actinomyces.
   - *A. israeli.*
   - *A. naeslundii.*

Extended Caries Hypothesis

A few authors divided the caries process into three reversible stages, viz. dynamic stage, acidogenic stage and the aciduric stage. This process is known as extended caries hypothesis.

Dynamic Stage

Many micro-organisms collected on tooth surfaces can produce acids from sugary foods, subsequently demineralising the dental hard tissues. However, if the acid production is mild, homeostatic mechanisms in the plaque may easily restore the mineral balance. The net mineral gain in favor of teeth is 'remineralization'. This dynamic environment brings the microflora to a stage whereby bacteria and hard tissues remain in stable stage.

Acidogenic Stage

When sugar intake is frequent or salivary secretions are less effective, the decrease in pH becomes severe and frequent. This change in the environment may enhance the acidogenicity and acidurance adaptation of plaque bacteria. The biochemical mechanisms underlying the acid-induced adaptation may involve the following mechanisms:

- An increase in proton impermeability of the cell membrane.
- Induction of proton-translocating ATPase activity that expels proton from cells.
- Induction of the arginine deiminase system that produces alkali from arginine or arginine-containing peptides.
- Induction of stress proteins that protect enzymes and nucleic acids from acid denaturation.

Microbial acid-induced adaptation (phenotypic change of the microflora) as well as acid-induced selection (genotypic change of the microflora) will cause a shift in the acidogenic potential of the microflora; subsequently demineralization/remineralization balance is disturbed over an extended period of time leading to initiation/progression of dental caries.

Aciduric Stage

Acidic environment temporarily impairs bacterial growth ability and that the acid-impaired bacteria need a considerable time to recover their growth ability. The normal flora will be eliminated and replaced by more aciduric bacteria, such as mutans streptococci and lactobacilli leading to a net mineral loss and caries progression.

At the aciduric stage, acid-induced selection by acid-impairment and growth competition are the major reasons for the shift in the composition of the microflora. The basic biochemical reactions remain the same.

RELATION OF STREPTOCOCCI TO CARIES

Oral streptococci are considered as the main causative agents in carious process. The *Streptococcus mutans* have the maximum cariogenic potential and is described as follows:

Primary Acquisition and Transmission of *Streptococcus mutans*

The inoculation of the human oral cavity starts immediately after the tactile contact of child with the environment. The oral cavity of the toothless child contains only epithelial surfaces and the first colonizers are species, which do not require a non-shedding surface for their survival. Early colonizers include streptococci, Veillonella, Actinomyces, Fusobacterium and also a few gram-negative rods. Amongst them, *Streptococcus salivarius* mostly colonize the dorsum of the tongue. *Streptococcus sanguis* and the *Streptococcus mutans* are colonized only after the first tooth has erupted.

The acquisition of micro-organisms by the human body is by direct transmission from one host to another, or through some objects. Pathogens can also be transmitted by food and water. Saliva is regarded as the most important vehicle for transmission of mutans streptococci via physical contact. The mother is considered to be the most important source of infection for the child. The time period when children gain mutans streptococci in their oral flora is when the primary teeth are erupting, that is, between 6 months and 30 months of age. The probability of colonization with mutans streptococci is high when inoculation with mutans streptococci is frequent (the baby's diet includes frequent intake of refined carbohydrates).

Oral streptococci have the cariogenic potential and the feature which mainly relates to cariogenicity is that their rate of growth and acid production exceeds that of any other oral micro-organisms.

The other features supporting their role as cariogenic organisms are:

a. Rapid generation time as compared to other oral bacteria living in the same environment.

b. Acid producing qualities (terminal pH4), indicating high acidogenicity.

c. Ability to attain the critical pH required for enamel demineralization more rapidly than other oral bacteria.

d. Facilitate fermentation of carbohydrates available in human diet.

e. Facilitate plaque formation with the help of fermentable carbohydrates.

f. Ability to initiate and maintain microbial growth and also continue acid production at low pH.

g. Production of extracellular polysaccharides from sucrose.

h. Significantly correlates with progression of carious lesion.

i. Significantly correlates with incidence/prevalence of caries.

j. Effective in experimental caries in animals. (Immunization of animals with *Streptococcus mutans* significantly reduces incidence of caries.)

Classification of Oral Streptococci

Streptococci are gram-positive cocci, mostly arranged in chains. They form a part of human flora but some of them are held responsible to cause pyogenic infections and dental caries. Oral streptococci inhabit the oral cavity and upper respiratory tracts of humans and animals as commensals. These can cause opportunistic infections at oral or non-oral sites.

The genus streptococci are broadly divided into two groups, on the basis of oxygen requirements; Aerobes/facultative anaerobes and obligate anaerobes.

Further, facultative anaerobes are divided into three groups based on their hemolytic properties. Three types of hemolytic reactions are observed on blood agar medium. Out of three, hemolytic group comprises the viridans group. Earlier oral streptococci were thought to be a part of viridans group only. Soon biochemical and serological heterogeneity was reported amongst various species of oral streptococci and it was found that oral streptococci exhibited all the three hemolytic properties.

Conventionally, oral streptococci have been classified on the basis of:

I. Physiological characteristics.
II. Serological variables.
III. Biochemical testing.
IV. Genetic/molecular methods.

I. Physiological Characteristics

Various physiological attributes such as growth on gelation and its variations with temperature and pH have been evaluated to identify streptococci species.

Earlier authors could recognize seven species:

1. *S. salivarius.*
2. *S. mitis.*
3. *S. anginosus.*
4. *S. equinus.*
5. *S. pyogenes.*
6. *S. faecalis.*
7. *Pneumococci.*

Out of these seven, *S. salivarius* and *S. mitis,* were categorized as oral species.

A few authors divided streptococci into four groups following different physiological characteristics:

1. Pyogenic.
2. Viridans.
3. Lactic.
4. Enterococcus.

Classification based on physiological characteristics was not effective as many species shared similar characters but differed serologically and genetically. Thus, other parameters were investigated to aid in classification of oral streptococci.

II. Serological Variables

Oral streptococci have been divided on the basis of Lancefield serological antigens (A-V) and cell wall antigens (a-g).

Lancefield grouping was proved to be insignificant for streptococci. It was observed that physiologically heterogenous organisms could possess common Lancefield antigen, thus may have same serotype. Overlapping amongst these serotypes was recognized, making this classification ineffective.

III. Biochemical Testing

The application of biochemical tests has been widely used in identification and classification of streptococci.

The commonly used biochemical tests are:
a. Capability to produce acid from sugars.
b. Production of enzymes (glucosyltransferase, etc.).
c. Ability to hydrolyse esculine, etc.
d. Production of extracellular polysaccharides.

On the basis of biochemical characterization, various classifications were proposed. The accepted classification is given in Table 8.1.

Biotypes of *Streptococcus mutans* have also been classified on the basis of enzymatic activity (Table 8.2).

IV. Genetic/Molecular Methods

With advancements in technology, genetic make-up of the organisms has become the most accepted way of species categorization. Routinely used genetic methods of identification are:
a. Rapid quantitative DNA-DNA hybridization.
b. Ribotyping.
c. Polymerase chain reaction.
d. SDS-PAGE.

Table 8.1: Accepted classification on basis of biochemical characterization

Anginosus group (effective in purulent infections)	Mitis group (do not ferment sugar)	Mutans group (effective in caries)	Salivarius group (rare in infections, common in saliva)
S. anginosus	S. mitis	S. mutans	S. salivarius
S. constellatus	S. oralis	S. sobrinus	S. vestibularis
S. intermedius	S. sanguis	S. cricetus	S. thermophilus
	S. gordonii	S. rattus	
	S. parasanguis	S. downei	
	S. pneumoniae	S. macacae	
		S. ferus	

Table 8.2: Biotypes of *Streptococcus mutans*

	Valine aryl amidase	Acid phosphatase	α-galactosidase
Biotype 1	+	+	+
Biotype 2	+	+	−
Biotype 3	+	−	−
Biotype 4	+	−	+
Biotype 5	−	+	+
Biotype 6	−	+	−
Biotype 7	−	−	+
Biotype 8	−	−	−

Streptococcus mutans were divided into four genetic groups:

Genetic group	Strain	Antigenic group
Group I	10449, GS5	c
Group II	BHT, FA1	b
Group III	KIR, SL1	unknown
Group IV	E49	a

Common Characteristic Features of Species of Mutans Streptococci

   i. Alpha hemolytic or non-hemolytic on blood agar.
  ii. On sucrose containing agar, produce extracellular polysaccharides. Extracellular polysaccharides may be water soluble glucans and fructans or water insoluble glucan and fructans.
 iii. Appearance of colonies.
      • Colonies are frequently white, rough, heaped and detachable.
      • A drop of liquid (water soluble glucan) may appear on the top of the colonies.
  iv. Produce acid from a wide range of carbohydrates, viz. amygdalin, lactose, maltose, sorbitol, etc.
   v. Acid is not produced from starch, erythritol, etc.
  vi. Alkaline phosphatase and urease not produced.
 vii. Three polysaccharide antigen c, e, f present (k is also recognized).
viii. Cell wall peptidoglycan is Lysine-Alanine.

The various strains of *Streptococcus mutans*, their source, serotypes, sugar fermentation and antibiotic susceptibility is explained in Table 8.3.

Characteristic features of individual species of group mutans streptococci are:

a. *S. mutans*
   • Facultative anaerobe.
   • Gram-positive cocci in pairs and chains
   • Glucan produced from sucrose.
   • Mannitol, sorbitol, raffinose and inulin fermented.
   • Ammonia not produced from arginine
   • Polysaccharide antigen c, e, f, k.

b. *S. cricetus*
   • Isolated from hamster.
   • Rough and heaped colonies.
   • Reduced oxygen tension required for growth.
   • Mannitol, sorbitol, raffinose and inulin fermented.
   • Mostly non-hemolytic.
   • Polysaccharide antigen a.

c. *S. sobrinus*
   • Rough and irregular colonies (usually have a drop of liquid at the top or border).
   • Mostly non-hemolytic, some may be hemolytic.
   • Raffinose not fermented.
   • Ammonia not produced from arginine.
   • Hydrogen peroxide is produced.
   • Polysaccharide antigen d and g.

d. *S. rattus*
   • Originally isolated from rat (genus rattus).
   • Rough and heaped colonies due to production of glucans.
   • Glucan produced from sucrose.
   • Mannitol, sorbitol, raffinose, inulin fermented.
   • Polysaccharide antigen b.

e. *S. ferus*
   • Adherent and raised colonies with no liquid.
   • Mannitol, sorbitol are fermented; raffinose not fermented.
   • Ammonia not produced from arginine.
   • Water soluble liquid glucan is not produced.
   • Polysaccharide antigen c.

f. *S. macacae*
   • α-hemolytic strains.
   • White crumbly colonies.
   • Production of dextran on sucrose containing agar resulting in detachable colonies.
   • Polysaccharide antigen c.

Table 8.3: Strains of *Streptococcus mutans*, their source, serotypes, sugar fermentation and antibiotics susceptibility

Species	Source	Serotype	Aerobic growth	Hydrolysis of arginine	Raffinose	Melibiose	Production of H_2O_2	Bacitracin	Cell wall sugar
S. mutans	Human	c, e, f, k	+	-	+	+	-	-	Glucose, rhamnose
S. rattus	Rats	b	+	+	+	+	-	-	Galactose, rhamnose
S. cricetus	Rats	a	-	-	+	+	-	+	Glucose, galactose, rhamnose
S. sobrinus	Human	d, g	+	-	-	-	+	-	Glucose, galactose, rhamnose
S. ferus	Rats	c	-	-	-	-	-	+	Glucose, rhamnose
S. macacae	Monkey	c	-	-	+	-	-	+	Glucose, rhamnose
S. downei	Monkey	h	-	-	-	-	-	+	-

g. *S. downei*
- Large conical colonies, surrounded by white halo.
- Mannitol, melibiose are fermented; sorbitol, raffinose not fermented.
- Do not produce hydrogen peroxide.
- Not able to grow in the presence of bacitracin.
- Does not produce hydrogen peroxide.
- Ammonia not produced from arginine.
- Polysaccharide antigen h.

J Killian Clarke (1924) was the first microbiologist who identified mutans group as the causative agents for caries. Later various authors confirmed Clarke's views.

Strains of *Streptococcus mutans* (serotype c, e, f, k) and *Streptococcus sobrinus* (serotypes d, g) are the species most commonly found in humans, with serotype c strains being most frequently isolated followed by d and e. Recently serotype k is designated as the ninth serotype of mutans streptococci. Various studies have reported serotype distribution of *Streptococcus mutans* as serotype c (70–80%), serotype e (15–20%), serotype f being less than 5%. Serotype k is also less than 5%.

Pathogenicity and Virulence of Streptococcus Mutans

The term 'pathogenicity' refers to the features which determine the ability of a micro-organism to cause a disease. A few authors later modified the definition, adding significance of the immune system of the host. Accordingly 'pathogenicity' of a given micro-organism is expressed by the degree of damage caused by the micro-organism itself and also by the immune system in response to the pathogen. Pathogenicity is due to:
- Invasiveness (the ability to invade the host tissues).
- Toxin production (substances that damage and/or kill cells). (However, some bacteria and the viruses do not produce toxins, but kill/damage cells by their replication.)

'Virulence' on the other hand is the ability of micro-organism to cause infection; dependent on the degree of pathogenicity. The virulence of a micro-organism is determined by the following:
- Division rate.
- Quality and quantity of toxins produced.
- Speed of invasion.
- Body's resistance (immune system).
- Cellular features, such as motility, attachment, etc.

Usually two types of toxins are recognized:

- *Exotoxins* released by dividing bacterial cells; mainly produced by gram-positive bacteria.
- *Endotoxins* released after the death of bacterial cells; mainly produced by gram-negative bacteria.

The virulence factors of mutans streptococci are surface proteins, acid tolerance, acid production and production of glucosyltransferases, mutacin and intracellular polysaccharides. Certain other properties of the micro-organisms also influence virulence. *Streptococcus mutans* produce two extracellular proteases, possibly metalloproteases, capable of degrading both gelatine and collagen-like substrates. Whether these metalloproteases are produced by the micro-organism or not has not been properly documented. A few authors are of the view that the organism itself does not produce their protease. Many oral streptococci do produce sIgA protease, which impairs the host defence. Another important factor is the ability of mutans streptococci to rapidly adapt to the environment by microbial genetic phenomena (because of this property, *Streptococcus mutans* dominated in cariogenic dental plaque).

Following factors contribute to virulence characteristics of *Streptococcus mutans*:

   i. Adherences to tooth surfaces and other bacteria.

   ii. Rapidly metabolizing nutrients.

   iii. Acidogenicity and acid tolerance (aciduric).

   iv. Mutacin production.

I. Adherences to Tooth Surfaces and other Bacteria

Streptococcus mutans have the potential to convert sucrose to glucan and dextran. These streptococci produce large amounts of extracellular dextran, a glucose-containing polysaccharide. The cariogenic streptococci produced relatively large amount of glucose-containing polysaccharides, whereas the polysaccharides produced by the non-cariogenic strains were primarily of fructose-containing type. Cariogenic lactobacilli produce comparatively less polysaccharide containing both glucose and fructose.

It could not be established that levan producing *Streptococcus salivarius*, found in abundance (5×10^8/ml saliva) in saliva, has any role in progress of caries. *Streptococcus salivarius* has been observed to be cariogenic in some animal studies and not in humans. These bacteria are supposed to reinforce mucinous dental plaque formation. Gibbons and Banghart (1967), however, have reported strain of *Streptococcus salivarius* initiating caries in gnotobiotic rats, thus indicating that some levan producing streptococci do have a cariogenic potential.

The bacterial adhesion may modulate susceptibility and resistance to dental caries. Adhesion of *Streptococcus mutans* correlates with high caries experience, however, adhesion of *Actinomyces naeslundii* LY7 correlates with low caries index.

Streptococcus sanguis on the other hand also produces glucan, though it is less adherent than that of *Streptococcus mutans*. The cariogenic potential has been confirmed in animals and not in humans, though found in abundance in human plaque.

Another potentially pathogenic factor is the ability of micro-organisms to synthesize and degrade intracellular polysaccharides (function by which the organisms continue fermentation and produce acid in the absence of exogenous carbohydrate). The synthesis and degradation of intracellular polysaccharides may play an important role in the ability of various bacteria in initiation and progress of caries.

Bacterial proteins that help in adherence are:

- Antigen I/II family.
- Adhesin.
- Fimbrial adhesion.
- Glucan binding protein.

Initial attachment of *Streptococcus mutans* to tooth pellicle is mediated by antigen I/II (adhesin) and Glycosyl transferase (Gtf). Agglutinins present in saliva contribute to the process of *Streptococcus mutans* adhesion. Sucrose is broken down into fructose and glucose by glycosyltransferases. Fructose and glucose get metabolized, resulting in lactic acid formation, which accumulate over the surface. Glucose is stored as a glucan polymer (dextran). *Streptococcus mutans* adhere to glucans produced by other bacteria in plaque.

Additionally, other surface proteins having an affinity to glucan [glucan binding proteins (Gbps)] contribute to biofilm generation. Four types of glucan-binding proteins, viz. [Gbps A], Gbps B, Gbps C and Gbps D, differ in their affinity to glucan.

II. Rapidly Metabolizing Nutrients

Streptococcus mutans utilize dietary sucrose to enhance colonization of the oral cavity. The quantity of this organism in the oral cavity can be increased/reduced by increasing/decreasing the dietary intake of sucrose. *Streptococcus mutans* act on sucrose resulting in production of glucans/levans which results in plaque formation and also acids which results in demineralization of tooth structure.

Sucrose-6-glucosyltransferase dextran sucrase, an enzyme produced by *Streptococcus mutans* converts sucrose to dextran. Dextran has the property of causing clumping of bacteria producing their aggregates.

Oral micro-organisms derive nutrients from saliva and gingival crevicular fluid. Additionally, exogenous substrates are provided intermittently in the diet. Thus, there is enormous diversity in substrates available and in the metabolic activities of the organisms which colonize the oral cavity.

Carbohydrates get metabolized by multiple sugar metabolism (MSM) system present in bacterial cytoplasm. These get transported via the phosphoenolpyruvate (PEP), an important enzyme in this pathway. Fluorides inhibit the functioning of this enzyme (emphasizing the role of fluorides in caries prevention).

Glucosyltransferases (Gtfs) and fructosyltransferases (Ftfs) catalyse the synthesis of water-soluble and water-insoluble glucan and fructan polymers from sucrose. Streptococcal Gtfs have two common functional domains. The amino-terminal portion (catalytic domain) is responsible for the cleavage of sucrose and the carboxyl-terminal portion (glucan binding domain) is responsible for glucan binding. *Streptococcus mutans* produce one Ftf and three Gtfs. Gtf B is related to insoluble glucan synthesis, Gtf C related to soluble and insoluble glucan, whereas Streptococci sobrinus has four Gtf genes. Gtf D relates to soluble glucan synthesis. Out of four Gtfs, Gtf-I produces water-insoluble glucans, while the other three produce water-soluble glucans.

Mutans defective in either or both Gtf B and Gtf C genes required for insoluble glucan synthesis, exhibited reduced levels of smooth surface carious lesions.

Mutans defective in the Gtf D gene required for synthesizing water-soluble glucan also produced significantly fewer smooth surface lesions.

It is established that Gtf B and Gtf C are essential for extra polysaccharide (EPS) matrix formation; whereas Gtf B is mainly responsible for *Streptococcus mutans* aggregation.

III. Acidogenicity and Acid Tolerance (aciduric)

It is established that pH below 5.5 (critical pH) results in the dissolution of calcium phosphate (hydroxyapatite) of the tooth enamel. Promotion in the growth of aciduric bacteria, further lowers the pH and promotes progression of the carious lesion.

The mutans streptococci metabolize sucrose to lactic acid more rapidly than other oral bacteria. This might be related to the enzyme systems catalysing the metabolism of sucrose. These metabolic reactions render the dental plaque acidic and the mutans streptococci continue metabolisms even at low pH. It has been established that mutans streptococci are more acid tolerant than other oral bacteria, with the exception of *lactobacilli*. The property of acid tolerance (or acidurance) is related with the membrane's H^+ (proton) - translocating adenosine triphosphatase (ATPase) of these organisms.

Various hypothesis explain the survival of aciduric bacteria in acidic environment. The most accepted is the 'pump proton hypothesis'. According to this hypothesis when the pH outside the cell is lowered, an increased proportion of protons will enter into cytoplasm lowering the intracellular pH. *Streptococcus mutans* maintain the intracellular pH slightly higher the external pH by activating and driving the proton motive force across the membrane. It is maintained by proton extension via membrane associated adenosine triphosphatase (ATPase) and acid end product efflux. The activity of the ATPase increased fourfold to low pH. Summarizing, the events are:

- Extrusion of protons through cell membrane.
- Membrane ATPase hydrolyze ATP molecules.
- Hydrolysis of one ATP, results in extrusion of H^+.
- H^+ results in elevation of cytoplasmic pH.
- When pH decreases, ATPase activity increases four-folds.

IV. Mutacin Production

Many bacteria produce bacteriocins (an antibacterial peptide), which interfere with the growth of other micro-organisms. The genes involved in the synthesis and modification of bacteriocins are often carried by a plasmid. Bacteriocins are frequently named according to the bacterial species producing them, such as bacteriocin produced by mutans streptococci is called mutacin. Mutacin production is usually not plasmid encoded. If bacteriocin activity is plasmid encoded, it confers bacteriocin immunity to the micro-organism. It is documented that strains producing increased amounts of mutacin colonize more easily.

Typing of Mutans Streptococci

Typing of micro-organisms is performed to evaluate whether certain strains are associated with specific clinical disease conditions and also to characterize the heterogeneity of infection, i.e. whether subjects are colonized by one or multiple types of the micro-organism. Evaluation criteria for typing methods include typeability (ability to give an outcome for every isolate included), reproducibility (ability to give the same result when repeating the analysis) and discriminatory (ability to differentiate between unrelated strains).

Two types of typing systems routinely recognized are phenotyping and genotyping.

a. Phenotyping

The method relied on measurement of characteristics expressed by the micro-organisms, viz. bacteriocin production/sensitivity, serotyping and biotyping, etc.

i. Bacteriocin production/sensitivity

Bacteriocins are proteinaceous substances produced by the bacteria that inhibit the growth of other bacteria. The typing is performed by measuring the inhibitory effect on bacterial growth of certain indicator strains and by measuring the sensitivity of the bacteria to bacteriocins from other strains.

ii. Serotyping

A total of eight serotypes of *Streptococcus mutans* have been recognized. Serotyping by immunodiffusion, immunofluorescence or immunoelectrophoresis has been widely applied for typing of mutans streptococci.

iii. Biotyping

The mutans streptococci have been classified as 6 biotypes (I to VI) according to the ability to ferment four carbohydrates (mannitol, sorbitol, raffinose and melibiose) and to deaminate arginine.

Phenotyping is relatively inexpensive; the typeability of mutans streptococci isolates is high, however, reproducibility and discriminatory powers are poor.

b. Genotyping

These methods have a higher discriminatory ability and reproducibility since the DNA of the micro-organisms are studied under these methods. The methods are plasmid analysis, restrictive endonuclease analysis (REA), restrictive fragment length polymorphism (RFLP), pulsed field gel electrophoresis (PFGE) and arbitrarily primed polymerase chain reaction (AP-PCR).

i. *Plasmid analysis*

Plasmid analysis was the first DNA-based technique applied on mutans streptococci. Since plasmids are infrequently detected in mutans streptococci(only 5%), it is not preferred method in typing these bacteria.

ii. *Restrictive endonuclease analysis (REA)*

In restrictive endonuclease analysis (REA), bacterial chromosomal DNA is cut with a restriction endonuclease and separated by gel electrophoresis. The restriction endonucleases are enzymes that cut the DNA chain at specific recognition sequences. After separation by gel electrophoresis, gels are stained and detected under UV light. REA has been utilized for evaluation of mutans streptococci isolates.

iii. *Restrictive fragment length polymorphism (RFLP)*

The chromosomal DNA of the micro-organisms are separated and labeled with either DNA or RNA probes. In ribotyping an isolate, the fragments are hybridized with the rRNA probe. When detecting the hybrids, every fragment containing a ribosomal gene will be highlighted. The ribotyping of mutans streptococci has been applied mainly in studies on transmission of mutans streptococci.

iv. *Pulsed field gel electrophoresis (PFGE)*

In pulsed field gel electrophoresis (PFGE), the orientation of the electric field across the gel is changed periodically (pulsed), thus larger bacterial DNA fragments can be analyzed than by restrictive endonuclease analysis. PFGE is considered the best amongst molecular typing methods, with excellent discriminatory power and reproducibility; however, it has not been applied for typing of mutans streptococci.

v. *Arbitrarily primed polymerase chain reaction (AP-PCR)*

Arbitrarily primed polymerase chain reaction (AP-PCR) is the least laborious method of genotyping *Streptococcus mutans*. AP-PCR is accepted method of typing mutans streptococci. It can be performed with a very small sample volume. Amplification results in an array of DNA fragments, often termed random amplified polymorphic DNA (RAPD), that can be resolved by gel electrophoresis. This method requires no previous knowledge of the DNA to be analyzed.

Incubation of *Streptococcus mutans*

The accepted method of incubating *Streptococcus mutans* is: The inoculated tubes are placed in anaerobic incubator at 35°C for 48 hours. The air is to be removed by evacuating once to 50 mm Hg for 2 minutes and replaced with a gas mixture of 90% N_2–10% CO_2 ($\pm$ 5% N_2 and CO_2 respectively has also been documented in the literature). The oxygen concentration of the chamber is maintained at 0.0006% by successive evacuation. The anaerobic condition can also be created by using Gas Pack anaerobic system.

Under aerobic culture, *Streptococcus mutans* require complex amino acids for their growth, such as supplements of uracil, glutamic acid, glutamine, aspartic acid, etc. Certain amino acids like leucine, valine, or isoleucine inhibit the growth of mutans under the anaerobic atmosphere.

Isolation and Culture of Streptococcus mutans

For the isolation of *Streptococcus mutans*, several media have been developed. The selective media used for isolation of *Streptococcus mutans* along with the constituents are given in Table 8.4. The media used are:

i. Mitis Salivarius Agar

Mitis salivarius agar was earlier used medium for the isolation of Streptococcus sp, viz. *Streptococcus mitis*, *Streptococcus salivarius* and also enterococci. Advantage of mitis-salivarius agar is that it allows the isolation of the species even when present in low numbers relative to total population.

Soon it was modified as the MSB agar (mitis salivarius-bacitracin), which is frequently used for the isolation and count of total streptococci and *Streptococcus mutans*. Sucrose causes *Streptococcus mutans* to form colonies with a characteristic morphology which facilitates its identification, while the other microflora are suppressed by the high sucrose concentration. *Streptococcus salivarius*, which forms large colonies is inhibited by the bacitracin. Although it is considered a selective culture medium, *Streptococcus mutans* recovery in this medium is much slower than mitis salivarius agar. This medium inhibits the growth of serotype a streptococcus.

ii. MSKB (Mitis salivarius, sorbitol, kanamycin bacitracin)

The inhibitive effect of sorbitol on *S. mitis*, *S. anginosus* and Candida contributed to a higher selectivity of MSKB compared to MSB. However, the percentage recovery of *Streptococcus mutans* was reduced in this medium as compared to MSB medium.

iii. GSTB (Glucose, sucrose, tellurite, bacitracin)

The medium is inferior in sensitivity and selectivity as compared to TYCSB, even though it could yield greater recoveries of *Streptococcus mutans* and less of non-*Streptococcus mutans* than MSB.

iv. TYCBS (Tryptone, yeast, cystine agar with bacitracin and sucrose)

The medium achieves maximum concentration of the *Streptococcus mutans* while suppressing the growth of other micro-organisms. TYCBS is effective in recovery of mutans serotype c and sobrinus d/g. TYCBS is highly sensitive and selective for enumerating very low levels of *Streptococcus mutans*. Later TYS 20B was developed to overcome the laborious process

Media	Constituents per 1 liter of culture media
MSB	90 g mitis salivarius dehydrated agar; 1.0 ml 1.0% potassium tellurite, 20% w/v sucrose; 0.2U distilled water.
MSKB	90 g mitis salivarius dehydrated agar; 1.0 ml 1.0% potassium tellurite; 20% w/v sorbitol; 1.0 µgm kanamycin monosulfate; 0.1U/ml bacitracin distilled water
GSTB	5 g trypticase peptone; 5 g yeast extract, 5 g K_2HPO_4; 20 g granulated agar; 0.5 ml of a salt solution (mixed with 1.5 g $MgSO_4.7H_2$; 0.19 g $MnSO_4.H_2O$; 0.068 g $FeSO_4. H_2O$; 5% w/v D-glucose anhydrous; 5% w/v sucrose; 1.0 ml 1.0% potassium tellurite; 0.3U/ml bacitracin; distilled water)
TYCBS	0.2 g L-cystine HCl monohydrate;15 g bacto peptone; 5 g yeast extract; 0.1 g Na_2SO_3; 0.1 g NaCl; 1.0 g $Na_2HPO_4.7H_2O$; 2.0 g $NaHCO_3$; 20 g $C_2H_3O_2Na._3H_2O$ 20% w/v sucrose; 15 g granulated agar; 0.2 U/ml bacitracin; distilled water
TYS20B	30 g trypticase-soy broth; 10 g yeast extract, 11 g granulated agar; 20% w/v sucrose; 0.2 U/ml bacitracin; distilled water.

Table 8.4: Selective media for *Streptococcus mutans* and their constituents

and cost involved in the manufacture of TYCBS agar. But this media supports the greater number of non-*Streptococcus mutans* colonies.

RELATION OF LACTOBACILLUS TO CARIES

Earlier lactobacilli were believed to be the causative agent for dental caries, which remained accepted for many years.

The factors which supported the cariogenic potential of lactobacilli were:

- Isolated in high numbers from carious lesion.
- Number in plaque positively co-related with caries.
- Produced caries in germ-free rats.
- Induced low pH.
- Produced lactic acid at pH<5.
- Maintained growth at low pH.
- Capable of producing extracellular polysaccharides.

It was established that plaque of carious environment contained elevated levels of lactobacilli as compared with plaque from non-carious surfaces. A rise in lactobacilli count in the oral cavity preceded the onset of dental caries. However, lactobacilli as exclusive agent in caries development could not be authenticated.

Features which do not favor lactobacilli as the causative agent in caries are:

- Low affinity of lactobacilli for teeth.
- Colonize dorsum of tongue, vestibular mucosa and hard palate better than tooth surface.
- Initiation of caries in children even in the absence of lactobacilli.

The lactobacilli fail to qualify as the exclusive microbial agent for dental caries; however, they do reinforce caries progress since lactobacilli are acidogenic and more aciduric than any other oral microbiota.

Lactobacilli alone might not be able to readily localize and create dental plaque in gnotobiotic animals. They may preferentially accumulate along with streptococci assisting in caries process.

Human carious lesions are initiated predominantly in pits, fissures and inter-proximal spaces where plaque harbours cariogenic micro-organisms. Accumulation of lactobacilli in these areas may also be an important factor in development/progress of dental caries.

RELATION OF ACTINOMYCES TO CARIES

Actinomyces are gram-positive, rod shaped, facultative anaerobes. Actinomyces colonies form fungus like branched network of hyphae. Some species of actinomyces has been implicated in primary root caries, secondary enamel caries and periodontal disease.

Classification of Actinomyces

The genus actinomyces belongs to family Actinomycetaceae. The members of this genus are parasitic or at least common salistic in nature. Their presence is recognized in oral cavity, mainly around teeth and pharynx. Actinomyces are gram-positive pleomorphic rods. The oxygen requirement of Actinomyces species is as follows:

- *Actinomyces viscosus*—facultative anaerobe (may require extra carbon dioxide).
- *Actinomyces israeli*—anaerobic.
- *Actinomyces naeslundii*—facultative anaerobe
- *Actinomyces odontolyticus*—facultative anaerobe.
- *Actinomyces bovis*—anaerobic.

Actinomyces viscosus and *Actinomyces naeslundii* have been widely implicated in root caries lesions. The species were studied further utilizing DNA-DNA hybridization studies. Two genospecies (1 & 2) of *A. naeslundii* were identified. *A. naeslundii* serotype I was reclassified as *A. naeslundii* genospecies 1; whereas *A. naeslundii* serotype II and III were reclassified as *A. naeslundii* genospecies 2 (genospecies 2 is more prevalent in infected dentin than genospecies 1). A few authors, recently, reclassified *A. israeli* serotype II as

A. gerencseriae; A. israeli predominantly serotype I remained as A. israeli. Predominantly, serotype strains of A. gerenscseriae and A. israeli have been isolated from root caries lesions.

Incubation of Actinomyces

Earlier brain heart infusion agar with blood supports the growth of Actinomyces species.

The most accepted medium for the growth of Actinomyces strains in CFAT medium; the composition of which is as follows:

- Trypticase soy broth   30 gm
- Agar   15 gm
- Cadmium fluoride   13 mg
- Potassium tellviate   80 mg
- Basic fuschin   2.50 mg
- Defibrinated sheep blood   50 ml
- Glucose   5 gm

Almost all strains grow in this medium except two strains. The medium is effective both for *Actinomyces viscosus* and *Actinomyces naeslundi*.

MICRO-ORGANISMS AND CARIOUS SURFACES

It is established that the human plaque is a biofilm with numerous aerobic and anaerobic micro-organisms. The micro-organisms present in various carious surfaces are:

I. Micro-organisms in Pit and Fissure Caries

The following micro-organisms are most prevalent in pit and fissure caries:

- *Streptococcus mutans.*
- *Streptococcus sanguis.*
- *Lactobacilli.*
- *Actinomyces.*
  - The pit and fissure caries have the highest prevalence of micro-organisms.
  - The pits and fissures provide excellent mechanical shelters for micro-organisms.
  - The relative proportion of *Streptococcus mutans* determines the cariogenic potential.

- Complex communities dominated by filamentous bacteria such as those in gingival crevice, fail to develop in pit and fissure habitat.
- The appearance of *Streptococcus mutans* in pit and fissure is usually followed by caries.
- Sealing the pits and fissures just after tooth eruption may provide resistance to caries.

II. Micro-organisms in Smooth Surface Caries

The micro-organisms most prevalent in smooth surface caries are:

- *Streptococcus mutans.*
- *Streptococcus salivarius.*
  - The proximal enamel surfaces especially immediately gingival to the contact area are the most susceptible (relatively free from the effects of mastication, tongue movement and salivary flow, etc.) to plaque accumulation.
  - Plaque accumulation on these surfaces depends upon oral hygiene, configuration of interdental col, functional/masticatory movements of teeth, etc.
  - Rough surfaces (poor quality restoration or a structural defect) facilitate plaque accumulation and such plaque is also difficult to clean.
  - Proximal surfaces of young children are in crevicular spaces and are less favorable habitats for *Streptococcus mutans*.
  - Often the gingival aspect of the facial and lingual smooth enamel surface that is supragingival but gingival to the occlusogingival height of contour is neither rubbed by the bolus of food nor cleaned by the toothbrush. Presence of caries in these surfaces is usually indicative of a caries active individual.

III. Micro-organisms in Root Caries

The micro-organisms most prevalent in root caries are:

- Actinomyces spp. viz. *A. viscosus*, *A. odonto-lyticus*, *A. naeslundi*, *A. israeli*, *A. bovis*, *A. gerensceriae* (Actinomyces are the early colonized micro-organisms of root caries).
- Streptococci spp. viz. *S. mutans*, *S. sanguis*, *S. salivarius*.
- Other filamentous rods.

Caries originating on the root is alarming since:
- Comparatively rapid progression.
- Often asymptomatic.
- Rapid progress, close to pulp.
- Difficult to restore, especially in hidden areas.
  - The proximal root surfaces are usually concave especially near the cervical line and remain unaffected by the conventional oral hygiene procedures.
  - The cervical areas especially when exposed to the oral environment (as a result of gingival recession), favor initiation of caries.
  - The facial and lingual root surfaces (particularly near the cervical line) remain unaffected by oral hygiene measures.
  - Root caries is more common in older individuals because of decreased salivary flow and poor oral hygiene due to lowered digital dexterity and decreased self motivation.

IV. Micro-organisms in Subgingival Area

The subgingival areas mostly harbour the following micro-organisms:
- *Lactobacillus spp.*
- *Streptococcus mutans.*
- *Actinomyces naeslundii.*
- *Actinomyces viscosus.*
- Other filamentous rods.
  - Metabolites released from plaque penetrate the epithelial lining of the sulcus.
  - The capillaries dilate and become permeable resulting in the leakage of blood plasma into the tissue.

- Some metabolites have chemotactic properties that induce infiltration of WBC's into the region.
- The gingival inflammatory reaction results in release of plasma like fluid containing immunoglobulin, PMN's, albumins, etc. (These immunologic materials may change characteristics of the adjacent plaque by removing the susceptible organisms.).
- New niches then become available because of loss of some species and availability of new ones.

Microflora of Root Caries

Root caries or caries on the root surface are mostly seen on proximal surfaces as compared to the facial surfaces. Usually mandibular molars are involved followed by mandibular premolars and canines. Primary root caries occurs in the absence of a restoration while secondary root caries occurs adjacent to the pre-existing restoration. In countries where scaling and root planning are commonly performed leading to exposure of dentin, the root caries initiate from dentin rather than cementum. Gingival recession and mechanical injury to the periodontium also play a part in exposing root surface to demineralization.

Root caries are especially prevalent in the geriatric population due to several factors which include:
- Decreased salivary flow (xerostomia) may lead to an acidic environment, subsequently promoting demineralization of tooth surfaces.
- Diminished manual dexterity leading to poor oral hygiene.
- Chronic medical conditions; for example, diabetes (patients with diabetes are more susceptible to dental caries).

A variety of bacteria contribute to root surface caries. The stage of lesion is important, as it would correspond to the presence of different bacteria. A unique bacterial flora exists on the roots as compared to the crown.

Several studies have indicated that the oral microflora gets modified with advancing age, introducing non-oral bacterial species such as staphylococci and enterobacteria. This might be due to impairment of the immune system. It is established that the root surface is more vulnerable to the demineralization process than enamel because cementum begins to demineralize at pH 6.7, which is higher than the enamel's critical pH of 5.5. Various studies have confirmed the diversity of root caries microbiota. Among gram-positive isolates, actinomyces spp are present in abundance especially (*A. naeslundii*). Other micro-organisms present include *Streptococcus mutans, lactobacilli, Bifidobacterium, Veillonella* spp and also enterococci. A few authors have also reported staphylococci (mainly *S. haemolytism* and *S. hominis*) from active as well as arrested carious lesions; whereas *S. epidermidis* reported from active lesions only.

Streptococcus mutans and *Streptococcus sobrinus* were not associated with active carious lesions; whereas *Streptococcus sanguis* have been reported to be associated with arrested and active lesions both.

Recent studies have demonstrated the presence of *Bifidobacterium, Scardovia* and *Parascardovia* in initiating root caries along with *mutans streptococci, lactobacilli* and *yeasts*.

Earlier scientists could identify 20 different strains of gram-positive filamentous organisms (most common-Rothia dentocariosa) including Actinomyces strains. Other strains resembling Actinomyces were also detected. They opined that Actinomyces strains could be associated with root surface lesions.

Sumney, et al (1974) confirmed *Streptococcus mutans* as a significant component of the flora; however, Actinomyces were also recognized amongst the 11 strains identified.

Syed, et al (1975) analyzed bacterial flora of softened dentin, deep carious lesions and also of root surface plaque. They hypothesized that *Actinomyces viscosus* being in large numbers should be considered as the main cause of root surface caries. Analyzing quantitatively they opined that *Streptococcus mutans* can also be responsible for causing caries. Their studies identified a range of bacteria viz. Streptococci, Enterococci, Bifidobacterium, *Actinomyces odontolyticus* and Veillonella. Lactobacillus, however, was not identified.

Ellen, et al (1985) observed that root surfaces harbouring *Lactobacillus* and *Streptococcus mutans* in their plaque had an increased risk of developing root surface caries.

Brown, et al (1987) observed significantly higher numbers of *Streptococcus mutans* at the initial lesion sites. They further opined that successive bacterial flora harbour as the root surface lesions progressed. The comparisons of the caries-free with the carious root samples showed that the caries-free sites had significantly higher number of Actinomyces than did carious root lesions. This was not consistent with earlier studies, which placed emphasis on Actinomyces as a primary cause for root surface lesions.

A few authors observed significantly higher number of *Streptococcus mutans* associated with soft lesions. No significant difference was detected in caries-free and carious surfaces.

The correlation between presence of *Streptococcus mutans* and Lactobacillus and the increased risk of root surface caries was accepted by that time. However, a few studies confirmed the presence of *Streptococcus sanguis* in significantly higher proportions on sound roots than on carious surfaces (Emilson, et al. 1987).

Brailsford, et al (2001) found that aciduric bacteria (grow at 4.8 pH) comprised 21.6% of the total microflora in root surface caries. The dominant bacteria were Actinomyces and lactobacilli. The aciduric bacteria (dominant actinomyces) comprised 10.7% in clinically sound root surfaces. In individuals without root caries, the aciduric bacteria comprised only 1.4% of the total microflora of clinically sound root surfaces. The authors correlated low pH actinomyces with root caries.

Shen, et al (2002) in their study on ethnic Chinese observed the presence of predominant groups of organisms viz. *Streptococcus* spp., *Lactobacillus* spp., *Staphylococcus* spp. and *Actinomyces* spp.

The bacterial profile of root caries in elderly patients has also been analyzed in couple of studies. The authors observed the presence of mainly *Selenomonas* and *Veillonella*. The microbiota of caries free surfaces included *Fusobacterium nucleatum*, *Polymorphum*, *Leptotrichia*, etc. *Lactobacilli* were absent; however, *Actinomyces spp.* were conspicuous. The microbiota of the carious surfaces were dominated by *Actinomyces spp.*, *lactobacilli*, *Streptococcus mutans*, *Enterococcus faecalis*, etc. The bacterial profiles of carious samples might vary from subject-to-subject. Aas, et al (2008) in their study observed that high concentration of mutans streptococci may be present on tooth surfaces without lesion development and caries can develop in the absence of this species. They suggested that acidogenic and aciduric bacteria other than mutans streptococci, including 'low-pH'non-mutan streptococci and Actinomyces might be responsible for the initiation of caries.

A few authors, in their studies have observed that species other than *Actinomyces* and *Streptococcus mutans* may play a key role in initiation of root caries. No particular bacteria appeared to be consistently involved in the pathogenesis of root caries. There might not be any association between *Actinomyces* and root caries, which is in contrast to conclusions from earlier studies. Similarly, while certain reports have associated *Streptococcus mutans* with root caries, these studies have observed limited role. Conversely, *Lactobacillus* spp. were notably associated with most carious root samples. Subject-to-subject variation concerning the microbial etiology of root caries has been established.

Ellen, et al (1985) carried out longitudinal microbiological investigation of a hospitalized population of older adults with a high root surface caries risk. They observed percentage of total cultivable flora comprising the suspect pathogens was much lower than anticipated. *Streptococci*, *Actinomyces* and *Veillonellae* represented greater than 50% of the flora. The counts were very low, even in comparison where MSA was also used to enumerate *streptococci* in gingival margin plaque.

Percentages of *A. viscosus* and *A. naeslundii* were comparable with earlier studies; however, much lower for established root caries lesions. *Actinomyces viscosus* was certainly the most frequently isolated and often the most numerous of the microorganisms present; proportionally it was not higher in carious than in caries-free situation. It is interesting to note the high correlation between *S. mutans* and Lactobacillus counts; *Streptococcus mutans* has been reported to be at higher level, whereas lactobacilli have been conspicuously absent from most of the reports on the root caries microflora. Preza., et al (2009) and couple of other authors were of the view that along with *Actinomyces* and *Streptococcus mutans*, other micro-organisms, viz. *Fusobacterium nucleatum*, *Polymorphum*, *Gemella morbillorum* and *Candida spp.* were also responsible for root caries. They could not observe any association between Actinomyces and root caries which is in contrast to conclusions from earlier studies. They observed *Lactobacillus spp.* and *Pseudoramibacter alactolyticus* to be notably associated with carious root surfaces. They also confirmed the presence of subject-to-subject variation concerning the microbial etiology of root caries.

Differences between Sound and Carious Root Surfaces

In sound root surfaces, dental plaque contains a microbial ecosystem in which non-mutans bacteria (non-mutans Streptococci and Actinomyces) are the primary micro-organisms that help to maintain the stability of the tooth surface and keep the dynamic balance between demineralization and remineralization. However, in carious root surfaces, acid selection of low pH non-mutans bacteria aids in the demineralization of cementum. Once the acidic environment is established, mutans streptococci and other aciduric bacteria may promote lesion formation by sustaining the acidic environment.

Commonly encountered bacterial and fungal strains of root caries lesions are given in Table 8.5.

The inferences of studies are summarized as:

- Root surface lesions can be initial lesions or advanced lesions. In initial lesions, higher proportions of *Streptococcus mutans* have been observed.

Table 8.5: Commonly encountered bacterial and fungal strains of root carious lesions

I. Aerobic bacteria
1. *Gram-positive*
   a. Gram-positive cocci
   Streptococcus spp.
      i. *S. intermedius*
      ii. *S. miitis*
      iii. *S. oralis*
      iv. *S. salivarius*
      v. *S. sanguis*
      vi. *S. vestibularis*
   Staphylococcus spp.
      i. *S. aureus*
      ii. *S. caprae*
      iii. *S. capitis*
      iv. *S. epidermidis*
      v. *S. haemolyticus*
      vi. *S. hominis*
      vii. *S. saccharolyticus*
      viii. *S. simulans*
      ix. *S. warneri*
   Micrococcus spp.
2. *Gram-negative*
   a. Gram-negative cocci (Neisseriae spp)
      i. *N. falvescens*
      ii. *N. mucosa*
      iii. *N. sicca*
      iv. *N. subflava*
   b. Gram-negative rods
      i. *Haemophilus parainfluenzae*
      ii. *Escherichia coli* (facultative anaerobe)

II. Anaerobic bacteria
1. Gram-positive
   a. Gram-positive cocci
      i. *Peptococcus* spp.
      ii. *Peptostreptococcus* spp.
      iii. *Gemella morbillorum*
   b. Gram-positive rods
      i. *Actinomyces* spp.
      ii. *Bifidobacterium* spp.
      iii. *Lactobacillus* spp.
      iv. *Propionibacterium* spp.
2. Gram-negative
   a. Gram-negative cocci
      i. *Veillonella* spp.
   b. Gram-negative rods
      i. *Bacteroides caccae*

III. Fungal strains
   a. *Candida* spp.
      i. *C. albicans*
      ii. *C. lusitaniae*
      iii. *C. pelliculosa*
      iv. *C. pulcherrima*

- Earlier studies placed emphasis on Actinomyces; however, certain studies have shown that this might not be the primary cause of root surface lesions. The presence of both *Streptococcus mutans* and Lactobacilli are predictive of the development of root surface lesions.
- Marked variation has been observed between the microflora from superficial plaque and that of the underlying lesion. Lactobacilli and other gram-positive rods were significantly higher in the deeper lesions, suggesting that bacterial succession occurs during the development of lesions.
- It is also confirmed that where there is high loss of minerals, the bacteria flora is dominated by either (a) *Actinomyces naeslundii* or (b) a combination of *Strepto-*

coccus mutans and *Lactobacilli*. Where there is a lesser loss of minerals, the microflora becomes more complex and diverse and includes *Actinomyces* spp., *Streptococcus mutans*, *Streptococcus mitis*, *Veillonella* spp., *Lactobacilli* and gram-negative rods.

- It is important to note that while *Streptococcus mutans* and Lactobacilli are associated with carious roots, they are also present on sound root surfaces.
- The bacterial flora in carious samples are highly diversified and differ from individual to individual. It might not be possible to identify single causative agent of root caries.

Microflora of Secondary Caries

The caries around a restoration is termed secondary or recurrent caries. The caries may be present at the surface surrounding the restoration or extend underneath or along the margins.

In secondary caries, the bacteria from oral environment get access into anaerobic environment of lacuna along the tooth-restoration interface. The microleakage and the cracks at the margins of the restoration are the main factors for the ecological niche of micro-organisms. The bacterial fermenta-tion of dietary carbohydrates accumulated at the rough margins produce more acids. Mutans streptococci have been isolated in high numbers from the surface of recurrent caries; however, a more diverse microflora has been isolated from the deeper layers. Interestingly the type of restoration may influence the development of microflora and affect recurrent caries. For example, if amalgam is replaced by glass ionomer cement, the same may leach fluoride into the immediate environment and exert an anti-bacterial effect. The observed variations in the numbers and types of organisms present in the dentinal lesions, coupled with the relative scarcity of lactobacilli and mutans streptococci, raised the possibility that other, less acido-genic micro-organisms could be involved in the recurrent dentinal caries.

Organisms like *Streptococcus mutans*, *Streptococcus salivarius*, other streptococci, viz. *S. Sanguis*, *S. gordonii*, *S. Milleri*, *S. Oralis*, *S. mitis* and Actinomyces species, viz. *A. naeslundii*, *A. viscosus* and *A. israelii* are commonly encountered in secondary caries.

Actinomyces odontolyticus, *micrococcus* species and *Lactobacillus* species, viz. *L. casei* and *L. plantarum* caused acid production in sucrose broth by isolates from recurrent caries lesions. Mo, et al (2010) analyzed the microflora of secondary caries around Class I and Class II composite and amalgam fillings and observed micro-organisms, viz. Prevotella, Veillonella, Lactobacilli, Streptococci mutans and Neisseriae. Other micro-organisms such as *actinomyces*, *peptostreptococcus*, *fusobacterium* and *porphyromonas* and occasionally *capnocytophaga* were also isolated though less prevalent. The proportion of obligate anaerobes were much greater than that of facultative anaerobes. The filling materials do affect the flora of secondary caries. It is observed that the variety of microbes under composite fillings was much greater as compared to amalgam.

Lactobacilli were found in relatively low numbers in root caries, viz. *L. gasseri*, *L. fermentum* and *L. salivarius*. Among Gram-negative isolates, *Prevotella spp* were found to be predominant, viz. *P. nigrescens*, *P. denticola*, *P. buccae* and *P. oralis*. They were associated with active and arrested root carious lesions. *Selenomonas spp.* (*Selenomonal flueggei*, *Selenomonas noxia* and *Selenomonas sputigena*) were the second most prominent isolates among gram-negative bacteria. *Capnocyto-phaga spp* has also been isolated. *C. gingivalis* and *C. ochracae* have the potential to ferment a range of carbohydrates and can demineralize cementum and dentin.

Capnocytophaga and other gram-negative rods are able to degrade protein under acidic conditions and may be important factors in the breakdown of dentin. Campylobacter spp (*Campylobacter rectus*, *Campylobacter showae*) were found to be associated with active lesions. The microbiota on root surfaces usually resembles marginal plaque associated with gingivitis.

Microflora of Arrested Caries

An arrested dentinal lesion differs from an active lesion (Table 8.6) by its darker pigmentation, absence of visible bacteria within the tubule and impermeability to dyes and isotopes. Sarnat and Massler (1965) identified following three layers in an arrested lesion (Table 8.7).

a. A narrow surface layer, brown in color and leathery in consistency.

b. The widest layer in the lesion, dark brown in color and hard in consistency.

c. Sclerotic layer is very hard, white and often harder than normal dentin.

Occasionally bacteria may be present in the most superficial layer. The dense condensation at the surface forms a narrow, homogenous calcified border approximately 2.0–5.0 m in width. The main bulk of lesion consists of dark pigmented and hard dentin. There might be increase in the diameter of the tubules along with irregular shape and width. Almost all tubules in the area harbour bacteria. The bulk of bacterial masses fills the lumen and can be visible in decalcified sections. A bacteria-free zone of almost normal appearance corresponding to deep calcified layer lies below this layer. The deep sclerotic zone has the highly calcified contents of the tubules and normal-appearing intertubular areas. Most of the tubules show a wide peritubular zone. No bacteria are observed in either the sclerotic zone or the normal dentin below.

The arrested lesion characteristically shows higher degree of mineralization. The possible ways by which the minerals may get accumulated in these lesions can be:

i. The surface layer may get mineralized from the salivary source absorbing calcium and phosphate.

ii. Secondly, the minerals dissolved by bacterial acids in the upper layer get reprecipitated to form large crystals in the area just below. These altered cyrstals are less soluble than original apatite crystals.

Table 8.6: Active carious lesion in dentin

Zones	Intratubular	Peritubular		Intertubular	
		Inner	Outer	Inorganic	Organic
• Necrotic	Some tubules filled with bacteria	Absent	Present but faint	Almost entirely absent	Present
• Upper zone of decalcified layer	Lumen enlarged (Bacteria abundant)	Absent	Present only in part	Bacterial invasion Absent but not entirely	Bacterial invasion Present
• Deep zone of decalcified layer	Bacteria-free	Absent in parts	Present	Absent but not entirely	Present as in normal
• Sclerotic zone	Calcified	Present	Present	Present	Present
• Normal dentin	Calcified material present (Protoplasm)	As in normal	As in normal	As in normal	As in normal

Source: Sarnat and Massler (1965)

Table 8.7 Arrested carious lesion in dentin

| Zones | Intratubular | Peritubular | | Intertubular | |
		Inner	Outer	Inorganic	Organic
• Surface layer	Some bacteria	Absent	Calcified	Heavily mineralized	Mineralized
• Upper zone of pigmented layer	Bacteria and coalesced bacterial bodies inside enlarged lumen	Very thin	Present	Present (mineralized)	Present (mineralized)
• Deep zone of pigmented layer	Bacteria-free	Wider	Normal	Normal	Normal
• Transitional zone	No bacteria (some lumen calcified)	Normal	Normal	Normal	Normal
• Sclerotic dentin	Lumina filled with calcified material	Normal	Normal	Normal to hyper-mineralized	Normal to hyper-mineralized

iii. Thirdly, sclerosis by intratubular calcification and obliteration of tubules of deeper layers underneath the lesion. Probably the minerals are mediated by odontoblastic processes through blood supply.

The characteristic change in bacterial morphology is observed in arrested lesions. In these lesions, the bacteria get coalesced into homogenous masses, showing signs of degeneration and disintegration. The bacteria present in the arrested lesion are degenerated and non-viable. The lesion shows deep pigmentation. The degenerated bacteria or the degradation products of their proteins and nucleic acids are the possible source of pigmentation. Bacteria are rarely observed in the deeper layers of arrested lesion. Schupback, et al (1992) in their histopathological study of arrested lesion described three zones, viz.

i. Formation of inner barrier as a result of tubular sclerosis in the area between carious and sound dentin.

ii. Formation of an outer barrier by a compact highly mineralized surface.

iii. An area of mineralization extending from the outer barrier towards the root canal in the demineralized dentin.

The microbiological aspects of caries process is summarized as:

• Caries is a worldwide disease with multiple etiology.

• Caries initiation and progression is dependent on the host diet and the ability of the oral flora to metabolize nutrients. Fermentation of carbohydrates leads to acid production, which further decreases the pH of the oral cavity and ultimately promotes tooth decay via demineralization of the enamel.

• The composition of the oral microflora has a significant impact on the progression of caries, often associated with *Streptococcus mutans*. Three of the most characterized virulence properties exhibited by this organism are: adhesion, acidogenicity and aciduricity. The organism has the property of acid tolerance.

• *Streptococcus mutans* can alter the rate of metabolic activity by lowering the pH, which is required for glycolysis in an acidified environment. Certain uncharac-terized genes involved in metabolic processes are also organized under acidic environment.

- *Streptococcus mutans* maintains an alkaline intracellular compartment by altering the composition of its cell membrane and also end product efflux via lactic acid, increasing the expression of proton pumps.

- The cellular DNA repair occurs through actions of a RecA-dependent and RecA-independent pathway, the latter of which utilizes uvrA and an apurinic-apyrimidinic endonuclease. All these proteins are regulated under acidic conditions.

- Increased expression of lactoylglutathione lyase effectively detoxifies methyglyoxal (an end product of glycolysis). An enzyme (pdhA) involved in pyruvate metabolism is also regulated.

- Biofilm organisms exhibit increased acid-tolerant characteristics when compared with their planktonic counterparts. Cell density is monitored via quorum sensing, which utilized a two-component regulatory system. The deletion of these regulatory systems results in acid-sensitive pheno-types and decreased cariogenic potential.

Bibliography

1. Aas JA, Griffen AL, Dardis SR, Lee Am, Leys EJ, Olsen I, Paster BJ and Dewhirst FE. Bacteria of dental caries in primary and permanent teeth in children and young adults. J. Clin. Mircobiol.: 2008;46:1407–17.

2. Aas JA, Paster BJ, Stokes LN, Olsen I and Dewhirst FE. Defining the normal bacterial flora of the oral cavity. J. Clin. Microbiol.: 2005;43:5721–32.

3. Ahn SJ, Wen ZT, Brady LJ and Burne RA. Characteristics of biofilm formation by *Streptococcus mutans* in the presence of saliva. Infect. Immun.: 2008;76:4259–68.

4. Ahn SZ and Burne RA. Effects of oxygen on biofilm formation and the AtlA autolysin of *Streptococcus mutans*. J. Bacteriol.: 2007;189:6293–302.

5. Aires CP, Del Bel Cury AA, Tenuta LM, Klein MI, Koo H, Duarte S and Cury JA. Effect of starch and sucrose on dental biofilm formation and on root dentin demineralization. Caries Res.: 2008;42:380–6.

6. Alam S, Brailsford SR, Whiley RA and Beighton D. PCR-based methods for genotyping viridians groups streptococci. J. Clin. Microbiol.: 1999;37:2772–6.

7. Alvares O. A mixed-bacteria ecological approach to understanding the role of the oral bacteria in dental caries causation: An alternative to *Streptococcus mutans* and the specific-plaque hypothesis. Crit. Rev. Oral Biol. Med.: 2002;13:108–25.

8. Arif N, Sheehy EC, Do T and Beighton D. Diversity of Veillonella spp. From sound and carious sites in children. J. Dent. Res.: 2008;87:278–82.

9. Arirachakaran P, Benjavongkulchai E, Luengpailin S, Ajdic D and Banas JA. Manganese affects *Streptococcus mutans* virulence gene expression. Caries Res.: 2007;41:503–11.

10. Arthur RA, Cury AA, Graner RO, Rosalen PL, Vale GC, Pes Leme AF, Cury JA and Tabchoury CP. Genotypic and phenotypic analysis of *S. mutans* isolated from dental biofilms formed *in vivo* under high cariogenic conditions. Braz. Dent. J.: 2011;22:267–74.

11. Arthur RA, Waeiss RA, Hara AT, Lippert F, Eckert GJ and Zero DT. A defined-multispecies microbial model for studying enamel caries development. Caries Res.: 2013;47:318–24.

12. Azevedo MS, van der Sande FH, Romano AR and Cenci MS. Microcosm biofilms originating from children with different caries experience have similar cariogenicity under successive sucrose challenges. Caries Res.: 2011;45:510–7.

13. Badet C and Thebaud NB. Ecology of lactobacilli in the oral cavity:A review of literature. The Open Microbiology Journal: 2008;2:38–48.

14. Banas JA. Virulence properties of *Streptococcus mutans*. Front. Biosci.: 2004;9:1267–77.

15. Bayrak S, Okte Z and Fidanci UR. Relationship between caries and dental plaque composition. Am. J. Dent.: 2011;245:45–8.

16. Becker MR, Paster BJ, Leys EJ, Moeschberger ML, Kenyon SG, Galvin JL and Bosches SK. Molecular analysis of bacterial species associated with childhood caries. J. Clin. Microbiol.: 2002;40:1001–9.

17. Beighton D. A simplified procedure for estimating the level of *Streptococcus mutans* in the mouth. Br. Dent. J.: 1986;160:329–30.

18. Beighton D. Can the ecology of the dental biofilm be beneficially altered? Adv. Dent. Res.: 2009;21:69–73.

19. Beighton D. The complex oral microflora of high-risk individuals and groups and its role in the caries process. Community Dent. Oral Epidemiol.: 2005;33:248–55.

20. Belda-Ferre P, Alcaraz LD, Cabera-Rubio R, Romero H, Simon-Soro A, Pignatelli M and Mira A. The oral metagenome in health and disease. ISME J.: 2011;6:46–56.

21. Berkowitz RJ and Jones P. Mouth-to-mouth transmission of the bacterium *Streptococcus mutans* between mother and child. Arch. Oral Biol.: 1985;30:377–9.

22. Biradar B and Devi P. Quorum sensing in plaque biofilms: challenges and future prospects. J. Contemp. Dent. Pract 2011, 12; 479–85.

23. Botha SJ, Boy SC, Botha FS and Senekal R. Lactobacillus species associated with active caries lesions. J. Dent. Assoc. S.Afr.: 1998;53:3–6.

24. Boue D, Armau E and Tiraby G. A bacteriological study of rampant caries in children. J. Dent. Res.: 1987;66:23–8.

25. Bowden GHW, Nolette N, Ryding H and Cleghorn BM. The Diversity and distribution of the predominant ribotypes of *Actinomyces naeslundii* genospecies 1 and 2 in samples from enamel and from healthy and carious root surfaces of teeth. J. Dent. Res.: 1999;78:1800–9.

26. Bowen WH and Koo H. Biology of *Streptococcus mutans*-derived glycosyltransferases: role in extracellular matrix formation of cariogenic biofilms. Caries Res.: 2011;45:69–86.

27. Bradshaw DJ and Lynch RJ. Diet and the microbial aetiology of dental caries: new paradigms. Int. Dent.J.: 2013;2:64–72.

28. Bradshaw DJ, Mckee AS and Marsh PD. Effects of carbohydrate pulses and pH on population shifts within oral microbial communities *in vitro*. J. Dent. Res.: 1989;68:1298–1302.

29. Brailsford SR, Lynch E and Beighton D. The isolation of *Actinomyces naeslundii* from sound root surfaces and root carious lesions. Caries Res.: 1998;32:100–6.

30. Brailsford SR, Shah B, Simons D, Gilbert S, Adams SE, Clarke B, Allison C, Ines I and Beighton D. The predominant aciduric microflora of root caries lesions. J. Dent. Res.: 2001; 80:1828–33.

31. Brailsford SR, Tregaskis RB, Leftwich HS and Beighton D. The predominant Actinomyces spp. Isolated from infected dentin of active root caries lesions. J. Dent. Res.: 1999;78:1525–34.

32. Brambilla E, Cagetti EG, Belluomo G, Fadini L and Garcia-Godoy F. Effects of sonic energy on monospecific biofilms of cariogenic microorganisms. Am. J. Dent.: 2006;19:3–6.

33. Buchen L. Microbiology: the new germ theory. Nature: 2010;4678:492–5.

34. Burne RA. Oral streptococci. Products of their environment. J. Dent. Res.: 1998;77:445–52.

35. Byun R, Nadkarni MA, Chhour KL, Martin FE, Jacques NA and Hunter N. Quantitative analysis of diverse Lactobacillus species present in advanced dental caries. J. Clin. Microbiol.: 2004;42:3128–36.

36. Caufield PW, Cutter GR and Dasanayake AP. Initial acquision of mutans streptococci by infants : evidence for a discrete window of infectivity. J. Dent. Res.: 1993;72:37–45.

37. Caufield PW, Li Y, Dasanayke A and Saxena D. Diversity of lactobacilli in the oral cavities of young women with dental caries. Caries Res.: 2007;41:2–8.

38. Caufield PW, Schon CN, Saraithong P, Li Y and Argimon S. Oral lactobacilli and dental caries: A model for niche adaptation in humans. J Dent Res 2015; 94: 110S–118S.

39. Caufield WP, Li y, Dasanayoke A, S Axena D. Diversity of Lactobacilli in the oral cavities of young women with dental caries. Caries Res.: 2007;41:2–8.

40. Chhour KL, Nadkarni MA, Byun R, Martin FE, Jacques NA and Hunter N. Molecular analysis of microbial diversity in advanced caries J. Clin. Microbiol.: 2005;43:843–9.

41. Chu CH, Mei L, Seneviratne CJ and Lo EC. Effects of silver diamine fluoride on dentin carious lesions induced by *Streptococcus mutans* and *Actinomyces naeslundii* biofilms. Int. J. Paediatr. Dent.: 2012;22:2–10.

42. Claesson MJ, van Sinderen D and O'Toole PW. Lactobacillus phylogenomics—towards a reclassification of the genus. Int. J. Syst. Evol. Microbiol.: 2008;58:2945–54.

43. Clarke JK. On the bacterial factor in the aetiology of dental caries. Br. J. Exp. Pathol.: 1924;5:141–7.

44. Clarridge III JE and Zhang Q. Genotypic diversity of Actinomyces species: Phenotype, source and disease correlation among Genospecies. J. Clin. Microbiol.: 2002;40:3442–8.

45. Colby SM and Russell RR. Sugar metabolism by mutans streptococci. Soc. Appl. Bacteriol. Symp. Ser.: 1997;26:S80–88.

46. Colby SM, McLaughlin RE, Ferretti JJ and Russell RRB. Effect of inactivation of gtf genes on adherence of Streptococci downei. Oral Miucrobiol. Immunol.: 1999;14:27–32.

47. Corby PM, Lyons-Weilder J, Bretz WA, Hart TC, Aas JA, Boumenna T, Goss J, Corby AL, Junior HM, Weyant RJ and Paster BJ). Microbial risk indicators of early childhood caries. J. Clin. Microbiol.: 2005;43:5753–9.

48. Dashper SG and Reynolds EC. Effects of organic acid anions on growth, glycolysis and intracellular pH of oral streptococci. J. Dent. Rews.: 2000;79:90–6.

49. Dashper SG and Reynolds EC. Lactic acid excretion by Streptococcus mutans. Microbiology: 1996;142:33–39.

50. Davey ME and O'toole GA. Microbial biofilms: from ecology to molecular genetics. Microbiol. Mol. Biol. Rev.: 2000;64:847–67.

51. de Soet JJ, Nyvad B and Kilian M. Strain-related acid production by oral streptococci. Caries. Res.: 2000;34:486–90.

52. de Soet JJ, van Dalen PJ, Pavicic MJand de Graff J. Enumeration of mutans streptococci in clinical samples by using monoclonal antibodies. J. Clin. Microbiol.: 1990;8:2467–72.

53. de Soet JJ, van Loveren C, lammens AJ, Pavicic MJ, Homburg CH, ten Cate JM and de Graaff J. Differences in cariogenicity between fresh isolates of Streptococcus sobrinus and Streptococcus mutans. Caries Res.: 1991;25:116–22.

54. Dewhrist FE, Chen T, Izard J, Paster BJ, Tanner AC, Yu WH, Lakshmanan A and Wade WG. The human oral microbiome. J. Bacteriol.: 2010;192:5002–17.

55. Dige I, Raarup MK, Nyengaard JR, Kilian M and Nyvad B. Actinomyces in initial dental biofilm formation. Microbiology: 2009;155:2116–26.

56. Dorita P, Olsen I, Aas JA, Willumsen T, Grinde B and Paster BJ. Bacterial profiles of root caries in elderly patients. J. Clin. Micro.: 2008;46:2015–21.

57. Douglass JM, Li Y and Tinanoff N. Association of mutans streptococci between caregivers and their children. Pediatr. Dent.: 2008;30:375–87.

58. Durso SC, Vieira LM, Cruz JN, Azevedo CS, Rodrigues PH and Simionato MR. Sucrose substitutes affect the cariogenic potential of Streptococcus mutans biofilms. Caries Res.: 2014;48:214–22.

59. Edwardsson S. Bacteriological studies on deep areas of carious dentin. Odontol. Revy. Suppl.: 1974;32:1–143.

60. Ellen RP, Banting DW and Fillery ED. Streptococcus mutans and Lactobacillus detection in the assessment of dental root surface caries risk. J. Dent Res: 1985a; 64: 1245–49.

61. Ellen RP, Banting DW and Fillery ED. Longitudinal microbiological investigation of a hospitalized population of older adults with a high root surface caries risk. J. Dent Res: 1985b; 64: 1377–81.

62. Facklam R. What happened to the streptococci: overview of taxonomic and nomenclature changes. Clin. Microbiol. Rev.: 2002;15:613–630.

63. Falkow S. Molecular Koch's postulates applied to bacterial pathogenicity- a personal re-collection 15 years later. Nat. Rev. Microbiol.: 2004;2:67–72.

64. Falsetta ML, Klein MI, Colonne PM, Scott-Anne K, Gregoire S, Pai CH. Gonzalez M, Watson G, Krysan DJ, Bowen WH and Koo H. Symbiotic relationship between Streptococcus mutans and Candida albicans synergizes the virulence of plaque-biofilms in vivo. Infect. Immun. 2014; 82:1968–81.

65. Fejerskov O, Nyvad B and Larsen MJ. Human experimental caries models: Intra-oral environmental variability. Adv. Dent. Res.: 1994;8:134–43.

66. Florio FM, Klein MI, Pereira AC and Goncalves RB. Time of initial acquisition of mutans streptococci by human infants. J. Clin. Pediatr. Dent.: 2004;28:303–8.

67. Forssten SD, Bjorklund M and Ouwehand AC. Streptococcus mutans, caries and simulation models. Nutrients: 2010;2:290–8.

68. Georgios a, Vassiliki T and Sotirios K. Acidogenicity and acidurance of dental plaque and saliva sediment from adults in relation to caries activity and chlorhexidine exposure. Journal of Oral Microbiology. 2015, 7: 26197-http://dx.doi.org/10.3402/jom.v7.26197

69. Giacaman RA, Araneda E and Padilla C. Association between biofilm-forming isolates of mutans streptococci and caries experience in adults. Arch. Oral Biol.: 2010;55:550–4.

70. Gibbons RJ. Bacterial adhesion to oral tissues: a model for infectious diseases. J. Dent. Res.: 1989;68:750–60.

71. Goadby KW. Micro-organisms in dental caries. Dental Cosmos: 1900;42:201–6.

72. Gold OG, Jordan HV and Van Houte J. A selective medium for *Streptococcus mutans*. Arch. Oral Biol.: 1973;18:1357–64.

73. Gonzalez-Cabezas C Li Y, Gregory RL and Stookey GK. Distribution of cariogenic bacteria in carious lesions around tooth-colored restorations. Am. J. Dent.: 2002;15:248–51.

74. Guggenheim B. Extracellular polysaccharides and microbial plaque. Int. Dent. J.: 1970;20:657–78.

75. Hall V, Talbot PR, Stubbs SL and Duerden BI. Identification in clinical isolates of actinomyces species by amplified 16S ribosomal DNA restriction analysis. J. Clin. Micro.: 2001;39:3555–62.

76. Hamada S and Salde HD. Biology, immunology and cariogenicity of *Streptococcus mutans*. Microbiol. Rev.: 1980;44:331–84.

77. Hardie JM. The microbiology of dental caries. Dent. Update: 1982;9:199–200, 202–4, 206–8.

78. Haukioja A, Soderling E and Tenovuo J. Acid production from sugars and sugar alcohols by probiotic lactobacilli and bifidobacteia *in vivo*. Caries Res.: 2008;42:449–53.

79. Haukioja A, Yli-Knuuttila V, Loimaranta K, unwehand AC, Meurman JH and Tenovuo J. Oral adhesion and survival of probiotic and other lactobacilli and bifidobacteria *in vitro*. Oral Microbiol. Immunol.: 2006;21:326–32.

80. Hoshino E. Predominant obligate anaerobes in human carious dentin. J. Dent. Res.:1985;64: 1195–8.

81. Hwang G, Marsh G, Gao L, Waugh R and Koo H. Binding force dynamics of *Streptococcus mutans* glucosyltransferase B to *Candida albicans*. J Dent Res 2015;94:1310–7.

82. Igarash T, Yamamoto A and Goto N. PCR for detection and identification of *Streptococcus sobrinus*. J. Med. Microbiol.: 2000;49:1069–74.

83. Inaba T, Ichihara T, Yawata Y, Toyofuku M, Uchiyama H and Nomura N. Three-dimensional visualization of mixed species biofilm formation together with its substratum. Microbiol. Immunol.: 2013;57:589–93.

84. Jakubovics NS, Yassin SA and Rickard AH. Community interactions of oral streptococci. Adv. Appl. Microbiol.: 2014;87:43–110.

85. Joen JG, Rosalen PL, Falsetta ML and Koo H. Natural products in caries research: current (limited) knowledge, challenges and future perspective. Caries Res.: 2011;45:243–63.

86. Jordan HV. Cultural methods for the identification and quantitation of *Streptococcus mutans* and lactobacilli in oral samples. Oral Microbiol. Immunol.: 1986;1:23–30.

87. Kamiya RU, Napimoga MH, Rosa RT, Hofling, JF and Goncalves RB. Mutacin production in *Streptococcus mutans* genotypes isolated from caries-affected and caries-free individuals. Oral Microbiol. Immunol.: 2005;20:20–4.

88. Kang MS, Oh JS, Lee HC, Lim HS, Lee SW, Yang KH, Choi NK, Kim SM. Inhibitory effect of *Lactobacillus reuteri* on periodontopathic and cariogenic bacteria. J. Microbiol.: 2011;49:193–9.

89. Keltjens HM, Schaeken MJ, vander Hoeven JS and Hendriks JC. Microflora of plaque from sound and carious root surfaces. Caries Res.: 1987;21:193–9.

90. Khoo G, Zhan L, Hoover C and Featherstone JD. Cariogenic virulence characteristics of mutans streptococci isolated from caries-active and caries-free adults. J. Calif. Dent. Assoc.: 2005;33:973–80.

91. Kleinberg I. A mixed-bacteria ecological approach to understanding the role of the oral bacteria in dental caries causation: an alternative to *Streptococcus mutans* and the specific plaque hypothesis. Crit. Rev. Oral Biol. Med.: 2002;13: 108–25.

92. Klinke T, Kneist S, de Soet JJ, Kuhlisch E, Mauersberger S and Forster A. Acid production by oral strains of *Candida albicans* and lactobacilli. Caries Res.: 2009;43:83–91.

93. Kokare CRF, Chakraborty S, Khopade AN and Mahadik KR. Biofilm: importance and applications. Ind. J. Biotech.: 2009;8:159–68.

94. Kolenbrander PE Andersen RN, Blehert DS, England PG, Foster JS and Palmer RJ. Communication among oral bacterial. Microbiol. Mol. Biol. Rev.: 2002;66:486–505.

95. Kolenbrander PE, Palmer RJ, Periasamy S and Jakubovics NS. Oral multispecies biofilm development and the key role of cell-cell distance. Reviews: 2010;8:471–80.

96. Kolenbrander PE. Oral microbial communities: biofilms, interactions and genetic systems. Annu. Rev. Microbiol.: 2000;54:413–37.

97. Kooh H, Falsetta ML and Klein MI. The exopolysaccharide matrix: a virulence determinant of cariogenic biofilm. J. Dent. Res.: 2013;92:1065–73.

98. Kooh H, Xiao J and Klein MI. Extracellular polysaccharides matrix–an often forgotton virulence factor in oral biofilm research. Int. J. Oral Sci.: 2009;1:229–34.

99. Krzysciak W, Jurcak A, Koscielniak D, Bystrowska B and Skalniak A. The virulence of *Streptococcus mutans* and the ability to form biofilms. Eur. J. Clin. Microbiol. Infect. Dis.: 2014;33:499–515.

100. Kulkarni GV, Chan KH and Sandham HJ. An investigation into the use of restriction endonuclease analysis for the study of transmission of mutans streptococci. J. Dent. Res.: 1989;68:1155–61.

101. Kuramitsu HK and Wang BY. The whole is greater than the sum of its parts: dental plaque bacterial interactions can affect the virulence properties of cariogenic *Streptococcus mutans*. Am. J. Dent.: 2011;24:153–4.

102. Kuramitsu HK. Virulence factors of mutans streptococci: role of molecular genetics. Crit. Rev. Oral Biol. Med.: 1993;4:159–76.

103. Lang C, Bottner M, Holz C, Veen M, Ryser M, Reindl A, Pompejus M and Tanzer JM. Specific Lactobacillus/mutans Streptococcus co-aggregation. J. Dent. Res.: 2010;89:175–9.

104. Leitao TJ, Tenuta LM, Ishi G and Cury JA. Calcium binding to *Streptococcus mutans* grown in the presence or absence of sucrose. Braz. Oral Res.: 2012;26:100–5.

105. Lembo FL. Longo PL, Ota-Tsuzuki C, Rodrigues CR and Mayer MP. Genotypic and phenotypic analysis of *Streptococcus mutans* from different oral cavity sites of caries-free and caries-active children. Oral Microbiol. Immunol.: 2007;22: 313–9.

106. Lemos JA and Burne RA. Regulation and psychological significance of ClpC and ClpP in *Streptococcus mutans*. J. Bacteriol.: 2002;184: 6357–66.

107. Li J, Helmerhorst EJ, Leone CW, Troxter RF, Yaskell T and Haffajee AD. Identification of early microbial colonizers in human dental biofilm. J. Appl. Microbiol.: 2004;97:1311–8.

108. Li Y and Caufield PW. The fidelity of initial acquisition of mutans streptococci by infants from their mothers. J. Dent. Res.: 1993;74:681–5.

109. Li Y, Ge Y, Saxena D and Caufield PW. Genetic profiling of the oral microbiota associated with severe early childhood caries. J. Clin. Microbiol.: 2007;45:81–7.

110. Liao S, Bitoun JP, Nguyen AH, Bozner D, Yao X and Wen ZT. Deficiency of PdxR in *Streptococcus mutans* affects vitamin B_6 metabolism, acid tolerance response and biofilm formation. Molecular oral microbiology. 2015, 30, 255–68.

111. Lima KC, Coelho LT, Pinheiro IV, Rocas IN and Siqueira JF Jr.. Microbiota of dentinal caries as assessed by reverse-capture checkerboard analysis. Caries Res.: 2011;45:21–30.

112. Liu YL, Nascimento M and Burne RA. Progress toward understanding the contribution of alkali generation in dental biofilms to inhibition of dental caries. Int. J. Oral Science: 2012;4:135–40.

113. Llena-Puy MC, Montanana-Llorens C and Forner-Navarro L. Cariogenic oral flora and its relation to dental caries. ASDC J. Dent. Child.: 2000;67:42–6.

114. Loesche WJ and Syed SA. The predominant cultivable flora of carious plaque and carious dentin. Caries Res.: 1973;7:201–16.

115. Loesche WJ. Role of *Streptococcus mutans* in human dental decay. Microbiol. Rev.: 1986;50: 353–80.

116. Maddi A and Scannapieco FA. Oral biofilms, oral and periodontal infections and systemic disease. Am. J. Dent.: 2013;26:249–54.

117. Mantzourani M, Fenlon M and Beighton D. Association between Bifidobacteriaceae and the clinical severity of root caries lesions. Oral Microbiol. Immunol.: 2009;24:32–7.

118. Mantzourani M, Gilbert SC, Sulong NH.N.H., Sheehy SC, Tank S, Fenlon M and Beighton D. The isolation of Bifidobacteria from occlusal carious lesions in children and adults. Caries Res.: 2009;43:308–13.

119. Marsh PD. Are dental diseases examples of ecological catastrophes? Microbiology: 2003; 149:279–94.

120. Marsh PD. Dental plaque as a biofilm:the significance of pH in health and caries. Compend. Contin. Educ. Dent.: 2009;30:76–78, 80, 83–7.

121. Marsh PD. Dental plaque as a microbial biofilm. Caries Res.: 2004;38:204–11.

122. Marsh PD, Head DA and Divine DS. Ecological approaches to oral biofilms: Control without killing. Caries Res. 2015;49:46–54.

123. Marsh PD. Microbiology of dental plaque biofilms and their role in oral health and caries. Dent. Clin. North Am.: 2010;54:441–54.

124. Marsh PD. The role of microbiology in models of dental caries. Adv. Dent. Res.: 1995;9:244–54.

125. Matsui R and Cvitkovitch D. Acid tolerance mechanisms utilized by *Streptococcus mutans*. Future Microbiol.: 2010;5:403–17.

126. Matsumoto M, Tsuji M, Sasaki H, Fujita K, Nomura R, Nokano K, Shintani S and Ooshima T. Cariogenicity of the probiotic bacterium Lactobacillus salivarius in rats. Caries Res.: 2005;39:479–83.

127. Mc Carthy C, Synder ML and Parker RB. The indigenous oral flora of man. I:The newborn to the 1-year-old infant. Arch. Oral Biol.: 1965;10: 61–70.

128. McNeil K and Hamilton IR. Effect of acid stress on the physiology of biofilm cells of *Streptococcus mutans*. Microbiology: 2004;150: 735–42.

129. Metzker ML. Sequencing technologies—the next generation. Nat. Rev. Genet.: 2010;11:31–46.

130. Mo SS, Bao W, Lai GV, Wang J and Li MY. The microflora analysis of secondary caries biofilm around class I and class II composite and amalgam fillings. BMC Infectious Diseases: 2010;10:241.

131. Modesto M, Biavati B and Mattarelli P. Occurrence of the family Bifidobacteriaceae in human dental caries and plaque. Caries Res.: 2006;40:271–6.

132. Motegi M, Takagi Y, Yonezawa H, Hanada N, Terajima J, Watanabe H and Senpuku H. Assessment of genes associated with *Streptococcus mutans* biofilm morphology. Appl. Environ. Microbiol.: 2006;72:6277–87.

133. Mullany P, Hunter S and Allan E. Metaghenomics of dental biofilms. Adv. Appl. Microbiol.: 2008;64:125–36.

134. Musnon MA, Banerjee A, Watson TF and Wade WG. Molecular analysis of the microflora associated with dental caries. J. Clin. Microbiol.: 2004;42:3023–39.

135. Nakano K and Ooshima T. Serotype classification of *Streptococcus mutans* and its detection outside the oral cavity. Future Microbiol.: 2009;4:891–902.

136. Nakano K, Lapirattanakul J, Nomura R, Nemoto H, Alaluusua S, Gronroos L, Vaara M, Hamada S, Ooshima T and Nakagawa I. *Streptococcus mutans* clonal variation revealed by multilocus sequence typing. J. Clin. Microbiol.: 2007;45: 2616–25.

137. Napimoga MH, Hofling JF, Klein MI, Kamiya RU and Goncalves RB. Transmission, diversity and virulence factors of *Streptococcus mutans* genotypes. J. Oral Science: 2005;47:59–64.

138. Nascimento MM, Gordan VV and Garvan CW, et al. Correlations of oral bacterial arginine and urea catabolism with caries experience. Oral Microbiol. Immunol.: 2009;24:89–95.

139. Nascimento NM, Hofling JF and Goncalves RB. *Streptococcus mutans* genotypes isolated from root and coronal caries. Caries Res.:2004;38:454–63.

140. Nunn ME, Braunstein NS, Krall Kaye EA, Dietrich T, Garcia RI and Henshaw MM. Healthy eating index is a predictor of early childhood caries. J. Dent.: 2009;88:361–6.

141. Nyvad B and Kilian M. Microflora associated with experimental root surface caries in humans. Infection and Immunity: 1990;58:1628–33.

142. Nyvad B, Crielaard W, Mira A, Takahashi N and Beighton D. Dental caries from a molecular microbiological perspective. Caries Res.: 2013;47:89–102.

143. Nyvad B, Machiulskiene V and Baelum V. Reliability of a new caries diagnostic system differentiating between active and inactive caries lesions. Caries Res.: 1999;33:252–60.

144. Ozaki K, Matsuo T, Nakae H, Noiri Y, Yoshiyama M and Ebisu S. A quantitative comparison of selected bacteria in human carious dentin by microscopic counts. Caries Res.: 1994;28:137–45.

145. Paes Leme AF, Koo H, Bellato CM, Bedi G and Cury JA. The role of sucrose in cariogenic dental biofilm formation. New insight. J. Dent. Res.: 2006;85:878–87.

146. Palmer CA, Kent R. Jr., Loo CY, Hughes CV, Stutius E, Pradhan N, Dahlan M, Kanasi E., Arevalo Vasquezz SS and Tanner AC. Diet and caries associated bacteria in severe early childhood caries. J. Dent. Res.: 2010;89:1224–9.

147. Pennisi E. A mouthful of microbes. Science: 2005;307:1899–901.

148. Peterson SN, Snesrud E, Schork NJ and Bretz WA. Dental caries pathogenicity: a genomic and metagenomic perspective. Int. Dent. J.: 2011;61: 11–22.

149. Pinto AC, Melo-Barbosa HP, Miyoshi A, Silva A and Azevedo V. Application of RNA-seq to

reveal the transcript profile in bacteria. Genet Mol. Res.: 2011;10:1707–18.

150. Preza D, Olsen I, Aas JA, Willumsen T, Grinde B and Paster BJ. Bacterial profiles of root caries in elderly patients. J. Clin. Microbiol.: 2008;46:2015–21.

151. Preza D, Olsen I, Willumsen T, Boches SK, Cotton SL, Grinde B and Paster BJ. Microarray analysis of the microflora of root caries in elderly. Eur. J. Clin. Microbiol. Infect. Dis.: 2009;28:509–17.

152. Rendueles O, Kaplan JB and Ghigo JM. Antibiofilm polysaccharides. Environ. Microbiol.: 2013;15:334–46.

153. Robinson WG, Old LA, Shah DSH and Russell RRB). Chromosomal insertions and deletions in *Streptococcus mutans*. Caries Res.: 2003;37:148–56.

154. Rogers AH. Evidence for the transmissibility of human dental caries. Aust. Dent. J.: 1977;22:53–6.

155. Ruby J and Goldner M. Nature of symbiosis in oral disease. J. Dent. Res.: 2007;86:8–11.

156. Russell RR. Changing concepts in caries microbiology. Am. J. Dent.: 2009;22:304–10.

157. Russell RRB. How has Genomics altered our view of caries microbiology? Caries Res.: 2008;42:319–27.

158. Sakamoto M, Umeda M and Benno Y. Molecular analysis of human oral microbiota. J. Periodont. Res.: 2005;40:277–85.

159. Sansone C, Van Houte J, Joshipura K, Kent R and Margolis HC. The association of mutans streptococci and non-mutans streptococci capable of acidogenesis at a low pH with dental caries on enamel and root surface. J. Dent. Res.: 1993;72:508–16.

160. Sanui T and Gregory RL. Analysis of *Streptococcus mutans* biofilm proteins recognized by salivary immunoglobin A. Oral Microbiol. Immunol.: 2009;24:361–8.

161. Schadt EE, Turner S and Kasarskis A. A window into the third-generation sequencing. Hum. Mol. Genet.: 2010;19:227–40.

162. Schupbach P, Osterwalder V and Guggenheim B. Human root caries; microbiota in plaque covering sound, carious and arrested carious root surfaces. Caries Res.: 1995;29:382–95.

163. Schupbach P, Osterwalder V and Guggenheim B. Human root caries: microbiota of a limited number of root caries lesions. Caries Res.: 1996;30:52–64.

164. Seemann R, Bizhang M, Kluck I, Loth J and Roulet JF. A novel *in vitro* microbial-based model for studying caries formation—Development and initial testing. Caries Res.: 2005;39:185–190.

165. Seneviratne CJ, Zhang CF and Samaranayake LP. Dental plaque biofilm in oral health and disease. Chin. J. Dent. Res.: 2011;14:87–94.

166. Shen S, Samaranayake LP and Yip HK. Coaggregation profiles of microflora from root surface caries lesions. Archives of Oral Biology: 2005;50:23–32.

167. Shen S, Samaranayake LP and Yip HK. *In vitro* growth, acidogenicity and cariogenicity of predominant human root caries flora. J. Dent.: 2004;32:667–78.

168. Sheng J and Marquis RE. Malolactic fermentation by *Streptococcus mutans*. FEMS Microbiol. Lett: 2007;272:196–201.

169. Shimotoyodome A, Kobayashi HJ, Tokimitsu I, Hase T, Inoue T, Matsukubo T and Takaesu Y. Saliva-promoted adhesion of *Streptococcus mutans* MT8148 associates with dental plaque and caries experience. Caries Res.: 2007;41:212–8.

170. Shu M, Wong L, Miller JH and Sissons CH. Development of multi-species consortia biofilms of oral bacteria as an enamel and root caries model system. Arch. Oral Biol.: 2000;45:27–40.

171. Sigurjons HJ, Mangusdottir MO and Holbrook WP. Cariogenic bacteria in a longitudinal study of approximal caries. Caries Res.: 1995;29:42–45.

172. Simmonds RS, Tompkins GR.and George RJ. Dental caries and the microbial ecology of dental plaque: a review of recent advances. NZ. Dent. J.: 2000;96:44–9.

173. Smith EG and Spatafora GA. Gene regulation in *Streptococcus mutans*: complex control in a complex environment. J. Dent. Res.: 2012;91:133–41.

174. Socransky SS and Manganiello SD. The oral microbiota of man from birth to senility. J. Periodontol.:1971;42:485–96.

175. Soderling EM, Marttinen AM and Haukioja AL. Probiotic lactobacilli interfere with *Streptococcus mutans* biofilm formation *in vitro*. Curr. Microbiol.: 2011;62:618–22.

176. Soderling EM. Xylitol, mutans streptococci and dental plaque. Adv. Dent. Res.: 2009;21:74–8.

177. Splieth C, Bernhardt O, Heinrich A, Bernhardt H and Meyer G. Anaerobic microflora under

Class I and class II composite and amalgam restorations. Quintessence Int.: 2003;34:497–503.

178. Sumney DL and Jordan HV. Characterization of bacteria isolated from human root surface carious lesions. J. Dent. Res.: 1974;53:343–51.

179. Svensater G, Borgstrom M, Bowden GH and Edwardsson S. The acid-tolerant microbiota associated with plaque from initial caries and healthy tooth surfaces. Caries Res.: 2003;37:395–403.

180. Syed SA, Loesche WJ, Pape HL and Grenier E. Predominant cultivable flora isolated from human root surface caries plaque. Infection and Immunity: 1975;11:727–31.

181. Takahashi N and Nyvad B. Caries ecology revisited : Microbial dynamics and the caries process. Car. Res.: 2008;42:409–18.

182. Takahashi N and Nyvad B. The role of bacteria in the caries process:ecological perspectives. J. Dent. Res.: 2010;90:294–303.

183. Takahashi N, Washio J and Mayanagi G. Metabolomic approach to oral biofilm characterization. J. Oral Biosci.: 2012;54:138–43.

184. Tanner ACR, Milgrom PM, Kent R Jr, Mokeem SA, Page RC, Riedy CA, Weinstein P and Bruss J. The microbiota of young children from tooth and tongue samples. J. Dent. Res.: 2002;81:53–57.

185. Tanzer JM, Linvingston J and Thompson AM. The microbiology of primary dental caries in humans. J. Dent. Educ.: 2001;65:1028–37.

186. Tanzer JM, Thompson A, Sharma K, Vickerman MM, Haase EM and Scannapieco FA. *Streptococcus mutans* out-competes *streptococcus gordonii* in vivo. J. Dent. Res.: 2012;91: 513–9.

187. Tanzer JM. Dental caries is a transmissible infectious disease: The Keyes and Fitzgerald revolution. J. Dent. Res.: 1995;74:1536–42.

188. Teanpaisan R, Piwat S and Dahlen G. Inhibitory effect of oral lactobacillus against oral pathogens. Lett. Appl. Microbiol.: 2011;53:452–9.

189. Thomas RZ, Zijnge V, Cicek A, de Soett JJ, Harmasen HJ and Huysmans MC. Shifts in the microbial population in relation to in situ caries progression. Caries Res.: 2012;46:427–31.

190. Van Ruyven FO, Lingstrom P, van Houte J and Kent R. Relationship among mutans streptococci, "low-pH" bacteria and Iodophilic polysaccharide-producing bacteria in dental plaque and early enamel caries in humans. J. Dent. Res.: 2000;79:778–84.

191. Wade WG. Unculturable bacteria—the uncharacterized organisms that cause oral infections. J.R. Soc. Med.: 2002;95:81–83.

192. Wan AKL, Seow WK, Walsh LJ and Bird PS. Comparison of five selective media for the growth and enumeration of *Streptococcus mutans*. Aust. Dent. J.: 2002;47:21–6.

193. Wang BYT, Deutch A, Hong J and Kuramitsu HK. Proteases of an early colonizer can hinder *Streptococcus mutans* colonization *in vitro*. J. Dent. Res.: 2010;90:501–5.

194. Waterhouse JC and Russell RRB. Dispensable genes and foreign DNA in *Streptococcus mutans* strains. Microbiology: 2006;152:1777–88.

195. Waterhouse JC, Swan DC and Russell RRB. Comparative genome hybridisation of *Streptococci mutans* strains. Oral Microbiol. Immunol.: 2007;22:103–10.

196. Waters MS, Kundu S, Lin NJ and Lin-Gibson S. Microstructure and mechanical properties of in situ *Streptococcus mutans* biofilms. ACS Appl. Mater. Interfaces: 2014;6:327–32.

197. Welin-Neilands J and Svensater G. Acid tolerance of biofilm cells of *Streptococcus mutans*. Appl. Environ. Microbiol.: 2007;73: 5633–8.

198. Whiley RA and Beighton D. Current classification of the oral streptococci. Oral Microbiol. Immunol.: 1998;13:195–216.

199. Wolff D, Frese C, Maier-Kraus T, Krueger T and Wolff B. Bacterial biofilm composition in caries and caries-free subjects. Caries Research: 2013;47:69–77.

200. Wolff MS and Larson C. The cariogenic dental biofilm: good, bad or just something to control? Braz. Oral Res.: 2009;23:31–8.

201. Xiao J and Koo H. Structural organization and dynamics of exopolysaccharide matrix and microcolonies formation by *Streptococcus mutans* in biofilms. J. Appl. Microbiol.:2010;108: 2103–13.

202. Yan W, Qu T, Zhao H, Su L, Yu Q, Gao J and Wu B. The effect of c-di-GMP (3'-5'-cyclic diguanylic acid) on the biofilm formation and adherence of *Streptococcus mutans*. Microbiol. Res.: 2010;165:87–96.

203. Yang F, Zeng X, Ning K, Liu KL, Lo CC, Wang W, Chen J, Wang D, Huang R, Chang X, Chain PS, Xie G, Ling J and Xu J. Saliva microbiomes distinguish caries-active from health human populations. ISME J.: 2012;6:1–10.

204. Yli-Knuuttila H, Snall J, Kari K and Meurman JH. Colonization of Lactobacillus rhamnosus GG in the oral cavity. Oral Microbiol. Immunol.: 2006;21:129–31.

205. Zaremba ML, Stokowska W, Klimiuk A, Daniluk T, Rozkiewicz D, Cylwik-Rokicka D, Waszkiel D, Tokajuk G, Kierklo A and Abdelrazek S. Micro-organisms in root carious lesions in adults. Advances in Medical Sciences: 2006;51:237–40.

206. Zaura E, Keijser BJ, Huse SM and Crielaard W. Defining the healthy "core microbiome"of oral microbial communities. BMC Microbiol.: 2009;9: 59.

207. Zaura E. Next-generation sequencing approaches to understanding the oral microbiome. Adv. Dent. Res.: 2012;24:81–5.

208. Zheng X, Zhang K, Zhou X, Liu C, Li M, Li Y, Wang R, Li Y, Li J, Shi W and Xu X. Involvement of gshAB in the interspecies competition within oral biofilm. J. Dent. Res.: 2013;92:819–24.

209. Zhu WM, Liu W and Wu DQ. Isolation and characterization of a new bacteriocin from *Lactobacillus gasseri* kt7. J. Appl. Microbiol.: 2000;88:877–86.

210. Zijnge V, van Leeuwen MBM, Harmsen HJ, Degener JF, Abbas F, Thurnheer T and Gmur R. Oral biofilm architecture on natural teeth. PLoS ONE: 2010;5:9321.

9

Histopathology of Dental Caries

Dental caries is an established multi-factorial disease. Multiple factors, such as the interaction of bacteria, diet, saliva and host response, influence initiation and progression of dental caries. The decalcification of enamel is followed by enzymatic lysis of organic structures leading to localized destruction, subsequently the caries. Low salivary pH promotes the growth of aciduric bacteria followed by proliferation of acidogenic bacteria creating an inhospitable environment for the protective oral bacteria. The environmental balance shifts in favor of cariogenic bacteria, which further lowers the salivary pH and the cycle continues. The fluctuations in pH cause net loss or gain of mineral content from the tooth. The development of dental caries depends upon the balance between this loss (demineralization)/gain (remineralization) of mineral contents.

Over the years, the histological research regarding the demineralization and remineralization processes in the initial lesion of the enamel became a priority of the researchers. The most common gold standard used for the assessment of carious lesions is the histological evaluation of hard tissue sections. Mature human dental enamel has a high degree of mineralization making structural studies somewhat more difficult than other tissues. Since the carious process involves demineralization of inorganic content and the decalcification procedure necessary for cutting thin sections may result in complete loss of enamel; therefore, special methods are used. There are several methods used to study dental caries which include ground sections, micro-radiography, scanning electron microscopy (SEM) and transmission electron microscopy (TEM), histochemistry radioisotopes and Confocal Laser Scanning Microscopy (CLSM).

In optical microscopy, the enamel and dentinal lesions are examined on ground sections (approximately 100 μm thick), using the ordinary and polarized light. The demineralization of the enamel and also the way of progression of caries on different surfaces of the teeth can also be studied. Polarized light is mostly used for evaluation of caries. The polarized light is more sensitive for contrasting normal from carious enamel than absorption-based techniques.

Normal Structures and Properties of Hard Tissues of Tooth

The normal histological aspects of a tooth structure are described in brief so as to understand the pathological deviations.

1. Enamel

It is an extremely hard and highly mineralized, translucent tissue covering the anatomical crowns of teeth. Enamel consists of the following:

a. Inorganic matter (95–97%).

Principal constituents:

Calcium	34.5–37.1%
Phosphorus	17.1–18%
Carbonate	2–2.8%
Magnesium	0.2–0.6%

Trace elements:

Sodium	0.2%
Potassium	0.05%
Iron	0.02%
Chlorine	0.30%
Fluoride	0.02%

b. Organic matter (0.2–0.8%) mainly glyco-proteins, carbohydrate matrix, Type I collagen.

c. Water (1.2–4%).

d. Rest is oxygen.

Structure Elements

a. *Enamel rods:* Enamel rods are the organizational units of enamel. These are polygonal, long, slender prisms having irregular five or six sides with diameter of 4 μm. Earlier authors described enamel rods as hexagonal and prism like in cross-section with a keyhole or paddle-shaped pattern. Presently, the enamel pattern is described as cylindrical rods embedded in the interrod enamel. The apatite crystals are arranged approximately parallel to the long axis of the rods in their bodies or heads and deviate about 65° from this axis as they fan out into the tails of the prisms.

b. *Prism sheath:* It is the least calcified portion of the enamel rod which is richer in organic substance than rest of the rods.

c. *Interprismatic substance:* A relatively softer, glossy and homogeneous portion of enamel, less than 1 μm in width present between the enamel prisms.

d. *The striae of Retzius:* They represent the poorly calcified portion of enamel, extending from the dentino-enamel junction towards the tooth surface. Their meeting point at enamel surface forms grooves encircling the tooth known as Perikymata (Fig. 9.1).

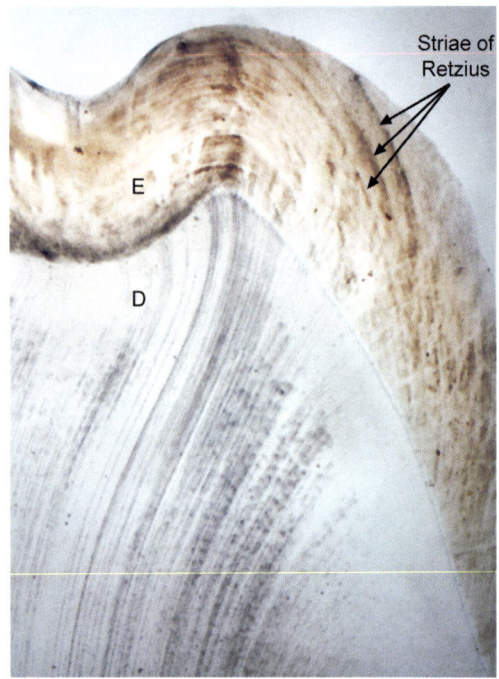

Fig. 9.1: Longitudinal ground section of tooth showing the position of striae of Retzius in the enamel layer (E). D: Dentin

e. *Enamel lamellae:* These are thin, leaflike structures that extend from the enamel surface towards the DEJ; rarely extending into dentin. The lamellae consist of organic material with little mineral content (Fig. 9.2).

f. *Enamel tufts:* These are the hypocalcified enamel rods and interprismatic substances that originate at the dentino-enamel junction (DEJ) and extends into the enamel for about 1/3rd–1/5th of its total thickness.

g. *Enamel spindles:* The spindle like structures, projecting from dentino-enamel junction (DEJ) into enamel; approximately 100 μm (inside), they appear as continuation of dentinal tubules. The direction of the odontoblastic processes and spindles in the enamel corresponds to the original

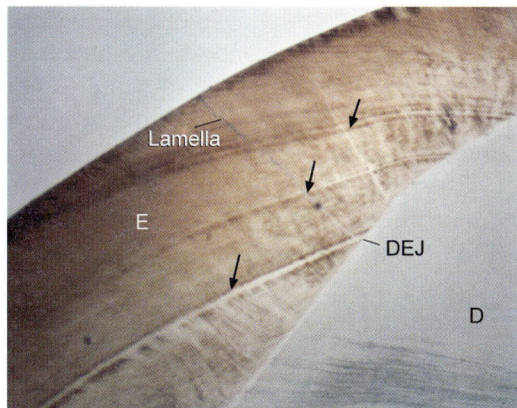

Fig. 9.2: Longitudinal ground section of tooth showing striae of Retzius (arrows). An enamel lamella can be seen running from the outer surface to the dentino-enamel junction (DEJ). E: Enamel; D: Dentin.

direction of the ameloblasts and is at right angle to the surface of dentino-enamel junction (DEJ).

h. *Hunter and Schreger bands:* The Hunter and Schreger bands are the optical phenomena produced by the changes in direction between adjacent groups of rods. These are the dark and light alternating zones that can be reversed by altering the direction of incident illumination. These bands are seen most clearly in longitudinal ground sections viewed by reflected light and are found in the inner 2/3rd of the enamel.

i. *Enamel membranes:* These are of two types:
   a. *Developmental:* Primary and secondary enamel cuticles.
   b. *Acquired:* Pellicle, Materia alba and plaque.

2. Dentin

Dentin is a calcified connective tissue which is penetrated by definitely arranged small canals containing protoplasmic processes belonging to cells which remain outside the tissue in pulpal cavity. Dentin consists of:

a. Inorganic matter 61.0–73.0%
   Principal constituents:
   Calcium 33.0–35.4%
   Phosphorus 16.0–18.0%

Carbonate	3.8–4.6%
Magnesium	0.9–1.1%

Trace elements:

Sodium	0.20%
Potassium	0.07%
Iron	0.02%
Fluorine	0.02%
b. Organic matter	20.3–22.4%
c. Water	10.8–15.7%

d. Oxygen (remaining part).

Structural elements

a. *Dentinal tubules:* These are minute S-shaped tubules radiating perpendicularly from pulp chamber and extending to the outer surface of dentin. These tubules end perpendicular to the dentino-enamel junction or dentino-cemental junction (Fig. 9.3).

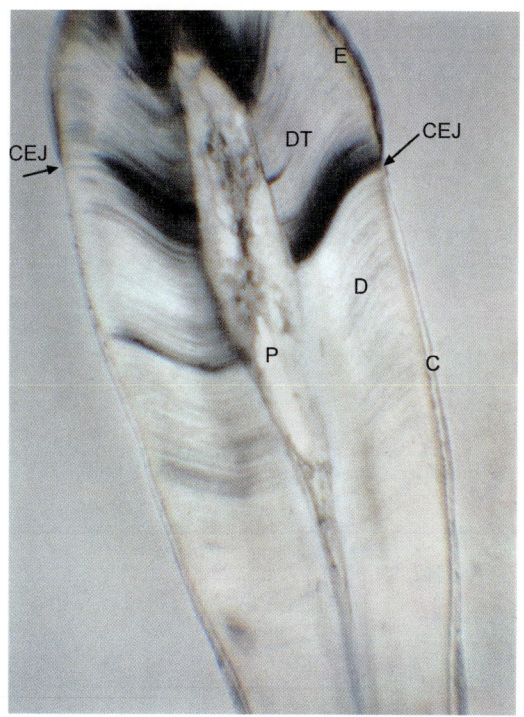

Fig. 9.3: Longitudinal ground section of tooth showing the S-shaped primary curvature of the dentinal tubules (DT) in the crown and their straight course in the root. Cemento-enamel junction (CEJ) depicting an edge to edge relation. E: Enamel; D: Dentin; P: Pulp; C: Cementum.

b. *The dentin matrix:* The dentin matrix is homogeneous and an elastic substance, containing dentinal tubules. The matrix consists mainly of collagenous fibrils, embedded in an organic cementing medium in which organic salts are deposited.

c. *Sheaths of Neumann:* A deeply stained area around the dentinal tubules was observed and was named Sheath of Neumann. Later, it was found to be the portion of dentinal matrix forming the immediate walls of dentinal tubule.

d. *Interglobular dentin:* These are areas of imperfectly calcified dentinal matrix formed due to incomplete fusion of calcospherites during dentinal development.

e. *Tomes' granular layer:* A granular area seen just below the surface of root dentin in ground section under transmitted light (Fig. 9.4).

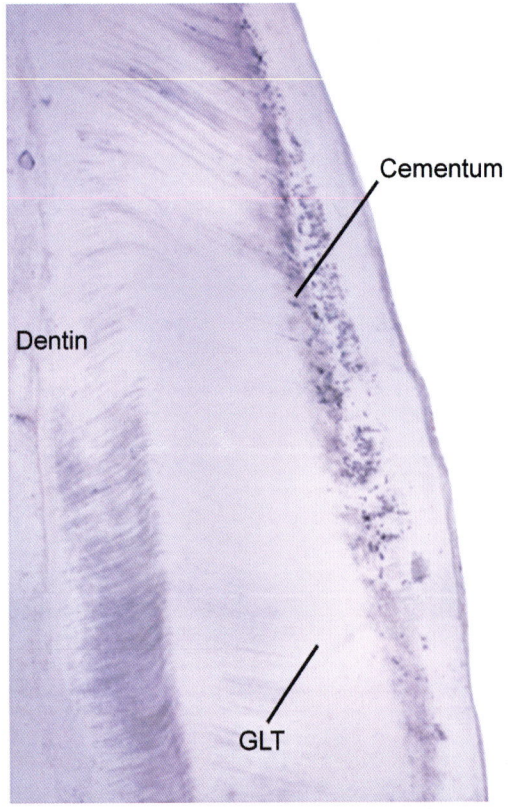

Fig. 9.4: Longitudinal ground section of middle third portion of tooth showing GLT, granular layer of Tomes

f. *Incremental lines of von Ebner:* The lines run at right angles to the dentinal tubules and mark the normal rhythmic, linear pattern of dentin deposition in an inward and rootward direction.

g. *Contour lines of Owen:* These are incremental layers of dentin produced by the disturbance in calcification of that layer at the time of its development. These are analogous to accentuated striae of Retzius in enamel.

h. *Mantle dentin:* It is the first formed dentin in the crown close to the dentino-enamel junction (DEJ). It is less mineralized and approximately 15 µm wide. It is bounded by a zone of interglobular dentin.

i. *Predentin:* It is the first deposited layer of unmineralized matrix (thickness varies 10–50 µ) and lines the innermost (pulpal) portion. It consists of both collagenous and non-collagenous components.

j. *Dead tracts:* Dentinal areas characterized by degenerated odontoblastic processes; may result from injury caused by caries, attrition, erosion or cavity preparation. They appear black in transmitted light and white in reflected light (Fig. 9.5).

k. *Secondary dentin:* It is the dentin formed after the completion of root formation and represents the slow and continuous deposition of dentin.

l. *Transparent dentin or sclerotic dentin:* It is formed due to vital reaction of dentin to irritation, e.g. caries in which, the odontoblastic processes undergo fatty degeneration and become a barrier for progression of caries.

m. *Tomes' Fibers:* These are the protoplasmic projections of the odontoblasts found in the dentinal tubules.

3. Dentino-enamel Junction

Kohliker (1855) was amongst the earlier authors who provided the histological view of the dentino-enamel junction (DEJ). When imaged microscopically, the researchers

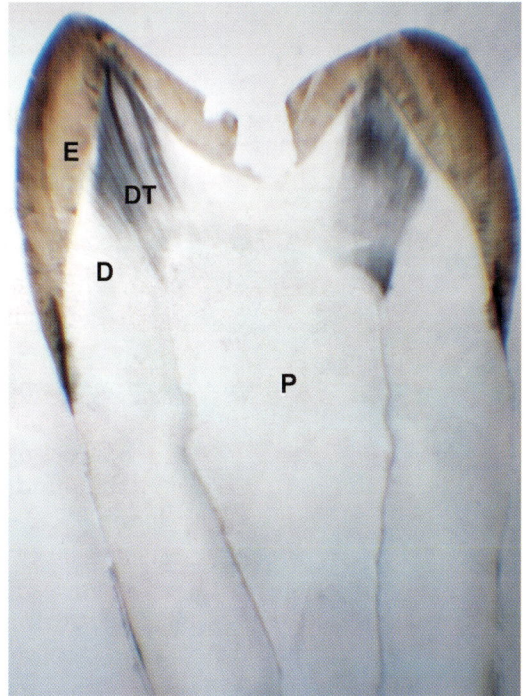

Fig. 9.5: Longitudinal ground section of tooth showing dead tracts (DT) in dentin (D) caused by crowding and degeneration of odontoblasts. E: Enamel; P: Pulp.

observed a simple line. The DEJ is thought to represent the original position of the basal membrane between ameloblasts and odontoblasts, where they contact in the embryological tooth bud.

With the emergence of Transmission electron microscope (TEM), a precise morphological description of the junction could be achieved. The DEJ has a hierarchical microstructure with a three dimensional scalloped appearance along the interface. The studies have indicated that DEJ is not restricted to a thin interface and is a transitional zone with spatiotemporal gradient in both tissues. Specifically collagen fibrils in the transitional zone were either perpendicular to the plane of the junction or converged towards enamel. These coarse fibrils forming bundles of 80–120 nm in diameter appeared to be similar to the "von Korff fibers". Under Scanning electron microscope (SEM), the junction

represents a series of ridges which increases adherence between dentin and enamel. This ridging is more developed in coronal dentin where occlusal stresses are greatest.

The junction between dentin and enamel is often scalloped with convexities directed towards dentin and concavities towards enamel (Fig. 9.6). This region has high proportion of inter-prismatic substance, considerable crossing and branching of dentinal tubules, enamel spindles and persistence of some of the organic substance (dentino-enamel cuticle). These factors make DEJ as the most vulnerable site for spread of caries.

Micro raman spectroscopy and confocal microscope have been proved to be useful in investigating the functional width and molecular structural differences across the DEJ. The width of the DEJ has been found to be dependent on the intra tooth location, with 12 μm width at the occlusal side and 6.2 μm at cervical side which might be related to its function.

4. Cementum

There are two types of cementum according to origin and structure:

a. *Acellular cementum:* The cementum present on the coronal and middle part of root, which is without any cellular content.

b. *Cellular cementum:* The first formed cementum present in the apical third of the root (Fig. 9.7).

Structural Elements

a. *The matrix:* It consists of fine fibers, connected to each other by a calcified connecting substance.

b. *Incremental layers of cementum (Lines of Salter):* The periods of rest following the activity period result in an incremental appearance of cementum in sections. The width between these layers is responsible for the thickness of cementum on a particular root surface.

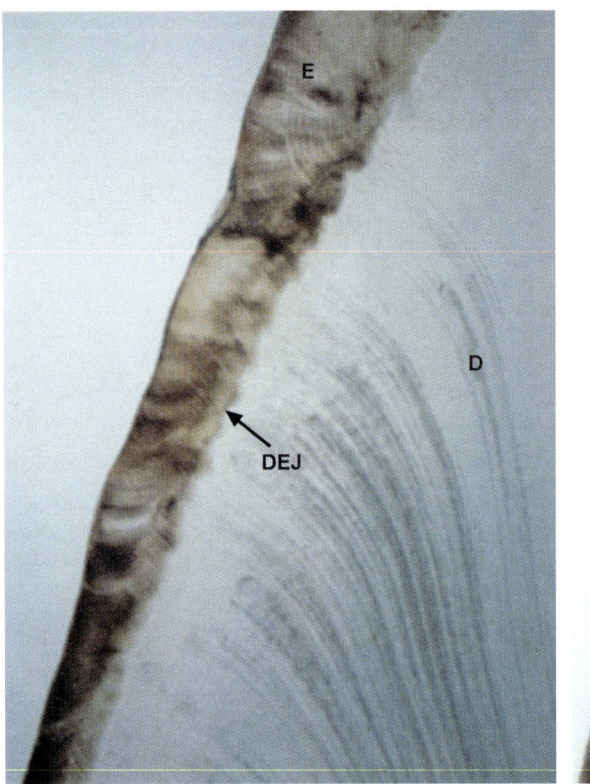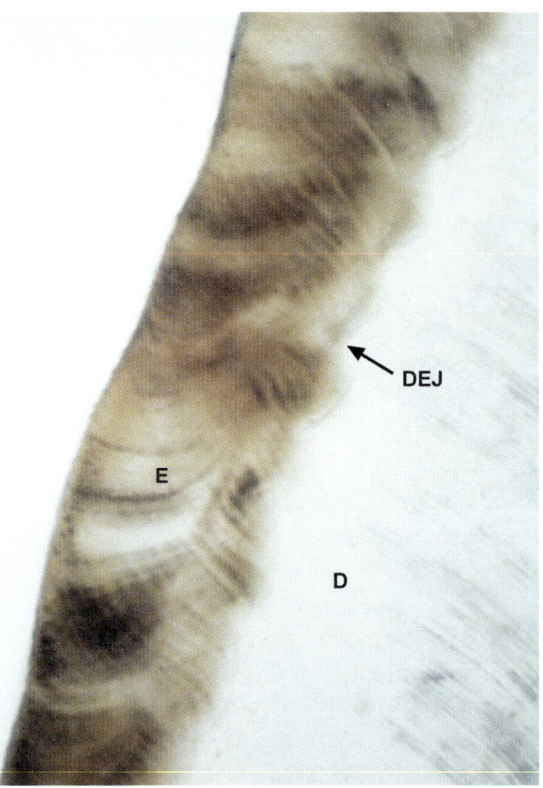

Fig. 9.6: Longitudinal ground section of tooth showing dentino-enamel junction (DEJ) as a scalloped outline. The convexities of the scallops are directed towards the dentin (D). E: Enamel

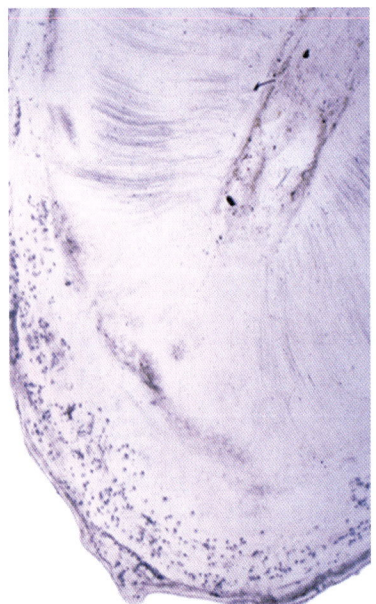

Fig. 9.7: Longitudinal ground section showing apical third of tooth. Cementocytes are present in the cellular cementum

c. *Cementocytes and lacunae:* The cells of cementum are called cementocytes and they are present in the irregular spaces known as lacunae (not present in acellular cementum).

d. *Sharpey's fibers:* These are the fibers of periodontal ligament, embedded in cementum and serve to attach the tooth to the surrounding bone.

5. Cemento-enamel Junction

It is the interface between the cementum and the enamel at the cervical region of the tooth. It generally presents as a smooth surface; with cementum overlapping enamel in 60–65% of cases; both ending in a butt joint in 30% cases and without meeting each other in 5–10% of cases (Fig. 9.8).

The enamel prisms, near the cemento-enamel junction (CEJ), directed approximately

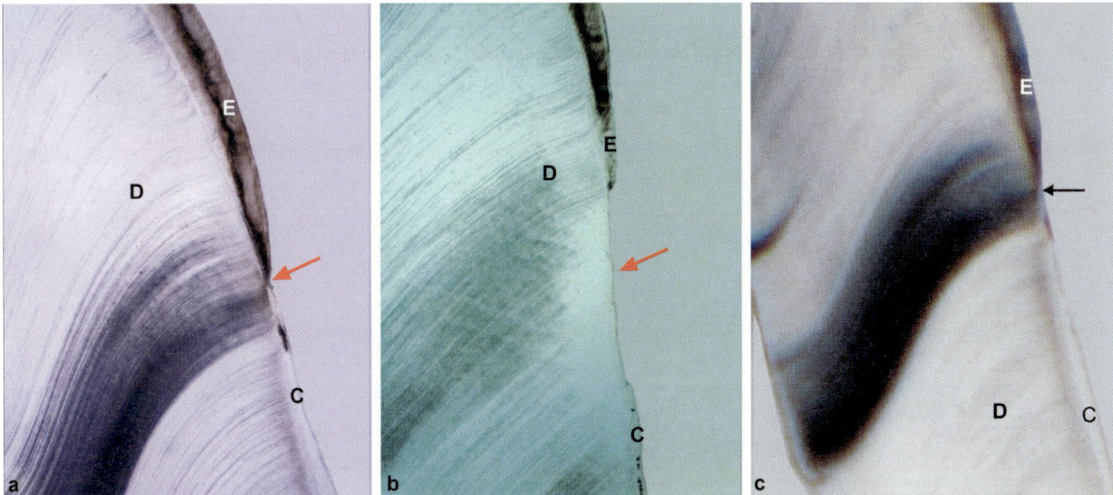

Fig. 9.8: Longitudinal ground sections of teeth depicting cemento-enamel junction a. edge to edge relation, b. gap junction, c. cementum overlapping enamel. (E: Enamel; D: Dentin; C: Cementum)

90° to the long axis of the tooth. Occasionally, the prisms are inclined occlusally on one side, while on the opposite side, they may be directed apically. In longitudinal sections the prisms assume parallel wave-like courses in a plane parallel to the cut surface. The sections of enamel in the stage of prism differentiation exhibits enamel prisms in the region of CEJ occupying occluso-angular relationship with the dentin. Occasionally, the enamel rods near the CEJ may lie in an arc, the peripheral end of which is directed towards the root apex. Prisms directed apically and occluso-angularly may occur at various places along the CEJ of the same tooth.

The CEJ is an important site where gingival fibers attach to a healthy tooth. In young adults, the CEJ of permanent teeth is protected by the gingival tissues. However, with increasing age, continuous passive eruption along with the recession of the gingiva, results in a shift of the gingival sulcus towards the CEJ. These changes expose the CEJ to the oral environment, thus making it vulnerable to pathological changes such as root caries, abrasion/erosion of dentin and sensitivity. The CEJ has become an area of clinical interest, especially for elderly dentate population because of the prevalence of root surface lesions involving the CEJ. The inter-relationship of mineralized tissues that composed the CEJ has been classified into four different categories: enamel overlapped by cementum, edge to edge contact of cementum and enamel, cementum overlapped by enamel and gap between cementum and enamel that exposes the dentin. The rare occurrence of enamel overlapping cementum, is difficult to explain from an embryological standpoint, because cementum formation begins after enamel formation is completed. A few authors regarded this novel morphology as an optical illusion that arose due to the thickness of ground sections; however, the similar morphology has been confirmed by various authors in their studies on primary and permanent teeth.

6. Cemento-dentinal Junction

The cemento-dentinal junction (CDJ) forms a biological and structural link between cementum and dentin. It is 2.0–3.0 μm wide, fibril-poor layer, full of proteoglycans (mucopolysaccharides and core proteins). The fibrils intermingling between cementum and dentin occur only in a few places (Fig. 9.9).

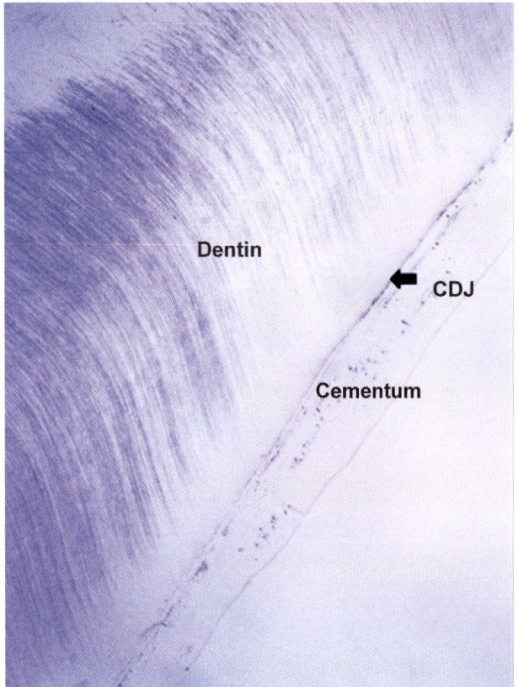

Fig. 9.9: Longitudinal ground section of tooth showing cemento-dentinal junction (arrow)

The cemento-dentinal junction (CDJ), is also known as the interzonal layer, intermediate cementum, collagen hiatus and Hopewell-Smith's hyaline layer.

The mineral contents of this zone are less as compared to either cementum or dentin; therefore, the mechanical properties are inferior. The inferior mechanical properties facilitate reducing the stress concentrations between the two mechanically dissimilar tissues. It contains hydrophilic and lower mineral content constituents, such as collagenous and non-collagenous proteins. This region of altered composition facilitates biological and biomechanical functions in addition to providing the structural integrity. The proteoglycans mainly contribute to its structural integrity under wet conditions.

It is established that the type of first formed cementum and the fibril density of the CDJ varies in different types of teeth. The distribution of individual cementum types relates to the past functional demands. In initial acellular cementogenesis, the first collagen of root dentin is deposited about 1.0 mm from the basal lamina of the epithelial sheath. The intervening gap contains dentinal ground substance and only a few, sparsely distributed collagen fibrils. At the initial dentin mineralization, the mineralization does not involve this surface layer, which mineralizes later to form the CDJ. With a breakdown of the sheath, proteoglycans on which primitive principal fibers are attached appear in the unmineralized superficial dentin layer.

In the cellular cementum, only a small number of intrinsic or extrinsic fibers penetrate the CDJ to reach the dentin surface. In addition, the CDJ is more irregular in cellular cementum than acellular cementum.

A few authors have suggested that cementum is attached to root dentin by the intermingling of collagen fibrils from both cementum and dentin. However, it is now believed that the CDJ is a narrow zone, 2.0–3.0 μm wide, containing proteoglycans with enamel- and bone-related proteins and this adhesive layer forms the primary attachment between cementum and dentin and that the intermingling of the collagen fibrils was less important. This layer was mistaken to be the intermediate cementum and the hyaline layer of Hopewell and Smith in the past; however, it has been demonstrated as a distinct tissue.

Certain important proteins crucial to periodontal regeneration, like bone morphogenic protein-2 and osteogenin 4 are also reported to be present in this tissue. The overall function of CDJ could aid absorption and distribution of occlusal loads between cementum and dentin before release into alveolar bone. Prolonged exposure of cementum to a microbial environment during periodontitis causes structural and compositional changes in cementum and also in the CDJ. In periodontitis, the bacterial destruction can be traced from the surface of cementum through CDJ and at times, till dentin. The effects of damage on cemental surface may be seen as areas of hypo- or hypermineralization and areas of resorption due to alterations in organic and inorganic components. The bacterial toxin traverses cementum, reaches CDJ and causes destruction of the unmineralized collagen which is present in abundance at CDJ. Collagen at the CDJ junction is particularly susceptible to denaturation because this interface is rich in unmineralized collagen. The area of destruction where collagen is lost appears as vacuoles under the microscope and is known as "pathologic granules". The destruction of fibres at CDJ could cause weakening of the CDJ in periodontitis affected teeth. More so, the tissues of a weakened junction may not withstand mechanical periodontal procedures resulting in complete removal of cementum, thus exposing dentin.

HISTOPATHOLOGY OF ENAMEL CARIES

The carious enamel was first visualized microscopically by Miller in 1890. He explained the process as dissolution of the interprismatic substance, subsequently bacteria forcing their way between the loosened prisms. Later, Williams (1923) described the carious process as dissolution of the interrod substance making the resultant material less resistant to the acid attack. A few authors (Beust, 1925) were of the view that since carious enamel resists acid action, caries cannot purely be because of acid action. GV Black (1936) described that the acid was formed by micro-organisms which cover the enamel surface and never enter the enamel until the enamel rods are loosened. Appelbaum (1943) showed that the incremental lines (lines of Retzius) became more visible in incipient caries. The calcium salts disappear by acid action and exhibits organic framework clearly. Gottlieb (1944) described undermining enamel caries, explaining it by the fact that the deeper layers of the enamel are less calcified than the superficial ones. The four stages can be differentiated in the progress of enamel caries: (i) the organic framework is thickened; (ii) the process invading the prisms making them more acid resistant while the prism sheaths turn black; (iii) the prism sheaths disappear while the isolated prisms remain and (iv) a necrotic mass replacing the enamel structure.

The carious process may vary slightly, depending upon the occurrence of the lesion on smooth surfaces or in pits or fissures. Accordingly, caries in enamel is discussed under two headings:

a. Smooth surface caries.

b. Pit and fissure caries.

a. Smooth Surface Caries

On smooth surface of tooth, the smooth chalky white area of decalcification manifests as the initial macroscopic evidence of incipient caries. The white spot enamel surface is hard and shiny and cannot be distinguished from the surface of adjacent sound enamel using the sharp explorer point. These surface lesions may appear brownish and are described as brown spots. This largely depends on the degree of exogenous material absorbed by the porous region and amount of water in the structure. The demineralization occurs due to increase in porosity of enamel and is related to relative refractive index (RI) of enamel (1.62), air (1.0) and water (1.33). In subsurface lesion, the pores are filled with a watery medium. As the pores are air dried, air replaces the water. As the differences of refractive indices are increased, the lesion looks more opaque and hence becomes more evident.

Enamel rods run parallel or even converge slightly from the entrance of cavity to dentino-enamel junction (DEJ). Thus, caries penetrate along the axis of enamel rods. In longitudinal ground sections, defect appears as cone shaped with the apex of the triangle directed towards the dentin and base towards the surface of the tooth (Fig. 9.10).

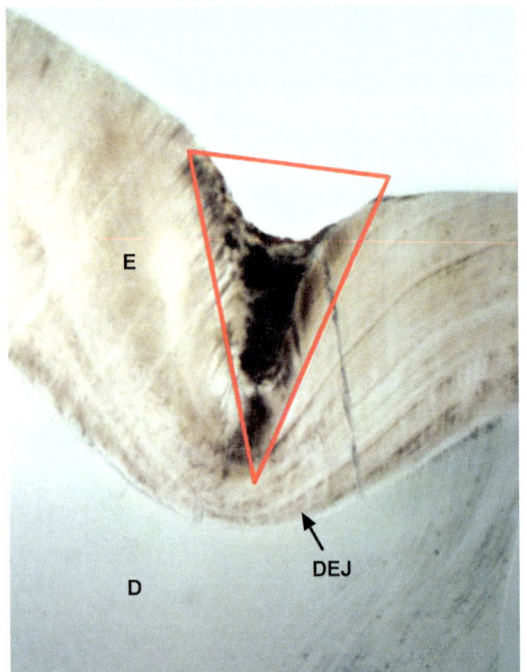

Fig. 9.10: Longitudinal ground section of tooth depicting early enamel caries; triangular in shape with the apex towards the dentino-enamel junction (DEJ) and base towards the enamel (E: Enamel; D: Dentin)

Transmission electron microscope (TEM) has revealed that the initial change is the loss of interprismatic or inter-rod substance of enamel resulting in increased prominence of the rods. The prisms are considered more susceptible to early attack as the initial change of roughening of ends of the enamel rods has been observed. The transverse striations of the enamel rods may be attributed to changes occurring in the rods between calcospherites. Another change in early enamel caries is the accentuation of the incremental striae of Retzius and Perikymata (external manifestation of striae of Retzius). The appearance of the calcification lines is an optical phenomenon due to the loss of minerals which causes the organic structures to appear more prominent.

b. Pit and Fissure Caries

The occlusal fissures are deep invaginations of enamel surface. These may vary in shape such as broad or narrow funnels, constricted hour glasses and inverted Y-shaped invaginations. The carious process in this region is same as in smooth surface caries except in anatomical and histological structure variations. The carious lesion usually initiate at both sides of the fissure wall rather than at the base which can be visualized as chalkiness, yellow, brown or black discoloration. Further, early dentin involvement frequently occurs as the enamel in the bottom of the pit or fissure may be very thin; however, some pits and fissures are shallow and have relatively thick layer of enamel covering their base. In both types, the enamel rods flare laterally in the bottom of the pits and fissures. The carious lesion characteristically forms a triangular or cone-shaped defect with its apex at the outer surface and its base towards the dentino-enamel junction (DEJ) as it follows the direction of the enamel rods. The general shape of the lesion is just the opposite of that occurring on smooth surfaces as the enamel rods diverge from the surface to the dentino-enamel junction. The arrangement of enamel rods and dentinal tubules almost invariably causes an immense involvement of tooth structure when the lesion reaches the DEJ (Fig. 9.11).

Histochemical Assessment

Wislocri and Sognnaes used different histochemical tests to study the formation of early carious lesions. The tests are as follows:

a. *The Ninhydrin test:* This test depends on the reaction of aqueous solution of triketohydrindene hydrate (ninhydrin) on organic materials in neutral solutions. The development of blue violet color indicates the presence of amino acids, free or bound peptides or proteins. The reaction is negative initially; whereas, in advanced lesions the reaction is positive. It is concluded that the protein structures are not broken down in the initial carious lesions.

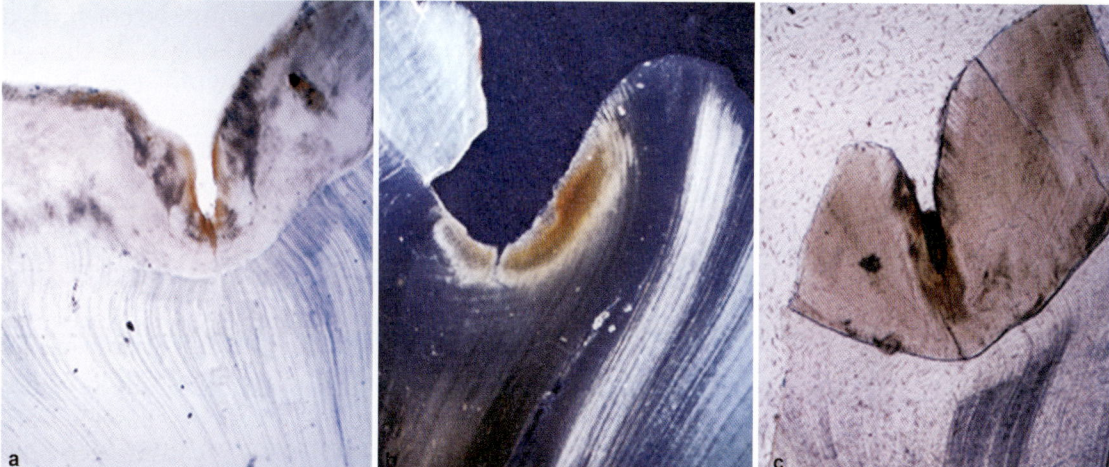

Fig. 9.11: Pit and fissure caries under a. Light microscope; b. Dark field microscope c. Phase contrast microscope

b. *The Morgan-Elson test:* This test primarily detects the presence of glucosamines. It was strongly positive in initial lesions. It was concluded that the organic structure contains a hexosamine (derived from mucopolysaccharides) that gives the positive test and rapid depolymerization of the acid mucopolysaccharides in enamel occurs during the initial lesions.

c. *Silver nitrate test:* Silver nitrate test was used to examine the path by which normal enamel is penetrated by bacterial products. Silver nitrate penetrated the normal as well as carious enamel along the organic pathways. In carious enamel, the permeability is increased.

Silver nitrate does not break proteins; therefore, organic framework of enamel need not to be broken down for the causation of initial carious lesions. The acid mucopolysaccharide around the rod prisms is dissolved before the breakdown of proteins.

Ultrastructure of Enamel Caries

Johnson (1967) exhaustively studied the electron-microscopic and transmission electron microscopic structures of both the inorganic and organic phases of the carious enamel.

Inorganic phase: In areas of advanced carious destruction of enamel, the organizational pattern of the tissue is usually more readily recognized than in the corresponding sound tissue. The location of rod sheaths becomes evident because of the loss of mineral matter and rod and inter-rod areas show reduced density of mineral distribution. These observations indicate that a generalized demineralization has occurred in the affected area with the establishment of an apparent system of microchannels between the crystallites and sometimes may be within the crystallites. Remaining crystallites are usually altered in their structure and morphology. Some present a hollow center in cross-sectional views, while others may show transverse perforations of irregular shape producing bizarre forms never observed in sound tissues.

Organic phase: The organic matrix of demineralized carious enamel often presents architecture similar to that of the sound tissue. Rod sheaths are frequently prominent in outline and not markedly altered in structure. Carious enamel may exhibit an increase in organic material as judged by the density of its distribution within the tissue. This observation probably reflects an influx of organic molecules from oral fluids.

Zones of Enamel Caries

Earlier authors used polarizing microscope to analyze the possible zones of carious process in enamel. The following four zones of enamel caries beginning from the enamel surface towards the dentinal side of the lesion have been proposed (Fig. 9.12).

Zone 1: The Surface Layer

The surface layer ranges from 20 to 100 µm. It is thinner in active lesions and thicker in inactive ones. Quantitative studies of the surface layer indicate that partial demineralization equivalent to about 1–10% loss of mineral salts has taken place and the pore volume of the surface zone is less than 5%.

After imbibing with a medium like water whose refractive index is less than that of the enamel, although the porous subsurface zone is seen to be positively birefringent, the surface zone retains a negative birefringence. This relatively unaffected surface zone is also identifiable on microradiographs as sharply demarcated from the underlying radiolucent regions of the lesion. Thus the surface zone, when examined by polarizing microscope, has been defined as the zone of negative birefringence, superficial to the positively birefringent body of lesion. It is the most unaffected zone due to the great resistance of the surface zone to decalcification because of the greater degree of mineralization of the surface (hypermineralized surface) and increased concentration of fluoride in the surface enamel where the pore volume is less than 5%.

- Surface layer relatively immune to caries due to hypermineralization (higher fluoride contact and saliva contact).
- Pore volume less than body of the lesion.
- Partial demineralization.

Zone 2: The Body of Lesion

This zone lies below the relatively unaffected surface layer. It is the largest portion of the incipient lesion in a demineralizing phase. In polarized light, the zone shows pore volume of 5% in spaces near the periphery to 25% in the center of the intact lesion.

When a longitudinal ground section is examined in quinoline with transmitted light, the body of lesion appears relatively translucent compared with sound enamel. This zone, unlike normal enamel, is positively birefringent when examined in water, denoting significant degree of mineral loss. However, the striae of Retzius within this region are well marked and therefore enhanced in contrast to sound enamel. The interprismatic areas provide access to the rod (prism) cores, which are then preferentially attacked. Bacteria may be present in this zone if the pore size is large enough to permit their entry. Studies using TEM and SEM demonstrate the presence of bacteria invading between the enamel rods (prisms) in the body zone.

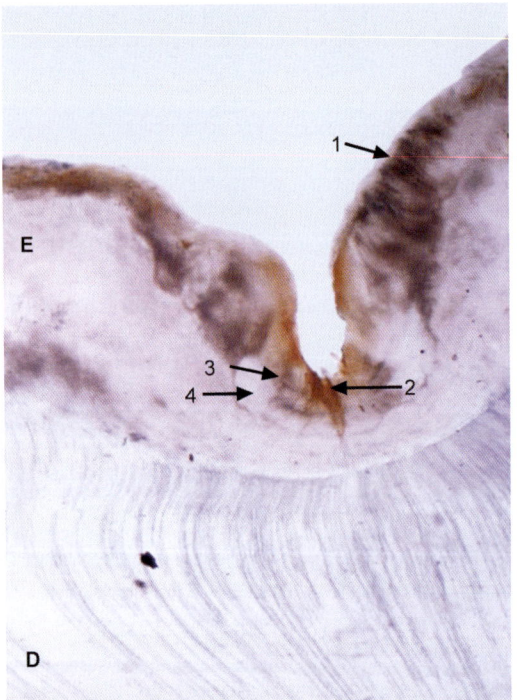

Fig. 9.12: Longitudinal ground section of tooth depicting zones of enamel caries. 1. Surface zone; 2. Body of lesion; 3.Dark zone; 4.Translucent zone.(E: Enamel; D: Dentin)

- In demineralization phase, it is the longest zone (Dark zone, or zone 3, is largest in remineralization phase).
- Large pores (pore volume 5–25%).
- Usually bacteria enter pores.
- Striae of Retzius well marked (striae of Retzius is the initial point of entry of caries into rod/prism core of enamel).

Zone 3: The Dark Zone

The dark zone lies beneath the body of the lesion and adjacent/superficial to the translucent zone. This zone appears dark brown in ground sections examined by transmitted light after imbibition with quinoline. Polarized light studies have shown that the dark zone has pore volume of 2–4%.

Dark zone shows positive birefringence in contrast to the negative birefringence of sound enamel. Hence, it is often referred to as the positive zone. These effects have shown to be due to the presence of very small pores in the zone besides the relative large pores that are present in the translucent zone. Therefore, when a ground section is examined in a mounting medium such as quinoline, the relatively larger molecules of medium are unable to penetrate the micro pore system of the dark zone. Since the micro pores remain filled with air or vapour, light is scattered on passing through the zone, causing brown discoloration of the dark zone. In a similar manner, the presence of a medium or low refractive index within micro pore system is responsible for the reversal of birefringence when examined in polarized light. If a ground section is examined under an aqueous medium having small molecule which penetrates the micro pores, the dark zone is no longer seen. There is some speculation that the dark zone is not really a stage in the sequence of the breakdown of enamel; rather, the dark zone may be formed by deposition of ions into an area previously only containing large pores. It must be remembered that caries is an episodic disease with alternating phases of demineralization and remineralization. Experimental remineralization has demonstrated increase in the size of the dark zone at the expense of the body of the lesion. There is also a loss of crystalline structure in the dark zone, suggestive of the process of demineralization and remineralization. The size of the dark zone is probably an indication of the amount of remineralization that has recently occurred.

- Many tiny pores block light transmission (smaller air/vapor filled pores make the region opaque).
- Loss of crystalline structure suggests process of demineralization and the remineralization occurring in this zone.

Zone 4: The Translucent Zone

The translucent zone lies at the base of enamel lesion and is recognized as the zone of alteration from normal enamel. Only half of lesions demonstrate this zone at their advancing front, which is seen only when longitudinal ground section is examined in clearing agent having refractive index (RI) identical to that of enamel, e.g. quinoline (RI=1.62). The name refers to its structureless appearance when perfused with quinoline solution and examined with polarized light. The spaces or pores created in the tissue in this stage of enamel caries are located at prism boundaries and other junctional sites. In this zone, the pores or voids form along the enamel prism (rod) boundaries, presumably because of the ease of hydrogen ion penetration during the carious process. When these boundary area voids are filled with quinoline solution, which has the same RI as enamel, the features of the area disappear. By means of polarized light it has been shown that this zone is slightly more porous than sound enamel, having pore volume of 1% compared with 0.1% in sound enamel. There is no evidence of protein loss in the translucent zone. It has been reported that carious attack may preferentially remove magnesium and carbonate rich minerals from translucent zone.

However, in arrested lesions, the internal porosity is reduced and the dark zone and body of lesion also decrease in size.

- Deepest zone, represent advancing front of enamel caries.
- Pores/voids form along the enamel prism (rod) boundaries (due to easy hydrogen penetration).
- Appears structureless when seen with polarized light (hence translucent).

Structural Changes of Enamel Crystals

High resolution electron microscope was used to observe the changes in enamel crystals in early carious lesions. In the demineralized zone, the crystals were mostly separated from each other, showing wide intercrystalline spaces. However, some crystals remained in close contact, keeping their original tightly packed arrangement. The transverse sections of the crystals frequently exhibited perforations in their centers, especially in those that had become separated from their neighbors and defects of various sizes on the lateral surfaces of these crystals. Frequently, the central perforations had apparently been opened by fusion with lateral defects.

Under high magnification, the inner density of the crystals appears inhomogeneous, showing a number of small electron-lucent spots, suggesting the start of dissolution. The enlargement of the perforations seemed to progress along the central dark line by involving the electron-lucent spots. Stereoscopic observation revealed that the central perforation had penetrated deep through the crystal, indicating the rapid dissolution progressed rapidly in this direction. In the regions with the presence of small spots, however, the enlargement of the defects also progressed involving the spots. The central dark line seems to be rather resistant to dissolution. One of the main factors for the central perforation of the crystals is thought to be the presence of especially large numbers of defective sites.

Natural Enamel Caries in Polarized Light Microscopy

Polarized light microscopy is more sensitive for contrasting normal from carious enamel than absorption-based techniques. One of the most influential contributions to the field of caries pathology came from the interpretation of birefringence of carious enamel under polarized light microscopy. Birefringence from enamel comes from the mineral (intrinsic birefringence, with negative sign) and the non-mineral volumes (form birefringence, with positive sign); so that the image of enamel in polarized light microscopy (the observed birefringence) is a result of the sum of these two types of birefringence. A mathematical approach to interpret enamel birefringence to obtain structural information at histological points has also been purposed.

Features of Different Enamel Carious Zones

De Medeiros RCG, et al (2012) presented histopathological features of human enamel caries by comparing the two different approaches to interpret enamel birefringence (Table 9.1). First by the use of immersion media with various refractive indices and molecular sizes (air, aqueous and oil media) in ground sections of the same lesion and second by the application of a mathematical approach for the analysis of pore sizes and volume. Enamel birefringence in different immersion media (air, water and quinoline) was interpreted by both qualitative and quantitative approaches, the former lead to an underestimation of the depth of enamel caries mainly when the criterion of validating sound enamel as a negatively birefringent area in immersion in water was used (a current common practice in dental research). They found that the optical properties of enamel play a significant role in the diagnosis of dental caries. The criteria of diagnosing normal enamel as translucent (in transmitted and reflected light) and negatively birefringent tissue in a single immersion

Table 9.1: Carious zones of enamel

Zones	Pore size/distribution	Mineral loss	Birefringence	X-ray absorption (with respect to unaffected enamel)
Zone 1 Surface layer	Intact enamel with higher density of pores	~10%	Negative	Approximating unaffected enamel
Zone 2 Body of the lesion	Decreased number of pores. Homo-geneous pore size distribution between 50 and 200 μm	~24%	Positive	Reduced (~75% of unaffected enamel)
Zone 3 Dark zone	Homogeneous pore size distribution between 50 and 200 μm	~6%	Positive	Approximating unaffected enamel
Zone 4 Translucent zone	Prevalence of larger pores (above 100 μ)	~1%	Negative	Slightly reduced (~93% of unaffected enamel)

medium needs revision. Regarding the histopathological features from polarized light microscopy, new efforts are needed to get a description that can be applied universally and comply with mineral volume measured by microradiography. One way of getting this might be by the more detailed interpretation of birefringence.

Histological Study on Biochemical Volumes

Sousa, et al (2005) compared the biochemical data (derived from interpretation of enamel birefringence) to diffusion/permeability at histological points of natural enamel caries and normal enamel and concluded as follows:

- Natural enamel caries presents a higher than normal organic content with a profile that decreases from the surface layer inward;
- Surface layer of natural enamel caries presents a mean mineral content lower than that of the body of the lesion and normal enamel;
- Surface layer of natural enamel caries presents alpha D (water volume more easily available for diffusion) values lower than that of the body of the lesion, similar to that of normal enamel and lower than

that of the surface layer of artificial enamel caries.

Hence, mineral, water and organic volumes are considered to predict permeability at histological zones of enamel caries, a new insight for studying remineralization and infiltration of enamel caries related to natural and artificial caries lesions.

Nanostructure of Carious Enamel

Smooth surface caries has been studied extensively, not just because of its epidemiological importance, but also because a relatively simple geometry facilitates studies and experimental modeling. Lesions have been studied in many ways, including macroscopic examination, hard tissue histology, light microscopy, SEM, TEM, microradiography, micro and nano indenta-tion, histochemical, microbiological and chemical analyses and X-ray imaging techniques. These methods have provided an in depth information as regard to various zones identified in carious process.

Electron microscopy has been used to observe microstructural changes such as clefts or channels in incipient lesions and to identify demineralization and remineralization induced changes to individual crystallites, but generally only after they have been removed from their original spatial organizational positions and associations with their neighbors. Detailed understanding or mapping of the entire lesion at the level of individual crystallites and porosities remain elusive.

Various authors have used differences in optical birefringence caused by the submicroscopic pores produced during demineralization to divide the smooth surface lesion into the four histological zones as mentioned above. However, this classification does not describe changes in crystallite structure or organization. Furthermore, smaller and deeper pores are not recognized by birefringence. As an early carious lesion may be only 0.1–0.2 mm in total thickness and because features within a moderate lesion may be <0.1 mm thick, increased point density is needed to study the four zones generally used to describe smooth surface caries. The combination of small angle X-ray scattering (SAXS) with real-space scanning allows for the investigation of a tooth's nano-structural components over extended areas through the acquisition of thousand scattering patterns.

SAXS is capable of delivering structural information about macromolecules or crystallites and of repeat distances in partially ordered systems as small as a few nanometers in size and up to several hundred nanometers. This range is well suited to study hydroxyapatite crystallite and collagen periodicities, the primary components of tooth structure.

The combination of SAXS with real-space scanning allows for the investigation of nano-structural components of tooth over extended areas through the acquisition of over thousand scattering patterns.

Deyhle H, et al (2011) used scanning SAXS with raster-scan step sizes of 20×20 μm^2 which allows the identification and comparison of morphological differences within and among carious zones with respect to structural organization.

The second zone, body of lesion, has higher anisotropy. In the third zone, anisotropy is decreased, indicating that re-deposition processes give rise to at least partially isotropic structures. It appears that, despite caries-induced destruction, the structural anisotropy of the affected enamel in fourth zone is preserved. The retention of organization, despite demineralization, has important implications for the potential to not only remineralize the demineralized enamel, but to do so in the original organizational form at the nanostructural level.

The fact that both orientation and anisotropy of the SAXS signal from carious enamel closely resembled those from unaffected regions reinforces the notion that naturally occurring demineralization and remineralization produce an anisotropic structure that retains the original nanoscale organization. This current SAXS data, demonstrating the preservation of orientation in carious lesions, independent of degree of demineralization or pore morphology over 20–200 nm, advances the understanding of the effects of demineralization and remineralization cycles at the crystallite level.

Saini R, et al (2007) identified microscopic changes at surface and subsurface levels in different carious lesions by using Confocal Laser Scanning Microscope (CLSM) and Image analyzer (light microscopy). In all the samples seen under Confocal Laser Scanning Microscopy, sound enamel and dentin did not show autofluorescence. Autofluorescence distribution from carious area depicted the extent of demineralization in the tissue. The marked differences between control sound enamel and dentin and carious area of the samples showed that a correlation existed between the zone of autofluorescence, demineralization and carious dentin that was softened due to carious process.

Marzuki and Masudi (2008) examined histopathological and morphological changes in dentinal tubules of dentin caries stained with alizarin red using Confocal Laser Scanning Microscopy. The serial images of dentinal tubules were taken and optimum images of three-dimensional structures were reconstructed using software of CLSM. Histopathological changes of dentinal tubules in human carious teeth showed areas of demineralized dentin, translucent zone and normal area. The dentinal tubules were thin and had numerous branches. They concluded that confocal microscopy study is a useful adjunct to reveal histopathological changes in dentinal tubules affected by carious lesions.

Magnus L, et al (2013) evaluated the concentrations of calcium, inorganic phosphate and fluoride in carious dentin and in different layers of sound dentin. Calcium and phosphate were analyzed using a colorimetric method with arsenazo III and molybdate reagents and fluoride was analyzed using a specific electrode. Lower amounts of calcium and inorganic phosphate were seen in carious dentin as compared to sound dentin. These results were found to be consistent with the pathology of dental caries, which is characterized by mineral loss.

Lee, et al (2013) analyzed the expression of MMP-13 in crown and root of normal and carious dentin by western blot analysis. MMP-13 expression was found to be increased with severity of caries in root dentin. They concluded that increase in MMP-13 expression plays an important role in caries progression.

HISTOPATHOLOGY OF DENTINAL CARIES

Dentin provides general form to the tooth. It is 2.0–2.5 mm thick in crown and 1.0–1.5 mm thick in roots; characterized as a hard tissue with tubules throughout its thickness. It contains within its tubules the processes of the specialized cells, the odontoblasts. Odontoblasts, located at the peripheral zone of the pulp adjacent to the pre-dentin account for the vitality of dentin. Caries in dentin begins along the dentino-enamel junction with the rapid involvement of greater

number of dentinal tubules. These dentinal tubules act as tract leading to the dental pulp (Fig. 9.13). The micro-organisms may also travel along these tubules. According to Arnold, et al (2000), the demineralization of dentin causes a patho-morphological reaction of the dentin pulp complex in response to the carious attack, resulting in peritubular, intratubular and reactive dentin deposition within the dentinal tubules and pulp chamber. The caries progressing into dentin have been shown differently by earlier authors.

Fusayama and co-workers divided carious dentin into two zones based on 10 seconds staining with a 0.5% solution of basic fuschin. The outer or first carious layer corresponds to the zone of decomposed dentin and the bacterial invasion stains red with fuschin. The inner or second carious layer does not take up the fuschin stain on short exposure. Histochemical techniques using the Mallory-Azan stain were used to distinguish between the outer layer which stains red and the inner layer which stains blue. In the outer carious dentin the cross-linkage is reduced. These biochemical findings suggested that remineralization can occur only in the inner layer where the collagen denaturation is reversible, depending on the pH.

Dentinal caries have been divided into following four zones based on staining characteristics. These zones may assist clinicians during caries removal.

a. Pink.

b. Light pink.

c. Transparent.

d. Apparently normal dentin.

However, this division of zones remained unclear, visualizing as to what characteristics of the lesion are stained or how staining is related to microstructural features of various carious zones. Not all stainable dentin is infected and also the absence of stain does not ensure bacterial elimination.

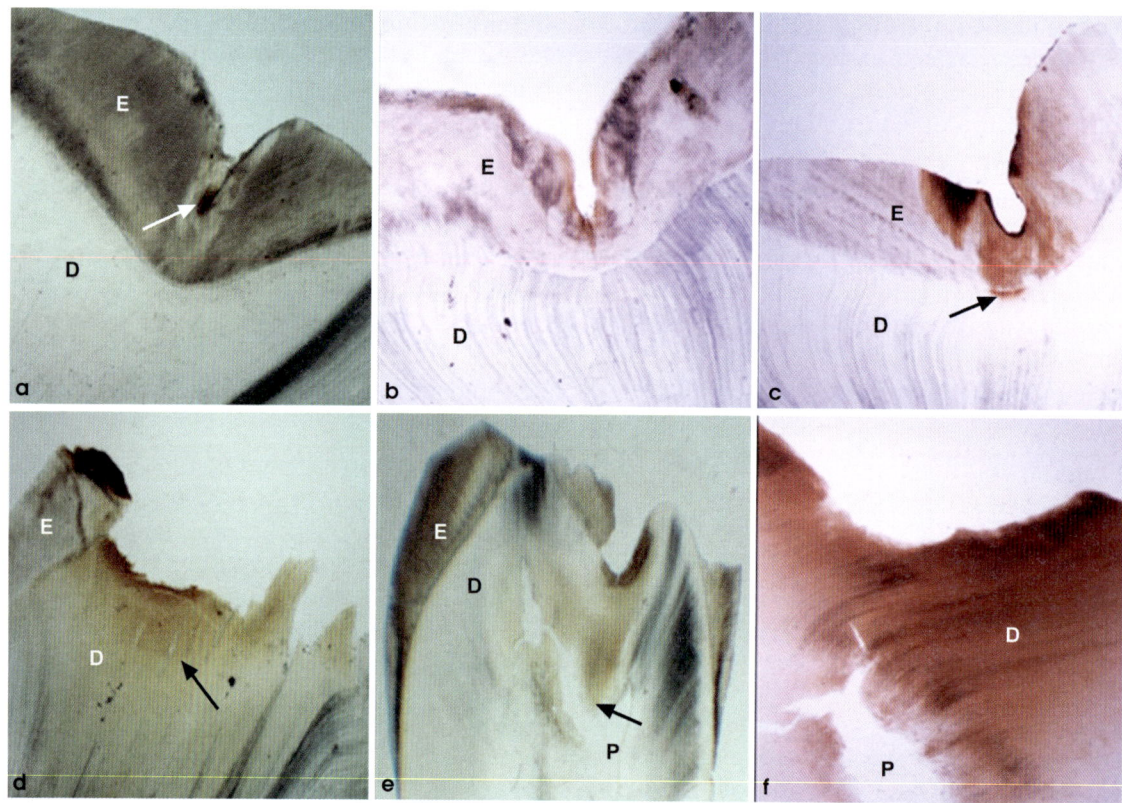

Fig. 9.13: Longitudinal ground sections of teeth with different stages of progression of occlusal carious lesions (a) occlusal pit; (b) early enamel caries; (c) advanced enamel caries with early involvement of dentin (arrow); (d) caries involving the dentin; (e and f) carious lesion penetrating the dentin and extending towards pulp. (E: Enamel; D: Dentin; P: Pulp)

Later, Arnold, et al (2003) classified carious dentin into the following six zones:

a. Softened dentin.

b. Demineralized dentin.

c. Bacterial invasion into the tubules.

d. Translucency zone of dead tracts.

e. Hypermineralized translucent zone.

f. Secondary dentin.

However, classification of carious dentin into two different layers—caries infected dentin (CID) and caries affected dentin (CAD) is accepted.

Caries infected dentin (CID) is a superficial layer, full of pathogenic bacteria and bacterial by-products. It is characterized by destruction of mineral matrix or crystal. This stage could not be remineralized due to high levels of decalcification or demineralization. On histological evaluation of this layer, degraded collagen fibers with disruption of cross-links were observed. The discontinuation of cross-links indicated an irreversible stage of collagen, or denatured collagen and thus, demonstrating the unremineralizable nature of this layer. Caries affected dentin (CAD) constituting the inner zone is partly but highly heterogeneously demineralized. This zone is free of bacteria and is remineralizable due to the presence of sound collagen fibers and presence of hydroxyapatite crystals. This zone should ideally be preserved during tooth preparation.

Active Caries of Dentin

The carious process after invading enamel, reaches dentino-enamel junction (DEJ) and spread laterally. The spread into dentin is orthograde due to its histology and mineralization. The progress and speed of caries in dentin is characterized by following five zones starting from pulp to DEJ (Fig. 9.14).

Zone 1: Zone of Fatty Degeneration of Tomes' Fibers

This zone is present at the most pulpal end of dentinal caries. Due to the irritation from bacterial products, the fats get deposited in the Tomes' fibers. When stained with Sudan red; two types of fat lipids are evident in this zone: one from the bacterial products and other derived from the dissolution of the intratubular dentin. The peritubular and intertubular dentin remain intact. The term 'fatty degeneration' is misnomer, as there is no fatty degeneration of Tomes' fibers;

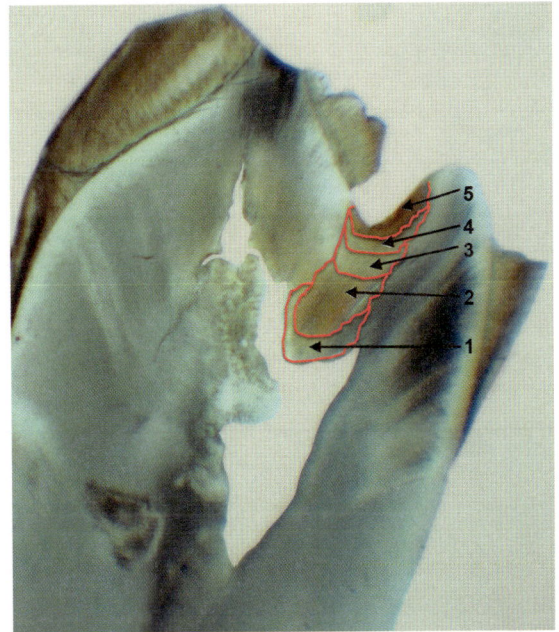

Fig. 9.14: Longitudinal ground section of tooth depicting zones of dentinal caries. (1) Zone of fatty degeneration of Tomes' fibers, (2) Zone of dentinal sclerosis, (3) Zone of decalcification, (4) Zone of bacterial invasion, (5) Zone of decomposed dentin

however, there is deposition of fat in Tomes' fibers.

- Characterized by presence of a layer of fat globules (stains red with Sudan red stain).
- Fat layer leads to impermeability of the dentinal tubules—trying to prevent further invasion of carious lesion.
- Also favors sclerosis of dentin in zone 2.

Zone 2: Zone of Dentinal Sclerosis

This zone is characterized by deposition of mineral salts in the dentinal tubules leading to the calcification of intratubular dentin. It is a reaction of vital dentinal tubules and vital pulp so as to seal off the healthy tooth structure from the diseased one and also prevent further penetration of the micro-organisms into healthy tooth. The formation of sclerotic dentin is minimal in rapidly advancing caries and is more evident in chronic caries. When viewed under transmitted light it is transparent; whereas, in reflected light it is dark. The peritubular and intertubular dentin are evident in this layer. The translucent dentinal tubules will be localized precisely beneath the demineralized enamel surface and will appear even before the enamel demineralization has reached the dentino-enamel junction.

- Calcification of dentinal tubules as a reaction of vital pulp to carious invasion so as to prevent invasion of micro-organisms.
- Sclerotic dentin appears white in transmitted light.

Zone 3: Zone of Decalcification of Dentin

This is a narrow zone preceding the bacterial invasion. The peritubular dentin is absent in some areas of the inner part of this zone; whereas, it is intact in the outer part. In intertubular dentin the collagen is normally present and the inorganic contents are mostly dissolved. The decalcification commences from the lateral walls of the tubules leading to their distension as they get filled with microbes in next zone. In early stage of caries, when only a few of the tubules are involved, micro-organisms may be found penetrating these tubules before there is any clinical evidence of carious process—'the pioneer bacteria'. Examination of individual tubules has shown almost pure form of bacteria, i.e. one tubule may be filled with cocci, while the adjacent tubules may contain only bacilli or spirocheates.

A few authors have enumerated the total bacterial population present in carious human dentin by using fluorescent in situ hybridization. A mean of 7.34×10^6, 5.23×10^6 and 1.69×10^6 bacteria/mg in superficial, middle and deep zones respectively has been documented. In the advancing zone, a mean of 0.34×10^6 total bacteria/mg dentin was recorded.

- Initially only walls of dentinal tubules get decalcified.
- Bacteria present in individual dentinal tubules are in pure form (i.e. either completely cocci or completely bacilli and not in mixed variety).
- Presence of 'pioneer bacteria' before there is any clinical evidence of caries.

Zone 4: Zone of Bacterial Invasion

In this zone, bacterial invasion of the decalcified, intact dentin occurs. Abundance of bacteria are present in the enlarged lumens of dentinal tubules or intratubular dentin. In the early stages, acidogenic bacteria are in abundance and in deeper layer—proteolytic bacteria replace the acidogenic bacteria. This zone supports the hypothesis that initiation is by acidogenic bacteria and the progression is by proteolytic ones. Acidogenic bacteria utilize carbohydrates while proteolytic bacteria utilize dentinal protein for their metabolism. Even the intertubular dentin is invaded by bacteria in advanced carious lesions. Inner peritubular dentin is completely absent and the outer peritubular dentin is present only in parts. Inorganic content of

peritubular dentin is absent but not entirely; whereas, collagen fibers are present.

- Presence of micro-organisms; in early stages only acidogenic bacteria and in progress proteolytic bacteria predominate.

Zone 5: Zone of Decomposed or Necrotic Dentin

Due to the bacterial invasion of dentinal tubules in the zone 4, there is an increase in diameter of these tubules; which are further broken down and coalesced so as to form the ovoid areas of destruction—known as liquefaction foci of Miller. Also, thickening and swelling of sheath of Neumann may sometimes be noted at irregular intervals in this zone. The liquefaction foci are present parallel to the course of dentinal tubules. It is filled with necrotic debris that tends to expand with time resulting in compression and distortion of adjacent dentinal tubules, thus further increasing the carious lesions. Inner peritubular dentin is absent completely and the outer peritubular dentin is faintly present. Inorganic content of intertubular dentin is almost entirely absent; whereas, collagen is present in early stages. This zone is most distinct in advanced dentinal caries.

- No recognizable structure seen.
- Collagen and minerals seem absent.
- Correct number of bacteria dispersed in this decomposed granular matter.
- Most superficial zone of dentin caries.

Arrested Caries of Dentin

Caries can get arrested both in enamel and dentin. The mechanism and the conditions favoring caries arrest are similar for both enamel and dentin.

Since the structural composition of enamel and dentin differ, the histopathological features in arrested carious lesions also differ. The carious lesions of enamel get easily arrested as compared to dentin because the meshwork of organic fibers are much more in dentin than in enamel. The histopathological features of arrested dentinal caries are as follows:

a. Leathery Surface Layer

This layer simulates the necrotic layer of the active lesions; however, it is denser and more mineralized. It is homogeneous calcified border of approximately 2.0–5.0 μm in width. Dentinal tubules house foci of calcifications. Intratubular dentin in this layer contains some bacteria. Inner peritubular dentin is absent and the outer peritubular dentin is completely calcified. In intertubular dentin, inorganic contents are increased and even the collagen fibers are mineralized. Occasionally, bacteria are seen in 'lacunae' within intertubular matrix. Collagen fibers of intertubular area retained their banded appearance.

b. Pigmented Layer

The pigmented layer has following two distinct zones:

  i. **Upper zone:** This corresponds to the zone of bacterial invasion in active carious lesions. Intratubular dentin in this zone contains bacteria coalesced inside the enlarged lumens of dentinal tubules. Inner peritubular dentin is thinned out and the outer peritubular dentin is present as in normal dentin. Intertubular dentin remains and its collagen fibers are mineralized. Dentinal tubules are increased in diameter and their shape and width is irregular.

  ii. **Deep pigmented zone:** This corresponds to the zone of decalcification of dentin of the active carious lesion. The intratubular dentin is bacteria free but the lumens of dentinal tubules are enlarged. Inner peritubular dentin is widened and the outer peritubular dentin is normal. Intertubular dentin appears normal.

c. Transitional Zone

Between the pigmented zone and underlying sclerotic dentin, a bacteria free zone is present. Intratubular dentin in this zone is without bacteria. Some dentinal tubules are calcified while others are normal. Both peritubular and intertubular dentin appears normal.

d. Sclerotic Zone

This is the white opaque zone present on the most pulpal side of the lesion. The main feature is the homogeneous, dense calcifications of tubules which completely or almost completely occlude the lumen. The calcified tubules are continuous with the peritubular dentin. Peritubular dentin appears normal. Intertubular dentin may be normal or hypermineralized.

Histopathology of Carious Process in Secondary Dentin

The carious involvement of secondary dentin does not differ remarkably from the involvement of primary dentin, except that it is usually somewhat slower because the dentinal tubules are fewer in number and more irregular in their course, thus delaying the penetration of the invading micro-organisms.

Ultrastructural Changes in Dentinal Caries

Various authors have studied the micro-structure of dentin. The changes have been described in two phases—inorganic and organic phases.

  a. *Inorganic phase:* In hypermineralized pericanalicular zones, persisting crystallites are often found in relatively large numbers which represent the remnants of corresponding hypermineralized structures in sound tissue. Intercanalicular areas constitute only a sparse distribution of crystallites, reflecting extensive demineralization. Individual crystallites are seen either as narrow, dense profiles or as broad, less dense plate-like structures associated with remaining collagenous fibrils. Based on chemical analysis of the soft carious dentin, it has been suggested that persisting crystallites accumulate fluoride from their fluid environment as the lesion progressed.

b. *Organic phase:* In extensively demineralized soft carious dentin, the network of collagenous fibrils is found to be relatively intact, except in the most superficial areas of the lesion. Staining procedures revealed that most of the fibrils displayed banding characteristic of unaltered collagen. These findings support the hypothesis that proteolysis occurred after the tissue had been demineralized. The canals of carious dentin are usually filled with plenty of micro-organisms.

The replacement of odontoblastic process by amorphous material has been detected by electron microscopy. Crystals present in the amorphous material eventually occlude the tubules with minerals. Two types of crystals have been observed: plate like hydroxyapatite crystals and large rhomboidal crystals. They have been identified as whitlockite by electron diffraction. These crystals result from reprecipitation of ions dissolved from dentin during carious process.

Agematsu, et al (2005) studied the relationship between large tubules and dentinal caries in human deciduous teeth that showed different ranges of attrition but no macroscopical carious lesions. Longitudinal sections of the teeth had been observed under scanning electron microscope. Dense collagen fibers run parallel to its long axis and aggregates of small spherical bodies in each large tubule but without any marked attrition. In attritioned teeth, bacteria infiltrated the large tubules through exposed dentin. In teeth with advanced attrition, large tubules and surrounding matrix are difficult to be distinguished with higher bacterial invasion in both areas. Through these findings, they supported the hypothesis that large tubules played a role in pathway of caries in coronal dentin and suggested that early treatment of exposed dentin surfaces might help in caries prevention.

Zavgorodniy AV, et al (2008) investigated the ultrastructural changes in different zones of carious dentin by transmission electron microscope (TEM) and electron diffraction techniques. They observed decreased size of intertubular mineral crystallites as the carious lesion progressed. In the transparent zone of carious lesion, both intratubular and intertubular dentin consisted of nano-size apatite crystallites with smaller size in the intratubular dentin. They suggested that a 'dissolution and precipitation' mechanism is important in understanding the process of formation of intratubular dentin within the transparent zone induced by caries attack.

Pugach MK, et al (2009) investigated the physical and microstructural properties of carious dentin in four different zones, i.e. pink, light pink; transparent and apparently normal by atomic force microscopy (AFM) imaging for microstructure and by transverse digital microradiography (DMR) for mineral content. Microstructure changes, mechanical properties and mineral content have been found to be significantly reduced in these areas. Hydrated elastic modulus and mineral content from normal dentin to Caries-Detector-stained dentin ranged from 19.5 GPa to 1.6 GPa and from 42.9 vol% to 12.4 vol%, respectively. Thus, analysis of data suggested that the pink zone, which is commonly removed by the clinician, could contain residual mineral and thus, may be worth retaining.

HISTOPATHOLOGY OF ROOT CARIES

The study of histopathology of root caries is divided into caries of cementum and caries of root dentin.

a. Cemental Caries

The cemental caries is quite different from the enamel and dentinal caries as the cementum is composed of more organic and less mineralized components as compared to enamel and dentin (Fig. 9.15).

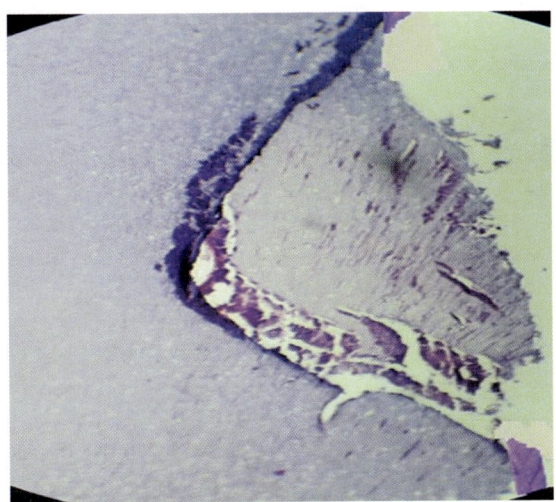

Fig. 9.15: The micropictograph of a carious tooth depicting small clefts traversing the cementum and extending into dentin

Active Caries

The attempt to describe the active carious lesions of root was made by Nyvad and Fejerskov. It was Schupbach P and his associates who gave the detailed description of the cemental caries in 1989. They described that active cemental caries histopathologically can have three patterns:

- *Pattern I:* This pattern is found most predominantly and is due to the high intensity acid attack in the oral cavity after exposure to sugars.

  It is characterized by the uniform demineralization of both cementum and its underlying dentin. The incremental lines of cementum are accentuated in these lesions. Cementum has higher degree of residual mineral components than the affected dentin.

- *Pattern II:* This pattern is generally present in the abraded, eroded or denuded surfaces either clinically or microscopically.

  This pattern is evident in roots exposed to mild acid attack. Initially, small clefts transversing the cementum and extending into dentin are present. These first get enlarged and then filled with microbes subsequently. These enlarged clefts with microbes form the microcavities exposing the peripheral dentin. Eventually, the exposed peripheral dentin gets covered by microbes and cementum borders get undermined by the micro-organisms. The destruction of cementum occurred stepwise along the fractures following incremental lines of cementum. In this pattern, no immediate bacterial invasion of peripheral dentin occurs.

- *Pattern III:* This pattern is least distinct and is found in the areas where demineralization and remineralization processes are going simultaneously, e.g. in the persons having high exposure to fluorides. In this pattern, a surface remineralized layer of 10–30 µm thickness is present. It is interrupted over well-defined areas of advanced demineralization. Uniform demineralization of cementum and peripheral dentin is the characteristic feature of these lesions.

b. Root Dentin Caries (Fig. 9.16)

i. Initial Lesions

The initial lesions have a mineralized surface layer of 10–20 µm over them. The multiple clefts present in the cementum enter the dentin along with their micro-organisms. These clefts spread laterally towards the pulp, fuse with each other to form the microcavities filled with microbes. As they enlarge further, the bacteria moved deeper towards the open dentinal tubules. A distinct clearly demarcated layer of complete demineralization can be distinguished from underlying intact dentin. The spread of caries occurs along the dentinal tubules through intertubular dentin.

ii. Advanced Lesions

Microradiographically advanced lesions of root dentin have shown various areas of both radiolucency and radiopacity with following two predominating patterns:

- *First pattern:* In this pattern, the radiolucent areas appeared as enlarged lesions with variable extent and depth along the

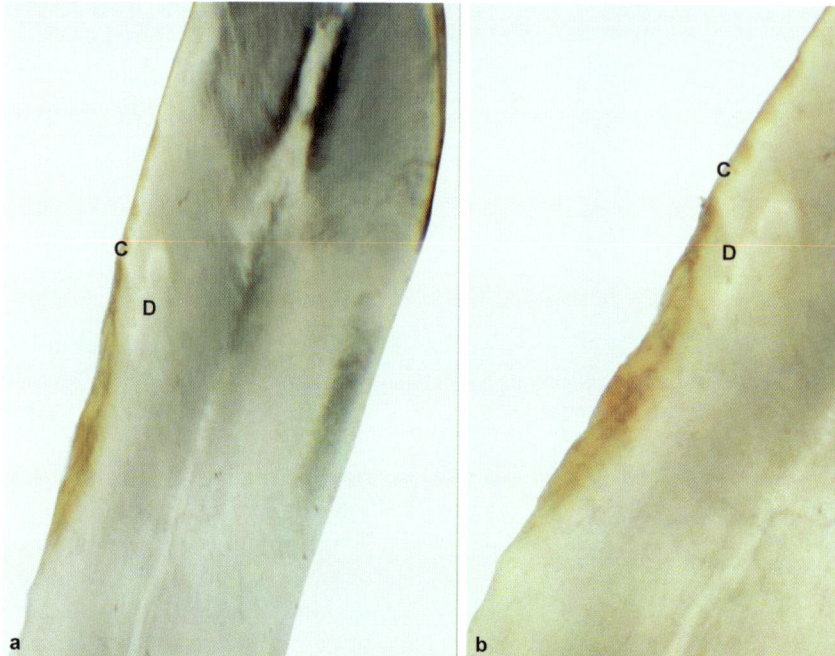

Fig. 9.16a and b: Longitudinal ground section of tooth depicting root surface caries lesion involving cementum (C) and dentin (D) with apparent considerable surface abrasion

exposed root surface. Some of the radiolucent areas are covered by the radiodense layer while others are not. In addition, radiodense layers were observed bordering the radiolucent areas over the inner dentin.

- *Second pattern:* In this pattern, only a single radiolucent saucer shaped area extending into dentin is present. Occasionally, this area is covered by the radiodense layer in parts. Rarely, a band-like radiopaque layer is present around the radiolucent lesion.

Histopathologically, the radiolucent and radiodense areas show the following features:

Radiolucent area
- Intertubular dentin is almost completely demineralized.
- Dentinal tubules and their lateral branches are occupied by micro-organisms.
- Peritubular dentin of those tubules is absent.

Radiodense area
- Accumulations of small needle like crystals throughout them.
- Massive spread of microbes is present.
- Microbes penetrating the dentinal tubules spread laterally, along the (parallel to) collagen fibers and reach adjacent tubules.
- Subsequently, the micro-organisms totally engulf the dentinal tubules.
- They, then form a radiodense band bordering the demineralized areas present towards inner dentin.

iii. *Arrested Lesions*
There are two types of arrested lesions in root dentin:
- *Truly/definitely arrested lesions:* These lesions are completely mineralized, with a distinct zone of tubular sclerosis. Dentinal tubules appear as solid rods embedded in partially demineralized dentin. The occlusion of dentinal tubules occurs with fine granular crystals.

Table 9.2: Comprehensive review of literature of the studies conducted on histopathology of dental caries

Author (Year)	Objective	Technique	Findings
Arnold WH (2000)	Investigation of the micro-morphology and progression of natural caries lesions in permanent teeth	Computer-assisted three-dimensional reconstruction technique and volumetric assessment using polarized light microscopy	There are usually more than one individual initial carious lesions at the approximal tooth surface
Banerjee A (2002)	Quantification of bacteria in human carious dentin	Fluorescent in situ hybridization	Increase in number of bacteria with increasing depth of carious lesions
Wany Y (2007)	Detection of the chemical profile of adhesive/caries affected dentin interface	Micro-raman microspectroscopy	Both the structure of collagen and mineral in the caries-affected dentin has been altered by the caries process
Saini R (2007)	Microscopic changes at surface and subsurface levels in different carious lesions	Confocal Laser Scanning Microscope (CLSM) and Image analyzer (light microscopy)	Sound enamel and dentin did not show autofluorescence Autofluorescence distribution from carious area depicted the extent of remineralization in the tissue
Zavgorodniy AV (2008)	To investigate the ultra-structural changes in the different zones of carious dentin	Transmission Electron Microscopy and Electron Diffraction Techniques	Dissolution and precipitation mechanism is important in understanding the process of formation of intratubular dentin within the transparent zone induced by caries attack
Marzuki (2008)	Detection of the histopatho-logical changes in dentinal tubules affected by carious lesions	Confocal microscopy	It is a useful adjunct to reveal histopathological changes in dentinal tubules affected by carious lesions
Pugach MK (2009)	Physical and micro-structural properties of carious dentin in the 4 different zones, i.e pink, light pink, transparent and apparently normal	Atomic force microscopy (AFM), transverse digital microradiography (TMR)	Found that the pink zone, which is commonly removed by the clinician, could contain residual mineral and thus may be worth retaining
De Medeiros RCG, et al (2012)	Differences in the histo-pathological features of enamel caries derived from a qualitative versus quantitative interpretation of enamel birefringence	Polarized light microscopy	The optical properties of enamel play a significant role in the diagnosis of dental caries
Magnus L, et al (2013)	To evaluate the concen-trations of calcium and inorganic phosphate	Colorimetric method with arsenazo III and molyb-date reagents	They found lower amounts of calcium and inorganic phosphate in carious dentin as compared to sound dentin

Contd..

Table 9.2: Comprehensive review of literature of the studies conducted on histopathology of dental caries (*Contd..*)

Author (Year)	Objective	Technique	Findings
Lee, et al (2013)	To analyze MMP-13 expression in crown and root of normal and caries dentin	Western blot analysis	MMP-13 was present in radicular dentin. MMP-13 was not expressed in the coronal dentin groups. MMP-13 expression was increased with caries progression in root dentin
Sousa, et al (2013)	Relation of biochemical data (derived from inter-pretation of enamel birefringence) to diffusion/permeability at histological points of natural enamel caries and normal enamel	Biochemical volumes	Mineral, water and organic volumes are considered to predict permeability at histo-logical zones of enamel caries, a new insight for studying remineralization and infiltration of enamel caries related to natural and artificial caries lesions
Deyhle H, et al (2014)	Identification and comparison of morpho-logical differences within and among carious zones with respect to structural organization	Scanning small-angle X-ray scattering (SAXS)	Both orientation and aniso-tropy of the SAXS signal from carious enamel closely resembled those from unaffected regions reinforce the notion that naturally occurring demineralization and remineralization produce an anisotropic structure that retains the original nano scale organization

- *Intermediate/mixed lesions:* These lesions show a mineralized surface layer and underneath this layer, a mineralization front advancing into demineralization zone is present.

Both of these lesions have common features which are enumerated below:

- Intertubular dentin is completely minerali-zed till surface.
- Their surface is covered with microbes.
- The dentinal tubules near the surface are packed with ghosts of micro-organisms.

Comprehensive review of literature of the studies conducted on histopathology of dental caries is mentioned in Table 9.2.

Bibliography

1. Agematsu H, Abe S, Shiozaki S, Usami A, Ogata S, Suzuki K, Soejima M, Ohnishi M, Nonami K and Ide Y. Relationship between large tubules and dentin caries in human deciduous teeth. Bull. Tokyo Dent. Coll.: 2005;46:7–15.
2. Angmar B, Carlstrom D and Glas J-E S. Studies on the ultrastructure of dental enamel. IV. The mineralization of normal human enamel. J. Ultrastr. Res.: 1963;8:12–23.
3. Arnold WH, Gaengler P and Saeuberlich E. Distribution and volumetric assessment of initial approximal caries lesions in human premolars and permanent molars using computer-aided three-dimensional reconstruction. Arch Oral Biol: 2000;45:1065–71.
4. Arnold WH, Konopka S, Kriwalsky MS and Gaengler P. Morphological analysis and chemical

content of natural dentin carious lesion zones. Ann. Anat. 2003b; 185: 419–424.

5. Banerjee A, Yasseri M and Munson M. A method for the detection and quantification of bacteria in human carious dentin using fluorescent in situ hybridization. J Dent.: 2002;30:359–63.

6. Barbosa de Sousa F, Dias Soares J and Sampaio Vianna S. Natural Enamel Caries: A Comparative Histological Study on Biochemical Volumes. Caries research: 2013;47:183–92.

7. Cloitre T, Panayotov IV, Tassery H, Gergely C, Levallois B and Cuisinier FJG. Multiphoton imaging of the dentin-enamel junction. J. Biophotonics: 2012;1–9.

8. Darling AI. Histopathology of enamel caries from birefringence: the surface layer. Br. Dent. J.: 1958; 105:119–35.

9. de Almeida Nevesa A, Coutinho E, Cardoso MV, Lambrechts P and Meerbeek B. Current Concepts and Techniques for Caries Excavation and Adhesion to Residual Dentin. J. Adhes. Dent.: 2011;13:7–22.

10. de Medeiros RCG, Soares JD and de Sousa FB. Natural enamel caries in polarized light microscopy: differences in histopathological features derived from a qualitative versus a quantitative approach to interpret enamel birefringence. Journal of Microscopy: 2012;246: 177–89.

11. Deyhle H, Bunk O and Muller B. Nanostructure of healthy and caries-affected human teeth. Nanomed Nanotechnol: 2011;7:694–701.

12. Deyhle H, White SN, Bunk O, Beckmann F and Muller B. Nanostructure of carious tooth enamel lesion. Acta Biomaterialia: 2014;10:355–64.

13. Fearnhead RW. Matrix-mineral relationships in enamel tissues. J. Dent. Res.: 1979;58:909–21.

14. Frank RM. Tooth enamel: current state of the art. J. Dent. Res.: 1979;58:684–94.

15. Gustafson G. The histopathology of caries of human dental enamel with special reference to the division of the carious lesion into zones. Acta. Odontol. Scand.: 1957;15:13–55.

16. Hardwick JL and Manley EB. Caries of the enamel and acidogenic caries. Br. Dent. J.: 1952;92:225–36.

17. Harrison JW and Roda RS. Intermediate cementum: development, structure, composition and potential functions. Oral Surg. Oral Med. Oral Pathol. Oral Radiol. Endod.: 1995;79:624–33.

18. Hashizume LN, Shinada K, Kawaguchi Y and Yamashita Y. Sequence of ultrastructural changes of enamel crystals and *Streptococcus mutans*

biofilm in early enamel caries *in vitro*. J. Med. Dent. Sci.: 2002;49:67–75.

19. Ho SP, Balooch M, Goodis HE, Marshall GW and Marshall SJ. Ultrastructure and nanomechanical properties of cementum dentin junction. J Biomed Mater Res 2004;68:343–351.

20. Hurlbutt M. Dental Caries: A pH mediated disease. CDHA: 2010;25:9–15.

21. Ichijo T, Yamashita Y and Terashima T. Observations on the structural features and characteristics of biological apatite crystals (2) Observation on the ultrastructure of human enamel crystals. J. Med. Dent. Sci.: 1992;39:71–80.

22. Ichijo T, Yamashita Y and Terashima T. Observations on structural features and characteristics of biological apatite crystals (9) Observation on dissolution of carious enamel crystals. J. Med. Dent. Sci.: 1994;41:1–13.

23. Johansen E. Microstructure of Enamel and Dentin. J. Dent. Res.: 1964;43:1007–20.

24. Johnson NW. Some aspects of the ultrastructure of early human enamel caries seen with electron microscope. Arch. Oral Biol.: 1967;12:1505–1521.

25. Johnson NW. Transmission electron microscopy of early carious enamel. Caries Res.: 1967;1:356–9.

26. Kidd EAM and Fejerskov O. What Constitutes Dental Caries? Histopathology of Carious Enamel and Dentin Related to the Action of Cariogenic Biofilms. J. Dent. Res.: 2004;83(Spec. Iss. C):C35-C38.

27. Larmas M. Dental cavities seen from the pulpal side:A non-traditional approach. J. Dent. Res.: 2003;82:253–256.

28. Nuca C, Bocskay S, Corneliu A and Laura-Daniela R. Study regarding the histological features of enamel caries. OHDMBSC: 2005;4:5–12.

29. Nylen MU. Matrix-mineral relationships—a morphologist's viewpoint. J. Dent. Res.: 1979;58: 922–9.

30. Odutuga AA and Prout RE. Lipid analysis of human enamel and dentin. Arch. Oral Biol.: 1974;19:729–31.

31. Palamara J, Phakey PP, Rachinger WA and Orams HJ. The ultrastructure of human dental enamel heat-treated in the temperature range 200 degrees C to 600 degrees C. J. Dent. Res.: 1987;66:1742–7.

32. Pratebha B, Sudhakar R, Manoj R. Cemento-dentinal junction in health and disease: A Light Microscopic Study. Int. J. of Oral and Maxillofacial Pathology: 2011;2:20–3.

33. Pugach MK, Strother J, Darling CL, Fried D, Gansky SA, Marshall SJ and Marshall GW. Dentin Caries Zones. Mineral structure and properties J. Dent Res.: 2009;88:71–6.

34. Sarnat H and Massler M. Microstructure of Active and Arrested Dentinal Caries.J. Dent. Res.: 1965; 44:1389.

35. Scott DB, Simmelink JW and Nygaard V. Structural aspects of dental caries. J. Dent. Res.: 1974;53:165–78.

36. Shellis RP, Hallsworth AS, Kirkham J and Robinson C. Organic material and the optical properties of the dark zone in caries lesions of enamel. Eur. J. Oral Sci.: 2002;110:392–5.

37. Stack MV. The organic content of chalky enamel. Br. Dent. J.: 1954;73–6.

38. Sullivan HR. The formation of early carious lesions in dental enamel Part I J Dent. Res.: 1954;33:218–30.

39. Tohda H, Takuma S and Tanaka N. Intracrystalline structure of enamel crystals affected by caries. J. Dent. Res.: 1987;66:1647–53.

40. Xu C, Yao X, Walker MP and Wang Y. Chemical/ Molecular Structure of the Dentin-Enamel Junction is Dependent on the Intra tooth Location. Calcif. Tissue Int.: 2009;84:221–8.

41. Yamamoto T, Domon T, Takahashi S, Islam MN and Suzuki R. The fibrillar structure of the cemento-dentinal junction in different kinds of human teeth. J. Perio. Res.: 2001;36:317–32.

42. Yamamoto T, Domon T, Takahashi S, Islam MN, Suzuki R and Wakita M. The structure and function of the cement-dentinal junction in human teeth. J. Perio. Res.: 1999;34,:261–8.

43. Zavgorodniy AV, Rohanizadeh R and Swain MV. Ultrastructure of dentin carious lesions. Arch Oral Biol.: 2008;53:124–32.

10

Diagnosis of Caries

The concept that dental caries is a multi-directional process rather than a systemic disease has been accepted since long. Early authors divided caries into three stages: caries of enamel, caries of dentin, and deep caries. They stressed the importance of diagnosis as the first step in the management of dental caries. Dr GV Black once stated,'Study of caries should be continuous, as it appears in the teeth of patients from day-to-day, with the view of becoming more familiar with its tendencies to spread on the surface of the enamel and the positions and directions of spreading'. Dr. Black developed a system for restoring decayed teeth knowing well the possible limitation of restorative approach in managing the dental caries.

Diagnosis literally means the determination and judgement of variations from the normal. The word 'diagnosis' is a Greek word, meaning specifically discriminating/distinguishing between two possibilities. In the present concept, this is interpreted as 'differential diagnosis'.

Diagnosis is defined as *the utilization of scientific knowledge in identifying a diseased process and to differentiate it from other diseased processes.*

Oxford dictionary defines diagnosis as *The identification of nature of an illness/problem by examination of the symptoms.*

The important and accepted definitions of diagnosis are:

McGhee: The correct determination, discriminative estimation and logical appraisal of conditions found during examination as evidenced by distinctive marks, signs and symptoms that are characteristic of health or disease.

Grossman: The process of identifying a disease by its signs, symptoms and results of various diagnostic procedures.

It is important to diagnose caries at its inception. Though it seems difficult, but the active carious lesion should be distinguished from inactive ones as soon as possible. The lesion should be diagnosed at the initial stage so that preventive treatment may be initiated to arrest lesion progression; also to increase the chances of success with non-operative or minimal operative interventions.

However, many authors are not in favor of intervention in early caries; they prefer giving chance to natural remineralization phenomenon. It is accepted that advanced techniques are required to distinguish between active and inactive lesions.

Requisites of Diagnostic Tests

The caries diagnostic test must be:
- Accurate.
- Sensitive (diseased tooth) and specific (sound tooth).

- Reproducible and reliable.
- Should not transfer any micro-organism from affected area to unaffected area.
- Should be cost effective.

Caries Detection Methods

1. Visual examination.
2. Tactile examination.
3. Radiographic methods.
   a. Conventional radiography.
      i. Periapical radiography.
      ii. Bitewing radiography.
   b. Xeroradiography.
   c. Modified radiographic techniques.
      i. Digital radiography.
      ii. Computer image analysis.
      iii. Subtraction radiography.
      iv. Computed tomography (CT) scan.
      v. Micro-computed tomography (micro CT) scan.
      vi. Cone beam computed tomography (CBCT).
      vii. Magnetic resonance imaging (MRI).
4. Electric resistance (electrical conductance and impedance).
   a. AC Ohmmeter.
   b. Caries meter-L.
   c. Vanguard electronic caries detector.
   d. Electronic caries monitor (ECM).
   e. Electrical impedance tomography.
   f. Alternating current impedance spectroscopy (CarieScan).
5. Optical detection methods.
   a. Optical caries monitor.
   b. Fiberoptic transillumination (FOTI).
   c. Digital imaging fiberoptic transillumination (DIFOTI).
   d. Ultraviolet illumination.
   e. Transillumination with near infrared light.
   f. Laser-induced fluorescence.
      Devices (with camera) using fluorescence principles
      i. Quantitative light-induced fluorescence (QLF).
      ii. Light induced fluorescence evaluation—diagnosis and treatment (LIFEDT) concept.
      iii. Newer cameras.
      Devices (without camera) using fluorescence principles
      i. DIAGNOdent.
   g. Visible luminescence spectroscopy.
   h. Terahertz imaging (TI).
   i. Multiphoton imaging (MPI).
   j. Optical coherence tomography (OCT).
   k. Polarized Raman Spectroscopy (PRS).
   l. Midwest caries ID (LED technology).
   m. Frequency-domain infrared photo thermal radiometry and modulated luminescence (PTR/LUM).
   n. Time-correlated single-photon counting fluorescence lifetime imaging microscopy.
6. Endoscopy/videoscopy.
7. Dye penetration methods.
8. Miscellaneous.
   a. Carbon dioxide laser.
   b. Infrared thermography.
   c. Ultrasonic imaging.
   d. Chemical analysis.
   e. Microradiography.
      i. Transverse microradiography.
      ii. Longitudinal microradiography
      iii. Wavelength independent microradiography.
   f. Energy dispersive X-ray element analysis
   g. Microhardness analysis.
   h. Iodine absorptiometry.
   i. Polarized light microscopy.

1. Visual Examination

Visual examination needs sufficient time and patience. The examination involves visually looking for surface roughness, opacification, discoloration and cavitation. The teeth are cleaned and dried with compressed air and illuminated under adequate light source. The limitation of using this method is discoloration of the pits and fissures, a common finding in normal healthy adult teeth (extrinsic stains) may simulate discoloration of caries. The individual's past history and the habits can help differentiate between these two discolorations.

2. Tactile Examination

The examination includes determining roughness/softness of the tooth surface with a sharp explorer. Both penetration and resistance to removal of an explorer tip (catch) have been interpreted as an evidence of caries. Probing is an age-old diagnostic aid; however, it has been criticized and questioned because of several reasons viz:

a. May transmit cariogenic bacteria from one site to another (one probe is used to examine different sites).
b. May produce irreversible traumatic defects in enamel, which further become susceptible to caries attack.
c. May not add any information to the visual examination.

d. The explorer tip may bind in a fissure because of reasons other than caries. The reasons can be:
 i. *Shape of the pit/fissure:* Small/rounded pits/fissures can bind the tip.
 ii. *Sharpness of an explorer:* A sharp explorer has a diameter of 200 microns at its tip and pressing the explorer may push the tip into enamel.
 iii. *Force of application:* Heavy pressure may lead to binding of the probe tip into enamel fissures.

Dental floss and tooth separators are also employed to detect proximal caries. After the tooth has been thoroughly cleaned, floss is inserted through the contact area and dragged occlusally against one proximal surface. If it shreds, one can suspect a proximal cavity; however, overhanging restorations on the proximal side may present similar features. This is to be looked into prior to flossing. Tooth separators and wedges aid in detecting the proximal caries visually by separating the teeth.

The commonly utilized visual-tactile criteria for detection of caries as proposed by various authors in the past are tabulated below:

Jackson D (1950)	There should be positive and clear evidence of enamel dissolution before the same is diagnosed as caries. 1. A clear mirror and sharp probe must be used for tactile examination. Ash's Sickle Probe No. 54 is used for pit and fissure lesions; whereas Ash's Probe No. 12 is used for proximal lesions. 2. The tooth must be dried thoroughly before examination. 3. A pit/fissure is counted as carious if, with a little pressure, the point sticks and requires a definite pull to be removed. The doubtful ones are not included. 4. Stained pits/fissures are not counted as carious unless they satisfy this test. 5. Stained or opaque light areas on other smooth surfaces are not counted as carious unless they show evidence of enamel dissolution. 6. Proximal lesions are considered 'carious', if Ash's No. 12 probe catches a roughened surface or a discontinuity. 7. Arrested caries is counted as carious, and exposed dentin in hypoplastic teeth is also counted as carious, only if there is positive evidence of softening.
Parfitt GJ (1954)	A slight discoloration with loss of luster on the enamel surface is considered as the first sign of caries.

Grade 1: Slight discoloration with loss of luster of the enamel surface.

Grade 2: Surface is roughened and pitted, a condition which can be detected by explorer point.

Grade 3: Further penetration and loss of tissue, causing pitting to reach the dentin.

Grade 4: Loss of dentin and cavitation.

Backers-Derks, et al (1961)

The clinical examination by mirror and explorer to detect proximal caries was discontinued because of poor accuracy.

The teeth were cleaned and dried with compressed air and examined under transmitted light. Caries was estimated in 4 different grades.

Grade I signifies a minute black line at the bottom of the fissure.

Grade II denotes a white zone along the margins of the fissure.

Grade III denotes the smallest perceptible break in the continuity of the enamel (cavity) with or without undermined margins.

Grade IV is a large cavity more than 3.0 mm wide.

McHugh, et al (1964)

Teeth were counted as carious if a probe stuck definitely in a pit/fissure after applying gentle pressure; designated as 'sticky fissure'. In addition, each carious cavity was given a "penetration score" on the following basis:

Score 1 = Sticky fissure.

Score 2 = Fissure or smooth surface cavity with softness at base and staining or opacity of the enamel.

Score 3 = Cavity with obvious dentin involvement in the proximal surfaces.

Score 4 = Cavity with pulp involvement.

Marthaler TM (1966)

Emphasis was given to visual examination. Probe was used only in case of doubt.

Grade 1: Slightly brown narrow line or [on smooth surfaces Class V] white spot with hard surface, smallest extent not exceeding 2.0 mm.

Grade 2: Clearly brown or black line or [on Class V lesions] white spot, smallest extent exceeding 2.0 mm; For Class III lesions [proximal of anterior teeth], the lesion has a dark brown discolored surface.

Grade 3: Cavity, discontinuity of the enamel surface.

Grade 4: Cavity with the narrowest extent of the entrance broader than 2.0 mm.

Moller IJ (1966)

Caries on smooth surfaces (buccal and lingual):

Grade I: A white opaque spot that keeps its luster after a short (3 seconds) period of drying.

Grade II: After being dried, the area appears white and chalky.

Caries in pits and fissures:

Grade I: Area is dark by incident as well as transmitted light; the lesion is confined to a small dark line.

Grade II: In addition to Grade 1, a white zone can be seen along the margins of the fissure, which appears dark in transmitted light.

Grade III: There is smallest perceptible break in the continuity of the enamel.

Radike AW (1968)

I. Frank lesions (lesions with cavitation): Visible presence of a cavitation.

   a. Cavitation as a result of discontinuity of the enamel surface caused by loss of tooth surfaces.

   b. Cavitation as a result of the caries process should be distinguished from fractures and smooth lesions or erosion and abrasion.

II. Lesions not showing cavitation: The criteria for detection of these lesions are categorized as:

A. *Detection of pit and fissure lesions of the occlusal, facial, and lingual surfaces.*

1. Area is carious when the explorer "catches" or resists removal after insertion into a pit or fissure with moderate to firm pressure and when accompanied by one or more of the following signs of caries:

   a. A softness at the base of the area.

   b. Opacity adjacent to the pit or fissure as evidence of undermining or demineralization.

   c. Softened enamel adjacent to the pit or fissure which may be scraped away with the explorer.

2. Area is carious if there is loss of the normal translucency of the enamel, adjacent to a pit, which is in contrast to the surrounding tooth structure. This condition is considered as an evidence of undermining. In some cases, the explorer may not catch or penetrate the pit.

B. *Detection of lesions on smooth surfaces (facial and lingual)*

1. Area is carious if surface is etched or if there is a white spot as evidence of subsurface demineralization, and if the area is found to be soft by:

   a. Penetration with explorer.

   b. Enamel can be scraped away with explorer.

2. Area is sound when there is apparent evidence of demineralization (etching or white spots) but no evidence of softness.

C. *Detection of lesions on proximal surfaces:* The procedures used for diagnosis of proximal surfaces varied considerably. Some examiners depend largely upon visual-tactile methods; whereas others on radiographs; a few have used the combination of these procedures. The inference is:

1. For area exposed to direct visual and tactile examinations, these are diagnosed as under "B" above for smooth areas.

2. For hidden areas not exposed to direct visual and tactile examinations:

   a. *Visual examination:* If the marginal ridge shows an opacity as evidence of undermined enamel, the proximal surface is carious.

   b. *Tactile examination:* Any discontinuity of the enamel in which an explorer will enter is carious if it also shows other evidence of decay, such as softness, shadow by transillumination, or loss of translucency.

   c. *Radiography:* Any definite radiolucency indicating a break in the continuity of the enamel surface is carious.

   d. *Transillumination:* A loss of translucency producing a characteristic shadow in a calculus-free and stain-free proximal surface is an adequate evidence of caries. It is used mostly for anterior teeth.

Moller IJ and Paulsen S (1973)

A. *Pits and fissures.*

   a. Discoloration not definite "sticking".

   b. Sticking with or without discoloration; no dentin involvement.

   c. Definite cavity with dentin involvement.

   d. Probable pulp involvement.

B. *Vestibular and lingual smooth surfaces.*

   a. White opaque area with loss of luster; no loss of substance.

   b. Discontinuity in the enamel; no dentin involvement.

   c. Dentin involvement.

   d. Probable pulp involvement.

C. *Proximal surfaces (diagnosed by means of radiographs).*

Murray J and
Shaw L (1975)
C1: A pit, fissure of smooth surface in which there is discoloration in both incident and transmitted light, with minute discontinuity in the enamel surface which does not allow definite "sticking" of the probe on gentle pressure.

C2: A cavity in a pit, fissure or a smooth surface in which a probe sticks with gentle pressure and requires a definite pull to be removed.

C3: A large open cavity, probably with pulpal involvement.

Howat AP (1981)
A. Visual method
   I. *Pits and fissures.*
     V1: Visibly intact enamel with one or both of the following; dark line at base of fissure and/or white discoloration on the walls.

     V2: Breakdown of walls of fissure with either visible open cavity or shadow or opacity beneath the enamel (evidence of undermining), less than 1.5 mm across the fissure.

     V3: Breakdown of walls of fissure with either a visible open cavity, or shadow or opacity beneath the enamel (evidence of undermining), greater than 1.5 mm across. the fissure.

   II. *Free smooth surfaces.*
     V4: White chalky opaque lesion, but intact surface.

     V5: Break in enamel with cavity less than 0.5 mm in diameter.

     V6: Cavity greater than 0.5 mm in diameter.

   III. *Mesio-distal surfaces.*
     V7: Shadow by transillumination, or loss of translucency.

     V8: Observable cavity.

B. Tactile method.
   I. *Pits and fissures.*
     T1: Sticky on probing; the probe requires a definite pull to be removed.

     T2: The explorer "catches" or resists removal with moderate to firm pressure, and adjacent softened enamel may be scraped away with the explorer.

     T3: The explorer "catches" or resists removal with moderate to firm pressure and is accompanied by softness at the base of the area.

   II. *Free smooth surfaces.*
     T4: A surface discontinuity, including defective (soft or brittle) enamel, tip of probe sticking superficially.

     T5: Cavity with a detectably softened floor.

     T6: Cavity detected by probing; probe sticking superficially.

   III. *Mesio-distal.*
     T7: Cavity detected by probing, with a detectable softened floor.

C. Visual-tactile method
   I. *Pits and fissures.*
     VT1: Fissure showing discoloration with incident as well as transmitted light and no definite stickiness.

     VT2: The explorer "catches" or resists removal in a pit or fissure with moderate to firm pressure, and is accompanied by opacity adjacent to the pit or fissure (evidence of undermining or demineralization).

     VT3: Visible cavity, probe penetrates dentin.

   II. *Free smooth surfaces.*
     VT4: White spots with loss of luster with hard intact surface.

     VT5: White spots with softness detected by penetration and scraping away of enamel by an explorer.

VT6: Break in enamel in a chalky or brown-stained area of diminished translucency less than 0.5 mm in diameter, with soft floor.

VT7: Definite cavity with soft floor, diameter greater than 0.5 mm.

III. *Mesio-distal.*

VT8: White or brown area of enamel seen by direct vision; dark area of enamel seen by transillumination, no visible cavity entered by the probe (mostly for anterior)

VT9: If the explorer detects roughness, softening, or surface discontinuity in a chalky or brown-stained area of diminished translucency.

WHO (1987) *WHO* (1997)	When a lesion in a pit or fissure, or on a smooth tooth surface, has a detectably softened floor, undermined enamel, or softened wall is categorized as 'caries'. A tooth with a temporary filling should also be included in this category. On proximal surfaces, the explorer should enter the lesion; in case of doubt, the lesion should not be recorded as caries. When a lesion in a pit or fissure, or on a smooth tooth surface, has a definite cavity, undermined enamel, or a detectably softened floor or wall is categorized as caries. A tooth with a temporary filling, or one which is sealed but also decayed, should also be included in this category. In cases where the crown has been destroyed by caries and only the tooth is left, the caries is presumed to have originated on the crown and is scored as crown caries only. The CPI probe should be used to confirm visual evidence of caries on the occlusal, buccal, and lingual surfaces. Doubtful cases are not recorded as caries.
Pitts NB and Fyfee HE (1988)	a. Initial caries: No detectable loss of tooth substance. For pits and fissures, there may be significant staining, discoloration, or rough spots in the enamel that do not catch the explorer, but where loss of substance cannot be positively diagnosed. For smooth surfaces, these may be white, opaque areas with loss of luster. b. Enamel caries: Loss of tooth substance in pits, fissures, or on smooth surfaces, but no softened floor or wall or undermined enamel. The texture of the material within the cavity may be chalky or crumbly, but there is no evidence that cavitation has penetrated the dentin. c. Caries of dentin: Detectably softened floor, undermined enamel, or a softened wall, or the loss has a temporary filling. On proximal surfaces, the explorer should definitely enter a lesion. d. Pulpal involvement: Deep cavity with probable pulpal involvement. Pulp should not be probed.
Pitts NB, et al (1997)	Code 1: Arrested dentinal decay: In case the surface has arrested lesion. Code 2: If the active caries is extended into dentin. Code 3: If the caries is extended into pulp.
Amarante, et al (1998)	Occlusal caries Grade 1: Caries characterized by white or brown discoloration without tooth substance loss. No radiographic findings. Grade 2: Little substance loss with break in the enamel surface or discoloring; caries restricted to enamel in the X-ray. Grade 3: Moderate tooth substance loss and/or caries in the external 1/3rd of the dentin radiographically. Grade 4: Considerable tooth substance loss and/or caries in the middle 1/3rd of the dentin radiographically.

Grade 5: Substantial tooth substance loss and/or caries in the internal 1/3rd of the dentin radiographically.

Similar grades were used for buccal and lingual surfaces and secondary caries.

Ekstrand, et al (1998)

0 = no or slight change in enamel translucency after prolonged air drying.

1 = opacity (white); hardly visible on the wet surface, but distinctly visible after air drying.

1a = opacity (brown); hardly visible on the wet surface, but distinctly visible after air drying.

2 = opacity (white); distinctly visible without air drying.

2a = opacity (brown); distinctly visible without air drying.

3 = localized enamel breakdown in opaque or discolored enamel and/or grayish discoloration from the underlying dentin.

4 = cavitation in opaque or discolored enamel, exposing the dentin beneath.

Nyvad, et al (1998)   Refer to Ch. 4 (Indices for Caries) pg. 73.

Fyfee, et al (2000)

1. White-spot lesion: Visual examination indicates intact surface; no clinically detectable loss of tooth substance, with a white or cream-colored area of increased opacity, presumed to be caries.
2. Brown-spot lesion: Visual examination indicates intact surface; no clinically detectable loss of tooth substance, with a brown/black discoloration, presumed to be caries.
3. Enamel cavity: There is a lesion with demonstrable loss of surface but no visual, clinical evidence of the lesion penetrating dentin.
4. Dentin lesion (uncavitated): There is a caries lesion into dentin but no visible evidence of cavitation.
5. Dentin cavity: There is a carious cavity into dentin.
6. Pulp involved: There is a carious cavity that involves the pulp.
7. Arrested dentinal decay: There is arrested caries in dentin.

ICDAS, I and II (2007-2009)   Refer to Ch. 4 (Indices for caries) pg. 73

Baurer, et al (1988)   Root Caries

Discrete, well-defined, and discolored cavitation on the root surface into which the explorer entered easily and displayed some resistance to withdrawal.

Beighton, et al (1993)

Root caries

The diagnosis of primary root caries was made by consideration of change in color, texture, and surface contour of the tooth.

The color of each lesion was categorized by visual comparison with a standard guide of four shades (yellow, light brown, dark brown, and black) which was prepared from photographs of primary root-caries lesions. The dimensions of each lesion, the occluso-gingival and mesiodistal lengths, and greatest loss of surface contour were measured with a periodontal probe marked with 1.0 mm intervals.

The texture of the lesion was classified into three grades: hard, leathery (assessed by means of a new Ash No.6 probe with moderate pressure but displaying resistance to its withdrawal), and soft lesions which were easily penetrated and displayed no resistance to withdrawal of the probe.

Rosen, et al (1996)   According to the location of the lesion: Caries lesions transversing the cemento-enamel junction and involving both the coronal and root portions of a tooth surface were classified as coronal caries.

	Cavitation: Lesions were classified as manifest caries as soon as the tooth structure has disintegrated as a cavity was formed. Discoloration: White or brown spot lesions on the crown and yellowish or brownish to black lesions on the roots were recorded as initial caries. Surface structure: The manifest lesions were classified as hard or soft and the initial lesions as smooth or rough.
Ekstrand, et al (2008)	Root caries. Texture of the lesion. • Hard (0). • Leathery (2). • Soft (3). Contour of the surface. • No cavitation or smooth cavity surroundings (1). • Cavitation with irregular border (2). Distance from the lesion to the gingival margin. • More than 1.0 mm from the gingival margin (1). • Less than 1.0 mm from the gingival margin (2). Color of the lesion. • Dark brown/black (1). • Light brown/yellowish (2).

Source: Ismail (2004)

Visual and tactile methods have been the hallmark of detection of carious lesions in the earlier studies. It is established as follows:

- The non-cavitated caries lesions are more prevalent than cavitated lesions in economically developed countries.
- Non-cavitated caries lesions are more likely to be restored compared with sound tooth surfaces.
- Non-cavitated lesions, especially on smooth tooth surfaces in young children, may serve as indicators of caries activity.
- Inclusion of non-cavitated lesions may provide a better understanding of the mechanism of action of fluoride, sealants, and other preventive agents.
- Inclusion of early signs of the caries process improves the precision of clinical trials of preventive agents.

Keeping in view these facts, emphasis is being given to diagnostic criteria, which can detect incipient carious lesions.

Disadvantages

- The visual tactile examination method, in all probability, may miss out an incipient lesion.
- The criterion for detection of caries is not standardized. The method of examination and criterion for diagnosis varies from individual to individual.
- Probing depth and pressure is controversial.

3. Radiographic Methods

The carious process leads to demineralization of the affected area of the tooth and that area appears radiolucent on the radiograph. The presence of radiolucency in the tooth substance is considered as caries. Radiographs have certain limitations; therefore, the combination of clinical examination along with the radiographic aid is considered mandatory for diagnosing caries. The mere presence of radiolucency may be misleading.

The following radiographic methods are used in routine:

a. Conventional Radiography

Conventionally, following two types of techniques are employed:

    i. Periapical radiography.

    ii. Bitewing radiography.

Other modalities like occlusal radiographs and panoramic radiographs are rarely employed in the detection of caries. Panoramic views are employed for having a broader view of the oral cavity. Moreover, the panoramic technique utilizes intensifying screen, which may hamper the finer details; whereas the occlusal technique does not determine the angulation of a tooth in that particular arch.

    i. *Periapical radiographs* are useful for detecting changes in and around the tooth tissues, such as extent of caries, cervical margins of the restoration, alveolar crest height, lamina dura as well as the size of the pulp chamber. The paralleling technique is considered superior to bisecting technique for detecting caries in both anterior and posterior teeth.

    ii. *Bitewing radiographs* are important to detect incipient lesions at the contact areas. With this technique, six to eight teeth in one radiograph can be visualized. The technique can be used for anterior as well as posterior teeth. The film is available in different sizes to suit the area to be radiographed. One long film can also be used to capture the area from first premolar to the last molar; however, conventional films provide better results.

Posterior bitewing radiographs are preferably utilized to detect interproximal caries. Recurrent caries at the cervical margins is best observed in bitewing films, since the central ray is directed along the plane of the cervical areas. Bitewing radiographs are useful in monitoring and evaluating the progress or arrest of dental caries.

Radiographic Appearance of Caries

Occlusal caries: Radiographs are not effective until the occlusal caries involves dentin. Once in dentin, the radiographic image shows a broad based thin radiolucent zone in the dentin with a little or no change apparent in the enamel (Fig. 10.1).

A significant manifestation of occlusal caries in dentin is the presence of a band of increased opacity at the base of carious lesion near the pulp chamber. The white band represents the calcification within the primary dentin; such a band may not be evident in buccal caries.

Limitations of radiographic interpretation of occlusal caries are:

- Difficult to detect caries in enamel because of superimposition of adjacent enamel over the fissures.
- Lesions involving buccal grooves of molars are superimposed over the occlusal area and can simulate occlusal lesions.
- A thin radiolucency at the dentino-enamel junction in occlusal caries, may be confusing with normal radiolucency in enamel and dentin.
- Difficult to distinguish between occlusal caries and the internal resorption.

Proximal caries: A considerable loss of mineral content is mandatory before it becomes visible on a radiograph. The initial

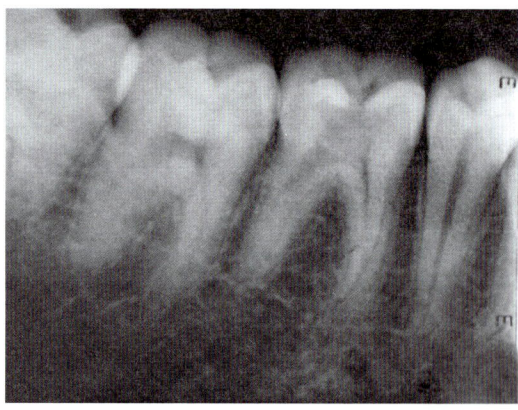

Fig. 10.1: Occlusal caries in mandibular first molar

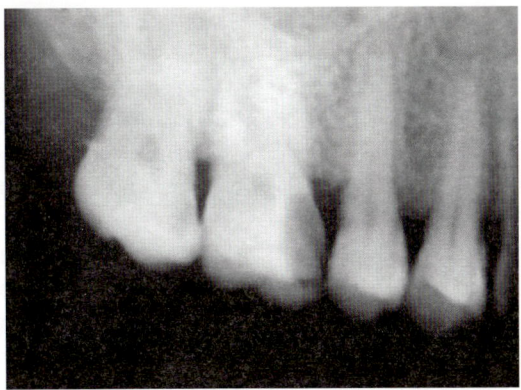

Fig. 10.2: Proximal caries in maxillary first molar

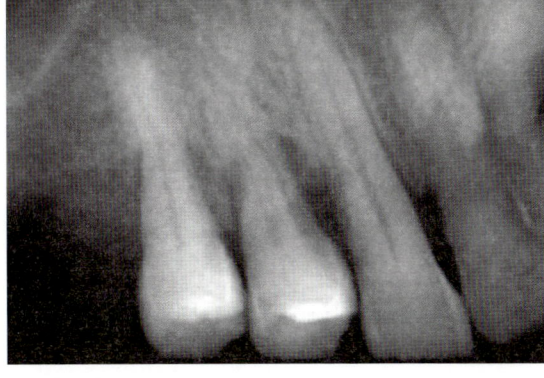

Fig. 10.3: Root caries in maxillary first premolar

loss of mineral content, may be distributed in the broad proximal area, is not evident in radiographs. The actual depth of the lesion is always deeper than may be seen radiographically (Fig. 10.2).

The white chalky appearance is the first evidence on the surface of enamel just below the contact point. The caries susceptible zone is 1.0 to 1.5 mm below the contact point, which is evident as a small radiolucent area below the contact area. With the advancing lesion, the radiographic image is like a diffuse triangle with the base at the surface of the tooth. Once the lesion crosses the dentino-enamel junction and invades into the dentin, the lesion appears as another triangle with the base at dentino-enamel junction. The pulp involvement is evident in advanced stages. Bitewing radiographs are preferred to detect proximal caries.

Root caries: Root lesions usually have ill-defined saucer-like appearances and are progressive in nature. These are usually observed within 2.0 mm area of cemento-enamel junction (Fig. 10.3). An exposed root surface is always at an increased risk of developing caries. Since root caries progresses more rapidly than enamel caries, early diagnosis becomes mandatory.

Recontouring of the defect followed by fluoride application can be helpful in preventing the initial lesions. Diagnosis of root

caries is not difficult, except in cases where the lesion is on interproximal surface (severe periodontal involvement lead to exposure of roots from all sides). Radiographic picture shows area of radiolucency in cementum alone or in cementum and dentin both. Pulp involvement can also be evident.

Secondary/recurrent caries: Caries that occurs adjacent to the restorations is known as secondary/recurrent caries (Fig. 10.4). It is established that secondary caries is the major cause of failure of restorations. Diagnosis of secondary caries is usually dependent on the clinical examination as the radiographs do not detect the lesion until only in advanced stages. There is no clinical parameter, which distinguishes between active and inactive

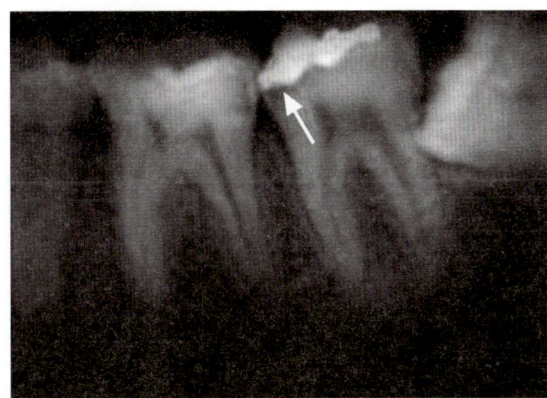

Fig. 10.4: Secondary caries below amalgam filling in mandibular second molar

lesions. The limitations in diagnosis of secondary caries are:

- Lesions between restoration and tooth surface cannot be visualized until reached to an advanced stage. Discoloration of margins can be due to extrinsic stains or corrosion products; hence, cannot be considered as a definite parameter for secondary caries.
- Radiographs can diagnose the cervical portion of the interproximal lesions, which is a prime site for secondary caries; however, radiolucency under composite restorations may be deceptive because the bonding agents are also radiolucent.
- It is often difficult to differentiate between secondary caries and caries which has been left during restorative procedures [residual caries]. Transillumination can be helpful for the diagnosis of discolored dentin, especially under tooth-colored restorations.

Hidden Caries

Hidden (occult/covert) caries is a term used to describe a carious lesion whereby the occlusal surfaces appear intact, and the radiographs show radiolucency in dentin. These caries develop through tiny enamel defects, progressing under seemingly intact tooth structure (Fig. 10.5). One of the reasons quoted is remineralization of the superficial enamel caries while the dentin is decaying underneath. Earlier authors were of the view that occlusal surface gets remineralized using fluorides and termed them "fluoride bombs" or "fluoride syndrome." They opined that fluoride encourages remineralization and slows down progress of the caries in the pit and fissure enamel, while the cavitation continues in dentin, and the lesion becomes masked by a relatively intact enamel surface. Later this hypothesis was challenged in a study which compared the prevalence of occult caries in two cities, one which was optimally fluoridated and the other non-fluoridated and observed 31% decrease in the prevalence of occult lesions in the fluoridated town. This finding was directly opposed to the fluoride hypothesis, and suggests that fluoride has minimal role in the pathogenesis of occult lesions. Current opinion regarding the pathogenesis of occult lesions is centered on traditional mechanisms of caries development. It is presumed that a proportion of these lesions began their course as fissure caries, which might have progressed to hidden caries because of remineralization of occlusal surfaces.

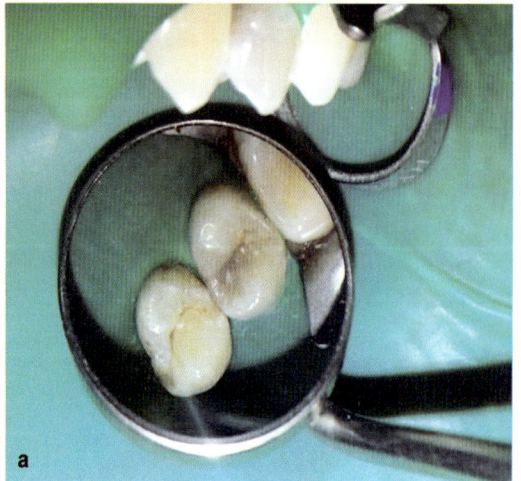 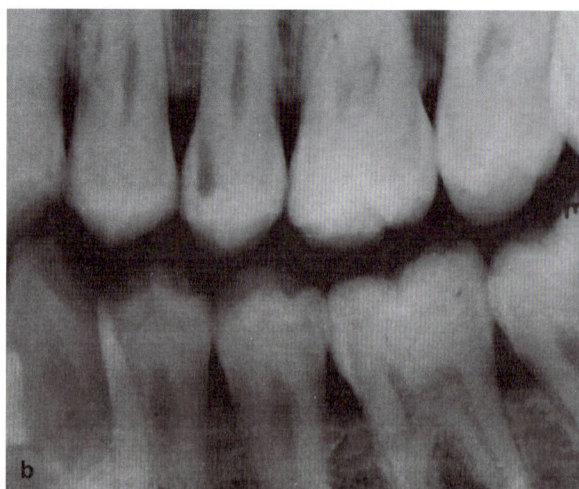

a   b

Fig. 10.5: Hidden caries in maxillary first premolar. (a) Clinical view, (b) radiographic view

The prevalence of hidden caries varies with an average of 3–5% in all teeth. In an investigation comprising 2,623, 14–15-year-old Scottish children, a prevalence of hidden caries observed was 0.8% in all premolars, 11.8% in lower molars, and 3.1% in upper molars. A recent study comprising over six thousand first and second permanent molars from adolescents reported that 6.3% of clinically sound maxillary molars and 12.9% of mandibular molars showed hidden dentin caries.

Along with hidden caries, there is one more entity named *pre-eruptive intracoronal resorptive lesions*. These defects were found on unerupted teeth as radiolucent areas. They are often found in dentin adjacent to the dentino-enamel junction in the occlusal aspects of the crown. As the lesion resembles the caries, they are often termed pre-eruptive caries. The nomenclature 'pre-eruptive' is controversial, since pre-eruptive teeth are completely encased in its crypt, and not likely to be infected with cariogenic micro-organisms.

It has been suggested that such lesions might have originated as a developmental anomaly in which part of the tooth failed to mineralize properly; however, soon it was disproved. The retentive nature of the cavitated lesions favors the caries development and the lesion becomes indistinguishable once it is exposed to the oral cavity.

The area of initiation of hidden lesion may explain why such areas are difficult to diagnose. It is thought that occlusal lesions may begin in two locations; first is an area superficially at or near the entrance to the fissure, where dietary substrates are readily available and the second is on the walls of the fissure near its base and hidden from direct view. Weerheijm, et al (1990) in their microbiological study reported that the bacterial profile within hidden lesion was mainly limited to *Streptococcus mutans* and lactobacilli, endorsing that these lesions are associated with micro-organisms as found in other carious lesions.

Limitations of conventional radiography

- Radiographs are two-dimensional image of a three-dimensional object.
- Overlapping of proximal contacts.
- The lesion depth may appear increased or decreased due to change in angulation.
- Difficulty in analyzing occlusal lesions.
- Radiolucency on radiograph can be because of caries or resorption or any other defect is difficult to analyze.
- The demineralized area on the buccal and lingual surfaces may appear as proximal carious lesion.
- Fracture of one lingual cusp may appear as radiolucent proximal lesion.
- Tilt of maxillary lateral incisors appears as caries on the mesial side of the lateral incisors.
- Cervical burn out areas may mimic cervical caries.
- Conventional radiography may not correlate the relationship between depth of the radiographic lesion and the clinical cavitation.

b. Xeroradiography

Xeroradiography technique uses xerographic copying techniques to record images produced by X-radiations. The technique has an additional feature called "edge enhancement" effect. Due to this effect, the tissues with subtle density differences are clearly visible.

In this technique, the image is recorded on an aluminium plate coated with a layer of selenium particles. These selenium particles are given a uniform electrostatic charge and are stored in a unit called 'conditioner'. When X-rays are passed on to the film, it causes selective discharge of the particles. This forms the latent image and is converted to a positive image by a process called 'development' in the processor unit. The main characteristics of xeroradiographic technique are the ability to have both positive and negative prints together. When positive current is applied to the film, negative particles are attracted and when negative current is applied, positive particles are attracted.

Xeroradiography is twice as sensitive as conventional D-speed films.

Xeroradiography was considered superior to conventional radiography; however, it has been established that the images were comparable to E-speed films of conventional radiography for diagnosing caries.

Advantages

- One-third of X-radiation is required.
- Real image is produced.
- Reflected light is used.
- No need for chemical processing in dark room.
- Economical/cost effective.

Disadvantages

- The electric charge over the film, many a times, causes discomfort to the patient since the humid environment of oral cavity acts as a medium for flow of current.
- Exposure time varies, as manufacturers do not indicate the exact thickness of the plate.
- The process of development cannot be delayed and is to be completed within 15 minutes.

c. Modified Radiographic Techniques

i. Digital radiography

Digital radiographic image may be obtained by digitization of a conventional film radiograph or by direct digital radiography. Radiovisiography (RVG) was the first digital radiograph introduced in oral radiography. Digital images are acquired either directly (using a sensor or imaging plate replacing conventional film) or indirectly (by scanning and digitizing a film-captured image) (Fig. 10.6).

Digital imaging systems are divided into two types:

- Real time (corded system).
- Photostimulated phosphor imaging (cordless system).

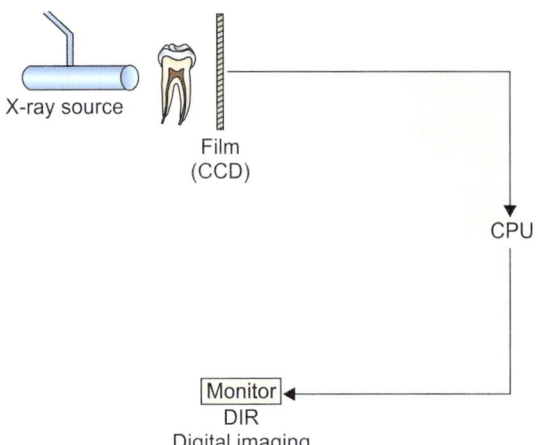

Fig. 10.6: Digital radiography

Real time (corded system)

The system employs conventional X-ray generating equipment but conventional film is replaced by either a CCD (charge coupled device) or a CMOS (complementary metal oxide semiconductor) sensor which is connected to the computer via a cable (or cord). The X-ray photons that reach the sensor are converted to light, by an intensifying or scintillation screen, which is picked by the CCD/CMOS and converted into an electrical charge which, once relayed to the computer, produces an almost instantaneous digital image on the monitor (hence the term Real time).

Different-sized intraoral as well as panoramic sensors are used. Intraoral sensor holders (with and without beam aiming devices), have been developed. When used clinically, the sensors need be covered with a protective plastic barrier for protecting from infection.

Photostimulated phosphor imaging (cordless system)

The system employs re-usable photostimulable phosphor imaging plates (PSPP) instead of film. The plates contain a layer of barium fluorohalide phosphor.

The phosphor layer absorbs and stores the X-ray energy that has not been attenuated by the patient. The image plate is then placed in a reader where it is scanned by a laser beam. The stored X-ray energy in the phosphor layer is released as light which is detected by a photomultiplier. From here the information is relayed to the computer and displayed as a digital image on the monitor. The time taken to read the plate depends on the particular system being used, and on the size of the plate, but usually varies between approximately 1 to 5 minutes.

The examples of digital radiography systems along with their image receptor size are:

- Radiovisiography (RVG)—19 × 28 mm (Trophy—Japan).
- Flash Dent (Villa—Italy)—20 × 24 mm.
- Sens-A-Ray (Regam—Sweden)—17 × 26 mm.
- Vixa (Gendex—Italy)—18 × 24 mm.

A range of intraoral plate sizes are available identical in size to conventional periapical films. Extraoral plates for panoramic and skull radiography are also available. The intra-oral plates are inserted into protective barrier envelops and can be used in conventional film holders. The extraoral plates are placed in conventional cassettes after the intensifying screens have been removed.

Advantages

- Lower dose of radiation required as both types of digital image receptors are more efficient than conventional films.
- No need for conventional processing, thus avoiding all hazards associated with handling of the processing solutions, including film faults.
- Easy storage and archiving of patient records.
- Easy transfer of images (teleradiology).
- Image enhancement and processing. Several image enhancement techniques are available, viz.
  - Inversion (reversal).
  - Alteration in contrast.
  - Embossing.
  - Magnification.
  - Coloring various tissues.

Disadvantages

- Long term storage of the images; although CDs may be helpful.
- Digital image not secured especially for longer times.
- Intraoral placement of sensors may be difficult.
- Loss of image quality and resolution on the hard copy print.
- Image manipulation may mislead the inexperienced operator.
- Image can be tampered by certain softwares.
- Expensive (especially panoramic systems).

ii. Computer image analysis

A number of computer softwares are available, overcoming the shortcomings of human eye and making the analysis easy. The observer variations in the interpretation of radiographs are well known. To avoid shortcomings of visual interpretation, softwares are being used for automated interpretation of digital radiographs. Automated analysis provides sensitive and objective observations, which may also permit the detection of small lesions that otherwise, may not be perceptible to naked eyes. Softwares are also available which can quantify the extent of carious lesions.

Advantages

- It provides sensitive and objective observation, especially of smaller lesions which otherwise may not be perceptible to naked eye.
- The lesion can be monitored.
- Small lesions can be quantified.

Disadvantages

- Exposure geometry need to be standardized.
- Specificity is less; however, sensitivity is better.

- Time consuming.
- Less economical (not cost effective).

Digital Image Analysis Using Fractal Dimension

Fractal dimension is a quantifiable value that characterizes shape. The dimension increases in number with the complexity of the structure. A fractal is a geometric shape, possessing characteristics of self-similarity or self-affinity. The image can be magnified during the image analysis and the shape/configuration of the magnified image can be quantified by deriving its fractal dimensions. It can be calculated by placing a grid of squares over the object and counting the number of squares through which any part of the object passes.

A few fractal analysis applications are being used to quantitatively evaluate the digital images to diagnose caries. Since the shape of the caries can be quantified, and the relationship between numerical value and condition of the lesion can also be demonstrated, this method is considered effective in diagnosing extent of caries.

The sensitivity and accuracy of Fractal dimensions has been observed to be greater than DIAGNOdent, especially for pit and fissure caries.

iii. Subtraction radiography

It is a technique in which the 'structured noise' is reduced in order to increase the detectability of different tissues/objects on the radiograph. The structured noises are the images, which are not of diagnostic value and interfere in routine interpretation of radiographs. Subtraction images can be obtained from photographic and electronic methods.

Digitization is achieved by taking a picture of the radiograph using high quality video camera. This is fed to a computer-imaging device, termed digitizer. Two standardized radiographs produced with identical exposure geometry are used. The first one is the 'Reference Image' and the subsequent images

are for comparison. The reference image is displayed on the screen. Then the subsequent images are superimposed. The difference between the original and the subsequent images will show as dark bright areas, which can be interpreted readily. It is emphasized that digitization does not increase the information available in the original radiograph. It turns the image into a form, which can be read by the computer.

Subtraction radiography is also considered superior to conventional film radiography for detecting proximal and recurrent caries. It is also useful in detecting the progress of re-mineralization and demineralization patterns of dentinal caries. The assessment of alveolar bone height in determining the progression of periodontal disease has been one of the major uses of subtraction digital radiography (Fig. 10.7a to d). The minimal thickness of bone that can be detected under optimal conditions has been found to be 0.12 mm; however, correct projection geometry is mandatory for detecting small lesions.

A subtraction image is a two-dimensional version of three-dimensional structures; however, tuned-aperture computed tomo-

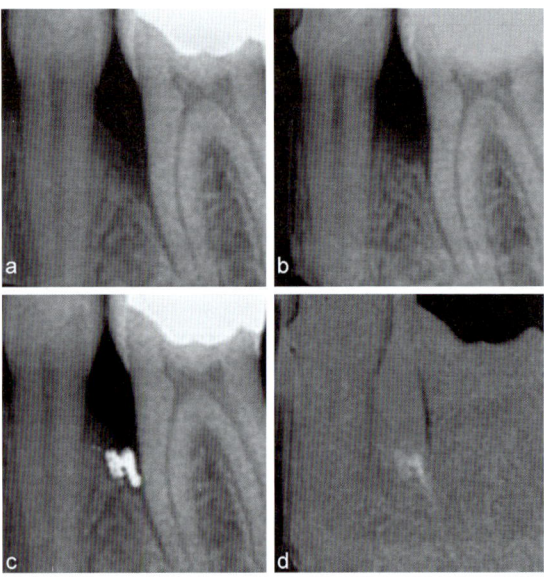

Fig. 10.7a to d: Interdental bone formation seen in digital subtraction radiography

graphy (TACT), have demonstrated three-dimensional display increasing the accuracy of detecting dental lesions.

iv. *Computed tomography (CT) scan*

A computed tomography (CT) scan is a non-invasive diagnostic test that uses X-rays and a computer to create three-dimensional images of the object. This cross-sectional imaging technique provided an in-depth insight into the object scanned.

Computed tomography (CT), also known as "computed axial tomography" produces cross-sectional images of any part of the body. Each cross-sectional image represents a "slice" of the area being imaged. These cross-sectional images are used for a variety of diagnostic purposes.

In a CT scan system, the X-ray source and the detector are situated at 180 degrees from each other; their 360 degrees movement around the patient, continuously detect information as the X-rays pass through the object. The computer further manipulates and integrates the acquired data and assigns numerical values based on the relative attenuation of the X-ray beam.

Attenuation coefficient: Every tissue of the body, viz. bone, teeth, soft tissues, etc. has a relatively constant attenuation value (blocking of X-ray beam as it passes across), and is known as tissue's attenuation coefficient. The attenuation value for bone is designated as +1000 HU (Hounsfield Unit), water is 0 HU, and air is –1000 HU. Bone and teeth appear white on the radiograph; soft tissues display gray shades and air appears black.

Windowing is the capacity of CT scan to focus on the field of interest. Tissues of interest can be assigned the full range of blacks and whites, rather than a narrow range of grey scale.

Refinements in detector technology lead to new CT scanners obtaining multiple slices in a single rotation. These scanners, called multislice CT or multidetector CT, provide thinner slices in a shorter period of time, subsequently getting detailed information.

Local Computed tomography (LCT) is another CT device introduced for caries detection. It is a portable device that uses an intraoral detector as image receptor.

The use of CT in caries diagnosis is limited because of high cost, excessive radiation, and not being user friendly.

v. *Micro-computed tomography (Micro-CT) scan*

Non-destructive techniques of analyzing mineral changes in dental tissues are being tried. The tissues can be evaluated of mineral loss/gain and also their kinetics.

Micro-CT is a variation of X-ray attenuation methods, which have been used to study demineralized lesions. Micro-CT is a modified version of the Computed Axial Tomography, but mostly applied for laboratory purpose. It is a non-destructive technique, which allows high spatial resolution of inner structures to be recorded. The principle of absorption of micro-CT consists in reconstructing the linear attenuation coefficient within the object; viewing the object at different angles. Differences in linear attenuation coefficient among tissues are responsible for X-ray image contrast, which allows the quantitative analyses. X-ray microtomography has emerged as one of the non-destructive 3D analytical techniques in hard tissue research, including caries research.

The micro-CT is mainly utilized for evaluation of mineral content in dental hard tissue. It also provides insights into the process of demineralization/remineralization of incipient lesions.

X-ray microtomography produces a 3D X-ray attenuation image of the scanned object, i.e. the resultant image is a true representation with no superimposition, as in intraoral radiographs. These advantages have made X-ray microtomography more popular as a means of measuring demineralization *in vitro*.

Since radiopacity corresponds well to mineral density in teeth, X-ray microtomography is well-suited in detecting demineralization characteristics of carious lesions.

The difference or change in mineral density is the basis of hard tissue research, vis-à-vis caries, and X-ray microtomography provides accurate approach as compared to conventional methods (Fig. 10.8).

vi. *Cone beam computed tomography (CBCT)*
Cone beam CT imaging was introduced with the aim to provide three-dimensional data with lower absorbed doses than the conventional CT and micro-CT. Cone beam CT is widely used in dentistry, particularly in caries diagnosis (Figs 10.9 and 10.10). The use of cone beam CT offers advantages over conventional tomography, viz. easier image acquisition, higher image accuracy, reduced artefacts, lower effective radiation doses, faster scan times and greater cost effectiveness. Rather than the fan-shaped beam emitted by conventional CT, cone beam CT emit a cone-shaped X-ray beam that can cover the region of interest.

Spiral CT was developed with an aim to decrease radiations. The spiral CT requires a continuously rotating X-ray tube head. The patient is advanced continuously while the equipment rotates, in a spiral movement, around the patient. The investigation time has been shortened to only a few seconds with a radiation dose reduction up to 75%.

Whatever type of scanner is used, the level, plane and thicknesses (usually between 1.5 mm and 6.0 mm) of the slices to be imaged are selected and the X-ray tube head rotates around the patient, scanning the desired part of the body and producing the required number of slices (usually in the axial plane).

The sequence of events of image formation can be summarized as follows:

- As the tube head rotates around the patient, the detectors produce the attenuation or penetration profile of the body being examined.

- The computer calculates the absorption at points on a matrix formed by the intersection of all the generation profiles for that slice.

- Each point on the matrix is called a pixel and typical matrix sizes comprise either 512 × 512 or 1024 × 1024 pixels. The smaller the individual pixel, the greater the resolution of the final image.

- The area being imaged by each pixel has a definite volume, depending on the thickness of the tomographic slice, and is referred to as a voxel.

- Each voxel is given a CT number or Hounsfield unit between + 1000 and – 1000, depending on the amount of absorption within that block of tissue.

- Each CT number is assigned a different degree of greyness, allowing a visual image to be constructed and displayed on the monitor.

- The patient moves along and adjacent sections are imaged.

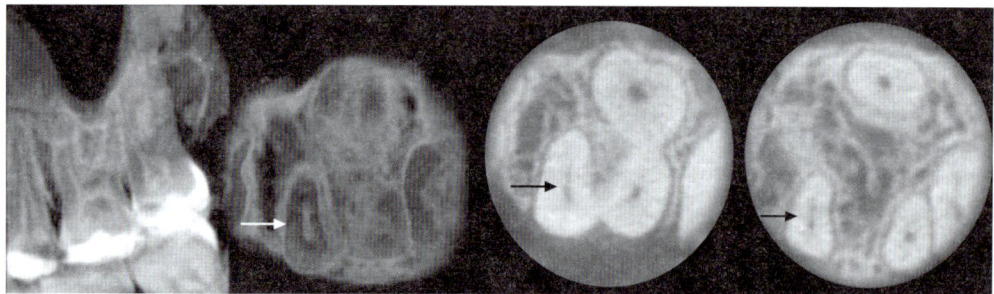

Fig. 10.8: Micro-CT images in evaluating caries

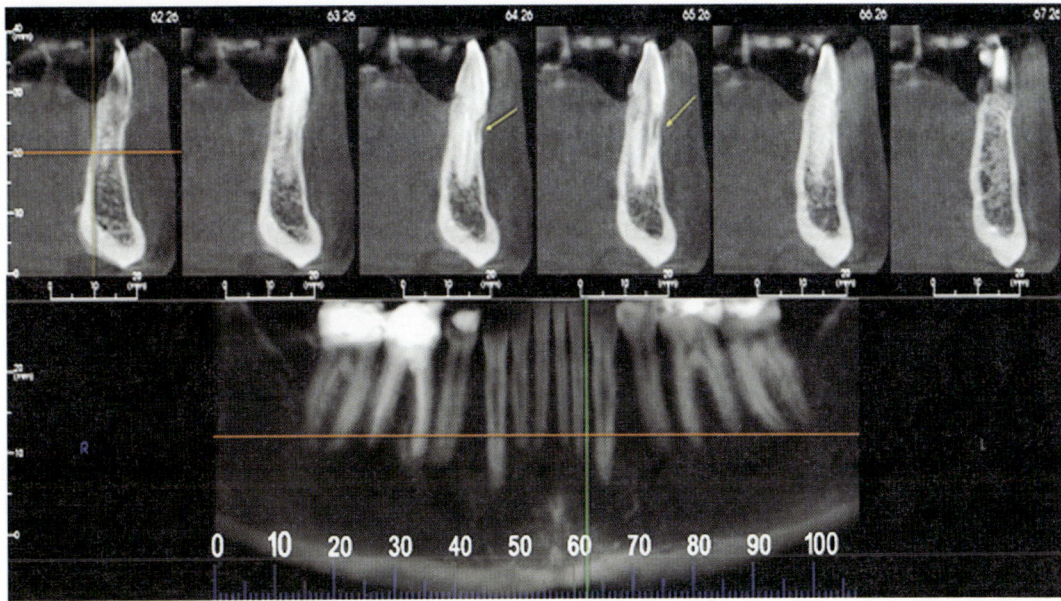

Fig. 10.9: Cross-sectional views of mandibular left canine showing hidden buccal cervical lesion extending up to the root canal

- The selected images are photographed subsequently to produce the hard copy pictures, with the rest of the images remaining on disc.

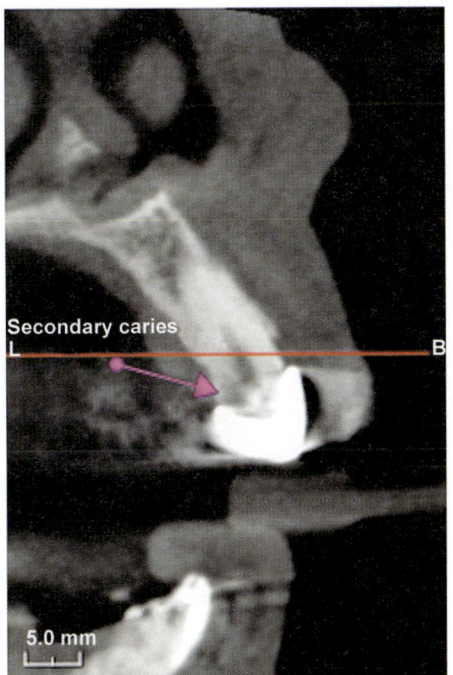

Fig. 10.10: CBCT image showing secondary caries

Disadvantages of CT scans
- Metallic objects, such as fillings may produce marked streak or star artifacts.
- Thin contiguous or overlapping slices may result in high dose.
- Inherent risks associated with contrast agents.
- The equipment is expensive.

The application of cone beam computed tomography (CBCT) in diagnosing dental caries is not established; however, CBCT has the definite advantage of inducing the least amount of radiation hazard. CBCT has been showing similar results when compared to charge-couple device (CCD) in detecting proximal recurrent caries.

vii. *Magnetic resonance imaging (MRI)*

This technology is not preferred for clinical application. In the laboratory, the technique is capable of producing accurate three-dimensional reconstructions of teeth and also the carious lesions. Conventional MRI is noninvasive diagnostic device used in soft tissues without using ionizing radiation. Conventional MRI cannot easily visualize teeth because of their high mineral content; minerals occupy 50% of dentin and 90% of enamel by volume. The conventional MRI techniques in dentistry have been restricted to imaging pulp, periodontal membrane and other surrounding soft tissues. The indirect imaging of enamel and dentin can be achieved through contrast produced by MRI-visible medium.

The Sweep Imaging with Fourier Transformation (SWIFT) MRI, a modified version of MRI, may overcome many limitations of the conventional MRI.

The mineral contents, especially of enamel, continuously pass through an alternate cycle of mineral loss and gain. During the progression of lesion formation, initially a local increase in liquid content with only moderate breakdown of the mineral structures occur. The increase is caused by the local production of acid by the bacterial inflammation and also by saliva penetrating into the lesion through the porous demineralized enamel layer. Advanced progression leads to an increasing decay of the mineral structures, subsequently lead to substantial breakdown and cavity formation. Both processes may cause an increase of the local MRI signal. MRI is not a preferred modality for detection of caries.

4. Electric Resistance (Electrical Conductance and Impedance)

It is established that sound tooth enamel is a good electrical insulator due to its high inorganic content. Enamel demineralization results in increased porosity of enamel. Saliva fills these pores and forms conductive pathways for electric current. The electric conductivity is directly proportional to the amount of demineralization. Electric resistance is measuring the electrical conductivity through these pores.

Since saliva is a better electrical conductor than enamel tissue, the conductivity increases with increase of demineralization. Electrical resistance is also measured during controlled drying. By drying the tooth surface, the resistance is determined by the tooth structure, avoiding electrical conductance by saliva. The higher values indicate well-mineralized tissue; whereas low values indicate demineralized tissue. The electrical conductivity of a tooth changes with demineralization even when the surface remains macroscopically intact.

Factors affecting Electrical Measurements

Following factors may have a significant impact on electrical measurements of teeth:

i. Porosity of the tissues

It is established that teeth undergo a maturation process after eruption; the process has a significant effect on porosity and hence, electrical properties. There may be variations among individuals or within the same individual; usually within one to one and a half year of eruption, the electrical impedance characteristics vary.

Porosity in the context of electrical measurement mean either the pore depth, the pore volume or the three-dimensional configuration of the pore (all three affect ionic migrations within dental hard tissues). Maturation of teeth also causes changes in the porosity of the dental tissues.

ii. Surface area of the electrode contact with the tooth

The surface area of the electrode contact with the tooth is a significant factor in electrical measurements. The two modes of electrodes, *site (point) specific* and *surface specific* produce different values for electrical properties; however, surface specific mode is conventionally used.

iii. Thickness of the tissues

Thickness of the tooth tissues, especially the variation of enamel thickness, affects electrical measurements.

iv. Hydration of the enamel

Hydration of the enamel does affect electrical measurements. The electrical measurement devices are designed to operate with a specific air-flow; however, the teeth should not be dehydrated prior to measurement. Standardized use of contact medium is preferred to achieve uniformity.

v. Temperature and concentration of ions in the fluid within the tooth

It is demonstrated that the temperature of the teeth affects the electrical conductivity. The concentration of ions in the fluids within the tissues, particularly within enamel, is also critical to electrical measurement values.

Advantages
- Very effective in detecting early pits and fissure caries.
- Effectively monitor the progress of caries.

Disadvantages
- Recognizes only demineralization and not caries specifically; hypomineralization (due to developmental defect or caries) will give similar readings.
- Presence of enamel cracks may lead to false positive diagnosis.
- Sharp metal probe may cause traumatic defects.
- Separate measurements are required for different sites making full mouth examination time consuming.

Devices using electrical conductance property are:

a AC Ohmmeter.

b. Caries meter-L.

c. Vanguard electronic caries detector.

d. Electronic caries monitor (ECM).

e. Electrical impedance tomography.

f. Alternating current impedance spectroscopy (caries scan).

a. AC Ohmmeter

AC Ohmmeter, though not in use these days, utilizes 500 Hz alternating current of frequency, to detect variation in electrical resistance at different areas of tooth. A dental explorer with 0.1 mm tip is placed over the tooth site and another metal sheet is kept in contact with cheeks, contralateral to the tooth to be measured.

b. Caries Meter-L

The caries meter-L, manufactured by two companies, G-C International Corp., Belgium and Onuki Dental Co. Ltd., Japan is a painless and safe modality for evaluating changes in mineral contents (Fig. 10.11). It works on the principle of electrical conductivity. Sine waves of 400 Hz are utilized to measure currents for the caries meter. The electrical impedance is indicated by four colored lights: green, yellow, orange and red. The inference can be drawn by change in color, subsequently the treatment decision (Table 10.1).

The measurements are taken using a probe tip and a clip attached to an oral electrode (cheek or lips). The tooth is dried using dry air and isolated by cotton rolls. Re-moistening, if required, is carried out with a drop of saline. A number of studies have observed sensitivity and specificity as 74% at the enamel caries; whereas 93% sensitivity and 63% specificity at dentin caries.

The information obtained from caries Meter-L is considered insufficient. The unorganized flow of air to dry the tooth and the area of saline contact medium made the technique less favorable. The display of 4 categories represented by color change may

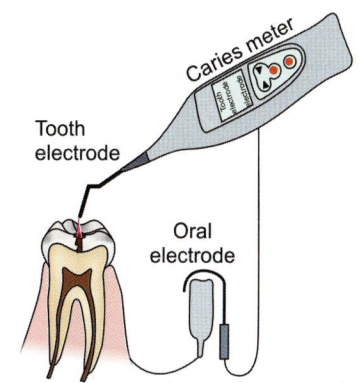

Fig. 10.11: Electronic caries meter

Table 10.1: Colors, indications, impedance values and treatment options

Color	Impedance values	Indication	Treatment options
Green	600 kΩ	Healthy tooth (no caries)	No treatment required
Yellow	Between 250 and 600 kΩ	Enamel caries	Observe for sometime: Use preventive methods
Orange	Between 15 and 250 kΩ	Caries extending into dentin	Remove caries and restore
Red	Below 15 kΩ	Caries invading tooth pulp	Root canal treatment

not exactly categorize changes in mineral contents of the tooth.

c. Vanguard Electronic Caries Detector

The Vanguard electronic caries detector, manufactured by Massachusetts manufacturing corporation, USA, overcame the inconsistency in the flow of air. The probe tip is placed centrally in the fissure and the superficial saliva is removed while taking the reading (in Caries Meter-L, the fissures are moistened with saliva). The measured conductance is converted to ordinal scale from 0 to 9. The readings are inversely related to the resistance and indicate increasing degrees of demineralization.

The device is valuable in measuring early lesion, as the porosity produced in enamel is responsible for the main drop in the resistance values; whereas dentin is markedly less resistant to the electric current. It is stressed that a single reading at one visit may not be able to measure the activity of the lesion; two, three or even more readings are taken and the mean is indicative of the change towards remineralization/demineralization process.

d. Electronic Caries Monitor (ECM)

Electronic Caries monitor employs a single fixed frequency (21 Hz, 23 Hz and 25 Hz) alternating current measuring the electric conductivity of tooth.

The initial design is close to the Vanguard Caries Detector. The electrical probe is placed onto the tooth site and the reference electrode on the lips. The ECM readings can be seen on a screen in front of the device, which may vary

in a range of about –1.00 to 13.00 (precisely -0.70 to 13.20), representing increasing electrical conductance. A higher reading means more decay (Table 10.2).

The ECM readings are site-specific. Substantial time is required in case the surface is to be measured at more than one point. Another limitation was the values measured were different in occlusal surface as compared to smooth surfaces.

ECM II

To overcome some of the limitations, electronic caries monitor (ECM) was improved as ECM II, which was battery operated.

The measurement values were expanded. The provision of the extended value (13.25) to include low resistance values, would act to monitor the progress of dentin lesions. An audible beep indicated that the circuit was completed between the probe tip and the hand-held connector. A double beep indicated when the stable conductance reading was reached. ECM IIb has also been launched. It consists of a probe tip connected to an alternating current supply. The digital display panel provides resistance measurement on a scale 0–2 MΩ. A conducting medium is used to obtain a surface-specific reading.

Table 10.2: Clinical interpretation of ECM values

Range	Clinical interpretation
–1.0 to 1.0	Sound enamel
1.01 to 3.00	Incipient caries
3.01 to 6.00	Enamel caries (up to DEJ)
6.01 to 8.00	Dentinal caries
8.01 to 13.00	Deep dentinal caries

ECM III

ECM III is being used to evaluate the effect of altering the protein content of enamel or etching the surface. ECM resistance readings decrease as the concentration and time of deproteinization increase. In evaluating root caries, the soft dentinal lesions and dark brown lesions depicted lower value than leathery lesions and light brown lesions respectively.

ECM IV

ECM IV depicts readings by three different procedures. The first is similar to Vanguard system; the second uses the "Continuous reading" procedure without applying air-drying, whereas third uses the "Standard ECM Scale" procedure. The total drying and measuring time is fixed at 5 seconds. At the end of the measuring cycle, the resistance value, in Ohm second units (Ω sec), across the total drying period is displayed. Higher readings indicate higher resistance and more caries.

The performance of ECM and the modified forms have been reported to be moderate; no obvious improvement could be observed with these newer models.

e. Electrical Impedance Tomography

Electrical impedance tomography (EIT), is based on the principle of electrical impedance spectroscopy (ECS). Unlike caries meter, which uses fixed frequency, EIT uses a range of frequencies and provide information on capacitance and impedance also.

f. Alternating Current Impedance Spectroscopy (CarieScan)

The alternating current impedance spectroscopy is used to quantify caries at an early stage. This device involves passing of an insensitive level of electrical current through the tooth to identify the presence and location of the decay. The frequency domain is based on a sinusoidal signal applied to the object at a given amplitude and frequency. The response waves are measured and the impedance is calculated by a transfer function relationship of the applied voltage and the acquired current. The CarieScan as claimed is not affected by optical factors such as staining or discoloration of the tooth; it provides a qualitative value based on the disease state rather than the optical properties of the tooth. The device is indicated for the detection, diagnosis, and monitoring of primary dental caries on occlusal and accessible smooth surfaces, which are not clearly visible to the human eye. It cannot be used to assess secondary caries, the integrity of a restoration, root caries, and the depth of an excavation.

Procedure: This device uses disposable tufted sensors for single use and the non-disposable test sensors for routine use. While tufted sensor brush contacts the tooth surface, a disposable metal clip is placed over the corner of the patient's lip, which connects to the CarieScan to complete the circuit. During measurement, a green color display indicates sound tooth tissue, while a red color indicates deep caries, and a yellow color associated with a range of numerical figures from 1 to 99 depicts severity of caries.

A modified version of CarieScan is the CarieScan-Plus, which is a wireless control system allowing data to be automatically captured, filed, and recalled electronically on a by-tooth, by-surface, by-date basis for dental health monitoring. This enhances communication with the patient and aid in preventive regime. Various studies comparing CarieScan with visual examination, bitewing radiograph, and DIAGNOdent reported CarieScan to have superior sensitivity and specificity (both 92.5%) over other methods.

5. Optical Detection Methods

It is recognized that the conventional methods are effective only if at least one-third thickness of enamel is involved. These methods relied on subjective interpretation and were insensitive to incipient caries.

The initial effects of the caries process (initial demineralization changes) result in an alteration in the optical properties of the affected dental tissues. Caries detection based on changes in a specific optical property are referred to as 'optical detection methods', or 'dental tissue optics'. The methods are based on the measurement of a physical signal, derived from the interaction of light with dental hard tissue.

Optical methods are based on the interaction of energy absorbed and emitted from the tooth. The energy interaction is in the form of a wave in the electromagnetic spectrum.

Caries process is the result of tilt of balance between the loss of mineral contents (demineralization) and the diffusion of mineral into the tooth (remineralization). The increase in demineralization is the start of carious process. The scattering of incident light is increased due to the structural change and appears as 'white spot'. The caries process leads to distinct optical changes that can be measured and quantified. Most of these methods use light in the visible and near-infrared region.

Let us understand four basic phenomena of the optical changes.

i. Scattering

Scattering is the process of re-distribution of light in different direction (Change of direction of photon without loss of energy). Particles suspended in the air or any other object scatter light. If the particles are only little larger than the wavelength of light, they scatter equally in all directions. The incident light is forced to deviate from a straight path when it interacts with small particles or objects in the medium through which the light passes. Scattering is highly wavelength sensitive; shorter wavelengths scatter much more than the longer ones. The caries detection methods employing wavelengths in the visible range of the electromagnetic spectra (400 nm to

700 nm) are limited by scattering. An incipient enamel lesion looks whiter than the surrounding healthy enamel because of strong scattering of light from the lesion.

ii. Absorption

It is accepted that light is absorbed and converted into heat. Dark colored objects absorb most of the light that falls on them. Absorption is defined as the process by which photons are stopped by an object and the wave energy is taken in by the same object. The energy lost is mostly converted into heat or into another wave which has less energy and hence longer wavelengths. Absorption of light in tissue is strongly dependent on the wavelength. Water is an example of a strong absorber in the infrared range.

iii. Fluorescence

Fluorescence is a phenomenon where the light is absorbed in a specific wavelength and then emitted in a higher wavelength. The energy absorbed is released by emission of light at a longer wavelength. The pattern of light absorption and remission in the dental tissues varies according to the excited wavelength. Autofluorescence, the natural fluorescence of dental hard tissue without the addition of other luminescent substances, is popular since long. Demineralization will result in loss of autofluorescence which can be quantified based on the differences in fluorescence between sound and carious enamel.

iv. Transillumination

The light passing through the tooth tissue can be used to analyze the carious lesions. Wavelengths in the visible range (400–700 nm) are limited by strong light scattering, making it difficult to image the tooth structure. The enamel is highly transparent in the near infrared range (750–1500 nm) due to weak scattering and absorption. When light illuminates the tooth, the scattering effect in the enamel caries results in less transparency. The detection of decreased light transmission is associated with carious lesion as compared to sound tissues.

a. Optical Caries Monitor

It is a non-invasive method based on the scattering of light by enamel crystals in relation to their surrounding environment. The scattering of light is quantified in enamel and also during the carious process. The clinical applications of optical caries monitor are established (preferred for smooth surface carious lesions).

The monitor consists of a light source, reference unit and a detection tip. The light is transported through a fiber bundle to the tip, which is placed against the tooth surface. The reflected light is collected and measured by the photo-diode of the different fibers in the tip.

ten Bosch, et al (1984) in their *in-vitro* study on bovine enamel showed that the output of the optical caries monitor correlated well with the mineral loss determined by micro-radiography or by chemical methods.

Advantages
- Facilitates quantification.
- Correlates with methods established for determination of mineral loss.

Disadvantages
- Useful only for carious lesions on smooth surfaces.

b. Fiberoptic Transillumination (FOTI)

It is accepted that there are different indices of light transmission for decayed and sound tooth structures. Illumination is delivered by means of fiberoptics from the light source to the tooth structure. The resultant changes in light distribution (light traverses the tooth) are recorded as an image. Since decayed tooth has a lower index of light transmission than the sound tooth structure, the decay areas exhibit as a darkened shadow.

Fiberoptic transillumination is mainly utilized for the detection of proximal caries. More so, it has been established to be more effective in the anterior region. The use in the posterior region is associated with some difficulty. In posterior teeth the light probe is positioned below the cervical margin of the tooth; light may not traverse properly (Fig. 10.12a and b).

The device consists of a halogen lamp and a rheostat which can produce light of variable intensity. The 150-watt lamp generates a maximum light intensity of 4000 lux. Two attachments are used alongside the 2.0 mm diameter cable; a plane mouth mirror mounted on a steel cuff and a 0.5 mm diameter

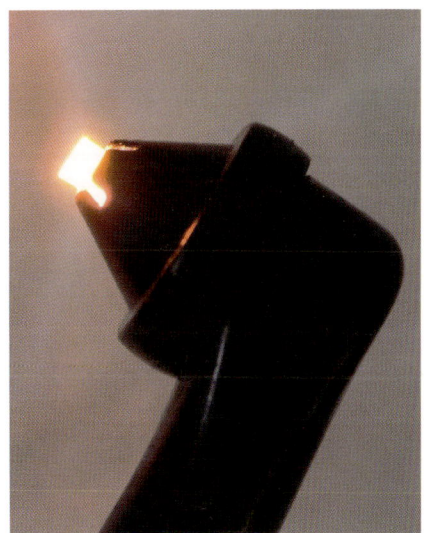

Fig. 10.12a: Fiberoptic tip

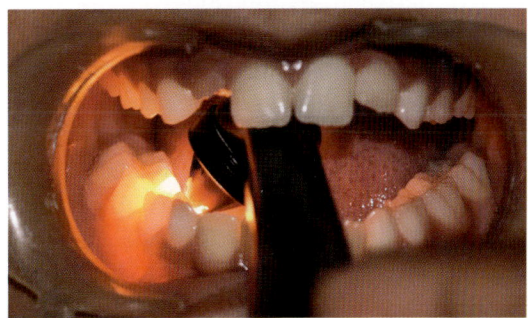

Fig. 10.12b: Fiberoptic tip positioned at the cervical margin of posterior teeth

fiberoptic probe. It produces a narrow beam of light for transillumination.

A shadow may be evident if there is a break in the integrity of the enamel and/or dentin. FOTI has been advocated as an adjunct to visual and radiographic methods. FOTI has led to mixed results in caries diagnosis because of high level of intra and inter-examiner variability.

Advantages

- Lesions, which remain undiagnosed radiographically, can be diagnosed easily.
- Simple and comfortable for the patients.
- No hazards of radiations.
- Less time consuming.

Disadvantages

- Record keeping is difficult.
- Subject to intra- and interobserver variations.
- Difficult to place the light probe in posterior regions.

c. Digital Imaging Fiberoptic Transillumination (DIFOTI)

Digital imaging fiberoptic transillumination (DIFOTI) method was developed in an attempt to overcome the shortcomings of FOTI by combining FOTI and a digital camera using charged couple device (CCD). Images so captured are transferred to a computer for analysis. The CCD projects instantaneous images, which can be compared for clinical changes between several images of the same tooth over a given period of time. In addition, illumination and other conditions that may affect the quality of the image can be easily controlled.

DIFOTI is being successfully used for the detection of incipient and recurrent caries. It enables the operator to confirm the presence of caries that cannot be seen radiographically, or felt by visual-tactile means.

It is important to note that DIFOTI images cannot indicate the depth of lesion penetration.

The device is highly sensitive; dark areas in DIFOTI images may sometimes be due to stains or calculi on tooth surface. It is suggested that prophylaxis should be carried out prior to the use of the device in order to increase the specificity.

DIFOTI is proved to be twice sensitive in detecting proximal lesions and three times sensitive in the detection of occlusal lesions. For buccal-lingual lesions, the sensitivity was 10 times that of conventional radiographs.

Diagnocam, a camera, using fiberoptic transillumination technology (excitation wavelength –780 nm) was introduced to capture pictures of the tooth surfaces at various angles; however, limited research is documented on its use.

Advantage

- CCD overcomes the disadvantages of FOTI.

Disadvantage

- Do not indicate the depth of the lesion.

d. Ultraviolet Illumination

Ultraviolet light has also been used to discriminate the carious and the sound tissue of the tooth. The fluorescence (UV illumination) of tooth tissue is decreased in areas of less mineral content, such as in carious lesions.

The caries lesion appears as a dark spot against a fluorescent background. The fluorescent effects have been used as a method for the detection of dental caries in smooth surfaces in humans as well as in research animals. The method is still not been developed into a quantitative method. This method was more sensitive than visual-tactile methods. However, protective measures against ultraviolet radiation were required both for patient and the examiner. The specificity was also a problem in distinguishing between a carious lesion and other hypomineralized areas.

Advantage

- More sensitive than visual-tactile method.

Disadvantage

- The carious lesion and the other areas of hypomineralization appear same.

e. Transillumination with Near-infrared Light

Wavelengths in the visible range (400–700 nm) are limited by strong light scattering, making it difficult to image through more than 1.0 mm or 2.0 mm of tooth structure. The methods employing wavelengths in the visible range (400–700 nm), such as laser fluorescence, quantitative light induced fluorescence (QLF), and digital imaging fiber-optic transillumination (DIFOTI) are highly limited by scattering. Methods that use longer wavelengths, such as near infrared spectra (780–1550 nm), can penetrate the tissues more deeply. This deeper penetration is desired for transillumination. It is established that enamel is highly transparent in the near-infrared light range (750–1500 nm) due to the weak scattering and better absorption in dental hard tissue. Therefore, this region of the electromagnetic spectrum is ideally suited to the development of new optical diagnostic tools based on transillumination.

The polarized light in the near-infrared range (1310 nm) gets depolarized by demineralized enamel and dentin. This rapid depolarization of polarized light by dental caries (demineralization) provides high contrast for imaging carious lesions (the dental tissues are highly birefringent; demineralization results in increase in light scattering and changes in birefringent).

The image can be captured, saved, and stored in digital format by use of transillumination with near infra-red light. This is a promising imaging technique for detecting the presence of caries and also the extent of its severity. The method is non-destructive, non-ionizing, and reportedly more sensitive to detect early demineralization than dental X-rays.

Detection of dental caries by transillumination is based on the fact that increased mineral loss in enamel leads to a two-fold increase in scattering coefficient. Caries thus appear as dark regions, since less light reaches the detector. When light illuminates the tooth, the strong scattering effect in the enamel carious lesions results in less transparency. The decreased light transmission associated with the lesion can be detected when compared to that of the surrounding sound tissue.

The transillumination method overcomes the limitations of radiographs, since it allows repeated projections. The location of the carious lesion and how the resolution differs when the resultant image has to traverse a thick part versus a thinner part of the tooth is also important. The ratio between the contrasts of images captured from both sides of the tooth can estimate the precise location of the carious lesions.

Advantages

- Less amount of back scattering.
- Can be easily differentiated from stains, pigmentation, and hypomineralisation (fluorosis).

Disadvantage

- May damage pulp.

f. Laser-induced Fluorescence

A few authors observed that normal teeth fluoresce under ultraviolet illumination and suggested that fluorescence might be useful in the determination of dental caries. A monochromatic light is used at 350 nm, 410 nm and 530 nm on carious and sound surfaces. In the carious lesions, the emission spectra shifts to more than 540 nm (red range of the electromagnetic spectrum). The largest difference between the carious and sound spectra is found at 600 nm. It is observed that when the enamel is illuminated with light in the blue-green range, the observable fluorescence occurs in the green-yellow range.

Infra-red fluorescence has also been utilized, which implies irradiating the tooth with a light wavelength of 700–15,000 nm. It has been established that the technique discriminates between sound and carious enamel and dentin. Further studies are required to determine if the fluorescence signal from exposure to infra-red irradiation is greater than that from other wavelengths. There may be potentially damaging effects on the dental pulp due to overheating from absorption of infra-red irradiation (the increased penetration and decreased scattering of infra-red irradiation). Specific coherent source of such irradiation have been relatively difficult to acquire, and detection involves the use of infra-red sensitive detectors.

The tooth is illuminated with a broad beam of argon-ion laser (blue-green light of 488 nm wavelengths) and the fluorescence observed in the yellow (540 nm) range. This fluorescence of enamel occurring in the yellow range (540 nm) is observed through a yellow high pass filter to exclude the tissue, scattering blue light. Demineralized areas appear dark than the healthy tissue. Fluorescent dyes such as fluorol, sodium fluorescein are also used to differentiate the areas of different mineral content. Demineralized tissues absorb dyes and fluoresce strongly. This is referred to as *dye enhanced laser fluorescence*. A quantified version of laser fluorescence in the form of micro-camera has been developed to capture the real image. A computer screen displays the real images of the teeth under examination.

Advantages

- Convenient and a relatively fast method.
- Incipient carious lesions (minute mineral loss) can be detected.
- Suitable for quantifying secondary caries (mineral loss around restorations).

Disadvantages

- Tooth surfaces and fissures being assessed should be clean and dry.
- No evidence present for the detection of proximal or secondary caries adjacent to existing restorations.

Devices (with camera) using fluorescence principles

i. *Quantitative light-induced fluorescence*
The quantitative light-induced fluorescence (QLF) is based on the principle that the autofluorescence differs with the change in the mineral content of the dental hard tissue. Increased porosity due to demineralization, result in loss of its natural fluorescence.

The QLF device uses a 50-watt xenon arc lamp and an optical filter producing blue light (290–450 nm wavelength), which is carried to the tooth. The fluorescence images are filtered and captured by a colored CCD camera (the device consists of intraoral color CCD camera, a computer and the custom software to capture and analyze the images).

When a lesion is present on the tooth surface, an increase in scattering is observed relative to the surrounding normal tissues. The contrast is increased whereby the lesion appears dark on the light green background of the tooth surface.

The fluorescence emitted is directly related to the mineral content of enamel. The change in enamel fluorescence is detected and measured. The image so produced is converted to black and white and after that the lesion site is rebuilt by extrapolation of fluorescence of healthy tissues around the lesion. The image can be used to quantify the size, depth and volume of the carious lesion. The parameters used are:

- Lesion depth—DF (percentage of fluorescence loss).
- Volume of the lesion—DQ (Area [in mm^2] × DF); provide extent of lesion.

The QLF-D Biluminator is a new type of QLF device. Fluorescence images are captured with a full sensor single lens reflex (SLR) camera.

Advantages

- Useful in detecting incipient lesions, secondary and root caries.
- Useful in detecting demineralization under orthodontic appliances/brackets, etc.

- Monitors extent of demineralization and remineralization.
- Provides quantitative parameters (lesion depth, area/volume).

Disadvantages

- Cannot differentiate between decay, hypoplasia or unusual anatomic features.
- Potential for operator bias, position of camera may vary.
- Inability to detect/monitor inter-proximal lesions.
- May be influenced by stains, fluorosis/hypomineralization etc.

ii. *Light-induced fluorescence evaluation—diagnosis and treatment (LIFEDT) concept*

Four different fluorescence versions can be observed based on the difference of fluorescence of dental tissues. The green fluorescence indicates healthy tissues; black green indicates infected dentin; bright red indicates the margin of infected/affected dentin; and acid green fluorescence indicates sound dentin. These different fluorescence signals aid in caries detection. This concept has been termed 'Light-Induced Fluorescence Evaluation—Diagnosis and Treatment (LIFEDT) concept'.

The principle is linked to the working of fluorescence based cameras. The basic procedure involved is the same and that is as follows:

- The occlusal surfaces of tooth are cleaned.
- Both can be observed in daylight or in a variety of modified forms.
- The reflected light from carious areas is noted and compared to healthy areas.
- System improves overall visual inspections.

The SoproLife camera works on the principle of LIFEDT has been launched to aid in caries detection. The camera captures the images in three different modes that is, daylight, diagnosis and treatment mode. Capturing in the daylight provides a white light image with a magnification of more than 50 times than the tooth surface. The other two modes of the camera work on the principle of autofluorescence. In the diagnostic mode, the camera uses a visible blue light frequency (wavelength 450 nm) to illuminate the surface of the teeth, and provides an anatomic image overlay of the green fluorescence image on the "white light" image. The green fluorescence is considered as an indicator of normal dental tissues; while carious lesions could be detected by variation in the autofluorescence of its tissues in relation to a healthy area of the same tooth. In addition to the green fluorescence, red fluorescence may also be seen in some diagnostic mode images. This red fluorescence may represent deep dentinal caries; however, at the same time it might be a false signal coming from the organic deposits covering the tooth. A correlation between the red signal and organic deposit has been observed. Hence, the red fluorescence signal in the diagnostic mode images should be validated. For validation, the area showing the red fluorescence be washed off with sodium bicarbonate or pumice, and if the fluorescence persists then only it is considered to be infected dentin. The fluorescence would not persist, if the source is organic deposits on the tooth surface. The third mode is the treatment mode, and the red fluorescence captured in this mode is considered as an indicator to differentiate between infected and affected dentin.

The loss of green fluorescence is termed *autofluorescence masking effect*. The black-green fluorescence indicates infected dentin and need to be excavated till acid green fluorescence is achieved. The acid green fluorescence is considered as an indicator of sound dentin. Thus, aiming to achieve acid green fluorescence might be used as a guideline for termination of excavation process. The bright red fluorescence indicates infected/affected dentin.

iii. *New cameras*

A new camera, the Soprococ, provides three modes: viz. daylight, caries and periodontal mode. VistaCam and vistaCam CL-IX work on the same principles with minor modifications.

Another camera based on light induced fluorescence phenomenon is VistaProof intraoral camera. With this device, different areas of dental surfaces can be seen (green fluorescence—sound tissue; red fluorescence—carious tissue). Softwares are available (viz. DBSWIN software) which can analyze the images in red fluorescence (to see the lesion extension). A numerical value, from 0 to 5, can be given to categorize the lesion extension.

Devices (without cameras) using fluorescence principles

i. *DIAGNOdent*

DIAGNOdent follows principle of fluorescence without the use of a camera.

DIAGNOdent recognizes changes affecting the tooth, such as early demineralization and initial carious lesions. The gadget is also useful in determining the amount of decalcification in different areas of the same tooth. Even the residual caries can be identified.

The instrument involves a laser diode (655 nm), with 1 mW power as the excitation light source, and a long pass filter (transmission > 680 nm) as the detector. A flexible tip is used to transfer light to dental tissues. The light passes through normal enamel without deflection; whereas in affected enamel, the light is diffracted and disposed. This results in autofluorescence due to fluorophores present in carious lesions. The fluorophores or the porphyrins (name suggested by certain authors) are derived from bacterial metabolism. The fluorescence so emitted is collected by nine concentric fibers and translated into numerical values (from –9 to 99).

Procedure

The tooth/teeth to be assessed should be thoroughly cleaned and dried. The refractive index is 1.33 for wet demineralized surfaces and 1.0 for dried demineralized surfaces;

making the opaque appearance of the caries clearly visible. As enamel is dried, light-scattering is increased, and a lower fluorescence can be measured. However, the performance (specificity and sensitivity) of the DIAGNOdent on dry tooth surfaces is not significantly different from that on moist surfaces.

The fluorescence of a sound surface of the tooth is measured, which is considered as the baseline value. This value is then subtracted electronically from the fluorescence of the site to be measured. Two different tips are used, one for occlusal site and the other for smooth surfaces. To achieve the maximum extension of caries on occlusal surfaces, one must tilt the instrument around the measuring site. This ensures that the tip picks up fluorescence from the slopes of the fissure walls, where the carious process often begins (Fig. 10.13a to c).

This system has a range of –9 and 99 with (–9 to 0) being the value of normal tooth. Initiation of caries is from 0 to 9; caries of enamel is from 10 to 17; and the rest is for dentinal caries depending upon the depth of caries. A new device, DIAGNOdent pen has also been introduced. The principle functioning is the same; however, tips are modified using sapphire fibers. The performance in proximal surfaces is found to be limited.

A couple of authors have observed DIAGNOdent as the most accurate device for the detection of occlusal caries. It is advisable

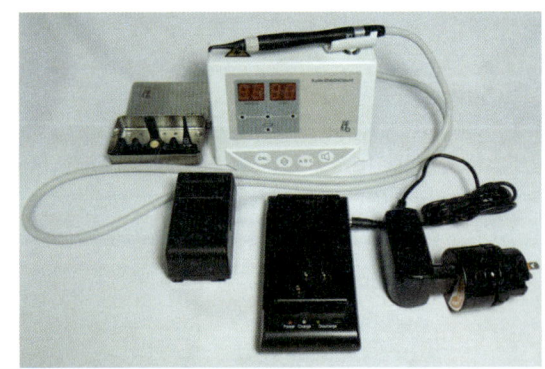

Fig. 10.13a: Kavo DIAGNOdent conventional unit

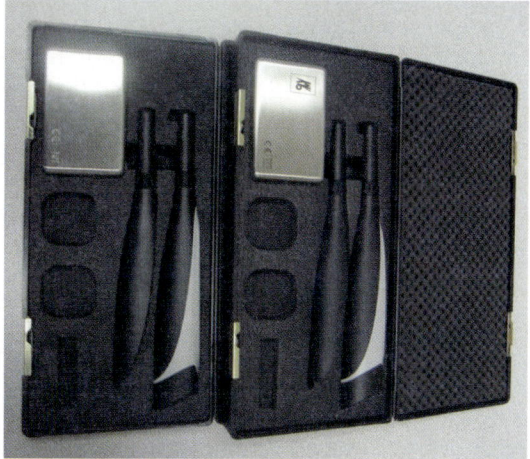

Fig. 10.13b: DIAGNOdent pen

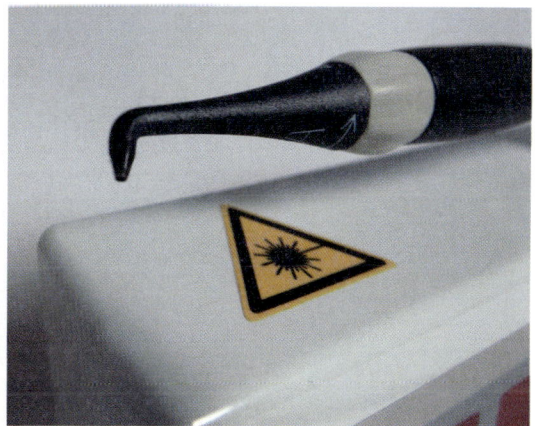

Fig. 10.13c: DIAGNOdent pen

to use these devices as a supplementary tool along with visual/radiographic methods.

Advantages
- 90% success rate.
- 0.92 sensitivity (more than electronic caries monitor).
- High reproducibility and reliability.
- Easy to use.
- Readily transportable.
- Non-invasive and painless.
- No operator bias.

Disadvantages
- May induce false readings in the presence of plaque and debris.

- Readings do not relate exactly to the amount of dentinal caries; presence of micro-organism also matters.
- Can't be used for recurrent caries.
- Staining, etc. may interfere with the results.

g. Visible Luminescence Spectroscopy
The visible emission spectra differ for decayed and non-decayed regions of teeth. Quasi-monochromatic light from a tungsten source dispersed with a grating monochromator is focused on the teeth. This is considered as a non-radiological, non-invasive clinical method to detect dental caries.

h. Terahertz Imaging (TI)
Terahertz waves (frequency = 10^{12} Hz: wavelength 30 mm) are being used in caries diagnosis. This wave-form provides reasonable resolution and also prevents loss of signal due to scattering. It was recognized earlier that photoconductive emitters could be used to generate and coherent picoseconds (10^{12} s) pulse, which would emit electromagnetic waves with a frequency in the terahertz range. The terahertz pulses can be produced on short timescale. A small portion of visible beam, when pass through the electro-optical medium, become elliptically polarized. The degree of this elliptical polarization is measured using optical photodetectors. By measuring the time taken by a terahertz pulse to travel through a medium/object, the thickness/depth and the refractive index can be determined.

The object is placed in the path of terahertz beam to record the image. Alternatively, the terahertz beam can be scanned over the surface of an object. Terahertz images have also been recorded using a CCD camera. Dental applications for this technique have been limited but promising. A longitudinal image of human tooth demonstrated the outline of the enamel-dentin junction as well as the dentin-pulp interface. Longitudinal sections further demonstrated increased terahertz absorption by early occlusal caries;

also ability to discriminate dental caries from idiopathic enamel hypomineralization.

The cost of the equipment, the complexity of the laser source, and the requirements for precise manipulation are some of the clinical limitations of using terahertz imaging.

Advantages

- Relative transparency of human tissue to terahertz rays.
- Low powers used for imaging (~ 1 W).
- Use of non-ionizing radiation.
- No alteration of electrical charge of the oral tissues.
- No adverse thermal effects.
- Low signal-to-noise ratio (facilitates clear imaging).

Disadvantages

- Complexity of the laser source
- Precise manipulation mandatory
- Care is required in image interpretation, since terahertz waves are strongly absorbed by water, a potential complication in the oral cavity.
- High cost

i. Multiphoton Imaging (MPI)

Caries detection systems such as QLF rely on the fluorescence signal observed when teeth are exposed to blue light (~ 488–514 nm). This causes sound tooth structure to fluoresce. Carious tooth tissue may also fluoresce, but the disruption in the tooth structure results in profound scattering, which may result in a little or no fluorescence. Consequently, sound tooth structure fluoresces at > 520 nm; whereas carious tooth tissue appears dark. It is not possible to collect light specifically from different depths within the tooth. Other methods, such as confocal microscopy, can be used to collect light from different depths but only within the outer 100 microns of the tooth. Information from deeper tissues is also desirable. Blue light tends to scatter substantially within carious lesions and therefore does not penetrate well through the lesion. At high intensity, blue light induces free-radical production, which may injure the pulp.

The choice of a longer wavelength of light for imaging reduces the scattering, allowing the light to penetrate more deeply within the tooth. This is the basis of multiphoton imaging (infrared light used at 850 nm), which makes clear image of the tooth.

In conventional fluorescence imaging, a single 'blue' photon is used to excite a fluorescent compound in the tooth. In the multiphoton technique, two infrared photons (with half the energy of the blue photon) are absorbed simultaneously. The probability of this happening is normally low, but by exposing the tooth to many more photons, it is possible to increase greatly the chances of two-photon absorption (the probability of two-photon absorption is proportional to the square of the light intensity). Generally, this means increasing the intensity of the light beam, which is also likely to generate heat within the tooth. To generate enough two-photon energy, a power of 2 kW would be required. A tooth may not survive this amount of heat. To minimize heat, ultrashort pulses of laser light are used at low power producing the same two-photon energy.

Ultra-short pulses (100 fs) of 850 nm laser light are generated at 200 MHz. The fluorescence resulting from two-photon excitation is recorded using given focal plane. The focal plane can be changed, from enamel towards the dentin. The sound tooth tissue fluoresces strongly; whereas, carious tooth tissue fluoresces to a much lesser extent. 3-D image inside the tooth depicts caries as a dark shadow form within a brightly fluorescing tooth.

Multiphoton imaging can collect information from up to 500 μm deep carious lesions. The technique has been performed only on extracted teeth. Its advantage lies in three-dimensional measurement of mineral loss. The low level of laser power is less toxic to pulp.

Advantages

- Provides 3-D image.
- A non-invasive method.
- Low speed of laser power is less toxic to pulp.
- Enhanced depth of penetration due to use of longer incident wavelength.
- Three-dimensional measurement of mineral loss possible.

Disadvantage

- It can cause harm to the tissues; however, ultra-short pulses can overcome this problem.

j. Optical Coherence Tomography (OCT)

Optical coherence tomography (OCT) was developed for imaging transparent and semi-transparent structures. Tooth tissues are considered semi-transparent. Initially OCT was used only in medical field. Baumgartner (2000) was among the early authors who used OCT in dental imaging. Most OCT techniques described for imaging dental tissues have used wavelengths of 840 to 1310 nm with imaging depths achieved from 0.6 to 2.0 mm.

Only *in-vitro* studies are available. The modified form of OCT, the polarized sensitive OCT (PS-OCT), can be correlated with the degree of demineralization and lesion severity. This is showing better results in assessing *in-vivo* carious lesions.

Optical coherence tomography (OCT) is based upon the principle of interference of light. When a light beam is split into two and then recombined, interference produces a pattern, the intensity of which is determined by the level of light in each beam. The OCT system uses Super Luminescent Diodes (SLDs) as a light source. These diodes produce light with a broad range of wavelengths, each of which will produce its own interference pattern. However, in certain circumstances, the merging of interference patterns may result in blurring of some signals. The signals that are not blurred are easily detected, facilitating optical section of the samples. The spectral bandwidth of the light (the difference between the shortest and longest wavelengths produced by the illumination source) determines the depth resolution of the technique. The intensity of the interference is a function of the scattering caused by the changes in tissue structure of the tooth. Variation in scattering measured in relation to depth from a single point on the tooth surface is designated as "A-scan". Taking several A-scans along a line produces information from a 'slice' of tooth tissue, which is the tomogram. The movement along the line of A-scans is known as the "B-scan", and, it takes from 30 to 60 seconds to acquire a 1 cm long B-scan. A-scan is produced when light from a suitable source passes through a beam splitter and divide it into two coherent beams of light. One beam is called the *sample beam* and the other, the *reference beam*. The sample beam penetrates the tooth and gets scattered according to the nature of the tissue. It is established that carious tissues scatter light to a greater extent than does sound tooth structure. Some of the sample beam will be scattered back towards the beam splitter. The reference beam travels to a movable mirror, where it is reflected back to the beam splitter. Here it is re-combined with the backscattered sample beam. The re-combined reference and back-scattered sample beams are focused onto a photodetector, where any degree of interference can be observed. In this way, changes in the scattering properties of the tooth as a function of depth can be recorded.

Analysis of caries lesions has been performed, and changes in signal are related to the degree of scattering and possibly the degree of mineralization. OCT is being used to assess the restoration-tooth interface for semi-transparent restorations. This may have implications for the non-invasive diagnosis of secondary caries, since as with all optical methods, the uptake of any stain confound the technique.

Advantages

- Clear image can be achieved.
- Quantitatively monitor the mineral changes in a caries lesion.
- Can determine severity of the lesion

Disadvantages

- False-positive results may be achieved due to back scattering.
- Limited to *in vitro* studies.

k. Polarized Raman Spectroscopy (PRS)

Polarized Raman Spectroscopy (PRS) measures light scattering as in optical coherence tomography. OCT imaging in regions of hypocalcification may show increased back-scattering, which could be misinterpreted as signs of early caries. To rule out such false-positive readings and increase the specificity of OCT, OCT is combined with PRS. PRS provides details on the composition (e.g. collagen in dentin vs inorganic apatite in enamel) and molecular structure of cells and tissues. The scattered photons after light scattering have the same energy and wavelength as the incoming excitation light. Approximately 1 in 10^7 photons scatters at an energy different from that of the incoming light. This energy difference is proportional to the vibrational energy of the scattered molecules within the sample and is known as the *Raman effect*. As with other optical methods, the properties of the scattered light within sound or porous carious regions determine the initial demineralization, vis-à-vis caries. In fluorescence-based techniques, there are a limited number of intrinsic fluorophores that can provide diagnostic information without the addition of external dyes. In contrast, PRS can provide information not only about bacterial porphyrins leached into carious regions, but also about the primary mineral matrix and, thus, the state of demineralization or remineralization of the tooth, without the need to add extrinsic dyes. PRS provides information on the composition and orientation of the mineral matrix, which are affected in caries process.

Advantages

- Non-invasive method analyzing bio-chemistry and molecular elements of white spot lesions.
- External dyes are not required.

Disadvantage

- Calculus, hypocalcification, and stains may lead to false-positive results.

l. Midwest Caries ID (LED technology)

Midwest Caries ID, developed on LED technology, detects differences of optical behavior of sound tooth and the tooth with changes in their mineral content. The Midwest Caries ID uses infrared and red light emitting diodes (LEDs) and a fiberoptic to distribute light to the given area of the object. A second fiberoptic collects light from that area to a photodetector that measures returned collected light. The photodetector then transmits the signal to a microprocessor that compares signal levels with defined parameters. When the detection is positive, the processor deactivates the green LED (pulses at a higher intensity than the red LED). When the detection is negative (healthy tooth area), the green LED is dominant (green illumination in healthy tooth tissues and red illumination in caries or demineralization). A buzzer also beeps with different frequencies to indicate the intensity of demineralization detected. The Midwest Caries ID can also be used for proximal caries by slightly angulating and moving the probe over the vulnerable proximal area. This modality is more convenient than the DIAGNOdent since it enables minimal dilution of the light signal from all surrounding structures. Inter-proximal detection using the Midwest Caries ID showed a sensitivity of 80% and specificity of 98%. However, this device can give false-positive signals in case of teeth with growth malformations in the enamel/dentin, teeth with thick, dark stains, hypermineralization, hypocalcification, dental fluorosis, and atypically shaped teeth due to alteration in the translucency of enamel. Light penetration is limited into the enamel and up to 3.0 mm in proximal area. If the probe is tipped too acutely when checking for proximal caries, deviated light reflection may provide false-positive results. Plaque and calculus etc. may also cause false-positive results. Rodrigues, et al (2011) however, in their study reported that Midwest caries ID could not differentiate enamel lesion from sound surfaces.

Advantage

- Intensity of demineralization can be measured.

Disadvantages

- May show false-positive results especially in teeth with growth malformations, hypermineralization, hypocalcification, dental fluorosis, etc.
- Plaque and calculus also cause false-positive results.
- Light penetration is limited (up to 3.0 mm in proximal area).

m. Frequency-Domain Photo-thermal Radiometry and Modulated Luminescence (PTR/LUM)

The combined frequency-domain laser-induced photo-thermal radiometry and modulated luminescence (PTR/LUM) is the recent development in caries diagnosis. The combined effect of PTR and LUM has been reported to be better than other related methods.

The technique is based on the photo-thermal response of a medium, resulting from optical radiation absorption from a low intensity laser beam. This is followed by optical-to-thermal energy conversion leading to slight rise in temperature. The PTR has depth-profilometric ability, i.e. it can penetrate and yield information of any scattering medium well beyond the range of optical imaging. In PTR applications to dental hard tissue, optical and thermo-physical properties and depth information are obtained in two distinct modes: (i) from near surface distances (5–500 µm) controlled by the thermal diffusivity of enamel and the modulation frequency of the laser beam intensity, and (ii) through mid-infrared emissions from considerably deeper regions. The PTR signal consists of both surface and subsurface responses of dental tissue; i.e. why it can distinguish between caries, stains on tooth surface, and developmental white spots, unlike the fluorescence device, such as QLF. Fluorescence techniques monitor radioactive emission variations between optically excited healthy and carious dental fluorophores; the mechanism utilized in DIAGNOdent instrument. The most fundamental difference lies in the fact that PTR/LUM is a depth profilo-metric technique; whereas DIAGNOdent and all other photonics-based technologies are not. PTR/LUM is sensitive to changes in both optical and thermal properties of the sample; whereas DIAGNOdent only senses differences in optical properties through the fluorescence changes. The combination of PTR and LUM techniques have the highest signal dynamic range in detecting very early demineralization, providing the best diagnostic results in caries diagnosis. A combination of PTR and LUM technique with combined specificity and sensitivity has been reported to be better than the DIAGNOdent, radiographic, and visual methods. A study that compared the caries diagnostic ability of PTR/LUM, DIAGNOdent, visual inspection, and radiographs with histological technique as the gold standard showed that the combined PTR/LUM method is superior to all other tested methods. Combining PTR and LUM showed a superior sensitivity and specificity over either PTR or LUM alone. A couple of authors have observed PTR/LUM technique reliable in detecting early proximal caries. The concept of PTR and LUM has been utilized in development of caries detection device called CANARY SYSTEM that has showed better sensitivity than conventional ICDAS readings (Fig. 10.14).

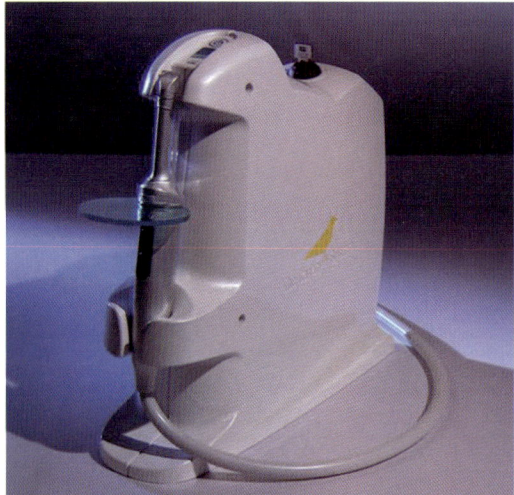

Fig. 10.14: Canary system for caries diagnosis

Advantages
- It is a depth profilometric technique while other photonic based technologies are not.
- It is sensitive to changes in both optical and thermal properties of the sample.
- It has the highest signal dynamic range in detecting very early demineralization.
- It is reliable and non-invasive.

Disadvantage
- Signal reception need be improved.

n. *Time-correlated Single-photon Counting Fluorescence Lifetime Imaging Microscopy*

The fluorescence lifetime imaging microscopy (FLIM) has also been used to distinguish the carious areas from sound dental tissue. A 488 nm excitation wavelength is required to perform time-correlated single-photon counting fluorescence lifetime imaging microscopy (TCSPC-FLIM) of dental tissues. The white-light generation source provides a flexible method of producing variable-bandwidth visible and pulsed light for TCSPC-FLIM. The method could discriminate diseased tissue from sound; however, stained tissue creates problems for evaluation.

Advantage
- Relatively safe compared to two-photon excitation method.

Disadvantage
- Time consuming.

The clinical applications, advantages and disadvantages of optical methods for detections of caries are summarized in Table 10.3.

6. Endoscopic/Videoscopic Methods

It is established that the difference in the fluorescence of sound and carious enamel is observed after illuminating the tooth with blue light (wavelength 400–500 nm). When this fluoresced tooth is viewed through a specific broadband gelatin filter, white spot lesions appear darker than the surrounding enamel. A white light source can also be connected to an endoscope by a fiberoptic cable so that the teeth can be viewed without a filter. This technique is referred to as 'white light endoscopy.'

Additionally, a camera can be used to store the image. The integration of the camera with the endoscope is called a videoscope. A miniature color video camera is mounted in a custom-made metal mirror holder. This is designed in such a way that the image of the surface of enamel can be viewed directly on a monitor. The videotapes are viewed by expert examiners who had also examined the teeth by conventional methods. It is established that the endoscopic examination can detect a greater number of initial carious lesions than do conventional methods.

Advantage
- Facilitate proper viewing (5- to 10-fold magnification achieved).

Disadvantages
- Time consuming (meticulous drying and isolation takes time).
- Costly.

7. Dye Penetration Method

Various types of dyes are being used to visualize an object from its routine background or if several objects have a similar

Table 10.3: The clinical applications, advantages and disadvantages of optical methods for detection of caries

Diagnostic method	Clinical application	Advantages	Disadvantages
Optical caries monitor	For detection of smooth surface caries	• Facilitates quantification • Correlates with methods established for determination of mineral loss	• Useful only for caries lesions on smooth surfaces
Fiberoptic transillumination (FOTI)	Mainly utilized for detection of proximal caries	• Non-ionizing • Gives instant images • Lesions, which remain undiagnosed radiographically, can be diagnosed easily • Simple and comfortable for the patients • No hazards of radiations • Less time consuming	• Record keeping is difficult • Subject to intra and inter observer variations • Difficult to place the light probe in posterior regions
Digital imaging fiberoptic transillumination (DIFOTI)	For detection of proximal, occlusal and smooth surface caries	• CCD overcomes the disadvantages of FOTI	• Do not indicate the depth of the lesion • Stains/calculus may create problems
Ultraviolet illumination	Carious lesion appear dark as compared to sound tissue	• More sensitive than visual-tactile method	• The carious lesion and the other areas of hypomineralization appear same
Transillumination with near-infrared light	Promising technique for detecting caries and measuring its severity	• Less amount of back scattering. • Can be easily differentiated from stains, pigmentation, and hypomineralisation (fluorosis)	• May damage pulp (not documented)
Laser auto fluorescence	Performs best in detecting smooth surface and occlusal pit and fissure caries	• Convenient and a relatively fast method • Incipient carious lesions (minute mineral loss) can be detected • Suitable for quantifying secondary caries (mineral loss around restorations)	• Tooth surfaces and fissures being assessed should be clean and dry • No evidence present for the detection of proximal or secondary caries adjacent to existing restorations
Quantitatively light-induced fluorescence (QLF)	Effectively monitor demineralization and remineralization of teeth *in vitro*. Also used to measure erosive potential of different mouthwash *in vitro*	• Useful in detecting incipient lesions, secondary and root caries • Useful in detecting demineralization under orthodontic appliances/brackets, etc	• It cannot differentiate between decay, hypoplasia or unusual anatomic features • Potential for operator bias (position of camera may vary)

Contd...

Table 10.3: The clinical applications, advantages and disadvantages of optical methods for detection of caries *(Contd..)*

Diagnostic method	Clinical application	Advantages	Disadvantages
		• Monitor extent of demineralization and remineralization • Provide quantitative parameters (lesion depth, area/volume)	• Inability to detect/monitor inter-proximal lesions • It may be influenced by stains, fluorosis/hypomineralization, etc • Has limited depth measurement
DIAGNOdent	Recognizes early changes affecting teeth (amount of decalcification in different areas of tooth)	• 90% success rate • 0.92 sensitivity (more than electronic caries monitor) • High reproducibility and reliability • Easy to use • Readily transportable • Non-invasive and painless • No operator bias	• May induce false readings in the presence of plaque and debris • Readings do not relate exactly to the amount of dentinal decay; presence of micro-organisms also matters • Cannot be used for recurrent caries • Staining, etc. also interfere with the results
Terahertz imaging (TI)	Dental applications for this technique are limited but promising	• Relative transparency of human tissue to terahertz rays • Low powers used for imaging ($\sim 1\ \mu W$) • Use of non-ionizing radiation • No alteration of electrical charge of the oral tissues • No adverse thermal effects • Low signal-to-noise ratio (facilitates clear imaging)	• Complexity of the laser source • Precise manipulation mandatory • Care is required in image interpretation, since terahertz waves are strongly absorbed by water, a potential complication in the oral cavity • High cost
Multiphoton imaging (MPI)	Currently the technique has been performed only on the extracted teeth	• Able to collect information up to 500 microns in depth • Provides 3-D image • A non-invasive method • Low risk of phototoxicity to the pulp due to low average speed of laser power used	• It can harm tissues; however, ultra-short pulses can overcome this problem

Contd...

Table 10.3: The clinical applications, advantages and disadvantages of optical methods for detection of caries *(Contd...)*

Diagnostic method	Clinical application	Advantages	Disadvantages
		• Enhanced depth of penetration due to longer incident wavelength used • Possibility of quantifiable measurement of mineral loss, as function of fluorescence loss, from a carious lesion in three dimensions	
Optical coherence tomography (OCT) and polarized sensitive OCT	Utilized in *in-vitro* studies. Polarized sensitive OCT useful for lesion severity and degree of demineralization	• Clear image can be achieved • Quantitatively monitor the mineral changes in a caries lesion • Can determine severity of the lesion	• False positive results may be achieved due to back scattering • Limited to *in-vitro* studies
Polarized Raman Spectroscopy (PRS)	Used in conjunction with OCT for better results	• A non-invasive method analyzing biochemistry and molecular elements of white spot lesions • External dyes are not required	Factors in the oral environment such as calculus, hypocalcification, and stain could lead to false positive results
Midwest caries ID (LED technology)	Preferred for proximal caries and measuring intensity of demineralization	• Intensity of demineralization can be measured	• False positive results in case of teeth with growth malformations, dark stains, hypermineralization, hypocalcification, dental fluorosis, etc. • Light penetration is limited (up to 3.0 mm in proximal area)
Frequency–domain photo thermal radiometry and modulated luminescence	Imaging of occlusal/proximal caries	• It is a depth profilometric technique while other photonic based technologies are not • It is sensitive to changes in both optical and thermal properties of the sample • It has the highest signal dynamic range in detecting very early demineralization	• Signal reception need to be improved

Contd...

Table 10.3: The clinical applications, advantages and disadvantages of optical methods for detection of caries *(Contd...)*

Diagnostic method	Clinical application	Advantages	Disadvantages
Time-correlated Single-photon Counting Fluorescence lifetime imaging microscopy	Differentiate between carious and sound regions by time-resolved fluorescence	• Relatively safe compared to two-photon excitation method	• Time consuming

appearance, dyes can discriminate them. The observation of the color can be qualitative or quantitative. For a qualitative assessment, the colored objects are differentiated from the noncolored ones. For a quantitative assessment, the intensity of color is to be determined. The total area, which is colored, can be compared with the uncolored areas. The intensity of color can be determined by absorption or fluorescence. Absorption measured by quantitating the decrease of light intensity; whereas fluorescence is measured by quantitating the increase of light intensity at a particular wavelength.

In caries diagnosis, qualitative examination is followed; observation of color change signifies presence of caries. The use of dye is based on the fact that development of microvoids leads to increase in porosity, which is considered as an early sign of caries process. The requisite characteristics of dyes are:

- Should be absolutely safe for intra- oral use.
- Should be specific and stain only the tissues it is intended to stain.
- Should be easily removed and not lead to permanent staining.

Dyes used for detection of enamel caries

Various dyes have been tried to detect enamel caries with varying success.

Procion dye stains enamel lesions but the staining becomes irreversible because the dye reacts with nitrogen and hydroxyl groups of enamel and acts as a fixative.

Calcein dye forms a complex with calcium and remains bound to the lesion. 'Fluorescent dye (Zyglo ZL-22)' has been used *in vitro*, which is not suitable for use *in vivo*. Ultraviolet illumination is required to visualize the dye.

Brilliant blue has also been used to enhance the diagnostic quality of fiberoptic transillumination.

Javaheri, et al (2010) evaluated the efficacy of two dyes, viz. caries detection and caries check and observed sensitivity of 74% and 71% respectively with 100% specificity for both.

Dyes are not recommended for diagnosing enamel lesions clinically.

Dyes used for Detection of Dentin Caries

Histopathologically, carious dentin is divided into two layers—outer layer of decalcification, which is soft and cannot be remineralized and the inner decalcified layer, which is hard and can be remineralized. Dyes have been tried to differentiate between these two zones of dentin caries. 0.5% Basic fuchsin in propylene glycol have been successfully used for the purpose; however, basic fuchsin dye was proved to be carcinogenic. Later, it was replaced by acid red and methylene blue. Methylene blue is also slightly toxic so acid red is preferred.

Quantification is not necessary because the dye is only used to identify carious dentin.

Sodium fluorescein has been used as a plaque-disclosing dye and was found to stain old plaque. This dye is currently used in ophthalmology for imaging retinal vessels, but it is not yet approved by the FDA for oral use. Sodium fluorescein has been tested as an alternative dye to be used in conjunction with laser fluorescence for detection of early caries.

Brooke, et al (1972) used calcium-binding reagent, calcein, which also becomes fluorescent upon chelation.

Fluorescent dye (Zyglo ZL-22) has been used in various studies as an aid in diagnosing incipient carious lesions. Zyglo ZL-22 consists of a solution of chlorinated hydrocarbons and other ingredients which act as a highly fluid and mobile carrier for a fluorescent dye.

Schaibany, et al (1996) compared the accuracy of diagnosis of carious lesions using caries detector dyes vs traditional tactile examination. They observed 75% of the occlusal carious lesions diagnosed by dye staining were missed with the tactile examination.

However, a few authors observed that the conventional tactile and optical criteria are satisfactory assessments of the caries status and the subsequent use of a caries detector dye may result in unnecessary tissue removal.

The dye penetration method is modified whereby iodine penetration is used for measuring enamel porosity of the incipient carious lesions. Potassium iodide is applied for a specific period of time to a well-defined area of the enamel and thereafter the excess is removed. The iodine, which remains in the micropores, is estimated indicating the permeability of enamel. This method seems complicated because for different areas, a separate calibration is required.

8. Miscellaneous

a. Carbon Dioxide Laser

Radiation of wavelength 10.6 μm (commonly used for CO_2 lasers), is strongly absorbed by water and can be vapourized instantaneously. The fact that most biological tissues contain large quantities of water makes them vulnerable to destruction by irradiation from a laser beam of this wavelength. The water in tissue is vapourized leaving a residue of carbon based material. The principle of carbon dioxide lasers to be used as a diagnostic tool is based on assumption that subsurface layer of early carious lesion has more organic content when compared with adjacent sound enamel. Photo-vaporization by a CO_2 laser of the organic material in the incipient carious lesion will leave a carbonized residue, which will appear black; the inorganic content of sound enamel with a minimum water content will be less affected.

b. Infrared Thermography

The thermal energy emitted by sound tooth structure is compared with that emitted by carious tooth structure. The technique, described by Kaneko, et al (1999) determines lesion activity rather than presence or absence of a lesion. The method uses indium/antimony thermal sensors, which can detect temperature changes in the order of 0.025°C. With a constant flow of air over the surface of the tooth, the change in temperature of the lesion is compared with that of the surrounding sound tooth structure. The source-to-sensor distance is 20 cm, and the time taken to capture the data for a lesion is up to 2 minutes. A reasonable correlation (0.67–0.79) between temperature changes and mineral loss and lesion depth has been established. The technique has not been used *in-vivo*, may be because of variations in the temperature of the oral cavity with respiration or fluid evaporation from other oral surfaces. The source-to-specimen distance is presently unsuitable for posterior teeth. Accessible smooth surface lesions have been used *in-vitro*, but there are no data on lesions which cannot be directly accessed. Additionally, the issue of lesion staining may also affect the heat transfer between the sound and carious tooth structure.

c. Ultrasonic Imaging

Ultrasonic, the use of sound waves, have been tried to detect early caries in enamel. Ultrasound has the frequency greater than 290 KHz. In contrast to X-ray imaging wherein the image is produced by transmitted radiation; in sonography, the image is produced by the reflected sound waves. The fraction of the beam that is reflected back to the probe is dependent on the acoustic impedance (density and the inherent acoustic velocity) of the tissue to be tested. Ultrasonic beam when directed perpendicular to the surface detects sub-surface defects; because the travel time of the sound waves is different in sound and defective surfaces.

Ultrasound waves are produced by an alternating voltage applied to a piezoelectric crystal. Sonic waves that are reflected back may cause a change in the thickness of the piezoelectric crystals, which produces electrical signal. This signal is processed, amplified and stored. Sound waves have to travel through a coupling medium to reach the target, i.e. tooth surface. The ideal coupling agent is one that has acoustic impedance similar to that of the target. This minimizes any reflection at the interface between the two media and maximizes the amount of ultrasound waves entering the specimen. Various acoustic coupling agents have been used for ultrasound evaluation of teeth, viz. mercury and aluminium rods bonded to the tooth surface containing water or glycerine. The use of water as a coupling agent did not permit ultrasound imaging in extracted teeth as deep as the dentin/pulp interface but was sufficient to detect enamel caries lesions. A few authors utilized ultrasound to determine the thickness of enamel; however, it was established that the method was not reliable. Yanikogv, et al (2000) histologically examined 20 proximal lesions in extracted teeth and demonstrated a sensitivity of 0.88 and specificity of 0.86. A few authors used different approach of ultrasound to detect caries. They used ultrasound waves which travel across the surface of the tooth along the interface between enamel and air, rather than through the tooth structure. In this way, ultrasound detects surface discontinuity present as a result of cavitated proximal lesions. It is established that ultrasonic caries detector could discriminate proximal caries from the sound surfaces. Ultrasound may be a quick and reliable tool for the detection of enamel caries. The use of longitudinal waves to measure demineralization in relation to the cementum-dentin junction is also useful.

Ultrasonics has remained in use for *in vitro* studies only.

d. Chemical Analysis

It is established that nutritional deficiencies are detected by analyzing the chemical composition of teeth. Use of microprobes and other techniques have indicated that trace elements are systematically and inhomogeneously distributed in enamel and dentin of teeth. Various trace elements are linked with the carious process. Exposure to environmental cadmium (Cd) has been linked to increased risk of caries. Inductively coupled plasma-mass spectrometry (ICP-MS) have been used to compare the presence/absence or amount of trace elements in healthy vs carious teeth. It is observed that mean concentration of Na, Al, Cr, Mn, Co, Cu, Zn etc. are in lower quantity in carious teeth as compared to the sound ones; however, Mg, Cd and Pb are observed to be higher in carious teeth than the healthy ones.

e. Microradiography

Microradiography is being used to quantify minerals in a given tissue. Three different microradiography techniques are used:

i. *Transverse microradiography (TMR):* Also known as contact microradiography; the samples are cut into thin slices (90 mm for enamel and 200 mm for dentin). The slices are placed on a piece of film and irradiated with monochromatic X-rays. The X-rays, so absorbed, are reflected in the optical density of the developed film. The densitometry is used to calculate the mineral content.

ii. *Longitudinal microradiography (LMR):* In this technique, longitudinal samples are prepared, cut parallel to the anatomical tooth surface (usually a thickness of 0.5 mm is taken). The microradiographic images are stored on the photographic plate. The absolute amount of mineral per unit area is calculated using densitometer.

iii. *Wavelength independent microradiography (WIM):* This method uses polychromatic high energy X-rays for determination of quantity mineral contents of the tissues. It measures the amount of mineral per unit area of enamel and dentin (thickness 0.3 to 0.6 mm). An improved X-ray film (0.04 mm size with resolving power of more than 3000 lines/mm) is used for images. Microradiography is considered as 'gold standard' that determines mineral density directly (via attenuation of X-ray energy by the minerals).

f. Energy Dispersive X-ray Element Analysis

The mineral content of sound and carious dentin varies. Energy dispersive X-ray element analysis (EDX) is based on the principle that the energy emitted in the form of X-ray photons when the electrons from external sources hit the atoms in a material generating characteristic rays of that element. The EDX detector measures the number of emitted X-rays versus their energy. A spectrum of the energy versus count of the X-rays is obtained and evaluated for qualitative and quantitative determination of the elements (mainly calcium and phosphorus) present in the specimen.

g. Microhardness Analysis

It is established that early caries lead to dissolution of enamel surface and enlargement of intercrystalline spaces. As the lesion progresses, the surface erosion becomes evident. The affected area is rough, chalky, dull and easily differentiated from the normal enamel. The subsurface demineralization or the surface erosion lead to changes in their hardness characteristics. Cross-sectional microhardness test is used to analyze the tooth with caries (demineralization) as compared to the sound tooth. The microhardness test is performed using Knoop indentoron, a microhardness tester (25 gm load is applied for 5 seconds at various angles). Two types of hardness measurement are recognized, (i) where the indentor load is perpendicular to the tooth surface (surface microhardness), and (ii) where indentor load is parallel to the tissues anatomical surface (cross-sectional microhardness). The microhardness test may not differentiate between caries demineralization and erosion due to external factors. Microhardness experiments are mainly carried out on enamel; their use in dentin may cause problems due to relaxation of dentin indentation with time due to drying shrinkage effect.

h. Iodine Absorptiometry

Iodine absorptiometry is regarded as a complement to other methods used to analyze mineral density. The advantage of iodine absorptiometry as compared to microradiography is that the non-destructive measurements can be carried out.

The sections are same as for longitudinal microradiography. The amount of absorbed photon radiation (photons of decayed I^{125} with an energy 27.4 KeV used to irradiate longitudinal section) is the measure of the amount of mineral per unit area. The method quantitatively analyzes the mineral loss.

Photon absorptiometry with radioactive iodine (I^{125}) and a non-image-forming detector is being used analyzing mineral content of enamel. During mineral loss, the transmission of the radioactive iodine through the mineralized tissue increases, which is recorded with high precision.

i. *Polarized Light Microscopy*

Polarized light microscopy is also used to analyze mineral loss and gain. The 20–80 µm sections are prepared and observed in polarizing microscope. The birefringence is calculated from the path difference, depending upon the variation in refractive index of the demineralized and the sound tooth surfaces. The measurement is indirectly for the porous areas of the tooth tissues (demineralization leads to more porosity and remineralization means decrease in that porosity). Polarized light measurements can provide quantitative information on the pore volume (porous) in the demineralized enamel and also the deep lesions.

Bibliography

1. Abalos C, Mendoza A, Jmienez-Planas A, Guerrero E, Chaparro A, Garcia-Godoy F. Performance of laser fluorescence for the detection of enamel caries in non-cavitated occlusal surfaces: clinical study with total validation of the sample. Am. J. Dent.: 2012;25: 44–8.

2. Alfano RR and Yao Ss. Human teeth with and without Dental caries studied by Visible Luminescent Spectroscopy. J Dent Res 1981; 60: 120–2.

3. Almqvist H, Wefel JS, Lagerlof F, Ekstrand J and Henrikson CO. *In vitro* root caries progression measured by 125I absoptiometry: Comparison with chemical analysis. J. Dent. Res.: 1988;67: 1217–20.

4. Alwas Danowska HM, Plasschaert AJ, Suliborski S and Verdonschot EH. Reliability and validity issues of laser fluorescence measurements in occlusal caries diagnosis. J. Dent.: 2002;30:129–34.

5. Ando M, Gonzalez Cabezas C, Isaacs RL, Eckert GJ and Stookey GK. Evaluation of several techniques for the detection of secondary caries adjacent to amalgam restorations. Caries Res.: 2004;38:350–6.

6. Ando M, Hall AF, Eckert GJ, Schemehorn BR, Analoui M and Stookey GK. Relative ability of Laser Fluorescence techniques to quantitate early mineral loss in vitro. Caries Res.: 1997;31:125–31.

7. Ando M, Stookey GK and Zero DT. Ability of quantitative light induced fluorescence (QLF) to assess the activity of white spot lesions during dehydration. Am. J. Dent.: 2006;19:15–8.

8. Angmar Mansson BE, al Khateeb S and Traonaeus S. Caries Diagnosis. J. Dent. Education.: 1998; 62:771–80.

9. Angmar-Mansson B and ten Bosch JJ. Advances in methods for diagnosing coronal caries—A review. Adv. Dent. Res.: 1993;7:70–9.

10. Angnes V, Angnes G, Batisttella M, Grande RH, Loguercio AD and Reis A. Clinical effectiveness of laser fluorescence, visual inspection and radiography in the detection of occlusal caries. Caries Res.: 2005;39:490–5.

11. Ansari G, Beeley JA, Reid JS and Foye RH. Caries detector dyes—an *in-vitro* assessment of some new compounds. J. Oral Rehab.: 1999;26:453–8.

12. Anttonen V, Seppa L and Hausen H. Clinical study of the use of the laser fluorescence device DIAGNOdent for detection of occlusal caries in children. Caries Res.: 2003;37:17–23.

13. Arends J and ten Bosch JJ. Demineralization and remineralization evaluation techniques. J. Dent. Res.: 1992;71:924–8.

14. Arnone D, Ciesla C and Pepper M. Terahertz imaging comes into view. Physics World: 2000;13:35–40.

15. Astvaldsottir A, Holbrook WP and Tranaeus S. Consistency of DIAGNOdent instruments for clinical assessment of fissure caries. Acta. Odont. Scand.: 2004;62:193–8.

16. Bab IA, Feuerstein O and Gazit D. Ultrasonic detector of proximal caries. Caries Res.: 1997;31: 322.

17. Bader JD and Shugars DA and Bonito AJ. A systematic review of the performance of methods for identifying carious lesions. J. Public Health Dent.: 2002;62:201–13.

18. Bader JD, Shugars DA. A systematic review of the performance of a laser fluorescence device for detecting caries. J. Am. Dent. Assoc.: 2004;135: 1413–26.

19. Bader JD, Shugars DA and Bonito AJ. A systematic review of selected dental caries diagnostic and management methods. J. Dent.Educ.: 2001;65:960–8.

20. Bamzahim M, Aljehani A and Shi XQ. Clinical performances of DIAGNOdent in the detection

of secondary carious lesions. Acta Odont. Scand.: 2005;63:26–30.

21. Bamzahim M, Shi XQ and Angmar-Mansoon B. Occlusal caries detection and quantification by DIAGNOdent and Electronic Caries Monitor: In vitro comparison. Acta. Odontol. Scand.: 2002;60:360–4.

22. Barberia E, Maroto M, Arenas M and Silva CC. A clinical study of caries diagnosis with a laser fluorescence system. J. Am. Dent. Assoc.: 2008; 139:572–9.

23. Barenie J, Leske G and Ripa LW. The use of fibre optics transillumination for the detection of proximal caries. Oral Surg., Oral Med., Oral Pathol.: 1973;36:891–7.

24. Bauer JG, Cretin S, Schweitzer SO and Hunt RJ. The reliability of diagnosing root caries using oral examinations. J. Dent. Educ.: 1988;52:622–9.

25. Bjelkhagen H, Sundstrom F, Angmar-Mansson B. and Ryden H. Early detection of enamel caries by luminescence excited by visible laser light. Swed. Dent. J.: 1982;6:1–7.

26. Bozkurt FO, Tagtekin D, Yanikoglu F, Fontana M, Cabezas CG and Stookey G. Capability of an ultrasonic system to detect very early caries lesions on human enamel. Marmara Dent. J.: 2013; 1:16–19.

27. Brooks SL and Miles DA. Advances in diagnostic imaging in dentistry. Dent.Clin.North Am.: 1993;37:91–111.

28. Caliskon Yanikoglu F, Ozturk F, Hayran O, Analoui M, Stookey GK. Detection of natural white spot caries lesions by an ultrasonic system. Caries Res.: 2000;34:225–32.

29. Cortes DF, Ekstrand KR, Elias-Boneta AR and Ellwood RP. An in-vitro comparison of the ability of fibre-optic transillumination, visual inspection and radiographs to detect occlusal caries and evaluate lesion depth. Caries Res.: 2000;34:443–7.

30. Costa AM, Paula LM and Bezerra AC. Use of DIAGNOdent for diagnosis of non-cavitated occlusal dentin caries. J. Appl. Oral Sci.: 2008;16: 18–23.

31. Crandell CE and Hill RP. Thermography in dentistry: a pilot study. Oral Surg., Oral Med., Oral Pathol.: 1966;21:316–20.

32. Crawley DA, Longbottom C, Cole BE, Ciesla CM, Arnone D, Wallace VP, Pepper M. Terahertz pulse imaging: A pilot study of potential application in dentistry. Caries Res. 2003;37:352–9.

33. Darling CL, Huynh GD and Fried D. Light scattering properties of natural and artificially demineralized dental enamel at 1310 nm. J. Biomed. Opt.: 2006;11:34023.

34. De Araujo FB, Rosito DB, Toigo E and dos Santos CK. Diagnosis of approximal caries: Radiographic versus clinical examination using tooth separation. Am. J. Dent.: 1992;5:245–8.

35. De Josselin de Jong E, Sundstrom F, Westerling H, Tranaeus S, TenBosch JJ and Angmar Mansson B. A new method for in vivo quantification of changes in initial enamel caries with laser fluorescence. Caries Res.: 1995;29:2–7.

36. DeJean KS, Caldas LD, Gois DN, Souza CS. Hidden dental caries: a study of diagnosis and prevalence. ClipeOdonto–UNITAU. 2009;1:7–13.

37. Eggertsson H, Analoui M, Vanderveen M, Gonzalez-Cabezas C, Eckert G and Stookey G. Detection of early interproximal caries in vitro using Laser Fluorescence, Dye-enhanced laser fluorescence and direct visual examination. Caries Res.: 1999;33:227–33.

38. Ekstrand KR. Improving clinical visual detection—Potential for caries clinical trials. J. Dent. Res.: 2004;83 spec No.C:C67–C71.

39. Ekstrand KR, Ricketts DN, Longbottom C and Pitts NB. Visual and tactile assessment of arrested initial enamel carious lesions: an in-vivo pilot study. Caries Res.: 2005;39:173–7.

40. Ekstrand KR, Ricketts DNJ, Kidd EAM, Qvist V and Schou S. Detection, diagnosing, monitoring, and logical treatment of occlusal caries in relation to lesion activity and severity: an in vivo examination with histological validation. Caries Res.: 1998;32:247–54.

41. Erten H, Uctasli MB, Akarslan ZZ, Uzun O and Baspinazr E. The assessment of unaided visual examination, intraoral canvas and operating microscope for the detection of occlusal caries lesion. Oper. Dent.: 2005;30:190–4.

42. Espelid I and Tveit AB. Diagnosis of secondary caries and crevices adjacent to amalgam. Int. Dent. J.: 1991;41:359–64.

43. Farah RA, Drummond BK, Swain MV and William S. Relationship between laser fluorescence and enamel hypomineralisation. J. Dent.: 2008;36: 915–21.

44. Ferreira Zandona AG, Analoui M, Beiswanger BB, Isaacs RL, Kafrawy AH, Eckert GJ and Stookey GK. An in vitro comparison between laser fluorescence and visual examination for detection of demineralization in occlusal pits and fissures. Caries Res.: 1998;32:210–8.

45. Ferreira Zandona A and Zero DT. Diagnostic tools for early caries detection. J. Am. Dent. Assoc.: 2006;137:1675–84.

46. Francescut P, Zimmerli B and Lussi A. Influence of different storage methods on laser fluorescence values: A two-year study. Caries Res.: 2006;40:181–5.

47. Fukukita H, Yano T and Fukumoto A. Development and application of an ultrasonic imaging system for dental diagnosis. J. Clin. Ultrasound: 1985;13:597–600.

48. Fyffe HE, Deery C, Nugent ZJ, Nuttall NM and Pitts NB. *In vitro* validity of the Dundee Selectable Threshold Method for caries diagnosis (DSTM). Comm. Dent. Oral Epidemiol.: 2000;28: 52–8.

49. Gimenez T, Piovesan C, Braga MM, Raggio DP, Deery C, Ricketts DN, Ekstrand KR and Mendes FM. Visual inspection for caries detection: A systematic review and meta-analysis. J Dent Res 2015;94:895–904.

50. Grondahl HG. Digital radiology in dental diagnosis: a critical review. Dentomaxillofacial Radiology: 1992;21:198–202.

51. Gungor K, Erten H, Akarslan ZZ, Celik I and Semiz M. Approximal carious lesions depth assessment with insight and ultraspeed films. Oper. Dent. 2005;30:58–62.

52. Gupta R, Chaudhary M, Patil S and Bohra S. Energy dispersive X-ray element analysis (EDX) and polarized light microscopic comparison between carious deciduous and permanent teeth. Int. J. Women Dent.: 2014;1:43–8.

53. Haak R, Wicht MJ, Hellmich M, Grossmann A and Noack MJ. The validity of proximal caries detection using magnifying visual aids. Caries Res.: 2002;36:249–55.

54. Hahn SK, Kim JW, Lee SH, Kim CC, Hahn SH and Jang KT. Micro-computed tomographic assessment of chemo-mechanical caries removal. Caries Res.: 2004;38:75–8.

55. Halse A, White SC and Espelid I and Tveit AB. Visualization of stannous fluoride treatment of carious lesions by subtraction radiography. Oral Surg., Oral Med., Oral Pathol.: 1990;69:378–81.

56. Hamilton JC. Should a dental explorer be used to probe suspected carious lesions? Yes—an explorer is a time-tested tool for caries detection. J. Am. Dent. Assoc.: 2005;136:1526, 1528, 1530.

57. Harase Y, Araki K and Okano T. Accuracy of extraoral tuned operative computed tomography (TACT) for proximal caries detection. Oral Surg., Oral Med., Oral Pathol.: 2006; 101:791–6.

58. Harorli OT, Barutcigil C, Akgul N and Bayindir YZ. Caries detector dyes: do they stain only the caries? J. Rest. Dent.: 2014;2:20–6.

59. Harris R, Nicoll AD, Adair PM and Pine CM. Risk factors for dental caries in young children: a systematic review of the literature. Comm. Dent. Health: 2004;21:71–85.

60. Heinrich-Weltzien R, Kuhnisch J, Oehme T, Ziehe A, Stosser L and Garcia-Godoy F. Comparison of different DIAGNOdent cut-off limits for *in-vivo* detection of occlusal caries. Oper. Dent.: 2003;28:672–80.

61. Heinrich-Weltzien R, Weerheijm KL, Kuhnisch J, Oehme T and Stosser L. Clinical evaluation of visual, radiographic and laser fluorescence methods for detection of occlusal caries. J. Dent. Child.: 2002;69:127–32.

62. Hibst R and Paulus R. Caries detection by red excited fluorescence: investigations on fluorophores. Caries Res.: 1999;33:295.

63. Hibst R and Paulus R and Lussi A. Detection of occlusal caries by laser fluorescence: Basic and clinical investigations. Medical Laser Application: 2001;16:205–13.

64. Hintze H, Wenzel A, Danielsen B and Nyvad B. Reliability of visual examination, fibreoptic transillumination and bite wing radiography and reproductibility of direct visual examination following tooth separation for the identification of cavitated carious lesions in contacting approximal surface. Caries Res.: 1998;32:204–9.

65. Ismail AI. Clinical diagnosis of precavitated carious lesions. Comm. Dent. Oral Epid.: 1997;25: 13–23.

66. Ismail AI. Visual and visuo-tactile detection of dental caries. J. Dent. Res.:83, Spec No.:C56-C66, 2004.

67. Jackson D. The clinical diagnosis of dental caries Br. Dent. J.: 1950;88:207–13.

68. Jeromin LS, Geddes G, White SC, Gratt BM. Xeroradiography for intraoral dental radiology: a process description. Oral Surg., Oral Med., Oral Pathol.: 1980;49:178–83.

69. Kidd EA, Ricketts DN and Pitts NB. Occlusal caries diagnosis: A changing challenge for clinician and epidemiologists. J. Dent.: 1993;21: 323–31.

70. Kielbassa AM. Current challenges in caries diagnosis. Quint. Int.: 2006;37:421.

71. Ko H-K, Kang S-M, Kim HE, Kwon H-K and Kim B-I. Validation of Quantitative light-

induced fluorescence-digital (QLF-D) for the detection of approximal caries *in vitro*. J Dent. 2015;568–75.

72. Kunin AA, Belenova IA, Ippolitov YA, Moiseeva NS and Kunin DA. Predictive research methods of enamel and dentin for initial caries detection. The EPMA Journal: 2013;4:19.

73. Lees S, Gerhard FB and Oppenheim FG. Ultrasonic measurement of dental enamel demineralization. Ultrasonics: 1973;9:269–73.

74. Lennon AM, Buchalla W, Switalski L and Stookey GK. Residual caries detection using visible fluorescence. Caries Res.: 2002;36:315–9.

75. Lippert F and Lynch RJM. Comparison of Knoop and Vickers surface microhardness and transverse microradiogrpahy for the study of early caries lesion formation in human and bovine enamel. Arch. Oral Biol.: 2014;59:704–10.

76. Longbottom C and Pitts NB. CO_2 laser and the diagnosis of occlusal caries: *in vitro* study. J. Dent.: 1993;21:234–9.

77. Longbottom C, Pitts NB, Reich E and Lussi A. Comparison of visual and electrical methods with a new device for occlusal caries detection. Caries Res.: 1998;32:298.

78. Lussi A. Comparison of different methods for the diagnosis of fissure caries without cavitation. Caries Res.: 1993;27:409–16.

79. Lussi A and Francescut P. Performance of conventional and new methods for the detection of occlusal caries in deciduous teeth. Caries Research: 2003;37:2–7.

80. Lussi A, Firestone A, Schoenberg V, Hotz P and Stich H. *In vivo* diagnosis of fissure caries using a new electrical resistance monitor. Caries Res.: 1995;29:81–7.

81. Lussi A, Hack A, Hug I, Heckenberger H, Megert B and Stich H. Detection of approximal caries with a new laser fluorescence device. Caries Res.: 2006;40:97–103.

82. Lussi A, Hibst R and Paulus R. DIAGNOdent: an optical method for caries detection. J. Dent. Res.:83, Spec No. C :C80-C83, 2004.

83. Lussi A, Imwinkelried S, Pitts N, Longbottom C and Reich E. Performance and reproducibility of a laser fluorescence system for detection of occlusal caries *in vitro*. Caries Res.: 1999;33:261–6.

84. Lussi A, Megert B, Longbottom C, Reich E and Francescut P. Laser fluorescence may increase diagnostic sensitivity in detecting class I caries. Journal of Evidence-Based Dental Practice: 2001;1:95–6.

85. Marsillac MWS and Vieira RS. Assessment of artificial caries lesions through scanning electron microscopy and cross-sectional microhardness test. Indian J. Dent. Res.: 2013;24:249–54.

86. Matos R, Novaes TF, Braga MM, Siqueira WL, Durate DA and Mendes FM. Clinical performance of two fluorescence-based methods in detecting occlusal caries lesions in primary teeth. Caries Res.: 2011;45:294–302.

87. McComb D and Tam LE. Diagnosis of occlusal caries: Part I. Conventional methods. Journal Canadian Dental Association: 2001;67:454–7.

88. Meller C, Heyduck C, Tranaeus S and Splieth C. A new *in vitro* method for measuring caries activity using quantitative light induced fluorescence. Caries Res.: 2006;40:90–6.

89. Major IA. Clinical diagnosis of recurrent caries. JADA: 2005;136:1426–33.

90. Meyer-Lueckel H, Wierichs RJ, Gninka B, Heldmann P, Dorfer CE and Paris S. The effect of various model parameters on enamel caries lesions in a dose-response model in situ. Journal of Dentistry 2015.

91. Mohamed A and Helal AF. Analysis of trace elements in teeth by ICP-M: Implications for caries. J. Phys. Sci.: 2010;21:1–12.

92. Moller IJ. Clinical criteria for the diagnosis of the incipient carious lesion. Adv. Fluor. Res. Dent. Caries Prev.: 1966;4:67–72.

93. Mount JH. Defining, classifying, and placing incipient caries lesions in perspective. Dent Clin N Am. 2005, 49:701–23.

94. Murray J and Shaw L. Errors in diagnosis of approximal caries on bitewing radiographs. Commun Dent. Oral Epidem. 1975;3:276–82.

95. Nair MK, Tyndall DA, Ludlow JB and May K. Tuned Aperture Computed Tomography and Detection of Recurrent Caries. Caries Res.: 1998;32:23–30.

96. Nyvad B. Diagnosis versus detection of caries. Caries Res.: 2004;38:192–8.

97. Nyvad B, Machiulskiene V and Baelum V. Reliability of a new caries diagnostic system differentiating between active and inactive caries lesions. Caries Res.: 1999;33:252–60.

98. O'Brien WJ, Vazquez L and Johnston WM. The detection of incipient caries with tracer dyes. JDR: 1989;68:157–8.

99. Parfitt GJ. A standard clinical examination of the teeth. Br. Dent. J.: 1954;96:296–300.

100. Penning C, Van Amerongen JP, Seef RE, Tencate JM. Validity of probing for fissure caries diagnosis. Caries Res.: 1992;26:445–9.

101. Pine CM and Ten Bosch JJ. Dynamics of and diagnostic methods for detecting small carious lesions. Caries Res.: 1996;30:381–8.

102. Pitts NB and Fyffe HE. The effect of varying diagnostic thresholds upon clinical caries data for a low prevalence group. J. Dent. Res.: 1988;67: 592–6.

103. Pitts NB and Stamm JW. International consensus workshop on caries clinical trials (ICW-CCT) final consensus statements: agreeing where the evidence leads. J. Dent. Res.:83, Spec No.C : C125-C128, 2004.

104. Pretty IA. Caries detection and diagnosis: novel technologies. J. Dent.: 2006;34:727–39.

105. Pretty IA, Ellwood PG, Davies RM, Worthington HW and Ellwood RP. The effect of illumination and focal distance on light induced fluorescence images *in vitro*. Caries Res.: 2006;40:73–6.

106. Radike AW. Criteria for diagnosing dental caries. In: Proceedings of the Conference on the Clinical Testing of Cariostatic Agents. Chicago: American Dental Association, 1968;87–8.

107. Ricketts DN, Kidd EA and Wilson RF. A re-evaluation of electrical resistance measurements for the diagnosis of occlusal caries. Br. Dent. J.: 1995;178:11–7.

108. Ricketts DN, Kidd EA, Smith BG and Wilson RF. Clinical and radiographic diagnosis of occlusal caries. A study *in vitro*. J. Oral Rehab. 1995;22: 15–20.

109. Rodrigues JA, Hug I, Neuhaus KW and Lussi A. Light-emitting diode and laser fluorescence-based devices in detecting occlusal caries. J. Biomedical Optics:16, 107003, 2011.

110. Rosen B, Birkhed D, Nilsson K, Olavi G and Egelberg J. Reproducibility of clinical caries diagnoses on coronal and root surfaces. Caries Res.: 1996;30:1–7.

111. Samarrai SE and Misbah MM. Diagnosis of initial carious lesion by clinical and conventional radiographic methods in comparison to direct digital radiography. Orthodontus, Pedodontus and Preventive Dentistry. J. Bajh Coll. Dent.: 2007;19:77–80.

112. Schmuck BD and Carey CM. Improved contact X-ray microradiographic method to measure mineral density of hard dental tissues. J. Res. Nati. Stand. Technol.: 2010;115:75–83.

113. Schwendicke F, Stolpe M, Meyer-Lueckel H and Paris S. Detecting and treating Occlusal caries lesions: A cost-effectiveness analysis. J Dent Res 2015;94:272–80.114.

114. Shakibaie F, George R and Walsh LJ. Applications of laser induced fluorescence in dentistry. Int. J. Dent. Clin.: 2011;3:38–44.

115. Sheehy EC, Brailsford SR, Kidd EA, Beighton D and Zoitopoulos L. Comparison between visual examination and a laser fluorescence system for in-vivo diagnosis of occlusal caries. Caries Res.: 2001;35:421–6.

116. Stookey G. Should a dental explorer be used to probe suspected carious lesion? No, use of an explorer can lead to misdiagnosis and disrupt remineralization. JADA: 2005; 136, 1527, 1529, 1531.

117. Stookey GK. Optical methods – quantitative light fluorescence. J. Dent. Res.:2004;83:C84-C88.

118. Stookey GK and Gonzalez-Cabezas C. Emerging methods of caries diagnosis. J. Dent. Educ.: 2001; 65:1001–06.

119. Tam LE and Mc Comb D. Diagnosis of occlusal caries: Part II. Recent Diagnostic Technologies. J. Can. Dent. Assoc.: 2001;67(8):459–463.

120. Tassery H, Levallois B, Terrer E, Manton DJ, Otsuki M, Koubi S, Gugnani N, Panayotov I, Jacquot B, Cuisinier F and Rechmann P. Use of new minimum intervention dentistry technologies in caries management. Aust. Dent. J.: 2013;58:40–59.

121. ten Cate JM. Remineralization of deep enamel dentin caries lesions. Aust. Dent. J.: 2008;53: 281–5.

122. Terrer E, Koubi S and Dionne A, Weisrock G, Sarraquigne C, Mazur A and Tassery H. A new concept in restorative dentistry: light-induced fluorescence evaluator for diagnosis and treatment: Part 1 – diagnosis and treatment of initial occlusal caries. J. Contemp. Dent. Pract.: 2009;10:86–94.

123. Terrer E, Raskin A, Koubi S, Dionne A, Weisrock G, Sarraquigne C, Mazuir A and Tassery H. A new concepts in restorative dentistry: LIFEDT-light induced fluorescence evaluator for diagnosis and treatment. Part 2—treatment of dentinal caries. J. Contemp. Dent. Pract.:2010;11: EO95–102.

124. Thylstrup A, Bruun C and Holmen L. In vivo caries models—mechanisms for caries initiation and arrestment. Adv. Dent. Res.: 1994;8:144–57.

125. Tonioli MB, Bouschilcher MR and Hillis SL. Laser fluorescence detection of occlusal caries. Am. J. Dent.: 2002;15:268–73.

126. Toraman M, Peker I, Deniz H, Bala O and Altunkaynak B. *In vivo* comparison of laser

fluorescence measurements with conventional methods for occlusal caries detection. Lasers Med. Sci.: 2008;23:307–12.

127. Vam de Rijke JW. Use of dyes in cariology. Int. Dent. J.: 1991;41:111–6.

128. Van Rijkom H and Verdonschot EH. Diagnostic method: For approximal caries compared: A meta-analysis. Caries Res.: 1995;29:364–70.

129. Verdonschot EH, Angmar-Mansson B, tenBosch JJ, Deery CH, Huysmans MCM, Pitts NB and Waller E. Development in caries diagnosis and their relationship to treatment decision and quality of care. Caries Res.: 1999;33:32–40.

130. Virajslip V, Thearmontree A, Aryatawong S and Paiboonwarachat D. Comparison of proximal caries detection in primary teeth between laser fluorescence and bitewing radiography. Pediat. Dent.: 2005;27:493–9.

131. Walsh LJ. The current status of laser applications in dentistry. Aust. Dent. J.: 2003;48:146–55.

132. Walsh LJ and Shakibaie F. Ultraviolet-induced fluorescence: shedding new ight on dental biofilms and dental caries. Aust. Dent. Pract.: 2007;18:56–60.

133. Weerheijm KL, de Soet JJ, de Graff J, van Amerongen WE: Occlusal hidden caries: a bacteriological profile. J Dent Child 1990;57:428–32.

134. Weerheijm KL, Van Amerongen WE and Eggink CO. The clinical diagnosis of occlusal caries: a problem. J. Dent. Child: 1989;56:196–200.

135. Wenzel A, Hintze H and Horsted-Bindslev P. Accuracy of radiographic detection of residual caries in connection with tunnel restorations. Caries Res.: 1998;32:17–22.

136. Wenzel A, Pitts N, Verdonschott EH and Kalsbeek H. Developments in radiographic caries diagnosis—A review. J. Dent.: 1993;21:131–40.

137. White GE, Tsamtsouris A and Williams DL. Early detection of occlusal caries by measuring the electrical resistance of the tooth. J. Dent. Res.: 1978;57:195–200.

138. Young DA and Featherstone JD. Digital imaging fiberoptic transillumination, F-speed radiographic film and depth of approximal lesions. JADA: 2005;136:1682–7.

139. Zandona AGF, Analoui M, Beiswanger BB, Isaacs RL, Kafrawy AH, Eckert GJ and Stookey GK. An *in-vitro* comparison between laser fluorescence and visual examination for detection of demineralization in occlusal pits and fissures. Caries Res.: 1998;32:210–8.

11

Caries Activity Indicators

Dental caries, undoubtedly, is one of the most common and oldest ailment of humankind. The initiation and progression of dental caries is often influenced by oral hygiene status coupled with morphological, biological and chemical factors. No single etiological factor could be ascertained till date. Why certain individuals are more prone to caries than others has always been a matter of concern for the researchers.

Caries activity tests are primarily undertaken to evaluate the susceptibility and aggression of the individual towards caries. Caries activity refers to the increment of new and recurrent lesions and also the progress of the already existing lesions over a period of time. Caries risk assessment infers predicting the future caries development before the clinical onset of disease. Caries activity measures the speed of progress of carious lesion; whereas caries susceptibility refers to the inherent tendency of the host to be afflicted by the caries. Caries activity tests measure the degree to which the local environmental challenges favor the probability of initiation of caries. An objective evaluation of caries activity requires quantification of factors associated with the pathogenesis of caries, viz. host, microflora and diet. Other associated factors such as morphology and chemical composition of

teeth, buffering capacity of saliva, early caries experience and certain systemic diseases also affect caries activity. Caries activity indicators are valuable adjunct for patient motivation in a preventive care program. Presently there is no ideal test in existence; although multiple tests have been documented.

Definitions

Risk: The probability of occurrence of an event within a certain period of time.

Risk indicators: Non-etiological factors that may point out caries risk but do not directly influence the caries process.

Caries risk: Risk of an individual developing a carious lesion.

Caries risk factors: The conditions or characteristics influencing the occurrence and progression of caries.

Caries susceptibility: The inherent tendency of the host (tooth) to be afflicted by caries process. This is the susceptibility (or resistance) of a tooth to a caries producing environment.

Caries activity: It is a measure of the speed of progression of a carious lesion or increments of new/recurrent carious lesions in an individual over a given period of time.

Caries risk assessment: The determination of the likelihood of the incidence of caries (i.e.

the number of new carious lesions) during a certain time period.

CARIES SUSCEPTIBILITY

It refers to the inherent tendency of the host and the target tissue, the tooth, to be afflicted by caries process. This is the resistance of a tooth to a caries-producing environment.

The caries susceptibility of a person can be measured on the basis of caries susceptibility tests and can be graded according to caries susceptibility index.

Caries susceptibility test: A test carried out to determine the likelihood of an individual to develop caries. Various parameters ascertaining caries susceptibility are evaluated under the tests.

Caries susceptibility index: Richardson (1961) conceived an index measuring caries susceptibility. Amount of caries developing during the given period of time divided by the amount of tooth surfaces at risk is the net caries susceptibility.

Procedure

All surfaces of a tooth and all teeth are taken into consideration. The anterior teeth are scored as four surfaces; whereas, posterior teeth are scored as five surfaces.

This way full permanent dentition will have 148 surfaces to be scored and full deciduous dentition will have 88 surfaces. The index involves examining the whole dentition and calculating the number of susceptible surfaces, number of carious and restored surfaces. Every surface which is not restored is considered susceptible.

Re-examination of same patient is carried out after 6–12 months and the number of new carious lesions is calculated. The number of new lesions developed during given period of observation divided by the number of susceptible surfaces determined during initial examination is the susceptible ratio (SR).

$$SR = \frac{\text{Number of new lesions developed during given period of observation}}{\text{Number of susceptible surfaces determined during first examination}}$$

Susceptibility index (SI) is calculated as:

$$SI = SR \times 100$$

The susceptibility index is expressed as percentage of susceptibility ratio, making the data more practical for survey purposes.

Factors Contributing to Caries Susceptibility

The main factors contributing to caries susceptibility are:

1. Dietary Pattern

It has been established that the frequency of carbohydrate intake and not the quantity affects the caries susceptibility of an individual.

Earlier it was confirmed that the ability of human oral flora to form intracellular polysaccharide from carbohydrates affects the caries susceptibility. Exhaustive studies have compared food habits, especially sugar intake in caries resistant and caries active group of individuals.

Comparing dietary pattern of cities and villages (sugar intake considered more in cities), it was observed that children belonging to cities had a significantly higher percentage of microbial intracellular polysaccharides forming colonies than did the village children.

A few authors have established that long duration breast-feeding children develop more caries and remain caries susceptible.

Coogan, et al (2008) evaluated *Streptococcus mutans* and lactobacilli from the dental impressions of various individuals to check their susceptibility. They observed that microbial growth on alginate impressions was directly related to caries activity and the salivary flow and amount of dietary fiber had inverse relation with caries susceptibility.

2. Saliva

The quantity and quality of saliva has always been considered an important parameter to assess the caries susceptibility. Individual with less flow of saliva (reason may be any) are more susceptible to caries. Certain enzymes, proteins and antibodies present in saliva make the individual less susceptible to caries.

Cristiane, et al (2009) evaluated the role of free amino acids in early childhood caries. They observed that proline was absent in caries-free individuals and glycine was absent in the individuals with high caries index.

Salivary carbonic anhydrase activity in saliva has also been evaluated by a few authors. Lower caries incidence was associated with high carbonic anhydrase activity (salivary buffer system).

Stuchell and Mandel (1983) quantified the lysozyme concentration in parotid, submandibular and sublingual saliva of caries resistant and caries susceptible adults. Concentration of lysozyme was higher in submandibular and sublingual than in parotid secretions and was significantly higher in unstimulated submandibular saliva. However, no significant difference in lysozyme concentration could be observed in caries resistant and caries susceptible individuals.

Concentration of lactoperoxidase, thiocyanate and preformed hypothiocyanite in parotid and submandibular saliva has also been evaluated; however, no significant difference in concentrations of three enzymes in caries susceptible and caries free individuals could be observed.

3. Morphology and Type of Teeth

It has been established that certain tooth surfaces are more prone to caries than others (susceptible surfaces to accumulate bacteria and subsequently acid production).

Brekhus (1931) in his study on young students, observed caries susceptibility in the following order:

- Upper and lower first molars—95%.
- Upper and lower second molars—75%.
- Upper second bicuspids—45%.
- Upper first bicuspids—35%.
- Lower second bicuspids—35%.
- Upper central and lateral incisors—30%.
- Upper cuspids and lower first bicuspids—10%.
- Lower central and lateral incisors—3%.
- Lower cuspids—3%.

Hyatt and Lotka (1929) studied caries susceptibility of various tooth surfaces and observed that occlusal surface was most commonly affected followed by mesial, buccal and lingual surface in descending order.

A few authors studied the caries susceptibility of jaw quadrants and observed higher caries susceptibility in maxillary teeth; however, right and left quadrants of both maxillary and mandibular arch exhibited bilateral distribution. The difference may be related to salivary buffering action being more pronounced in lower teeth.

4. Sex Variation

It is established that at same chronological age, girls have more number of permanent teeth than boys. Girls get their permanent teeth erupted at earlier age than boys. Girls are more prone to caries due to exposure of their teeth for longer duration of time than those of boys; however, many studies have reported equal and even reverse relations. It is also reported that girls, being more conscious in their oral hygiene, are less prone to caries. Many studies reported no difference in susceptibility between males and females.

Burrill (1943) studied caries susceptibility by means of bacterial and chemical determinations. By bacterial determination, it was found that between 13 and 18 years of age, males are more susceptible than females and between 18 and 21 years, females are more susceptible than males. Chemical determination showed that between 13 and

15 years, females are more susceptible than males and between 16 and 18 years, males and females had equal susceptibility and between 19 and 21 years, males are more susceptible than females.

5. Smoking

It is established that passive smokers are at higher risk of caries, may be because of higher level of salivary nicotine along with increased number of *Streptococcus mutans* and lactobacilli.

6. Microbial Variations

The quantity of *Streptococcus mutans*, lactobacilli and Actinomyces has been found to be much more in caries active individuals than others. Further certain serotype (e.g. Serotype-c of *Streptococcus mutans*) are in abundance in caries susceptible individuals.

7. Genetics

Schuler (2001) reported that caries incidence is affected by host factors that are related to enamel structure, immunologic response to cariogenic bacteria and/or composition of saliva. It is established that inherent disorders of tooth development with altered enamel structure increases the incidence of dental caries and also the altered immune response to cariogenic bacteria may increase the incidence of caries. Further, it is reported that there is weak association between HLA genetic pattern and dental caries.

8. Stress Factors

Stress is a psychophysiological response of an individual to a perceived threat. Stress in general is not what happens to someone, but how someone reacts to what happens.

Animal studies have shown increased susceptibility to caries when animals are exposed to different stresses like separation of mother from newborn litter, with-holding of food for longer period, etc.

Sutton (1962) attempted to co-relate acute dental caries with circumstances of stressful life events and observed that 96% of patients who suffered from acute caries had undergone some several mental stress.

It is established that association between perceived stress/emotions and prevalence of caries could be attributed to reduction in salivary flow, decreased resistance and changes in pH of oral environment.

It is hypothesized that in case of joy and appreciation, the DNA responds by releasing and unwinding its strands, thereby enhancing the immune system. In contrast when someone is in stress or fear, the DNA contracts and become shorter, depleting the immune system. This affects teeth and caries susceptibility.

9. Miscellaneous

Moschen, et al (1992) studied renal clearance in patients with high and low caries prevalence. They observed that calcium excretion was significantly greater in those individuals with low caries prevalence than in those with high prevalence.

Geographical Factors affecting the Susceptibility of Caries

Dental caries, being a multifactorial disease, may get affected by a little known factors such as latitude and altitude directly or indirectly. The associated factors of latitude and altitude include sunshine, rainfall, humidity and temperature. These factors are usually directly or indirectly related to one another. Chemical composition of water supply and urbanization are other factors indirectly associated with caries.

a. Sunshine which varies with latitude is one important factor related to dental caries. Ultraviolet B in sunlight reduces risk of dental caries which might be because of production of vitamin D, followed by induction of cathelicidin and defensins, which have antimicrobial properties.

The increase in temperature due to sunshine warrants increased demand for water consumption, which, help wash away food debris from oral cavity.

The measurement of sunshine is not simple. The possible hours of sunshine per year increase a little as one leaves the equator.

Sunshine duration depends on clouds and fog; locations with arid climate correlate with high sunshine duration values.

b. *Rainfall:* As the rainfall increases leaching of the minerals from soil especially fluorides will lead to reduction of fluoride concentration in crops. Rainfall is accompanied by heavy clouds which block sunlight.

Higher altitude areas receive more rainfall as compared to coastal areas.

c. *Relative humidity:* Relative humidity is a measure of the amount of moisture in the atmosphere in proportion to the amount to be tolerated without precipitation at a given temperature and barometric pressure. It was found that increase in relative humidity results in increase in caries incidence.

As humidity rises, the caries incidence rises too. This is because of the decreased demand of water intake in areas with high humidity levels. Relative humidity is higher near the coastal region.

d. *Temperature* varies almost entirely with latitude. Temperature modified the caloric requirements and water intake of human beings. Carbohydrate food is not only a quick, but a relatively cheap, source of caloric energy. Inhabitants of colder climates consume more carbohydrates as they provide quick warmth and energy.

The colder environment is further associated with decrease in water intake and therefore, caries incidence increases. The reverse phenomenon occurs in areas with high temperature.

The temperature near coastal area is higher as compared to land area.

The major factors involved in variation with latitude appear to be sunshine and temperature. These factors suggest that dental caries increase with latitude.

e. *Urbanization:* Urbanization also affects caries incidence because of consuming soft diet containing plenty of carbohydrates.

f. *Fluorides:* Fluoride in the drinking water during the time of tooth development results in formation of fluorapatite crystal, which are more caries-resistant. The degree of leachable fluoride in a hard rock terrain is more important in deciding fluoride content in water rather than mere presence of fluoride bearing minerals in the bulk rock/soils. Higher sodium and pH causing factors are the reasons for the release of fluoride into groundwater of coastal regions.

g. *Water hardness:* Water hardness is usually measured in terms of presence of calcium carbonate. An inverse relation was reported between caries incidence and the total water hardness. Sea water has higher water hardness as compared to fresh water sources.

The major factors involved in variations with distance from seacoast appear to be fluorides, total water hardness and relative humidity. Dental caries increase with distance from seacoast.

CARIES RISK ASSESSMENT

According to the American Academy of Pediatric Dentistry (AAPD) identifying risk factors for caries should be an essential component of ethical dental practice. Caries Assessment Tools (CAT) can be used that will assist clinicians not only with identifying individuals at risk but also help managing the preventive protocol.

Goals of Caries Risk Assessment

- Classify individuals into high/moderate/low risk after screening.
- Make patient aware of their risk for developing caries, motivating them for preventive care.
- Guide as regard to choice of restorative material.
- Help design a preventive program.
- Assess impact of caries control measures.

Factors Affecting the Evaluation of Caries Risk

- Morphology of teeth (shape/crowding of teeth, occlusal anatomical features, retentive areas, etc.).
- Chemical components of teeth (enamel maturation, salivation with fluoride, etc.).
- Biological factors (composition of plaque, microbial activity, etc.).
- Salivary factors (buffering capacity, immunological factors, oral clearance, etc.).
- Diet (frequency, amount and quantity of carbohydrates consumption, intake of any caries prone diet, etc.).
- Family caries experience or caries in childhood, etc.
- Systemic diseases influencing oral health.

The various models used for caries risk assessment (CRA) are:

a. CAMBRA (Caries management by risk assessment).
b. Cariogram.
c. Dundee caries risk model.
d. Caries risk assessment tools.
e. Traffic light matrix (TL-M) model.

a. CAMBRA (Caries management by risk assessment)

It is established that dental caries is a multifactorial disease which is influenced by lifestyle and host factors. Caries protective factors are biologic or therapeutic measures that can be used to prevent pathologic challenges posed by caries risk factors. Caries management by risk assessment (CAMBRA) is an evidence-based approach to prevent and treat the cause of dental caries at the earliest stages rather than to wait for irreversible damage to the teeth.

Ramos-Gomez, et al (2007) modifying the basic concept of managing caries at an early stage, identified risk factors and protective factors by interviewing and clinically examining of the children at definite age groups. Bacterial culturing is also included only for those children who exhibited certain levels or combinations of risk factors. This protocol helps recommend treatment and preventive care at an early age.

Various associations have developed different forms categorizing children into high risk, moderate risk and low risk levels. Two forms, one for 0–6 years old children and the other for 6 and above category are widely used. American Academy of Pediatric Dentistry favored categorizing children forms into 0–5 years and 5 years and above. The forms weigh the disease indicators, risk factors and protective factors, evaluating the balance between the risk and protective factors.

b. Cariogram

Brathall (1996) developed a computer based tool, the cariogram that depicts the interaction of caries provoking factors and the probability of developing new carious lesions. It is represented by a pie chart in 5 sectors: diet, bacteria, susceptibility, circumstances and chance that includes risk factors. The circumstances sector includes factors that do not participate directly in the development of caries but are risk predictors of dental caries, such as past caries experience and systemic diseases.

Cariogram depicts caries risk graphically. It illustrates the interaction of caries related factors. It also gives an indication of any chance to avoid caries. Cariogram is divided into five categories; each suggestive of the weightage of the factors related to the caries. Each category is assigned one color. Red infers amount of plaque and *Streptococcus mutans*; dark blue is diet factor (diet contents and frequency); dark green is what is left after taking care of the other factors; light blue is salivary factors, their secretions, buffer capacity etc., yellow is the combination of past caries experience and other related factors (Fig. 11.1).

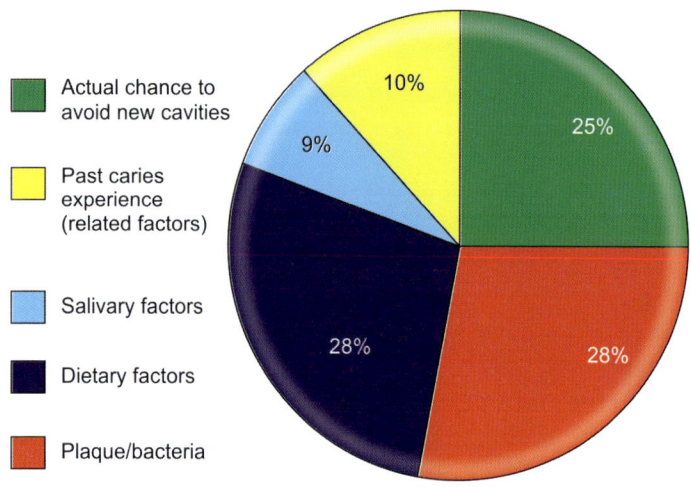

Actual chance to avoid new cavities

Past caries experience (related factors)

Salivary factors

Dietary factors

Plaque/bacteria

Fig. 11.1: Cariogram

The bigger the green color, the better is the dental health. Small green color depicts high caries risk. For other categories, smaller the percentage, better is the dental health. Chance to avoid caries (green color) and caries risk are expressed inversely. Small green color means less chances to avoid caries, i.e. high risk and large green implies the reverse, i.e. high chances to avoid caries.

All the five factors are calculated from patients' record and examinations. The scores so given are displayed graphically.

The program prompts the clinician to enter a weight (0 to 3, with '0' representing a low risk and '3' representing a high risk) for nine risk factors (caries experience, related general diseases, dietary contents, dietary frequency, plaque amount, *Streptococcus mutans*, fluoride, saliva secretion and saliva buffering capacity) and a clinical judgment score. An algorithm was constructed such that all the factors entered into the model could be weighed and the patient's chance of avoiding caries could be calculated. This is represented graphically. With this program, the clinician can demonstrate to the patient their susceptibility to caries risk. Additionally, the patient's caries susceptible risk features can be utilized for preventive measures.

c. Dundee Caries Risk Model (DCRM)

The caries risk factors of more than thousand infants born in 1994 were assessed and the data was collected under three categories, viz. socio-demographic variables, microbiological data and the clinical examination. The presence of caries can be detected at the age of three on the basis of risk indicators collected at age one. The main advantage of this model is that it can be used by non-dental personnel in a pediatric clinic as they are the first to see infants and young children.

d. Caries Risk Assessment Tools (CAT)

The caries risk assessment tool categorizes children into low, moderate, or high risk. These tools are designed for both dentists and the non-dental personnel. The categorization is carried out by parental interview, clinical examinations and also by microbiological analysis. When risk factors outweigh the protective factors, it indicates an increased likelihood for the development of caries and the child is considered as high risk. The use of risk assessment presents an ideal opportunity to design any preventive protocol for the individuals and also for the community. American Dental Association has suggested guidelines for caries risk assessment for various age groups (Table 11.1).

Table 11.1: Signs and management protocol of individuals based on caries risk assessment

Categories	Signs	Management
Low-risk	• Possess ideal tooth morphology • Not fond of cariogenic diet • No caries in the previous year • Good oral hygiene • Use of preventive measures • Regular dental visits • No medical history affecting salivary flow	• 1-year recall • Advise good oral hygiene • Regular use of a fluoridated dentifrice
Moderate-risk	• Number of carious lesion (at least one) in the last year • Deep pits and fissures especially in the molar region • Oral hygiene is only adequate • White spot lesions are present • Irregular dental visits; or undergoing orthodontic treatment	• 6-month recall • Following preventive regimes; fluoride applications, etc. • Dietary counseling • Use of pit-and-fissure sealants • Use of fluoride dentifrices • Motivate the individuals
High-risk	• Number of new carious lesions (more than two) in the last year • Poor oral hygiene • Consuming cariogenic diet • Irregular dental visits • Reduced salivary flow	• Pit-and-fissure sealants • Use of fluoride dentifrice • Following preventive regimes; fluoride applications, etc. • Routine visit to a dentist • Use of antimicrobial agents

AAPD Caries Risk Assessment Tool

AAPD developed CAT in 2002 based on risk factors organized into 3 general domains: clinical, environmental and general health considerations. But a recent CAT version divides risk categories into child history, clinical evaluation and supplemental professional assessment. Caries risk assessment form for 0–5-year-old is depicted in Table 11.2 and for more than six years is depicted in Table 11.3.

The AAP recommends the inclusion of the first caries risk assessment by child health professionals at age 6 months during well-child visits and that referrals to a dentist for the establishment of a dental home occur within 6 months of the eruption of the first primary tooth and no later than age 1 year. This is particularly critical for children considered at high risk for dental caries.

e. Traffic Light Matrix (TL-M) Model

A traffic light matrix (TL-M) model offers a systematic approach to the assessment of all the risk factors predisposing to caries. The model is based on the fact that the caries process is multifactorial and gets affected by social and environmental changes. The concept of using traffic light colors, viz. red, yellow and green to convey the different levels of risk has been tried earlier. The concept is based on the existing risk assessment models along with an assessment of patient motivation and lifestyle activities. It does not attempt to predict caries incidence; rather it acts as an early warning system alerting the clinician as regard to the presence of risk factors. The TL-M model allocates a threshold value for each risk category. If the results exceed the predetermined threshold values, the model alerts the clinician to a possible

Table 11.2: Caries-risk assessment form for 0–5 years old

Factors	Low risk	Moderate risk	High risk
Biological	-	• Child has special health care needs • Child is a recent immigrant	• Mother/primary caregiver has active caries • Parent/caregiver has low socioeconomic status • Child has >3 between meals sugar-containing snacks or beverages per day • Child is put to bed with a bottle containing natural or added sugar • Child has special health care needs
Protective	• Child receives optimally-fluoridated drinking water or fluoride supplements • Child has teeth brushed daily with fluoridated toothpaste • Child receives topical fluoride from health professional • Child has dental home/regular dental care	– – – –	– – – –
Clinical findings	– – –	– – –	• Child has >1 decayed/missing/filled surfaces • Child has active white spot lesions or enamel defects • Child has elevated mutans streptococci levels

problem. The model investigates sixteen risk factors and scores a red light, yellow light or green light for each risk factor depending upon predetermined criteria. The system uses a specially designed form to record risk factors and the test can be carried out either by a dentist or an auxiliary who has been trained to collect the data.

The second element (Matrix) of the TL-M model is designed to assess the patient's present disease status and attitude to maintain their own dental health. It is a very useful measure of the patient's ability or willingness to comply with treatment directives. Attitude towards dental health is scored as A, B or C on the vertical axis of the grid and the current disease status is scored as 1, 2 or 3 and is recorded on the horizontal axis.

Matrix Component of Traffic Light Matrix Model

Current disease status

1. No current disease.

2. Need for repair or maintenance.

3. Active disease.

Table 11.3: Caries-risk assessment form for ≥ 6 years old

Factors	Low risk	Moderate risk	High risk
Biological			• Patient is of low socio-economic status • Patient has more than 3 between meals sugar-containing snacks or beverages per day
Protective	• Patient receives optimally-fluoridated drinking water • Patient brushes teeth daily with fluoridated toothpaste • Patient receives topical fluoride from health professional • Additional home measures (e.g. xylitol, MI paste, antimicrobial) • Patient has dental home/regular dental care		
Clinical findings		• Patient has defective restorations • Patient wearing an intraoral appliance	• Patient has less than 1 or 1 interproximal lesions • Patient has active white spot lesions or enamel defects • Patient has low salivary flow

Attitude toward dental health

a. Yes.

b. May be.

c. No.

The sixteen risk factors, grouped under five headings, used in the TL-M model are:

Saliva

- Ability of minor salivary glands to produce saliva.
- Consistency of unstimulated saliva.
- pH of unstimulated saliva.
- Stimulated saliva flow rate.
- Buffering capacity of stimulated saliva.

Diet

- Number of sugar exposures per day.
- Number of acid exposures per day.

Fluoride

- Past and current exposure.

Oral Biofilm

- Differential staining.
- Composition.
- Activity.

Modifying Factors

- Past and current dental status.
- Past and current medical status.

- Compliance.
- Lifestyle.
- Socioeconomic status.

In order to formulate a preventive oriented treatment plan the patient's risk of developing caries first needs to be assessed.

The management protocol includes thorough examination, restoration and motivation as regard to preventive measures.

CRA is still in a developmental stage, hence no single model can be recommended for use in a clinical setting at this time. However, if used routinely in dental practice, there will be a shift in the dental treatment from a surgical to a preventive model.

CARIES ACTIVITY INDICATORS

Caries activity indicators are used to:
- Identify high-risk individual/groups.
- Determine the need for caries control measures.
- Monitor the effectiveness of oral health education programs.
- Determine optimal time for care of existing lesions.
- Determine the progress of the preventive measures undertaken.
- Select cases for the study of caries.
- Serve as an indicator of period of exacerbation.

Classification

The caries activity indicators are classified by various authors. The modified version of the accepted classification (Nikiforuk 1985) is:
1. Defense factor indicators
    a. Teeth based.
    b. Saliva based.
2. Host factor indicators.
    a. Socioeconomic status.
    b. Old hygiene status (plaque index, etc.).
    c. Ecology of microflora.
    d. Diet consumption (quality, frequency, etc.).

e. Age.
f. Medication.
3. Caries activity tests.
    a. Lactobacillus count test.
    b. Snyder test.
    c. Alban test.
    d. Salivary reductase test.
    e. Salivary buffer capacity test.
    f. Fosdick calcium dissolution test (Enamel solubility test).
    g. Dewar test.
    h. Mutans streptococci screening test.
        i. Plaque/toothpick method.
        ii. Saliva/tongue blade method.
        iii. *Streptococcus mutans* adherence test.
        iv. Dip slide test.
        v. Modified dip slide test.
    i. Plaque and saliva pH measurement test.
    j. Swab test.
    k. Electronic caries detector.
    l. Ora test.
    m. Predicting caries activity based on previous caries experience.
    n. Cariostat (CAT21 test).
    o. Cariscreen.

A few authors have divided these tests into 'tests which measure caries activity' and 'tests which measure caries susceptibility'. Ora test was kept as 'miscellaneous'.

1. Tests Which Measure Caries Activity

a. Lactobacillus count test.
b. Alban test.
c. Swab test.
d. Salivary buffer capacity test.
e. Mutans streptococci screening test.
- Plaque/tooth pick method.
- Saliva/tongue blade method.
- *Streptococcus mutans* adherence method.
- Dip slide method.

2. Tests Which Measure Caries Susceptibility

a. Snyder test.
b. Fosdick calcium dissolution test (enamel solubility test).

c. Salivary reductase test.

d. Dewar test.

3. Miscellaneous

a. Ora test.

The various indicators are described as:

1. *Defense factors indicators*

a. *Teeth based.*

    i. Newly erupted teeth are more susceptible to caries.

    ii. Crowded teeth are more prone to caries.

    iii. Fluorosed teeth, initially resistant to caries.

    iv. Existing carious teeth indicates probability of caries.

b. *Saliva based*

    i. Buffering capacity of saliva (bicarbonate is buffer): Neutralizes acidic environment, thereby reducing caries probability.

    ii. Salivary secretion rate: Less secretion, more prone to caries.

    iii. Certain medications reduce salivary flow, thereby increasing caries probability.

2. *Host factors indicators*

a. Socioeconomic status: Low socioeconomic group individuals more prone to caries.

b. *Oral hygiene status:* Poor oral hygiene prone to caries; plaque index value predicts caries.

c. *Microflora ecology:* Level of lactobacilli and streptococci indicates high caries risk.

d. Diet consumption: Frequency and quality of sugar intake influence caries probability.

e. *Age:* As the age advances, caries probability increases.

f. *Medication:* Certain medicines like anti-depressants, anti-psychotic drugs influence caries probability.

3. *Caries activity tests*

Caries activity tests are part of caries activity indicators which have been described by various authors. No single test fulfills all the requirements of these tests; however, these are useful for screening population and identifying caries prone individuals who need intensive motivation and preventive care. Earlier previous caries experience was considered as the strong predictor of caries risk; however, over the years caries activity was accepted as a strong predictor of caries risk.

The caries activity test should be:
- Accurate and sensitive.
- Simple and inexpensive.
- Less time consuming.
- Reproducible.
- Measurable.
- Applicable to any setting.

The commonly employed tests are:

a. Lactobacillus Count Test

This test introduced by Hadley (1933) is of a historical interest only. It quantitatively evaluates lactobacilli bacteria in the saliva. The lactobacilli colonies appearing on Tomato agar or Rogosa agar plates are counted; the increase signifies caries activity.

Procedure: The patient is asked to chew paraffin before breakfast and the saliva is collected in a bottle. A 1:10 dilution is prepared by pipetting 1.0 ml of this saliva sample into 9.0 ml tube of sterile saline solution. This is shaken and 1:100 dilution is made by pipetting 1.0 ml of 1:10 dilution into another 9.0 ml tube of sterile salt solution. The 0.4 ml of each solution dilution is spread on the surface of an agar plate (Rogosa agar is considered better than Tomato agar). The plates are labeled and incubated at 37°C for 3–4 days. A count of number of colonies is made by using quebec counter.

It is observed that the bacterial count up to 1000 is unimportant; between 1000 and 5,000 is indicative of slight caries activity; between 5,000 and 10,000 is moderate caries activity and count over 10,000 is associated with high caries activity (Table 11.4).

Advantages
- Simple, easy to carry out in a few minutes.
- Useful for screening larger groups.

Table 11.4: Lactobacillus count and caries activity

No. of lactobacilli/ml	Caries activity
0–1000	(+) little or none
1000–5000	(+) slight
5000–10000	(++) moderate
> 10,000	(+++) marked

Table 11.5: Color change and caries activity

	24 hours	48 hours	72 hours
Color	Caries activity	Caries activity	Caries activity
Yellow	Marked	Definite	Limited
Green	Continue test	Continue test	Caries inactive

Disadvantages
- Inaccurate for predicting onset of caries.
- Does not exclude the possibility of growth of other aciduric micro-organisms.
- Complex equipment required.
- Growth of colonies take longer time.
- Counting of colonies is tedious; can be biased.
- Results take several days.
- Costly.

b. Snyder Test
Modifying lactobacillus count test, Snyder introduced a relatively simple colorimetric test for the estimation of aciduric and acidogenic organisms in saliva. It also indicates the ability of salivary micro-organisms to form acids from the carbohydrate medium. The medium consists of casein, yeast extract, dextrose, agar and bromocresol green. When pH decreases (production of acids) to 4.0 or even less; the color changes from green to yellow. The rate of color change from green to yellow is indicative of the degree of caries activity.

Procedure: Saliva is collected as is given in lactobacillus test. A tube of Snyder glucose is melted and then cooled to 50°C. 0.2 cc of collected saliva is pipetted into 10 ml of medium and is incubated at 37°C for 72 hours. Rate of color change is noted at 24 hours, 48 hours and 72 hours (Table 11.5).

Advantages
- Test is relatively simple (serial dilutions are not required). An acceptable method of educating people.

- Color changes can be noted easily as compared to the counting of bacteria.
- Cost effective

Disadvantages
- Measure acidogenic potential of salivary organisms; may not be representative plaque micro-organisms.
- Color change might not be clear.
- Time consuming.

c. Alban Test
This test, a modified version of Snyder test, is recommended because of its low cost, simplicity, diagnostic and motivational values. This test eliminates the need for melting and cooking as the medium allows easy penetration of saliva and acids. The main features are:
- Sampling is simple as the patient expectorates directly into the tubes containing medium.
- Instead of simple color change, this test measures the depth of change of color yellow (Table 11.6).
- A new calibrated scoring provides better results.

Table 11.6: Depth of color change and caries activity inference

Color change	Inference
No color change	-
Color change beginning at the top of medium	+
One half color change from top to bottom	++
Three-fourths color change from top to bottom	+++
Total color change to yellow	++++

Procedure: 60 gm of Snyder test agar is placed in one liter of water and boiled over low or medium heat. When adequately melted, the molten agar is distributed in tubes, each tube containing 5.0 ml of the test medium. The tubes should be allowed to cool before storing them in the refrigerator. The cooling procedure prepares the tubes along with the test medium and are ready to be used when desired.

For the actual testing, the patient is asked to expectorate directly into the tube such that sufficient amount of saliva covers the test medium. A sterilized funnel facilitates the collection of saliva. The tubes are labelled and incubated at 37°C for 4 days. Observations are made for the color change (bluish green, pH 5.0 to definite yellow, pH 4 or less) and the depth of color change. According to Alban, the volume of saliva, the time of day at which the saliva is collected and the proximity of this time to the time of eating does not significantly affect the results.

Advantages
- Simple and inexpensive.
- Ideal for motivation and education.

Disadvantages
- More armamentarium required.
- Color change evaluation might be subjective.

The final recording after 72 or 96 hours of incubation is carried out as follows:
- Readings negative for the entire incubation period are labelled 'negative'.
- Readings are labelled 'positive' irrespective of the degree of positivity.

- Slower change or less color change compared to the previous test is labelled as 'improved'.
- Faster change or more pronounced change compared to the previous test is labelled as 'worse'.
- When readings are identical compared to the previous test, it is labelled as 'no change'.

d. Salivary Reductase Test

It measures the activity of the enzyme, reductase present in salivary bacteria using a dye 'Diazoresorcinol'.

Procedure

The saliva is collected conventionally by chewing paraffin and shifted in a plastic container. The sample is mixed with a fixed quantity of Diazoresorcinol dye, which color the saliva blue. The change in color after 30 seconds (immediately) and 15 minutes is taken as a measure of caries activity (Table 11.7). A kit, 'Treatex', is available to carry out this test.

Advantages
- No incubation required.
- Time saving (quick results).

Disadvantages
- Results vary with time after food intake and after brushing.

e. Buffer Capacity Test

The buffer capacity is quantitated using either a pH meter or color indicator. The test measures the number of milliliter of acid

Table 11.7: Time, change in color, score and caries activity

Color	Time	Score	Caries activity
Blue	15 minutes	1	Non-conducive
Orchid	15 minutes	2	Slightly conducive
Red	15 minutes	3	Moderately conducive
Red	Immediately	4	Highly conducive
Pink/white	Immediately	5	Extremely conducive

required to lower the pH of saliva, arbitrarily taking any interval; for example, say from pH 6.0 to pH 5.0. Alternatively, the amount of acid or base necessary to bring color indicators to their end point can be analyzed. The caries activity is inversely related to the buffering capacity of saliva. Individuals having considerable number of carious lesions; their saliva should have less acid-buffering capacity.

Advantage
- Simple.

Disadvantage
- Do not correlate adequately with caries activity.

f. Fosdick's Calcium Dissolution Test (Enamel solubility test)

The acid formed from patient's saliva and glucose is mixed with powdered enamel and kept for four hours. The amount in milligrams of powdered enamel dissolution is evaluated.

Saliva is stimulated by chewing gum (paraffin is avoided because glucose is needed for the test; in case paraffin cannot be avoided, additional glucose is added) and approximately 25 ml of saliva is collected. Part of saliva so collected is analyzed for calcium content. The rest is kept in a tube containing 0.1 gm of powdered enamel for four hours at body temperature. After that it is analyzed for calcium content. The caries activity is directly proportional to enamel dissolution.

Advantage
- Useful in limited studies.

Disadvantages
- Complex test, trained persons required.
- Accurate measurements difficult.
- Costly.

g. Dewar Test

Dewar modified the enamel dissolution test measuring pH of the saliva-glucose-enamel mixture (instead of calcium dissolution, only pH is measured). The procedure is not common, since it has not been listed clinically for correlating caries activity.

h. Mutans Streptococci Screening Test

The test measures the number of *Streptococcus mutans* colony forming units (CFU) per unit volume of saliva and also from plaque samples taken from different site of tooth (say occlusal, proximal, etc.). Incubation is carried out in Mitis Salivarius Bacitracin Agar (MSBA) medium. Bacitracin suppresses the growth of non-*Streptococcus mutans* colonies. It is hypothesized that level of *Streptococcus mutans* more than 10^5/ml of saliva is potentially positive for caries activity.

Advantage
- Simple quantitative method.

Disadvantages
- The quantity of *Streptococcus mutans* may vary in the same individual at different times.
- No definite correlation could be established between caries activity and the number of *Streptococcus mutans*.

The test was slightly modified depending upon the procedure of collecting samples and also the adherence capacity of mutans streptococci. Various modified forms are:

i. Plaque/toothpick method

The test involves screening of diluted plaque sample.

Procedure: Plaque samples are collected from the gingival third of the buccal tooth surfaces (one from each quadrant) and placed in Ringer solution. The sample is shaken and streaked across a mitis-salivarius agar plate. After incubating at 37°C for 72 hours, the cultures are examined and the total colonies in 10 fields are recorded. More than 8 colonies/10 fields signifies high caries activity and is given grade 3 (Table 11.8).

Table 11.8: Grading number of *Streptococcus mutans*

Colonies/10 fields	Grades/caries activity
None	1 (Low caries)
Less than 8	2 (Moderate caries)
More than or equal to 8	3 (High caries)

ii. *Saliva/tongue blade method*

The test estimates the number of *Streptococcus mutans* in stimulated saliva.

Procedure: The individuals chew a piece of paraffin wax for one minute. A sterile tongue blade is rotated in their mouth 10 times, so that both sides of the blade are thoroughly inoculated by the oral flora. The tongue blade is pressed into an MSB agar and incubated at 37°C for 48 hours. The numbers of colonies forming units are counted. This is a simplified method for field studies.

This test was developed for use with a large number of schoolchildren avoiding the necessity of collecting saliva.

iii. *Streptococcus mutans adherence test*

The test infers on the ability of *Streptococcus mutans* to adhere to glass surface.

Procedure: 0.1 ml unstimulated saliva is inoculated in MSB broth at 37°C for 24 hours. After bacterial growth, the medium is removed and the cells adhering to the glass surface are examined microscopically. This method is primarily used in epidemiological studies because of its simplicity (Table 11.9).

iv. *Dip slide test*

This is a simple and inexpensive test. Undiluted saliva is flowed over a plastic dip slide coated with agar. This slide is placed in a sterile tube and incubated for four days at 35°C. The color density is compared with a model chart. More than 10,000 colonies signify caries activity; whereas less than 1,000 colonies signifies no caries.

v. *Modified dip slide test*

This test estimates the count of three micro-organisms, namely mutans streptococci, lactobacilli and Candida.

Procedure: Five milliliters of paraffin-stimulated saliva sample is collected and poured over a three compartment slide containing Mitis-salivarius, Bouitrain agar, Rogosa agar and Sabourand dextrose agar. Slide is incubated in a 5% CO_2 incubator for 48 hours. The salivary mutans streptococci, lactobacilli and Candida counts are obtained.

Advantages

- The test is simple and useful for the early selection of patients.
- It is a valuable education aid for the motivation and dietary counseling among children.

i. *Plaque and Saliva pH Measurement Test*

The pH of plaque and saliva is measured using methyl red dye. The color of methyl red changed from yellow at pH 6.0 to orange at 5.2 and to red below pH 5.0. 0.1% solution of methyl red is applied topically on the suspected site and the glucose solution is sprayed over the area. The sites that turn red are recorded. This method is very simple, inexpensive and can be used at chair side. Plaque pH can be measured by radio-telemetry, which indicates continuous pH changes which may occur during various activities like eating or sleeping, etc. It is useful for research purposes also.

j. *Swab Test*

Principle method involved is the same as of Snyder test.

Table 11.9: Adherence of *Streptococcus mutans* and caries activity

Mutans adherence	Caries activity
No growth/adherence	−
Few small size deposits (1–10)	+
Scattered deposits smaller size (10–20)	+ +
Numerous large size deposits (>20)	+ + +

The buccal surfaces of teeth are swabbed with color applicator and subsequently incubated. The change in pH following 48 hours incubation is read on a pH meter; alternatively color change is read by use of color indicator (Table 11.10).

Advantages

- Collection of saliva not required.
- Useful in predicting caries increments, especially in children.

k. Electronic Caries Detector

This device works on the principle that intact enamel is resistant to passage of current as compared to porous enamel which contains saliva with all its electrolytes. Thus, teeth showing less resistance to electronic current have more probability of getting carious.

This method is more useful in detecting early pit and fissure lesions than the conventional probe. The positive correlation between the diagnosis made by commercially available electronic caries detector and the histologically determined depth carious lesion is confirmed by various authors.

l. Ora Test

The Ora test, developed by Rosenberg, et al (1989), evaluates oral microbial level, based on the rate of oxygen depletion by micro-organisms. Normally the bacterial enzyme, aerobic dehydrogenase transfers electrons or protons to oxygen. Once oxygen gets utilized by the aerobic organisms, methylene blue acts as an electron acceptor and gets reduced to leucomethylene blue, reflecting the metabolic activity of the micro-organisms.

Procedure

10 ml of sterile milk is rinsed in the oral cavity for 30 seconds and the expectorate is collected in a sterile container. 3.0 ml of this milk is transferred to a tube to which 0.12 ml of 0.1% methylene blue is added. The tubes are observed every 10 minutes for any color change and also the time of initiation of the color change. The higher the number of organisms, lesser is the time taken for the change in color.

Advantages

- Simple and less time consuming.
- Economical.

Disadvantage

Lack specificity.

m. Predicting Caries Activity based on Previous Caries Experience

Previous caries experience has been considered to be a reasonable indication for future trends; however, the assumption may prove negative because of awareness of preventive factors in later life (Table 11.11).

Procedure: A group of children of varying age groups are examined as regard to number of tooth surfaces restored/carious. The following surfaces are generally examined and given score one for each surface.

- Proximal surfaces of incisors.
- Proximal surfaces of first permanent molars.
- Buccal surfaces of upper first permanent molars.
- Lingual surfaces of lower first permanent molars.

Table 11.10: Range of pH and caries activity

pH	Caries activity
4.1 or > 4.1	Marked
4.2–4.4	Active
4.5–4.6	Slightly active
4.6 or > 4.6	Inactive

Table 11.11: Prediction of future caries activity

Group	Caries activity	Surfaces restored/caries (score)
Low caries active	Low	Zero
High caries active	High	>4

The children who had a score 4 or more were considered highly caries active, whereas those who had a score zero were considered low caries active. This method can be used for identifying children with high and low caries activity so as the preventive therapy can be initiated accordingly.

The serious drawbacks for using this method are:

- Considerable caries might have already occurred.
- Not applicable to the very young individuals.
- Requires lengthy examination process.

n. Cariostat (CAT 21 test)

The method, developed by Shimono and Sobue (1974), is a colorimetric test that determines the acidogenicity of oral micro-organisms in the plaque through changes in pH. Scoring is carried out by comparing the results (color) of the samples with 4-scale (0, 1.0, 2.0 and 3.0) reference color chart provided with the kit. A score of '0' designates low caries activity; '3.0' would be highest caries susceptibility.

Procedure

The buccal cervical surfaces of maxillary teeth of any quadrant are wiped twice with cotton swabs. The swab then shifted to a container, is incubated for 48 hours at 37°C. A color chart is provided and the scoring is carried out in daylight. A blue color infers pH 6.1 + 0.3; green 5.4 + 0.3; yellow-green 4.7 + 0.3 and yellow being 4.0 + 0.3.

Advantages

- Method is simple, effective and inexpensive.
- Can be used individually or at large scale.

o. Cariscreen

The Cariscreen Swab Sampling device is a self-contained ATP device for use with the Cariscreen Caries Susceptibility Testing Meter. It is used for screening for presence of dental caries. The sample is collected by swabbing the mid lingual surface of the lower anteriors from canine to canine. The Cariscreen meter in conjunction with the Cariscreen Swab measures adenosine triphosphate (ATP). The amount of light generated, after the contact of ATP with the unique liquid-stable uniferase/luciferin reagent, is measured with Cariscreen Meter. The reading will appear on the screen as a number of RLUs (Relative Light Units 1–9999). The values 0–1500 is considered as 'low risk'; whereas 1501–9999 is at 'high risk'.

Bibliography

1. Alaluusua S, Kleemola K ujala E, Gronroos L and Evalahti M. Salivary caries related tests as predictor of future caries increment in teenagers. A three year longitudinal study. Oral Microbiol. Immunol.: 1990;5:77–81.
2. Anna YA, Mary EM, Solveig F and Birkhed D. Assessment of caries risk in elderly patients using the cariogram model. J. Can. Dent. Assoc.: 2006; 72:459–63.
3. Arino M, Ataru ITO, Fujiki S, Sujiyama S and Hayashi M. Multicenter study on caries risk assessment in Japanese adult patients. J Dent, 2015. 07.010
4. Baca P, Parejo E, Bravo M, Castillo A and Liebana J. Discriminant ability for caries risk of modified colorimetric tests. Med. Oral Patol. Oral Cir. Bucal.: 2011;16:978–83.
5. Basavaraj P, Khuller N, Khuller R and Sharma N. Caries risk assessment and control. J. Oral Health and Comm. Dent.: 2011;5:58–63.
6. Beck JD. Risk re-visited. Comm. Dent. Oral Edpidemiol.: 1998;26:220–5.
7. Beck JD, Kohout F and Hunt RJ. Identification of high caries risk adults: attitudes, social factors and diseases. Int. Dent. J.: 1988;38:231–8.
8. Beighton D. A simplified procedure for estimating the level of *Streptococcus mutans* in the mouth. Br. Dent. J.: 1986;160:329–30.
9. Bhasin S, Sudha P and Anegundi RT. Chair side simple caries activity test: Ora test. Indian Soc. Pedo. Pre Dent.: 2006;24:76–9.
10. Bowden GH. Does assessment of microbial composition of plaque/saliva allow for diagnosis of disease activity of individuals? Comm. Dent. Oral Epidemiol.: 1997;25:76–81.

11. Bowen WH. Caries activity tests. Int. Dent. J.: 1969;19:267–72.

12. Brathall D and Hansal PG. Cariogram—a multifactorial risk assessment model for a multifactorial disease. Comm. Dent. Oral Epidemiol.: 2005;33:256–64.

13. Camling E and Emilson CG. Results with the caries activity test Cariostat, Compared to prevalence of mutans streptococci and lactobacilli. Swed. Dent. J.: 1989;13:125–30.

14. Campus G, Cagetti MG, Senna A, Blasi G, Mascolo A, Demarchi P and Strohmenger L. Does smoking increase risk for caries? A cross-sectional study in an Italian military academy. Caries Res.: 2011;45:40–6.

15. Crossner CG. Salivary Lactobacillus counts in the prediction of caries activity. Comm. Dent. Oral Epidemiol.: 1981;9:182–90.

16. Douglas AY, Fontana M and Wolf MS. Current concepts in Cariology. Dent. Clin. North Am.: 2010;54:527–32.

17. Esra UC, Necmi G and Mustafa A. Efficiency of caries risk assessment in young adults using Cariogram. Eur. J. Dent.: 2012;6:270–9.

18. Fontana M and Zero DT. Assessing patients' caries risk. J.A.D.A.: 2006;137:1231–72.

19. Fontana M, Young D and Wolff M. Evidence based caries risk assessment and management. Dent. Clin. North Am.: 2009;53:149–61.

20. Gabris K, Nagy G, Madlena M, Denes Z, Marton S, Keszthelyi G and Banoczy J. Associations between microbiological and salivary caries activity tests and caries experience in Hungarian adolescents. Caries Res.: 1999;33:191–5.

21. Hannigan A, O'Mullane DM, Barry D, Schafer F and Roberts AJ. A caries susceptibility classification of tooth surfaces by survival time. Caries Res.: 2000;34:103–8.

22. Holmen A, Stromberg U, Magnusson K and Twetman S. Tobacco use and caries risk among adolescents—a longitudinal study in Sweden. BMC Oral Health: 2013;13.

23. Ismail AI, Sohn W, Betz J, Tallez M, William JM and Lepkawski J. Risk indicators for dental caries using the international caries detection and assessment system (ICDAS). Comm. Dent. Oral Epidemiol.: 2008;35:55–68.

24. Jenson L, Budenz AW, Featherstone JDB, Romos Gomes FJ, Spolsky WW and Young BA. Clinical protocol for caries management by risk assessment. J. Calif. Dent. Assoc.: 2007;35:714–23.

25. Jung EH, Lee ES, Kang SM, Kwon HK and Kim B. Assessing the clinical validity of a new caries activity test using dental plaque acidogenicity. J. Korean Acad. Oral Health: 2014;38:77–81.

26. Kang SMJH, Jeong SH, Kwon HK and Kim B. Development of a new color scale for a caries activity test. J. Korean Acad. Oral Health: 2010;34: 9–17.

27. Klock B and Krasse B. A comparison between different methods for prediction of caries activity. Scand. J. Dent. Res.: 1979;87:129–39.

28. Koroluk I, Hoover JN and Komiyama K. The sensitivity and specificity of a colorimetric microbiological caries activity test (Cariostat) in preschool children. Pediatr. Dent.: 1994;16:276–81.

29. Krasse B. Relationship between caries activity and the number of lactobacilli in the oral cavity. Acta. Odontol. Scand.: 1954;12:157–9.

30. Kuhnisch J, Galler M, Seitz M, Stich H, Lussi A, Hickel R, Kunzelmann KH and Bucher K. Irregularities below the enamel-dentin junction may predispose for fissure caries. J. Dent. Res.: 2012;91:1066–70.

31. Kunte SS, Chaudhary S, Singh A and Chaudhary M. Evaluation and co-relation of the Oratest, colorimetric Snyder's test and salivary *Streptococcus mutans* count in children of age group of 6–8 years. J. Int. Society of Prev. and Comm. Dent.: 2013;3:59–66.

32. Li Y and Wang W. Predicting caries in permanent teeth from caries in primary teeth: an eight-year cohort study. J. Dent. Res.: 2002;81:561–6.

33. Muller-Bolla M, Courson F, Droz D, Peguier L and Velly AM. Definition of at-risk occlusal surfaces of permanent molars—a descriptive study. J. Clin. Pediatr. Dent.: 2009;34:35–42.

34. Nicholau B, Marcenes W, Bartley M and Sheiham A. A life course approach to assessing causes of dental caries experience: the relationship between biological, behavioural, socioeconomic and psychological conditions and caries in adolescents. Caries Res.: 2003;37:319–26.

35. Nishimura M, Oda T, Kazriya N, Matsumura S and Shimono T. Using a caries activity test to predict caries risk in early childhood. JADA: 2008;139:63–71.

36. Patalay A, Shubhada C and Nadiger SL. Oratest: A simple, chair-side caries activity test. J. Indian Soc. Pedod. Prev. Dent.: 1996;14:6–9.

37. Powell V. Caries risk assessment: Relevance to practitioner. JADA: 1998;129:349–53.

38. Reich E, Lussi A and Newbrun E. Caries risk assessment. Int. Dent. J.: 1999;49:15–26.

39. Rodis DMM, Matsumura S, Shimono T and Ji Y. Comparison of plaque samples and saliva samples using the CAT 21 test (Cariostat method). Pediatric Dent. J.: 2005;15:6–9.

40. Rooban T, Vidya K, Joshua E, Rao A, Ranganathan S, Rao UK and Ranganathan K. Tooth decay in alcohol and tobacco abusers. J. Oral Maxillofac. Pathol.: 2011;15:14–21.

41. Rosenberg M, Barki M and Portnoy SA. A simple method for estimating oral microbial levels. J. Microbiol. Methods: 1989;9:253–7.

42. Saxsena S, Pundir S and Aena J. Oratest: A new concept to test caries activity. J. Indian Soc. Pedod. Prev. Dent.: 2013;31:25–8.

43. Shimono T and Sobue S. A new calorimetric caries activity test. Dental Outlook: 1974;43:829–35.

44. Shimura N, Nakamura C, Hiranwama Y and Yonemitsu M. Anxiety and dental caries Comm. Dent. Oral Epidemiol.: 1983;11:224–7.

45. Snyder ML. A simple colorimetric method for the estimation of relative numbers of lactobacilli in the saliva. J. Dent. Res.: 1940;19:349–55.

46. Stromberg U, Holmen A, Mangusson K and Twetman S. Geo-mapping of time trends in childhood caries risk—a method for assessment of preventive care. BMC Oral Health: 2012;12:9.

47. Stromberg U, Magnusson K, Holmen A and Twetman S. Geo-mapping of caries risk in children and adolescents—a novel approach for allocation of preventive care. BMC Oral Health: 2011;11:26.

48. Suddick RP and Dodds W. Caries activity estimates and implications: insights into risk versus activity. J. Dent. Educ.: 1997;61:876–84.

49. Tamgadge S, Tamgadge A and Evie S. Caries activity indicators: Guide for dental practitioners. Int. J. Oral and Maxillo. Path.: 2013;4:34–42.

50. Thaweboon B, Thawboon S, Sopavanit C and Kasetsuwan R. A modified dip-slide test for microbiological risk in caries assessment. Southeast Asian J. Trop. Med. Public Health: 2006;37:400–4.

51. Twetman S, Fontana M and Featherstone J. Caries risk assessment—can we achieve consensus? Comm. Dent. Oral Epidemiol.: 2013;41:64–70.

52. Twetman S, Johansoon I, Birkhed D and Nederfors T. Caries incidence in young type 1 diabetes mellitus patients in relation to metabolic control and caries associated risk factors. Caries Res.: 2002;36:31–5.

53. Van Houte J. Microbiological predictors of caries risk. Adv. Dent.Res.: 1993;7:87–96.

54. Wyne AH and Guile EE. Caries activity indicators: A review. Ind. J. Dent. Res.: 1993;4:39–46.

55. Young DA, Featherstone JD, Roth JR, Anderson M, Autio-Gold J, Christensen GJ, Fontana M, Kutsch VK, Peters MC, Simonsen RJ and Wolff MS. Caries management by risk assessment implementation guidelines. J. Calif. Dent. Assoc.: 2007;35:799–805.

12

Prevention of Caries

Man's fight with 'disease' is a continuous process. Since time immemorial, researchers remained active finding causes and cures of various diseases inflicting human being. Over the years the dental ailments could not be recognized, since superstitions and ignorance have been engulfing the early population. The need to prevent a disease process or at least to slow down its effect on living tissues has always been a challenge for the medical professionals. Preventive dentistry is that branch of dental practice, 'which deals with establishment and maintenance of oral environment conducive for the preservation of sound and healthy stomatognathic system'. The rationale is to promote optimal health of the oral tissues and to prevent the future damages also.

In recent years with increasing oral health awareness, more people retain their natural teeth into old age. With the old age, there is increased susceptibility to periodontal problems, leading to gingival recession and root surfaces getting exposed to oral environment making them vulnerable to root caries. When secondary caries and root caries are considered, the aggregate caries increment may come to be higher, especially in older adults. The caries and its sequel, rather than periodontal disease, is the primary cause of tooth loss in our aging population.

Until recently, the preventive measures were based on the old theories of etiology of oral/dental disease; however, the knowledge of mechanism of initiation and progress of oral/dental diseases has expanded manifold now.

It is essential that every effort should be made to translate our present knowledge of etiological factors in oral diseases to preventive dentistry. This knowledge should then be transmitted to practicing dentists so as to enable them to refresh themselves regarding preventive aspects which can be involved in oral diseases.

There are significant differences between the developed and the developing countries as regard to the resources and the development of professional oral care services are concerned. These differences may affect the choice of priorities in health care and their practical implementation.

Preventive regimes are broadly divided into four components (Table 12.1).

- Primordial prevention is the prevention of risk factors, beginning with change in social and environmental conditions in which these factors are observed to develop and continue for high-risk children, adolescent and young adults.
- Primary prevention refers to those procedures applied prior to the inception

Table 12.1: Components of preventive regimes

Primordial prevention (preventing risk factors)	Primary prevention (pre-pathogenic)	Secondary prevention (pathogenic)	Tertiary prevention (post-pathogenic)

• Changing lifestyle
• Promote physical activities
• Modify food habits
	• Fluoride therapy
	  – Systemic
	  – Topical
	• Diet control
	• Plaque control
	• Sealants
		• Early diagnosis
		• Conservative restorations
		• Tissue biopsy
			• Fixed prosthesis
			• Permanent restorations

of a disease. This is also known as 'pre-pathogenic prevention', which is accomplished by avoidance of the factors responsible for inception of the disease.

- Secondary prevention is to diagnose and manage the disease in its early stages so that the subsequent damages are minimized. It is also named 'pathogenic prevention'.
- Tertiary prevention refers to utilizing restorative procedures to prevent any further damage from the disease. It is also designated as 'post-pathogenic prevention'.

General Guidelines for Preventive Regime

Following guidelines should be implemented in any preventive regime:
- Basic oral health care information should be provided to each and every individual.
- Motivation as regard to awareness of importance of prevention.
- Good oral hygiene as an essential part of the general body hygiene should be emphasized.
- Use of fluoride containing toothpastes (wherever required).
- An adequate non-cariogenic diet should be recommended.
- Use of other preventive measures.
- The guidelines should orient towards health promotion, health awareness, self-care and self-reliance.

PREVENTIVE CARE REGIME

The preventive care regime is divided into four levels:

- **Care level 1:** Aims at increasing awareness of oral health, educating and motivating the individuals to adopt preventive measures.
- **Care level 2:** Includes informing the people about the available preventive aids and their clinical use.
- **Care level 3:** Includes initial restorative procedures and removal of the etiologic factors.
- **Care level 4:** Deals with tertiary preventive regimes.

Care Level 1: Awareness, Education and Motivation

All individuals should be provided information as regard to role of healthy oral tissues in retaining a functional dentition for life. The information should emphasize upon the advantages of a clean and healthy mouth. The awareness is required for the health professionals also.

Promotion of self-assessment and self-care should be a part of general awareness. Self-care begins with regular self-assessment, i.e. evaluation of the condition of oral tissues by an individual to enable him to make a judgment on the need of extra self-care or professional assistance. The black spots over the teeth are common signs which indicate impending caries.

Education

There are many sources of information for educating the patient. The operator is the best source of information; however, a few sources also play an important role:

- *Mass media:* Television, radio and magazines, etc.
- Family and friends.
- Physician, schoolteachers, nurses, etc.
- Computers.
- Pamphlets.

Physicians, nurses and other health professionals are powerful opinion makers. Schoolteachers should be educated for effective oral care means; the knowledge they would dissipate to the students.

Patients should be informed about the importance of periodic checkups. Since most of the dental and oral lesions are painless in their initial stages and the patient is unaware of the disease in the oral cavity, it is the dentist who can guide the patient for proper treatment at an early stage.

Motivation

Motivation is an art of stimulating people to take a course of action usually desired by others. If the goal is desired by the person himself, that is known as self-motivation. Motivation is derived from the word 'motive'. Motive means an idea, need, emotion or organic state that prompts a man to act. It is defined as *the process of attempting to influence others to do your will through the possibility of gain or reward.*

Self-motivation can be— 'All those forces operating within the individual which impels him to act or not to act in certain ways'.

The factors, which may influence motivation are:

- Family circumstances.
- Literacy level.
- Negative personality.
- Social standards.
- Financial constraints.
- Peer groups.
- Emotional quotient.
- Psychological complexes.

Care Level 2: Introduction of Preventive Aids and their Clinical Use

The people are motivated and educated to know the availability of home care devices which can help prevent the oral diseases. These include mechanical and chemical means. Mechanical aid includes toothbrush and interdental cleaning aids (toothpick, dental floss, interdental brush). Chemical aids include chemoprophylactic agents like mouthwashes and toothpaste. The most common preventive aid is toothbrush. Individuals are motivated to adopt self-care preventive measures.

Care Level 3: Initial Restorative Procedures and Removal of Etiological Factors

The incipient lesions are treated immediately and the lesions are restored with remineralizing solutions so as to arrest the caries at this level. The associated factors promoting caries are also controlled at this stage.

Care Level 4: Tertiary Preventive Regimes

An extensive range of treatment modalities fall into this category. Tertiary care is usually provided to the resourceful people. Others are referred for better care in respective institutes.

For prevention of dental caries, the three-point strategy was evolved at National Caries Preventive Programs along with creating awareness among masses through motivation and education.

The preventive strategies are:

A. Control of caries inducing micro-organisms.
B. Modification of caries promoting diet.
C. Increasing the resistance of the teeth to decay.
D. Miscellaneous.

A. CONTROL OF CARIES INDUCING MICRO-ORGANISMS

It has been established that the plaque formation precedes the caries process. Plaque consists of a bacterial film that produces acids as a by-product of its metabolism. These acids have the potential to dissolve calcium and phosphate contents of the tooth substance; the process known as demineralization. The process of demineralization can be reversed (i.e. remineralization); if not, will lead to initiation of caries.

The deteriorative effect of dental plaque accumulation and metabolism is bidirectional, i.e. outward towards soft tissue causing periodontal disease and inward towards the tooth causing dental caries.

WHO defined dental plaque as 'a specific but highly variable structural entity resulting from sequential colonization and growth of micro-organisms on the surfaces of teeth and restorations consisting of micro-organisms of various strains and species embedded in the extracellular matrix, composed of bacterial metabolic products and substances from serum, saliva and blood.'

Plaque control measures are considered as the prime approach to prevent dental caries. It includes mechanical procedures as well as chemical agents, which retard plaque formation. Mechanical plaque control is indispensable to achieve optimum success and chemical measures are used only as an adjunct to mechanical means and not as a substitute.

The procedures of personal plaque removal by toothbrushing and/or flossing help maintain good oral hygiene. In addition, tooth-brushing is a proven caries preventive procedure, especially with the self-application of fluoride dentifrice.

The caries control protocol includes thorough plaque removal, use of fluorides and dietary counselling.

Professional tooth cleaning also has an important effect on caries reduction. Effective plaque removal reduces the development of new carious lesions.

The guidelines as regard to maintaining oral hygiene vis-à-vis preventing caries are as follows:

- Maintaining oral hygiene requires a lot of motivation. Instructions should include the available mechanical aids and their selection, based on the patients needs.
- Routine brushing with approved dentifrices.
- Thorough rinsing and flossing after every meal.
- During sleep, a decrease in salivary flow allows unrestricted plaque growth. Therefore, emphasize oral hygiene measures before bedtime.
- The routine flossing removes debris and bacterial plaque from the interproximal spaces.
- Rinsing should follow flossing and brushing. Rinsing is repeated until the expectorated rinse water is clear.

Methods of Plaque Removal

The plaque removal methods are categorized into following:

   I. Mechanical.

  II. Chemical.

 III. Miscellaneous.

I. Mechanical Plaque Control

The mechanical plaque control devices include:

a. Toothbrushes.
  - Manual.
  - Powered.
b. Dentifrices.
c. Auxiliary aids/interdental aids.
  - Dental floss.
  - Wooden/plastic sticks.
  - Interdental stimulators.
  - Interdental brushes.
  - Dental tape.
d. Oral irrigation.

a. Toothbrushes

Toothbrushes are the most widely used oral hygiene aid. Toothbrushes can effectively remove plaque by using correct brush and adequate techniques.

Generally toothbrushes vary in size, design as well as in length and arrangements of bristles. To standardize the toothbrush, ADA has suggested specification as:

- *Length:* 1 to 1.25 inches.
- *Width:* 5/16 to 3/8 inches.
- *Number of rows:* 2 to 4 rows.
- *Number of tufts:* 5 to 12 tufts per row.
- *Number of bristles:* 80 to 85 bristles per tuft.

The toothbrushes are classified on the basis of bristle material, its hardness and the manner of use. The types are:

Type 1: Bristle material used in toothbrushes

Two types of materials are routinely used: Natural (hog bristles) and artificial (nylon filaments).

Natural bristles easily get soften, lose their elasticity and may break; whereas artificial bristles last longer.

Type 2: Hardness of toothbrush bristles

The hardness of bristle is proportional to the square of the diameter of the bristle and inversely proportional to the square of bristle length. On the basis of hardness (diameter of bristle) of bristles, the toothbrushes are:

- Soft brush: 0.007 inch (0.2 mm).
- Medium brush: 0.012 inch (0.3 mm).
- Hard brush: 0.014 inch (0.4 mm).

Soft bristles are more flexible, can clean beneath the gingival margin and reach farther onto the proximal tooth surfaces. The hard bristles can cause trauma to soft tissues and abrasion of exposed root surfaces. The hard bristles will not be able to clean the interproximal areas due to poor adaptation to these contours.

The use of a hard toothbrush and vigorous horizontal brushing, along with abrasive dentifrices may lead to cervical abrasion of teeth. However, it is established that the action of brushing is more damaging than the hardness of the bristles. Even the amount of force used to brush is not critical for effective plaque control.

Type 3: Manner of use of toothbrushes

Generally the toothbrushes are used manually; however, powered brushes are also available.

i. **Manual toothbrushes:** The toothbrushing can be carried out manually using various techniques, viz. horizontal scrub, Bass, Stillman, Charters and Fones, etc.

- The horizontal scrub is the common method; however, may cause gingival and enamel damage if aggressive strokes are used.
- The Stillman's method is primarily used for massage and stimulation of the gingiva. 45 degree angle of the bristles along with vibratory/pulsating strokes are usually used. It is recommended in gingival recession.
- The Charters method also involves a 45 degree angle of the bristles using rotary/ vibratory motion forcing the bristles interproximally. It is generally recommended in orthodontic cases and fixed partial dentures and in patients who had periodontal surgery.
- Bass's method is generally recommended for adults since it effectively removes plaque and debris from the gingival sulcus. In this technique, the toothbrush is positioned in the gingival sulcus at a 45 degree angle to the tooth apices and a vibratory action (back and forth) cleans the sulcus. The technique is modified giving final 'sweep' toward the occlusal surfaces to remove debris subgingivally.
- Fones technique is preferred in children as they lack manual dexterity. The toothbrush is moved in a circular method over both the upper and lower teeth. In the anterior region, the teeth are placed in an edge-to-edge position and the circular motion is continued.
- Vertical technique involves a 90° angle of bristles to the long axis of the teeth. The

teeth are placed in an edge to edge position; brush the teeth with up and down stroke. Maxillary and mandibular teeth are brushed separately.
- Physiological method (Smith method) is based on the principle that the toothbrush should follow the physiological pathway that is followed by food when it traverses over the tissues during mastication.
- In roll technique, bristles are placed at 45 degree angle and lightly rolled across the tooth surface towards occlusal surface. This technique is preferred in children and adults with limited dexterity.

ii. *Powered toothbrushes:* Electrically powered toothbrushes were invented in early nineties. Powered toothbrushes are safe to use similar to manual toothbrushes. These brushes are recommended in persons with low manual dexterity or physical limitations. The larger handle is ideal for patients with arthritis or stroke victims who cannot grip the smaller toothbrush handles. Many varieties of powered toothbrushes are available, viz. Oral-B, Triumph, Philips Sonicare, etc.

Whichever toothbrush is used, the individuals should be taught to remove the plaque in a sequential order, without skipping any surface. The instructions should also include brushing the tongue to remove debris and bacteria. To maintain cleaning effectiveness, toothbrush should be replaced when bristle head shows fraying or wear patterns.

b. Dentifrices

A dentifrice is a substance used with a toothbrush for the purpose of cleaning the accessible surfaces of the teeth. It is the French word for toothpaste. The dentifrices are supplied in paste, powder, gel or liquid form (Fig. 12.1).

Ingredients

The main ingredients of dentifrice are:
- *Abrasives:* The common abrasive used in dentifrices is hydrated silica; however,

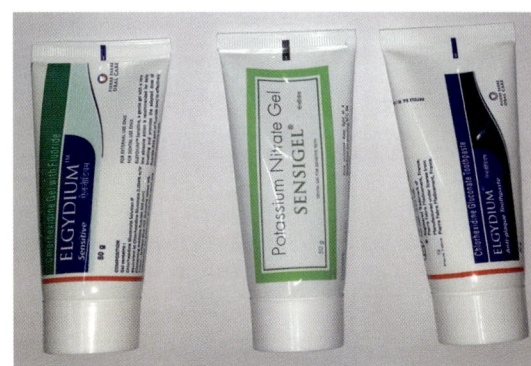

Fig. 12.1: Dentifrice

alumina and calcium carbonate have also been used.
- *Binding/thickening agents:* The binding/thickening agents control the viscosity of the toothpaste and provide creamy consistency. They are usually derived from cellulose; sodium carboxymethyl cellulose being the most commonly used. Carrageenans (seaweed derived), alginates are also used.
- *Humectants:* The Humectants are used to prevent loss of water and subsequent hardening of the paste, when it is exposed to air. They also provide a creamy texture. Glycerine and Sorbitol are commonly used humectants.
- *Solvents:* Water is the most common solvent used in toothpastes. It helps in dissolution and mixing of the ingredients.
- *Detergents (Surfactants):* Detergents lower the surface tension of the liquid environment so that the ingredients in the toothpaste can contact the teeth more easily. The foaming effect produced by the detergent removes debris and is beneficial in cleaning the teeth. The most widely used detergent is Sodium lauryl sulphate.
- *Flavoring agents:* Combinations of water-insoluble essential oils, such as peppermint, eucalyptus and menthol are usually used as flavoring agents in toothpastes.
- *Sweeteners:* The commonly used sweeteners are sodium saccharin, sorbitol and glycerin.

Xylitol as a sweetener also provides anti-caries activity.

- *Coloring agents:* Titanium dioxide usually provides color to the toothpastes.
- *Preservatives:* Preservatives prevent the growth of micro-organisms. The commonly used preservatives are sodium benzoate, methylparaben and ethylparaben.
- *Therapeutic agents:* Different types of therapeutic agents used in toothpaste are:
  - Anti-caries agents: Fluoride in the concentration of 0.10–0.15% is considered to be the most effective caries-inhibiting agent. The most common form used is sodium fluoride, but mono-fluoro-phosphate and stannous fluoride are also used.

    Sodium bicarbonate and calcium phosphate are other anti-caries agents used in toothpastes.
  - Anti-plaque agents: Triclosan and metal ions such as zinc and stannous are commonly used anti-plaque agents.
  - Anti-calculus agents: Pyrophosphate and zinc are used as anti-calculus agents.
  - Whitening agents: Along with abrasives, Dimethicones (cause a smooth surface on the tooth that prevents stain formation) and Papain (sulfhydryl protease, extracted from the Carica papaya plant) are used in toothpastes as whitening agents. Bromelain, a proteolytic enzyme derived from pineapple, is also used.

The composition of dentifrice is:

Ingredients	Weight %
Humectants	6–20
Water	0–50
Binders	0–12
Abrasives	18–50
Flavors	0.5–2.0
Sweeteners	0.2–1.0
Surfactants	0.5– 2.0
Fluorides	0.2–1.2

c. Auxiliary Aids/Interdental Aids

Many accessories/aids are used along with toothbrushing to achieve significant cleaning. The effective aids are:

1. Dental floss: The purpose of flossing is to remove plaque from the interdental areas. Unlike a toothbrush, which cleans the external surfaces of the teeth and gums, floss is an interdental cleaner. It is the most widely recommended tool for removing plaque from proximal tooth surfaces. Different types of floss are: waxed/un-waxed, mint/cinnamon, etc. It has been established that the plaque removing ability is the same with different types of floss. Various types of toothbrushes and floss are shown in Fig. 12.2.

Procedure

Flossing is carried out using either circular/loop method or spool method (Fig. 12.3).

- *Circle/loop method:* It is preferred for children or any individual with low manual

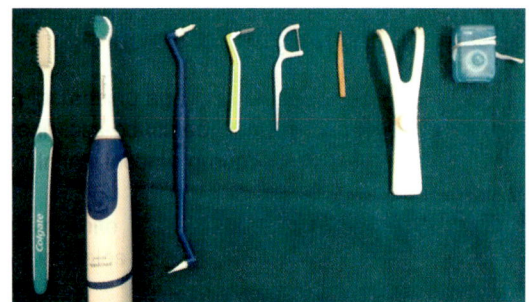

Fig. 12.2: Various types of toothbrushes and dental floss

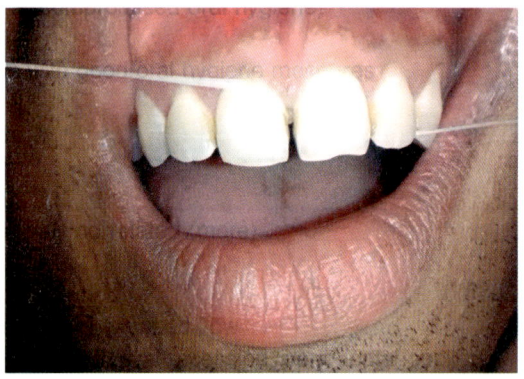

Fig. 12.3: Clinical use of dental floss

dexterity. A piece of floss approximately 18 inches long is tied at the ends to form a loop or circle. The patient uses the thumb and index finger to guide the floss interproximally through the contacts. The floss is gently eased between the teeth with a seesaw motion at the contact point. Once through the contact area, gently slide the floss up and down the mesial and distal marginal ridges directing the floss subgingivally to remove the debris.

- *Spool method:* Approximately 18 inches long floss is wound around the middle finger of one hand and around the middle finger of the opposite hand. After cleaning one surface, the used floss is moved or spooled to the other hand until all supragingival and subgingival areas have been cleaned.

A floss holder is also available which facilitates easy access to the interdental areas.

2. Wooden/plastic sticks: The wooden/plastic sticks are used as an adjunct to other interdental cleansing aids. The sticks are used to clean the embrasure areas, reshape the soft tissues to functional form and also increase keratinization of the interdental col.

The sticks are available with or without handle. These are triangular in shape and should be placed through the embrasure without touching or hurting the lingual papillae. The sides of the triangular stick remove the plaque from the proximal surfaces of the teeth in the depth of the embrasure. The base of the triangle rests on the gingiva.

Wooden sticks are usually used on the facial surfaces of anterior teeth. Wooden sticks should be discouraged in the presence of sub-gingival calculus; it may tear the junctional epithelium.

3. Interdental stimulators: Interdental stimulators are used to massage the gingiva; may remove some debris also. These are made of rubber, wood or plastic, which is attached to a handle. The stimulator is inserted from the facial or lingual aspect into an open inter-dental embrasure. Light pressure is exerted against the soft tissue and the handle is rotated gently. There should be sufficient space in the interdental embrasure to insert stimulators without injuring the soft tissue. The stimulator should be inserted gently, otherwise it may damage the epithelial attachments.

4. Interdental brushes: The interdental brushes are recommended for proximal cleaning of teeth with sufficient interdental spaces, concave root surfaces and furcation areas.

The interdental brushing is carried out using a small brush, which readily passes between the teeth when gentle pressure is exerted on the handle.

The brush is rotated and vibrated with wrist motion, which removes the accumulated soft materials in between the teeth; gingival massage is accomplished as well.

Cone shaped/cylindrical interdental unitufted brushes are also available which are useful especially in areas with large gingival embrasures. For best cleaning efficiency, the diameter of the brush should be slightly larger than the gingival embrasure so that the bristles can exert gentle pressure on the proximal surfaces and concavities of the root. Unitufted brushes are also helpful around dental appliances, including implants and orthodontic wires and brackets.

5. Dental tape: Dental tape is thicker than dental floss and is flattened like a ribbon. Strands of tape can be used to loosen retained debris over the proximal and the gingival surfaces. Since the tape is flattened like a ribbon, it presents a greater working area than floss. Tape should be carefully adapted to the curved surfaces of teeth because its edges are narrower and sharper than floss and can hurt the soft tissue.

d. Oral Irrigation

Oral irrigation with different solutions is an effective aid for removing debris from the inaccessible areas like interdental areas, pockets, furcations and also around orthodontic appliances and fixed prostheses.

Various irrigating solutions, viz. warm water, normal saline, iodine solutions, sanguinarine, essential oils, chlorhexidine, etc. have been used. A few authors observed transient bacteremia with water irrigation; however, it is considered an easy and safe irrigant.

II. Chemical Plaque Control

Mechanical measures are the primary methods for removal of debris and plaque. Chemical agents as plaque inhibitors have also been tried; however, these agents should not replace the mechanical measures. The chemical agents are used as an adjunct to mechanical techniques and should be prescribed according to the needs of the individual. The requisites of anti-plaque agents are:

- Should eliminate the pathogenic bacteria only.
- Should not develop resistance.
- Substantivity (the agent should remain in contact with the surface for a longer period).
- Safety to the oral tissues at the recommended concentration and dosages.
- Should not stain the teeth or alter the taste.
- Easy to use.
- Inhibits calcification of plaque.
- No adverse effect on teeth and restorations.
- Cost effective.

Classification of Chemical Plaque Control Agents

The chemical plaque control agents have been classified by various authors. These have also been categorized into generations by a few authors. The most accepted classification, used till date, was given by New Burn (1985). The classifications is as follows:

A. Antiseptic agents
1. Phenolic compounds and essential oils.
   - Phenol, thymol.
   - 2-phenyl phenol.
   - Hexylene-resorcinol.
   - Listerine.
   - Triclosan.
2. Quaternary ammonium compounds.
   - Cetyl pyridinium chloride.
   - Benzethonium chloride.
   - Domiphen bromide.
3. Oxygenating agents.
   - Peroxide.
   - Perborate.
4. Herbal extract.
   - Sanguinarine.
5. Bis-Biguanides.
   - Chlorhexidine.
   - Alexidine dihydrochloride.
6. Bis-Pyridines.
   - Octenidine dihydrochloride.
7. Pyrimidines.
   - Hexetidine.
8. Halogens.
   - Iodine, iodophors and fluoride.
9. Heavy metals.
   - Silver, mercury, zinc and copper.
B. Antibiotics.
   - Tetracycline.
   - Streptomycin.
   - Kanamycin.
   - Bacitracin.
   - Penicillin.
   - Spiramycin.
C. Enzymes.
   - Mucinase.
   - Pancreatase.
   - Protease-amylase.
D. Plaque modifying agents.
   - Ascoxal-T tablets (vitamin C, sodium percarbonate, copper sulphate).
   - Peroxidase.

E. Material interfering with bacterial colonization.
- Polystyrene membrane.
- Silicones.

The commonly used chemical plaque control agents are:
1. Chlorhexidine (Bisbiguanides).
2. Essential oil (Listerine).
3. Delmopinol (Decapinol).
4. Fluorides.
5. Metal ions.
6. Iodine.
7. Iodophors.
8. Chloroxylenol.
9. Natural products.
10. Enzymes.
11. Triclosan.
12. Oxygenating agents.
13. Quaternary ammonium compounds.
14. Sodium benzoate.
15. Antibiotics.

1. Chlorhexidine (Bisbiguanides)

Chlorhexidine gluconate has been traditionally used as a wound and skin cleaner.

It has also been successfully tried as the primary agent for chemical plaque control (Fig. 12.4). It is established that 0.2% chlorhexidine can inhibit development of dental plaque, subsequently diseases related to it.

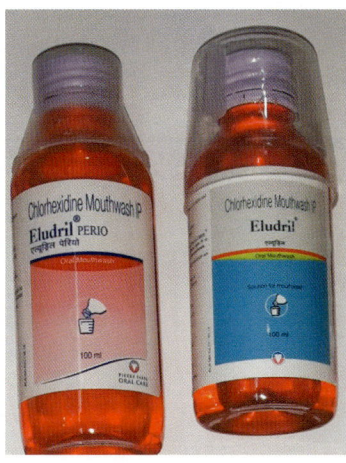

Fig. 12.4: Mouthwash

Chlorhexidine has a wide spectrum of activity encompassing gram +ve and gram –ve bacteria, viruses, yeast, fungi, etc.

The local antibacterial effect of chlorhexidine is because of its ability to interact with organic and inorganic components of the tooth surface. It gets adsorbed on to these surfaces and remains potent for a long period. This quality of prolonged contact time between the agent and the substrate is known as *substantivity*. Chlorhexidine is considered as the best agent as far as substantivity is concerned.

At low concentrations, the chlorhexidine agent is bacteriostatic and at higher concentrations, it is bactericidal.

The dicationic nature of chlorhexidine plays an important role, whereby one charged end of chlorhexidine molecule binds to the tooth surface and the other interacts with bacterial membrane of the micro-organism; the phenomenon known as 'Pin Cushion effect'. The pin cushion effect functions as follows:
- Disorients the lipoprotein structure.
- Alters the cell membrane's integrity.
- Destroys osmotic barriers.
- Increases the permeability of inner membrane and allowing the leakage of low molecular weight potassium ions.

At this bacteriostatic stage, the effects of chlorhexidine are reversible. As the concentration increases, leakage of low molecular weight components falls, reflecting coagulation and precipitation of cytoplasm by the formation of phosphate complexes such as adenosine triphosphate and nucleic agents. This bactericidal stage is irreversible.

Various formulations of chlorhexidine are available such as gels, sprays, varnishes, chewing gums, etc.

Chlorhexidine may produce some undesirable side effects, which include staining of teeth, restorations and even tongue. A few studies have observed alteration of taste, burning sensation, feeling of soreness, dryness of mouth, desquamation and increased supragingival deposits.

Chlorhexidine does not have any significant toxic effects on human beings, nor does it develops any resistance to oral micro-organisms.

2. Essential Oil (Listerine)

The phenol mouthwashes have been used since long. Listerine is one of the phenols, which is commonly used as a mouthrinse and as an irrigant (Fig. 12.5).

The composition of Listerine is as follows:

- Menthol   0.04%
- Thymol   0.06%
- Eucalyptol   0.09%
- Methyl salicylate   0.06%
- Benzoic acid   0.15%
- Ethyl alcohol   21.6 to 26%
- Color   Fast green to caramel

Listerine substantially reduced plaque scores as has been confirmed in various studies. When listerine with chlorhexidine was compared, it was observed that listerine was less effective in reducing plaque and gingival scores than chlorhexidine. Many studies have observed that most of the plaque bacteria were killed completely by a 10 second exposure to listerine. It has also been reported that bacteria and *Candida albicans* were reduced by a 30 second exposure to listerine.

Antiviral effect of Listerine has also been established. Being a phenolic preparation, it exerts a non-specific bacterial action. It penetrates the lipid component of cell wall of gram-negative bacteria, resulting in structural damage to the wall. It further halts several metabolic processes that are dependent on enzymes contained in the cell membrane.

The adverse effects of listerine are bitter taste, burning sensation and occasional staining of teeth. Listerine contains alcohol, thus, should not be used along with metronidazole/ tinidazole.

3. Delmopinol (Decapinol)

Delmopinol (Decapinol) is an ethanol derivative, which has been effectively tried in the inhibition of dental plaque. 0.2% Delmo-pinol has been successfully used as an adjunct to mechanical methods in reducing plaque.

Delmopinol hydrochloride is a surface active agent. It is established that delmopinol interferes with the plaque matrix formation and reduction of bacterial adherence, subsequently plaque adheres loosely to the tooth and can be easily removed by mechanical cleaning. Delmopinol is suitable as a pre-brush mouthrinse.

However, delmopinol, unlike chlorhexidine has a low antimicrobial effect. In addition, it has much lower substantivity than chlorhexidine.

The adverse effects of delmopinol include transient numbness of the tongue, alteration of taste perception, tooth and tongue discoloration and rarely mucosal soreness and erosion.

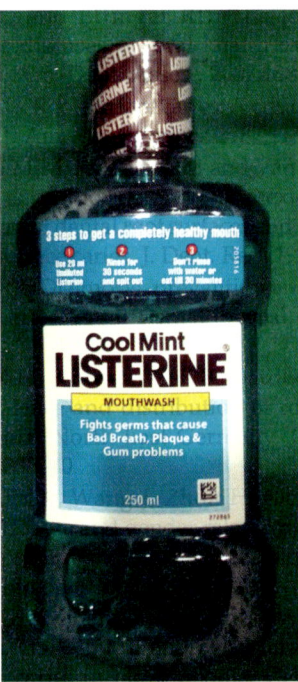

Fig. 12.5: Listerine mouthwash

4. Fluorides

The role of fluorides in the prevention of dental caries has been established. Stannous fluoride is the most effective amongst commonly available fluorides. A significant reduction in plaque in subjects brushing with 0.4% stannous fluoride has been observed. Sodium fluoride and stannous fluoride when used as a rinse, can reduce micro-organisms responsible for caries (Fig. 12.6). Subgingival irrigation with stannous fluoride was effective in those sites which were inaccessible to mechanical plaque control. However, stannous fluoride remains unstable in aqueous solution, so it is effective only when freshly prepared. Recently, stabilized tin ions are being used in toothpastes. Stannous gluconate and stannous pyrophosphate/citrate, both were effective against plaque.

5. Metal ions

a. Zinc

The potential of zinc ion as a plaque inhibitor has been recognized. Zinc salts have been tried as a dentifrice having cariostatic potential. Zinc citrate dentifrice is being effectively used as a plaque reducing agent.

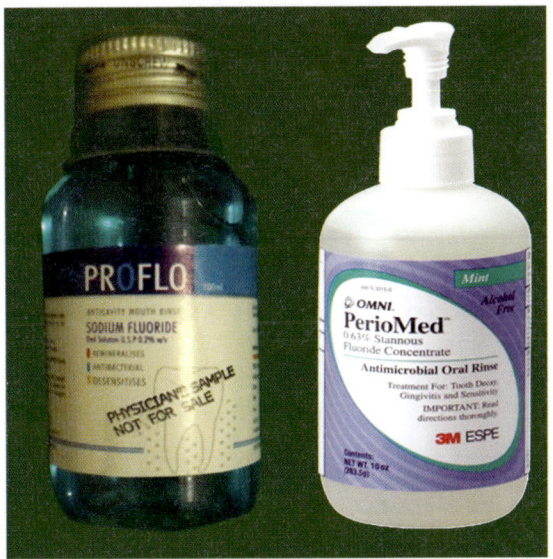

Fig. 12.6: Fluoride mouthrinse

b. Tin

Tin fluoride has been tried to modify the plaque bacteria. Tin ions bind to gram-negative bacteria, reversing its ability to adsorb on the tooth surface. Further, the accumulation of tin in bacteria may alter their metabolism and other physico-chemical characteristics.

c. Copper

Copper has also been shown to be a potent inhibitor of plaque formation. It inhibits glycolysis like other ions. It is usually used in mouthwashes or dentifrices. The adverse effects include unpleasant taste, staining potential and toxicity.

6. Iodine

Iodine is a powerful antiseptic with a wide spectrum of activity. It is effective against leptospira, entamoeba, fungi, yeasts and viruses, etc. 2.0% solution of iodine in 70% alcohol virtually sterilizes the skin in 30 seconds. However, it may produce skin sensitivity; so it should not be used in routine. It appears to have no significant antiplaque activity when used as 1% mouthwash.

7. Iodophors

Newer iodine compounds, such as iodophors are being tried in an attempt to overcome the shortcomings of iodine. Iodophors are complexes of iodine with surface active agents such as nonionic detergents, quaternary compounds and macromolecules. They are generally non-toxic, non-irritating, non-staining and miscible with water. They do not produce sensitivity when applied to mucous or skin surfaces. 0.5% povidone iodine before surgery significantly reduces surface bacteria.

8. Chloroxylenol

Chloroxylenol is a widely used and relatively non-irritant antiseptic. It is active against streptococci and less active against staphylococci and almost inactive against pseudomonas and proteus. Its activity may be reduced in the presence of blood or serum. The commercial preparation, Dettolin (1.02% chloroxylenol and menthol), is a routinely used mouthwash.

9. Natural products

a. *Sanguinarine*
A herbal extract extracted from the roots of the plant *Sanguinaria canadensis*, is a potent anti-plaque agent. Sanguinarine when used as a mouthwash is effectively retained by plaque. The antimicrobial and anti-inflammatory properties of sanguinarine have been established.

The antiplaque action of sanguinarine may be related to its bacteriostatic and bactericidal actions; i.e. it interferes with the adherence of certain bacteria to the tooth surface by blocking specific receptors either on the bacteria or on the tooth pellicle.

The antiplaque efficacy of sanguinarine was found to be less when compared with chlorhexidine. A few authors have observed no significant change in plaque ecology with sanguinarine.

Since sanguinarine contains 11.5% alcohol, it may produce burning sensation in the oral soft tissues. Its use should be avoided with the metronidazole/tinidazole preparations.

b. *Propolis*
It is another naturally occurring product derived from bees. It has shown antiseptic, anti-inflammatory and bacteriostatic action; however, its effectiveness is negligible therefore, not considered ideal for use as a mouthwash.

c. *Curcumin (turmeric)*
Curcumin (turmeric) shows anti-plaque and anti-microbial property comparable to chlorhexidine with better safety profile, commercially available as Turmix (Fig. 12.7a). It inhibits the growth of *Capnocytophaga*, *Porphyromonas gingivalis* and *Prevotella melaninogenica*. It shows better biocompatibility

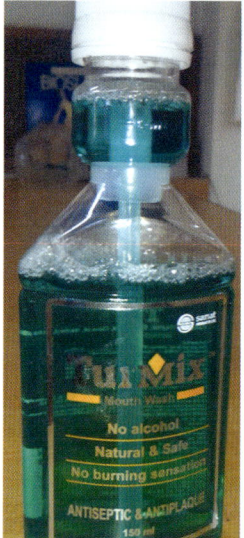

Fig. 12.7a: Turmix

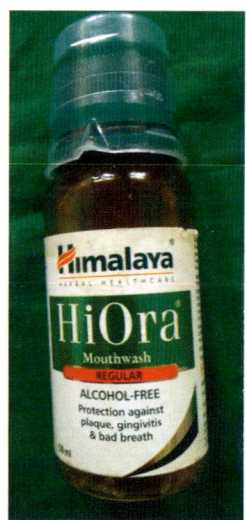

Fig. 12.7b: HiOra mouthwash

and acceptability by the subjects. It is free of side effects of bitter taste and staining which occur with the chlorhexidine group.

HiOra, a commercial product, also contains natural products like Belliric Myrobalan (Bibhitaki), Betel (Nagavalli) and Miswak (Pilu) (Fig. 12.7b).

10. Enzymes

Different enzyme preparations have been tried to inhibit organization of dental plaque.

They act by interfering with the mechanism of bacterial attachment and also breaking apart the existing plaque matrix. The commonly used enzymes are:

a. Mucinase.

b. Viokase.
- Trypsin.
- Chymotrypsin.
- Carboxypeptidase.
- Amylase.
- Lipase.
- Nucleases.

c. Lactoperoxidase–thiocyanate system.

d. Urea.

a. *Mucinase*

The mucinase-containing dentifrice has been observed to inhibit the mineralization of plaque deposits; indirectly might be responsible for disorganization of plaque bacteria.

b. *Viokase*

Viokase, a group of pancreatic enzyme preparation, are able to digest the toxic protein material that constitutes a favorable substrate for bacterial growth. Certain preparations have also been tried as chewing gums; however, because of unpleasant taste, they were discontinued. The enzymes with high proteolytic and low amylase activity have been proven more effective for plaque inhibition. A combination of enzymes might prove better. The enzymes may have deleterious effect on oral mucosa. The prepared enzyme preparations should not develop any resistance or produce adverse changes in the oral mucous membrane.

c. *Lactoperoxidase–thiocyanate system*

Lactoperoxidase and thiocyanate are both found in saliva naturally. Lactoperoxidase when combined with H_2O_2 (produced by oral bacteria or introduced by extraoral agents) at higher concentration, produce hypothiocyanite ion, which is toxic to bacterial metabolic system. This system includes glucose oxidase and amyloglucosidase. These degrade starch and glucose to hydrogen peroxide.

This preparation has shown promising results in inhibiting plaque formation. Zendium, a commercial toothpaste containing enzymes, has significant effect on reduction of gingivitis; however, their use as a mouthrinse provided contradictory results.

d. *Urea*

Urea is a potent protein. 30% urea as solvent significantly inhibits plaque maturation by dissolving the mucoproteinaceous material of plaque matrix.

11. *Triclosan*

Triclosan as an antibacterial agent, effective against both gram-positive and gram-negative organisms, has been used with several dentifrice formulations to inhibit plaque (Fig. 12.8).

Triclosan can interfere with bacterial metabolism and acid production even at a low concentration. No adverse effects are associated with its use; however, it has poor substantivity. Triclosan is combined with zinc citrate to improve its substantivity and also the antibacterial effect.

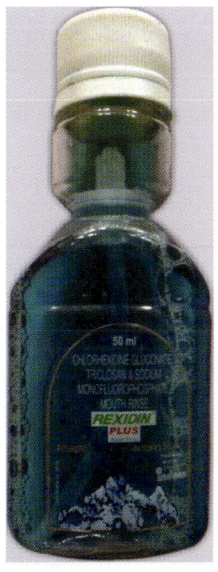

Fig. 12.8: Triclosan mouthwash

Significant improvement in gingival health is reported with the use of 0.5% triclosan and 1.0% zinc citrate. The commercially available toothpastes usually contain 0.2% triclosan with or without zinc citrate. Zinc citrate is more effective on existing plaque and triclosan inhibits plaque formation on clean surfaces. Triclosan exerts its effect by preventing adhesion of bacteria on the tooth surface, whereas zinc reduces the rate of bacterial proliferation in existing plaque.

The addition of co-polymers (polyvinyl methyl ether and maleic acid) to triclosan enhances retention of triclosan to tooth and mucous membrane. The combination significantly inhibits both supragingival plaque and subgingival plaque.

Triclosan has the unique property, known as 'double-barred effect'. It not only kills bacteria, but also neutralizes the product of bacteria, which can provoke inflammation.

12. Oxygenating Agents

The oxygenating agents are commonly used to suppress/control the infections caused by gram-negative anaerobes. The commonly used agents are: hydrogen peroxide, urea peroxide and an oxygen releasing enzyme glucose oxidase. They release oxygen with effervescence which is bacteriostatic. Hydrogen peroxide when combined with baking soda is used as a whitening toothpaste. Chlorine dioxide when added in toothpastes and mouthrinses may have some antiplaque effects.

The beneficial effects of oxygenating agents are:

- Antibacterial effect against anaerobes.
- Stimulate endogenous antibacterial activity in saliva.
- Promote healing.
- Enhance leukocyte functions at tooth/gingiva interface.

An ideal oxygenating agent should provide an optimum dose for the antibacterial effect, be stable, substantive and slowly release oxygen. Unfortunately, the clinical efficacy of routinely used oxygenating agents could not show promising result. Recently, Tetrapotassium peroxydiphosphate have been tried and shown better results. It is stable, very substantive to enamel surfaces and releases active oxygen slowly in the presence of salivary/plaque phosphates.

13. Quaternary Ammonium Compounds

Quaternary ammonium compounds are cationic antiseptics and surface active agents.

The commonly available quaternary ammonium compounds, viz. benzethonium chloride, benzalkonium chloride, cetylpyridinium chloride and domiphen bromide have a net positive charge which reacts with negatively charged phosphate groups of cell membrane of the micro-organisms. The cell wall gets disrupted leading to increase in permeability and subsequently the cell death. Quaternary amines are more effective against gram-positive than gram-negative organisms. Therefore, these antiseptics are beneficial against early developing plaque which contains predominantly gram-positive bacteria.

The effectiveness of quaternary ammonium compounds as compared to chlorhexidine is limited. The oral retention is twice that of chlorhexidine but desorption of quarternary ammonium compounds in saliva is much more rapid.

Cetylpyridinium chloride is being extensively used as an antiseptic. 0.05% cetyl pyridinium chloride is being used as a mouthrinse. It is considered safe and effective antiplaque agent in mouthrinse formulations.

Some undesirable side effects of quaternary ammonium compound mouthrinses are burning sensation of tongue and mucous membrane, yellowish brown discoloration of tongue and aphthous ulceration of the oral mucosa.

14. Sodium Benzoate

Sodium benzoate has been tried as a pre-brushing cleaning agent, since it effectively loosens plaque before brushing. A few authors, however, are of the view that the pre-brushing is not much effective. No side effects have been reported with its use.

15. Antibiotics

The bacterial nature of the dental plaque has its significant role in the etiology of caries. The use of antibiotics in the prevention of caries is still being established.

Characteristics of antibacterials to be used as an antiplaque

- Broad spectrum antibacterial activity.
- Substantivity to oral surfaces.
- Compatible with other ingredients of tooth-paste/mouthwash.
- Low toxicity and good taste.

Earlier authors used penicillin having potential to inhibit plaque formation; however, daily use of penicillin develops resistant strains and therefore discontinued.

Vancomycin, primarily active against gram-positive micro-organisms, has been routinely used in various formulations. The topical application of vancomycin may reduce micro-organisms. Later, it was observed that the anti-plaque effect of vancomycin is temporary and does not prevent plaque formation in persons who do not mechanically remove plaque.

Broader spectrum antibiotics, such as kanamycin, have also been tried. It is observed that 5.0% topical application of kanamycin, produced improvement in gingival inflammation. However, it did not eliminate gingivitis as it was not effective against anaerobic bacteria.

Macrolide antibiotics, like erythromycin and spiramycin, are moderately effective in reducing gingival inflammation.

The use of antibiotics as plaque control agents is not encouraged because of production of bacterial resistance and hypersensitivity reactions.

III. Miscellaneous

a. Biological Plaque Control

Biological plaque control, a novel therapeutic approach, is currently used as an adjunct to mechanical and chemical plaque control. It is mainly divided into two categories: Probiotics and vaccines.

i. **Probiotics:** Described in subsequent pages.

ii. **Vaccines:** Described in Chapter 13.

b. Photo Dynamic Therapy

Photo dynamic therapy is a painless, non-invasive photo-disinfection procedure that significantly improves bacterial inhibition. It is a non-antibiotic therapy that rapidly destroys gram –ve oral pathogens without pain, heat, or surgery.

It involves three components: Light, a photosensitizer and tissue oxygen. Light is utilized to activate a photosensitizing agent in the presence of oxygen. The exposure of the photosensitizer to light results in the formation of toxic oxygen species, causing localized photo damage and cell death.

A few authors observed that the photosensitizer was taken up into the biomass of the biofilm leading to cell death when used on old plaque biofilm formed on natural enamel surfaces. Also, the treated biofilms were much thinner with a little evidence of channels and a less dense biomass. The potential use of photo dynamic theory in the management of oral biofilms is established.

c. Herbal Products

Herbal products have recently been incorporated into dental field making it 'holistic' or complementary systems managing many oral ailments including caries. The products being 'natural', rather than 'synthetic' are regarded safer and part of healthy lifestyles.

i. *Chewing sticks*

Pencil-sized sticks, slightly longer than toothbrush, derived from the stems, branches and roots of certain plants have been traditionally used for maintaining oral hygiene in many Afro-Asian communities, especially among the rural population. It is commonly referred to as 'Datun' in south asian countries.

Most popular plants from which chew sticks can be obtained include *Salvadora persica* (miswak) and *Azadirachta indica* (Neem).

The plant fibres mechanically remove plaque and massage the gums.

Also, it stimulates salivation and thus has a better cleaning effect. Other than plaque removal, these plants possess other properties as antiseptic, antibiotic, antifungal, astringent, styptic, anti-inflammatory, sialagogue, antiviral and anticarious. The constituents of chewing sticks and their effects are tabulated in Table 12.2.

No cytotoxic effect has been noticed with the use of sticks. However, their bristles may penetrate in the gums. Since the bristles are situated along the long axis of their handle, the lingual and interproximal surfaces are more difficult to clean.

Table 12.2: Constituents of chewing sticks and their effects

	Effect
Fluoride	Wet tooth enamel, caries prevention
Tannin	Astringent effect
Resins	Forms a layer over enamel, protection against caries
Sodium bicarbonate	Mild abrasive and germicidal
Alkaloids	Antibacterial
Essential oils	Antiseptic effect
Vitamin C	Antioxidant, repair of tissues
Benzylthiocyanate	Viricidal, especially against HSV-1

ii. *Traditional herbs*

Various traditional herbs are being used in different preparations providing benefits to oral cavity. Aloevera has been reported to be a boon for dentistry owing to its antioxidant properties. It soothes gums and relieves pain. Clove oil reduces infection and acts as an obtundant relieving pain. Turmeric is an established anti-inflammatory. Tulsi (*Ocimum sanctum*) is used as an immunity booster and breath purifier. Chamomile is said to have anti-bacterial, anti-viral and anti-fungal effects. Myst is reported to have a strong cleaning and healing action. Eucalyptus oil is a known antiseptic. Echinacea is claimed to stimulate the immune response and to activate the leucocytes. Peppermint oil is reputed to possess analgesic, antiseptic and anti-microbial properties.

Green tea is used as a gargle to treat dental decay, halitosis, plaque formation, thrush and tonsillitis. It has been described as a new, safe and non-toxic product which is safe for children and pregnant women as well and is free from side effects of chemical mouthwashes.

d. *Oil Pulling Therapy*

Oil pulling or oil swishing, is a traditional Indian folk remedy that involves swishing oil in the oral cavity for achieving oral and systemic health benefits, viz. decrease in dental caries, dental plaque control, reduction of gingival inflammation, etc. One tablespoon of oil is recommended for rinsing for 15–20 minutes on an empty stomach, before drinking/eating anything in the morning. Various oils used for swishing are:

- Coconut oil.
- Corn oil.
- Rice bran oil.
- Palm oil.
- Sesame oil.
- Sunflower oil.
- Soyabean oil.

In ancient times, the practice of oil (*Thaila* in Sanskrit) pulling (*Aabarh* in Sanskrit) was a popular Indian ayurvedic treatment.

Oil pulling therapy with sesame oil has been used for many years. The modern version of oil pulling was coined by Ukranian physician, Dr. Karach, after he experimented swishing oil with the above-mentioned method and cured himself for a blood disease.

Oil pulling has been used to prevent decay, bleeding gums, oral malodour, dryness of throat, cracked lips and for strengthening teeth, gums and jaws.

Procedure

The steps followed are:

Step 1: In the morning on an empty stomach and before drinking any liquids (including water), pour exactly one tablespoon of coconut oil or sesame oil into the mouth.

Step 2: Swish the oil in the oral cavity and through your teeth without swallowing it, (like a mouthwash). Oil will start to get watery as your saliva mixes with it. Keep swishing.

Step 3: After sometime (say 10–15 minutes), oil mixed in saliva along with toxins of the body will make it thinner and will appear white. Spit out the oil into the toilet. If it looks yellow, that means the oil remained in the oral cavity for insufficient time (the swishing should be repeated).

Step 4: Finally rinse out oral cavity with warm saline and also with appropriate mouthwash. The oil pulling/swishing is carried out preferably before breakfast. It can be repeated 3 times a day to achieve better results; but always before meals on an empty stomach.

Mechanism of action

Swishing activates the enzymes and the enzymes draw toxins out of the blood. The oil must not be swallowed, because it has become toxic. As the process continues, the oil gets thinner and white.

The exact mechanisms of oil-pulling action are not known. It has been proposed that the viscosity of the oil can inhibit bacterial adhesion and plaque coaggregation. The other possible mechanism might be the saponification process that occurs as a result of alkali hydrolysis of oil by bicarbonates in saliva.

Sesame oil (contains sesamin and sesamolin) has been reported to increase both the hepatic mitochondrial and the peroxisomal fatty acid oxidation rate. Sesame seed consumption appears to increase plasma gamma tocopherol and enhance vitamin E activity which is believed to prevent cancer and heart disease. Sesame oil has been established to have antibacterial activity against *Streptococcus mutans*.

Oral health benefits

It prevents:
- Dental caries.
- Oral malodour.
- Bleeding gums.
- Dryness of the throat.
- Cracked lips.

General health benefits

It prevents:
- Thrombosis.
- Eczema.
- Intestinal infection.
- Diabetes.
- Bronchitis.
- Asthma.
- Headaches.
- Chronic skin problems.
- Growth of malignant tumors.

Table 12.3 enlists various plaque control agents with their mode of action.

B. MODIFICATION OF CARIES PROMOTING DIET

The relationship of diet and caries is an old phenomenon. Diet encompasses everything that is eaten, regardless of its nutritional value, whereas nutrition deals with those elements of the diet that are absorbed from the intestinal tract. Dietary factors exert local effects while nutritional factors effect systemically upon dentition.

Table 12.3: Chemical plaque control agents and their uses

Group	Examples of agents	Action	Used in
1. Antibiotics	Penicillin Vancomycin Kanamycin Niddamycin Spiramycin	Antimicrobial	Rarely used
2. Enzymes	Protease Lipase Nuclease Dextranase Mutanase	Plaque removal	Not used
	• Glucose oxidase • Amyloglucosidase	Antimicrobial	Toothpaste
3. Bisbiguanide antiseptics	Chlorhexidine Alexidine Octenidine	Antimicrobial	• Mouthrinse • Spray • Gel • Toothpaste • Chewing gum • Varnish
4. Quaternary ammonium compounds	Cetylpyridinium chloride Benzalkonium chloride	Antimicrobial	Mouthrinse
5. Phenols and essential oils	Thymol Hexylresorcinol Eucalyptol Triclosan Listerine	Antimicrobial Anti-inflammatory	• Mouthrinse • Toothpaste
6. Natural products	Sanguinarine	Antimicrobial	• Toothpaste • Mouthrinse
7. Fluorides	Sodium fluoride Sodium monofluoro phosphate Stannous fluoride Amine fluoride	Antimicrobial	• Toothpaste • Mouthrinse • Gel
8. Metal salts	Tin Zinc Copper	Antimicrobial	• Toothpaste • Mouthrinse • Gel
9. Oxygenating agents	Hydrogen peroxide Sodium peroxyborate Sodium peroxy-carbonate	Antimicrobial plaque removal	Mouthrinse
10. Detergents	Sodium lauryl sulfate	Antimicrobial plaque removal	• Toothpaste • Mouthrinse
11. Amine alcohols	Octapinol Delmopinol	Plaque matrix Inhibition	Rarely used

Sweetness of food and dental caries has long been interrelated. Pierre Fauchard, the founder of dental profession, has quoted that 'all sugary foods contribute to the destruction of teeth and those who use sugar frequently, rarely have good teeth'.

It was believed that acids formed from lodgement of food caused caries; and the teeth could be decalcified by placing in a mixture of saliva and sugar. The lactic acid and acetic acid was thought to be responsible for this decalcification.

The famous Miller's theory believes that acids are produced by the interaction of carbohydrates and saliva. This acid leads to the demineralization of enamel causing caries. It is observed that the patient with rampant caries frequently have sucrose containing foods.

Epidemiological Observation of Caries and Diet

General epidemiologic surveys are helpful in determining the possible causes and ways of preventing a disease.

Numerous reports have indicated that Eskimos living on their natural diet had low caries experience; however, their dental health declined after being exposed to high sugar diet.

The children who used to have different types of sugar containing refined foods had greater caries activity. The sugarcane and unprocessed wheat contained a 'protective agent' that is lost in the refinement of these foods also encourage caries.

It has been observed that the diet consumed up to 12 years might not confer any protection from caries during subsequent years.

Hereditary fructose intolerance (HFI) is a rare hereditary disease caused by an inborn error of metabolism whereby the patients do not possess liver enzyme (fructose-1-phosphate splitting aldolase B) required for ingestion of foods containing fructose. On the other hand, starchy foods (not containing fructose) are well tolerated. It has been observed that these patients are generally caries free as compared to equivalent age group of the general population.

The low prevalence of caries in persons with HFI indicates that starchy foods do not produce decay, whereas sugary foods cause caries. Highly significant differences in the proportion of *Streptococcus mutans* and lactobacillus were observed in the plaque of the HFI group and that of the control population.

A few authors have reported high caries incidence in diabetics (explained by slightly increased salivary glucose levels and reduced salivary flow); however, most surveys have shown a lower caries experience in diabetics. The severe restriction in sugar intake was considered the most likely cause of the lower caries experience in the diabetics.

Workers in sugar industries such as bakeries and candy factories are exposed daily to air polluted with sugar dust. They also consume relatively large amounts of sugar-containing foods during work. The higher caries risk of these workers has been confirmed. Further, the caries experience was higher in production-line workers compared with non-production-line workers in the industry.

Phenylketonuria is a rare inherited defect in which there is a deficiency of the liver enzyme, phenylalanine hydroxylase. These patients have to be given a high carbohydrate diet, otherwise severe mental deficiency can occur. Such patients usually exhibit higher caries experience.

Pediatric medicines are usually given in syrup form, which are sucrose based. The children taking such syrups have a higher caries experience than the control ones.

The Vipeholm study was conducted on mentally retarded children to evaluate the effect of sugar and fluorides on dental caries. The conclusions of the Vipeholm study were:
- Sugar consumption in between meals has a larger effect on increasing dental caries

activity than sugar consumption during meals, even if sugar is taken up to four times a day at meals.

- Consumption of sugar both between meals and at meals is associated with a marked increase in caries experience.
- The increase in caries activity, under uniform experimental conditions varies widely from person to person.
- The increase in caries activity disappears as soon as the sugar intake is withdrawn.
- Carious lesions do occur despite the avoidance of sugars.

The effect of substituting sucrose with either fructose or xylitol on dental caries has been evaluated in Turku sugar study. It is reported that substitution of sucrose by xylitol resulted in a lower caries experience. The plaque organisms are unable to metabolize xylitol to acids. However, substitution of sucrose by fructose does not cause a definite caries reduction.

It is established that substitution of sorbitol in sweets caused a substantial reduction in caries increment. Excessive use of sorbitol sweetened products, however, leads to an increased production of acids from sorbitol in plaque and an increased number of sorbitol fermenting microorganism in plaque.

Lycasin, a hydrogenated starch hydrolysate, when substituted with sucrose resulted in reduction in caries activity.

The cariogenic potential of various types of sugars and their pH values were evaluated. It is established that addition of 25% glucose, fructose, lactose or maltose caused significantly less caries than 25% sucrose.

The pH of plaque before, during and after intake of food is a guide to the cariogenic potential of that food. Plaque pH studies have been used to differentiate between the potential cariogenicity of different sugars and the different concentrations of sugars. The intake of cheese and sugarless chewing gums after sugary food prevents the fall in plaque pH.

Table 12.4: Relative cariogenicity of sweetening agents

Compound	Approximate sweetness relative to sucrose
Sugars	
Sucrose	1
Glucose	0.7
Fructose	1.2
Lactose	0.3
Maltose	0.4
Sugar compounds	
Trichlorosucrose	2000
Sucralose	600
Sugar alcohols	
Xylitol	1.0
Sorbitol	0.5
Sucralose	0.7
Erythritol	0.75
Lactitol	0.35
Sugar complex	
Hydrogenated glucose (lycasin)	0.75
Isomalt (palatinit)	0.5
Dipeptide/polypeptide	
Aspartame	180
Monellin	3000
Thaumatin	4000
Miscellaneous	
Saccharin	5000
Cyclamate	50
Acesulfame	130

The relative cariogenicity of sweetening agents is given in Table 12.4.

Sucrose has been termed the 'arch criminal of dental caries'. Being the most common constituent in our diet, it is a major cause of dental caries. A property of sucrose, which makes it more cariogenic, is its unique ability to enhance production of extracellular polysaccharides such as dextran in dental plaque. Dextran is not easily metabolized in plaque subsequently making it sticky. It also increases the bulk of plaque.

A few studies have observed sucrose to be more cariogenic while others indicated similar level of cariogenicity with all sugars. Practically substituting sucrose with glucose, fructose, or maltose for the prevention of dental caries is not much effective. Lactose and galactose are significantly less cariogenic than other dietary sugars.

Cariogenicity of Alternative Sweeteners

The commonly used alternative sweeteners are:

Sorbitol and Mannitol

Sorbitol is extensively used in foods manufactured for diabetics and as sweeteners in sugarless syrups. Mannitol is used mainly in chewing-gum. Sorbitol and mannitol are fermented slowly by plaque organisms, much slower than that of sucrose.

Xylitol

Xylitol is used in confectionery and tooth pastes. Xylitol modifies the synthesis of poly-saccharides from sucrose in *Streptococcus mutans,* thereby decreasing the ability of the cells to adhere to hard surfaces. Depression of mutans streptococci in plaque and/or saliva has been co-related with the regular use of xylitol. It is reported that total substitution of dietary sugar by xylitol resulted in very low caries incidence; however, a few authors reported insufficient evidence to prove that xylitol prevents caries.

Hydrogenated glucose (Lycasin)

Hydrogenated glucose as a syrup is sold under the trade name Lycasin. Lycasin is fermented slowly compared with sucrose and causes minimal depression of plaque pH. It is much less cariogenic than sucrose.

Isomalt

It is sold under the trade name Palatinit. Isomalt (Palatinit) causes a little acid production when incubated with oral streptococci. It is reported that use of isomalt resulted in lower plaque accumulation than sucrose. It is reported that intake of snacks containing 100% isomalt in between meals resulted in the decrease of mutans streptococci.

Sucralose

Sucralose is a non-toxic, intensively sweet agent that has been shown to be non-cariogenic. Sucralose is not fermentable. Cariostatic effect of sucralose is mainly because of its ability to inhibit glucosyl transferase (GTF) and fructosyl transferase (FTF).

Erythritol

Erythritol is the sugar alcohol produced from glucose. It is 70–80% as sweet as sucrose and is also non-hygroscopic. Erythritol is neither used as substrate for the lactic acid production nor for plaque formation. Reduction in caries has been reported using erythritol containing diet. Erythritol is a promising sugar substitute from the point of view of cariogenicity.

C. INCREASING THE RESISTANCE OF THE TEETH TO DECAY

Pit and Fissure Sealants

Pit and fissure sealants, as the name implies, are the agents, which seal the pits and fissures. Pits and fissures are the potential site for the initiation of caries and are mostly located on occlusal surfaces of posterior teeth, buccal/lingual surfaces of molars and on lingual surfaces of anterior teeth.

The pits and fissures are formed as a result of improper union of developmental lobes during the formation of tooth structure. Occlusal pits and fissures vary in shape but are generally narrow and tortuous with invaginations where bacteria and food debris are retained. The termination of pits and fissures has broadly been observed as:
- A shallow groove.
- Complete penetration of the enamel.
- Fissure may end blindly.
- End of the fissure opens into an irregular chamber.

Types of Fissures

Nagano (1960) classified pits and fissures into following forms (Fig. 12.9):

1. **V-type:** Wide at the top, gradually narrowing towards the bottom (mostly self cleansing and caries resistant).
2. **U-type:** The width is almost the same from top to bottom (mostly self cleansing and caries resistant).
3. **I-type:** An extremely deep and narrow slit, resembles a bottleneck (prone to caries).
4. **IK-type:** Extremely narrow slit associated with a large space at the bottom (prone to caries).
5. **Inverted Y-type:** Narrow on top, splitting into two (prone to caries).

The caries starts from the bottom in the V-type, half way down in the U-type and from the top in I-type, IK-type and inverted Y-type. The caries starts from the bottom in shallow pits and from top in deep pits.

Saliva may not readily reach the base of the fissures. An explorer tip or toothbrush bristle is too large to penetrate into the fissure, therefore the areas cannot be mechanically cleaned.

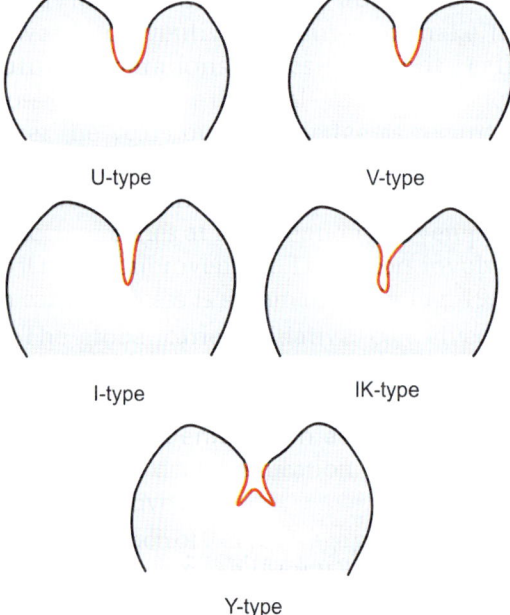

U-type   V-type

I-type   IK-type

Y-type

Fig. 12.9: Types of fissures

It has been documented that even fluorides are least effective in the prevention of pit and fissure caries. The possible reasons may be attributed to the inaccessibility of the fluorides at the base of pits and fissures.

Historical Evolution of Sealants

Before the advent of sealers, following techniques and procedures were tried to decrease the vulnerability of pits and fissures to caries.

i. Extension for Prevention

Earlier authors were of the view that the cavity preparations should be extended to eliminate non-carious fissures also. The principle known as *extension for prevention* is still being practiced, though to a lesser extent.

ii. Prophylactic Odontomy

Small amalgam restorations were placed in pits and fissures of newly erupted teeth before the appearance of clinical signs of caries. The process is no longer used.

iii. Fissure Eradication

The pits and fissures were reshaped into wide non-retentive grooves without any restoration. The dentin exposed by grinding would undergo secondary changes and become resistant to caries. These procedures could not gain popularity because of the reluctance of parents to get operative procedures performed on normal teeth and also the cost factor.

iv. Application of Impregnating Solutions

Ammoniacal silver nitrate solutions were flown onto enamel, increasing the resistance of the enamel surface. Zinc chloride and potassium ferrocyanide have also been reported to be effective in reducing caries. The impregnating solutions form protein complexes with the organic part of the tooth. The use of impregnating solutions was based on the belief that the primary route for the initiation of caries was by proteolytic action of organisms on the organic part of enamel. However, this concept was not endorsed by various authors.

v. *Application of Non-adhesive Dental Materials*

Zinc phosphate and copper cements were used to block pits and fissures; however, these materials had limited value due to their high solubility and poor retention.

A low viscosity material is applied to the pits and fissures in order to isolate them from the oral environment. The sealant acts as a physical barrier preventing oral bacteria and dietary carbohydrates from aggregating within the pits and fissures, subsequently preventing the acids causing caries.

Requirements of Sealant Material

The sealant may not fill the entire depth of the fissure but it should bond firmly at the fissure orifice. The enamel-sealant interface should not exhibit any microleakage so as to prevent nutrients from diffusing to organisms remaining in the fissures and also to prevent new organisms from entering into the fissures. Although, some bacteria sealed within the fissures may remain viable for extended periods of time, they cannot initiate caries if continuous source of fermentable carbo-hydrates is not provided.

The requirements of a sealant material are:
- Adhesion to enamel for longer duration.
- Easy manipulation.
- Free flowing, i.e. capable of entering narrow fissures by capillary action.
- Non-injurious to oral tissues.
- Rapidly polymerized.
- Low solubility in oral fluids.

Pits and Fissure Sealants Classification

1. Polymerization methods.
   - Self activation (mixing two components).
   - Light activation.
2. Based on generations.

- First generation—UV light cured.
- Second generation—self cure/chemically cured.
- Third generation—visible light cured.
- Fourth generation—fluoride releasing.
3. Based on presence/absence of filler.
   - Unfilled.
   - Filled.
4. Based on color.
   - Tinted.
   - Clear.
5. Resin systems.
   - BIS-GMA.
   - Urethane acrylate.

Sealant Materials

The commonly used sealant materials are:

i. *Cyanoacrylates*

Methyl-2-cyanoacrylate with or without filler particles has been used as sealant. The clinical studies showed mixed or negative results. The material is considered unsuitable because of difficult handling characteristics and solubility in oral fluids.

ii. *Polyurethane*

A polyurethane product, Epoxylite-9070, containing 10% disodium monofluoro-phosphate was used as a sealant. The material showed poor retention and solubility in oral fluids. A polyurethane resin containing amine fluoride has also been used; however, was not effective for longer duration.

The commercially available urethane dimethacrylate sealants are: 'Contact seal' (chemically cured) and 'Helioseal' (light cured).

iii. *Bisphenol-glycidyl-methacrylate*

Bisphenol-glycidyl-methacrylate is the resin component of conventional composite resin materials. Bisphenol-glycidyl-methacrylate was diluted with methyl-methacrylate or other co-monomers to improve flow characteristics to be used as a sealant. The mixture undergoes less polymerization shrinkage and has a lower coefficient of thermal expansion than methyl-methacrylate alone and likely forms and maintains firm bonds with enamel. The commercially available sealants are: Concise sealant, delton, NUVA-Seal IA, oralin, prisma-shield, visio-seal, duraphat, glass-ionomer cements.

Use of Sealants in Individual Care Programs

Any individual having teeth is at risk of developing dental caries and as a preventive protocol, should be considered for sealant applications (Fig. 12.10). The patients having caries in pits and fissures are also given sealant therapy. Such sealants are referred to as *Therapeutic sealants*.

Although the sealants are usually placed in children, it is established that age is no bar in placing sealants. The goal of preventing caries by use of sealants is best accomplished by applying sealants to young teeth and placing therapeutic sealants on others.

The following factors affect the decision of sealant placement:

a. Risk Assessment of Individuals

The individuals in a given population are assessed for being caries susceptible. Factors contributing for individual to be at risk

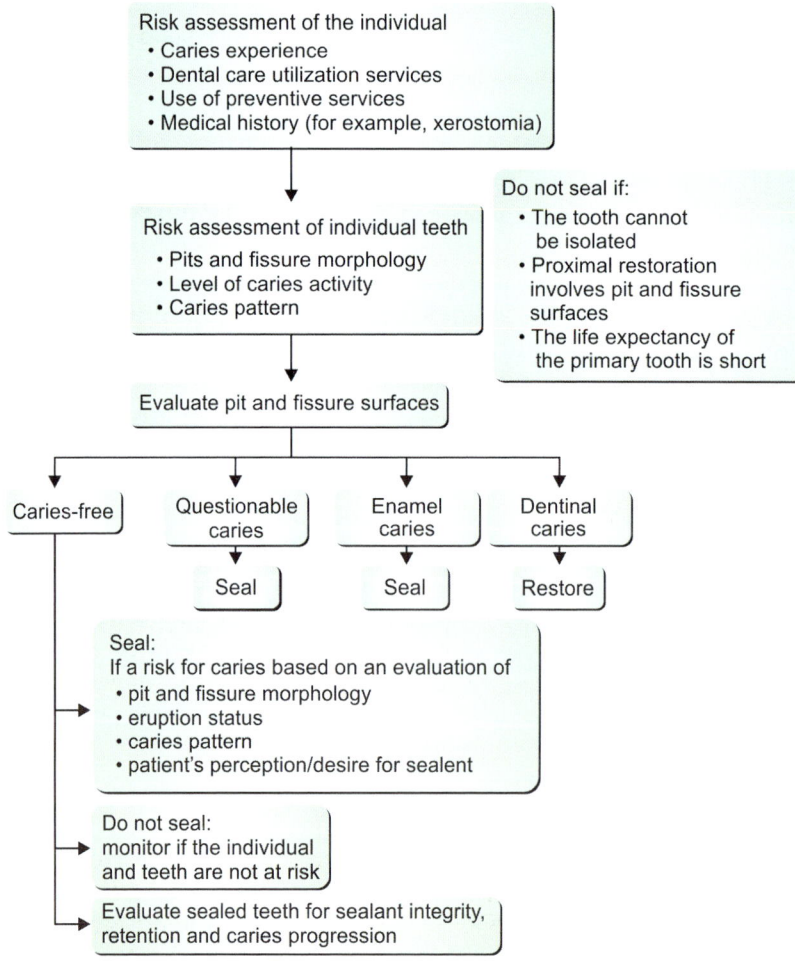

Fig. 12.10: Guidelines for sealant use in individual care programs

include history, previous dental care, use of preventive practices in family and systemic problems. Use of sweetened medicines, health status and lifestyle certainly influence an individual's caries risk.

b. Risk Assessment of Teeth

The individual's teeth at risk are to be assessed, e.g. level of caries activity, pit and fissure morphology and the caries pattern. The eruption status and the ability to isolate adequately are also the key factors required for effective sealing. Further, the distribution of caries provides a clear indication of susceptibility of different teeth. It is hypothesized that first and second permanent molars are at risk for pit and fissure caries. The decision for pit and fissure sealing depends upon whether the teeth are caries free or exhibiting enamel/dentin caries:

    i. Caries free teeth.

    ii. Teeth with enamel caries.

    iii. Teeth with dentin caries.

i. *Caries free teeth*

The decision to seal a caries free tooth is based upon the potential risk, which is influenced by pits and fissures morphology, eruption status, caries activity and also the questionable caries.

Pit and fissure morphology: The morphology of pits and fissures is a significant factor. Teeth with well coalesced pits and fissures and wide grooves do not require sealing; however teeth with deep pits and fissures are ideal candidates for sealants (Fig. 12.9). Permanent molars have the most susceptible pits and fissures. Premolars are much less susceptible to occlusal caries. The need for sealants in first and second deciduous molars is determined by pit and fissure morphology and the life expectancy of the tooth. Sealants are indicated on deciduous molars depending upon evidence of caries activity and/or deep fissures.

Eruption status: Earlier authors were of the view that the tooth should be sealed immediately after eruption. It is established that adequate isolation is essential for sealant retention and the success depends upon operator's ability to maintain a dry field. It is recommended that the sealant placement should be delayed until the tooth is sufficiently erupted.

The clinical and epidemiological data shows that the post eruptive age should not be used as a criterion for deciding whether a tooth should be sealed or not. The primary consideration should be the risk of the pits and fissures coupled with an individual's overall susceptibility to caries.

Caries activity: If the caries activity indicates susceptibility to caries, it is advised that the remaining caries free pits and fissures should also be sealed. If an individual demonstrates proximal caries activity, sealant is indicated for non-carious occlusal surfaces. The conservation of occlusal surfaces should be considered during restoration of proximal surfaces.

Questionable caries: Many a times it becomes difficult to distinguish sound pits and fissures, from those with just initiated caries in enamel. Such teeth (questionable caries) are considered at risk and appropriate for sealant application. A sealant placed over a carious lesion limited to enamel may prevent the progression of caries. The concept that the sealant is helpful in the diagnosis of questionable caries is no longer authentic.

ii. *Teeth with enamel caries*

The teeth with enamel caries demonstrate a white opaque appearance surrounding the pits or fissures. Current radiographic methods cannot detect enamel caries in pits and fissures until the lesion has reached the dentin. Sealants can be placed on enamel lesion to restrict the progress.

iii. *Teeth with dentin caries*

The progress of caries in the dentin usually results in the collapse of at least part of the overlying enamel producing an identifiable clinical cavity. However, certain cases exhibit intact surface enamel, thus making it difficult to detect dentinal caries. Pits and fissures with definite caries in dentin should be restored conservatively.

Sealant Application

The clinical technique for applying sealant involves the following steps:

1. Tooth Preparation

a. Prophylaxis

The tooth surface is cleaned using common dentifrices. Flavored, oil based or fluoride containing prophylaxis pastes are not recommended since they adversely influence the conditioning of enamel. The pumice slurry can be applied with either the rubber cup or bristle brush rotating at slow speed. After the prophylaxis, the tooth is thoroughly washed and inspected for residual pumice in the pits and fissures.

b. Isolation

The teeth are properly isolated. Saliva or crevicular exudate should not be allowed to contact the enamel prior to etching. A rubber dam offers the best means of isolation. Cotton rolls and saliva absorbers can provide a dry field but care should be exercised during change. If contamination occurs accidentally, the site should be isolated, cleaned and re-etched.

c. Acid etching

The isolated teeth are etched for 10–15 seconds with 37% phosphoric acid (the etchant is moved gently over the enamel surface with a cotton pellet or brush). The surface is washed using an air-water spray. Oil-free air is used to dry the teeth.

2. Sealant Application

The sealants commonly used are light cured composites. The usual procedure is to apply primer first followed by the flowable resin into the pits and fissures. The applicator tip is applied to the occlusal surface and the sealant is discharged through applicator. Excess sealant material outside the fissure is routinely removed.

It has been documented that small lesions sealed within the tooth structure do not advance. The etchant and sealing procedure produces an immediate bactericidal effect. Gross reductions occur in the number of viable bacteria in carious dentin of sealed teeth. Chemical and radiographic findings indicate that incipient lesions in sealed teeth will not progress further. Carious teeth, however, should be treated according to conventional operative techniques.

Caries Vaccination

The details of immunization of caries are discussed in Chapter 13.

D. MISCELLANEOUS: OZONE AND CARIES PREVENTION

Ozone is a gas composed of three atoms of oxygen and is the most powerful oxidant. Ozone filters the light spectrum high-up in the atmosphere and protects the living objects from the ultra-violet rays. Ozone is an unstable gas, which quickly gives up nascent oxygen. Due to the property of releasing nascent oxygen, it has been used to kill bacteria, fungi and also to inactivate viruses.

Edward Fisch (1950) first used ozone in dentistry.

Ozone therapy prevents dental caries by destroying the cariogenic bacteria. It disrupts the bacterial cell membrane by oxidation of their lipid and lipoprotein components, subsequently the bacteria dies. In case of incipient caries, ozone can kill bacteria in the demineralized tooth structure that otherwise can be remineralized using remineralization solutions. It can also be used to kill bacteria painlessly and even without anesthesia in a frank carious lesion. It is applied to the carious lesion in a controlled manner; killing the bacteria that have caused caries.

Ozone has shown promising results in preventing the pit and fissure caries and reversal of incipient caries through significant reduction in the number of micro-organisms. Small, non-cavitated lesions seem to respond better to ozone treatment, through a greater fall in number of micro-organisms than large cavitated lesions suggesting that the ozone-induced reversal of carious lesion depends on size and site of the lesion. It is considered suitable only for easily accessible surfaces.

It is opined that the microbiological kill rate of ozone increases with increase in the contact time (length of time the tissue is exposed to ozone before it disintegrates). It acts as a disinfectant when applied for 10–20 seconds and acquires sterilizing potential when contact time increases to 20–40 seconds. 40–60 seconds application of ozone has been found to reduce significantly the number of *S. mutans*, *L. casei* and *A. naeslundii*. It does not have any adverse effect on enamel and dentin substrate.

In addition to elimination of pathogens related to caries, ozone has a wide range of therapeutic actions. It restores proper oxygen metabolism, induces a friendly ecologic environment, increases circulation, activates immune system and stimulates humoral anti-oxidant system.

Technique

HealOzone (Kavo Ltd.) is a commercial apparatus that converts oxygen to ozone. Ozone exhibits its antibacterial action through permeating carious enamel and dentin, deactivating 99% of all bacteria. It further neutralizes all acids produced by bacteria.

Ozone is led to a hand piece fitted with a silicone cup. Differently shaped silicone cups are available that correspond to the form of various teeth and their surfaces. This ensures close contact between the silicone cup and the carious area of the tooth so that Ozone does not escape. It is directed through the silicone cup over the tooth for a minimum of 10 seconds. Ozone in the silicone cup is collected again and reconverted to oxygen by the apparatus. Ozone treatment of the carious lesion is completed within 2–3 minutes. Thereafter, a solution containing 2.0% sodium fluoride and 5.0% xylitol is applied to promote remineralization of the carious lesion.

Indications of Ozone other than Prevention of Dental Caries

- Managing cavitated lesions along with conventional conservative measures.
- Bleaching of discolored teeth.
- Desensitization of extremely sensitive teeth.
- Help in healing of soft tissue pathologies.

Contraindications of Ozone Therapy

- Pregnancy.
- Deficiency of glucose-6-phosphate-de-hydrogenase.
- Hyperthyroidism.
- Acute alcohol intoxication.
- Anemia.
- Active hemorrhage.
- Myocardial infarction.

Advantages

- No need of drilling.
- No need of injection.
- Minimally invasive.
- Safe and less time consuming.

Although no adverse side effects of ozone were reported; the cost of the equipment being high, its efficacy in preventing dental caries is still under research.

LASER AND CARIES PREVENTION

Lasers have been tried as a preventive modality since long. Various forms of lasers coupled with different protocols are still being used to prevent caries. Ruby lasers were among the first tried in early sixties, reporting the effectiveness of laser irradiation for the prevention of dental caries. A few authors used Nd:YAG (Neodymium-doped Yttrium

Aluminium Garnet) laser for caries prevention. Hicks, et al (1995) used Argon laser *in-vitro* and reported that laser irradiation enhanced the resistance of enamel to cariogenic challenge. CO_2 laser has also been used successfully in preventing caries.

Types of Lasers used in Caries Prevention

* Ruby.
* Neodymium (Nd:YAG).
* CO_2.
* Argon.
* Erbium (Er:YAG).

Mechanism of Action

Laser energy to be used as a tool for caries prevention must be absorbed and efficiently converted to heat without damage to underlying and surrounding tissues. Laser irradiation modifies the composition of dental tissues thus promoting an increase in resistance to demineralization.

Lasers can significantly alter the permeability and acid-solubility of enamel, subsequently promoting an increase in its resistance to demineralization. The irradiation of enamel with high-intensity laser may raise the surface temperature up to 1000°C. The temperature between 100 and 650°C lead to loss of water. At higher temperature, pyrophosphates (oxidation of phosphates) are formed and also promote formation of α and β-tricalcium phosphate (α-TCP and β-TCP).

A few parameters may affect laser-dental tissue interaction. These are:
* Wavelength of laser used.
* Pulse energy and its duration.
* Continuous/pulsed emission.
* Beam size of radiations.
* Delivery method.
* Repetition rate.
* Optical and thermal properties of the tissues to be irradiated.

The effects of laser irradiation mainly depend on the energy distribution inside the tissue. The temperature rise in the exposed area is the combined result of energy distribution and heat conductance of the tissue. This temperature rise subsequently modifies the physical and chemical structure of the irradiated tissue.

The exposure time and the amount of energy delivered are also important for the rise in temperature at the tooth surface. The concept of 'thermal relaxation time' (the time needed for temperature at a given depth to reach a temperature which is approximately 84 percent of the difference between the surface temperature and initial temperature), clarifies this phenomenon. The pulse duration is an important parameter for determining laser tissue interaction. If the pulse duration of the laser is the same or less than the thermal relaxation time for the tissue, the energy will remain static leading to rise in temperature. In case the pulse duration is much longer than the tissue's thermal relaxation time, the thermal energy will flow towards the centre, heating a large volume of the tissue, subsequently damaging the pulp. However, if the pulse duration is much shorter than the tissue's thermal relaxation time, the energy density will be too high causing ablation; subsequently facilitating removal of the tissue rather damaging the pulp.

Laser can also be used to detect caries because carious lesions will fluoresce differently from healthy tissues. In case of caries removal and cavity preparation, the laser must be absorbed by these tissues. Absorption of laser in enamel and dentin is weak in visible and near infrared ranges. Dentin absorption is low in the visible range, but the tissue scatters more than enamel due to its higher content of water and protein. In the region of Nd:YAG laser (1064 nm), the absorption coefficient of enamel is low; that is why many researchers use dyes or inks with Nd:YAG lasers to improve enamel absorption.

Water being the main absorber, makes these lasers effective in removal of intact enamel and dentin and also the carious lesions.

Inference of Laser Studies

- The Nd:YAG laser is one of the widely studied laser.
- It is established that laser irradiation, combined with topical fluoride treatment, can induce better resistance.
- It is hypothesized that laser irradiated enamel can retain fluoride longer than unlased enamel. However, it has been shown that combined laser irradiation and fluoride treatment can induce the transformation of hydroxyapatite to fluorapatite due to the heating caused by CO_2 (10.6 μm wavelength) laser irradiation, which enables fluoride to be incorporated into melted layers of enamel surfaces. Topical APF application promotes the dissolution of more soluble apatite crystals, forming large quantity of CaF_2 on the surface. Laser irradiation can retain fluoride ions longer than unlased enamel (mechanisms of this fluoride retention are still unknown).
- Various authors opined that laser irradiation can promote the formation of microspaces in enamel, which would facilitate the fluoride incorporation; moreover, laser irradiation can induce the formation of fluorapatite by incorporation of fluoride into the melted layers of the enamel surface.
- A few authors suggested that laser irradiation can increase fluoride diffusion through enamel and generate fluoride reservoirs.
- It is established that topical fluoride treatment following laser irradiation provided better caries resistance. Since heat was found to enhance the uptake of fluoride, it was speculated that the thermal effect of laser might be the main factor in promoting fluoride uptake and an increase in enamel resistance to demineralization.

Efficacy of Laser Application

Several studies have been carried out to evaluate effect of laser on enamel surface as regard to its microhardness and solubility. Different laser wavelengths used in these studies were Argon laser at 488–514 nm, CO_2 laser at 9300, 9600, 10600 nm and the Erbium laser at 2780 and 2490 nm.

Hsu, et al (2001) reported a significant reduction in enamel solubility following CO_2 laser irradiation and reported that there was significant synergism between laser and 0.2 ppm fluoride solution. The combined laser-fluoride treatment led to 98 percent reduction in mineral loss. In another study, Flaitz, et al (1995) showed that combining acidulated phosphate fluoride with argon laser irradiation resulted in a 50 percent reduction in lesion depth. A couple of other authors reported a significant reduction of white spotting or etching, using a zinc fluoride and argon laser combination. It was hypothesized that this treatment stabilises and restores its structural defects.

The efficacy of using argon laser irradiation combined with APF was investigated on primary teeth; the surface layer may contain fluoride-rich calcium and phosphate mineral phases that could act as reservoir for fluoride, calcium and phosphate, thus providing a certain degree of protection from caries. Westerman, et al (2003) reported that the micro-hardness of the enamel surface was higher when exposed to low argon laser irradiation only or in combination with APF. Featherstone, et al (1998) reported 70% inhibition of caries progression by using 9300 nm and 9600 nm laser comparable with the inhibition produced by the daily use of fluoride toothpaste. The subsurface temperature increase was minimal (<1°C at 2.0 mm depth) and there was no thermal damage to the pulp. A couple of authors have also confirmed that the CO_2 laser was efficient in reducing the subsurface enamel demineralization and its association with fluoride treatment may enhance the protective effect.

It is established that the erbium laser wavelength may have the potential to increase acid resistance, can reduce enamel solubility and increase caries resistance.

Although several studies have investigated the effect of different types of lasers used alone or in combination with topical fluoride application upon dental hard tissues, certain issues still need be investigated. It remains unclear, for example, whether topical fluoride application should be carried out before or after irradiating enamel. The lasers have different wavelengths and will interact differently with the tooth structure. These differences might affect the fluoride uptake in enamel. Laser irradiation may enhance or reduce the fluoride uptake and retention. Depending on these results, topical fluoride treatment protocol becomes important for optimum fluoride uptake.

While some studies have demonstrated the potential preventive effect of laser irradiation on sound enamel, the effect of irradiation on white spot lesions is still unclear.

Very few studies have compared the effect of different types of lasers on caries inhibition. Tsai, et al (2002) compared the effectiveness of CO_2 and Nd:YAG lasers on acid resistance of enamel, using different pulse duration, number of pulses/second, the wattage used and the pulse incident energy. The study concluded that enamel surfaces treated with either CO_2 or Nd:YAG lasers were eroded to shallower depths than untreated enamel.

An another study, compared the ablation effects of Nd:YAG and Ho:YAG (Holmium) laser irradiation on enamel and dentin. The author reported that the Holmium laser was more suitable for cutting enamel and dentin when compared to the Nd:YAG laser, which caused uncontrolled melting of tooth structure.

There is a definite need for more laser comparative studies not only to determine the most effective laser types in preventing caries but also to compare their performance clinically.

FLUORIDES AND CARIES PREVENTION

Fluoride has always been regarded as the cornerstone of modern preventive dentistry. The use of fluoride in both systemic and topical form has led to a remarkable decrease in dental caries worldwide. The Centers for Disease Control and Prevention (CDCP) has designated water fluoridation as the most important regime for caries prevention.

The use of fluorides has proved to be the most clinically effective caries preventing protocol based on large number of clinical trials. The ability of fluoride to prevent the progress of dental caries may involve reducing acid solubility of enamel, promoting enamel remineralization, inhibiting utilization of glucose by acidogenic bacteria and imparting bacteriostatic/bactericidal effects.

The topical fluorides, applied professionally or self applied, help increase the resistance of the teeth against dental caries.

It is established that baseline level of fluorides in saliva is around 0.02 ppm, which is not effective in preventing caries. The intake of fluoridated water along with use of fluoride products, may raise the salivary fluoride level to 0.04 ppm. This level of fluoride concentration in saliva is effective in minimizing caries process.

History of fluorides dates back to 1901, when Dr. Fredrick McKay of Colorado (USA) accidentally discovered that many of his patients had an apparently permanent stain on their teeth, which was referred to as 'colorado stain'. Various other authors confirmed the findings of Dr McKay.

It was established soon that the causative factor of such stains might be present in domestic water, especially during the period of teeth maturation.

Trendley H. Dean (1931) was amongst the first few authors who correlated mottled enamel with fluoride in water. Later, he proposed Dean's index for Fluorosis.

Dean (1941) in his study observed that individuals continuously living in a fluoride rich area had less caries as compared to the individuals who had lived in the same fluoride rich areas during calcification of teeth but shifted to non-fluoride areas thereafter. This led to hypothesis that the effect of fluoride was continuous even after calcification of teeth.

Mechanism of Action

The cariostatic potential of fluorides has been established; however, the exact mechanism involved is still debatable. Let us first clarify caries resistant concept vis-à-vis caries controlled concept.

Caries Resistant Concept

It was thought that fluoride had to be present during tooth development to provide 'caries resistance' to the teeth. Fluoride is the most electronegative of all the elements and has a strong affinity for exchange with hydroxyl ion in hydroxyapatite $[Ca_{10}(PO_4)_6OH_2]$. The electrostatic attraction between Ca^{2+} and F^- will be more as compared to that between Ca^{2+} and OH^-, making fluoridated apatite more crystalline. When fluoride is incorporated into the enamel, the crystals become less acid soluble. This is how fluorides make teeth more resistant to caries.

It is established that increased intake of fluoride during tooth formation raises the fluoride concentration in enamel and hence increases the acid resistance. The increased intake of fluorides from sources like drinking water, fluoride tablets, drops, lozenges, salt, milk, etc. was considered optimal solution for caries control.

The concept of incorporating fluoride during tooth development making it caries resistant was considered genuine. The worldwide decline in caries prevalence due to water fluoridation authenticated this concept; however, over the years, the researchers disagreed and presented different concept.

Ogaard B, et al (1991) conducted a study whereby the authors placed human and shark enamel slabs in removable appliances and covered them with orthodontic bands to allow plaque accumulation. Shark enamel was used as it is composed of pure fluorapatite (around 30,000 ppm fluoride). On microradiography, it was revealed that carious lesions formed in both substrates, although they were less severe in shark enamel. In addition to this, when human enamel treated with 0.2% NaF was used, it exhibited less mineral loss than shark enamel without any additional treatment. The study proved that structurally bound fluoride (shark enamel) was not very effective in inhibiting demineralization, whereas fluoride in solution (NaF rinse) led to high degree of protection. The inference of the study was that primary action of fluoride was topical due to its presence in the fluid phases of the oral environment.

Caries Controlled Concept

A few authors opined that the caries reducing effect of fluoride is primarily achieved during active caries development at the plaque/enamel interface. It alters the dynamics of demineralization/remineralization and also affects the plaque bacteria. The primary caries-preventive protocol remains the post-eruptive topical mechanism. It is established that best strategy to control caries is use of topical fluorides at low concentration. The adverse effects of systemic ingestion like fluorosis are also minimized.

The mechanisms of cariostatic potential of fluorides include:

   i. Inhibiting demineralization.

   ii. Enhancing remineralization.

   iii. Antibacterial action (inhibiting bacterial activity).

i. Inhibiting Demineralization

Fluoride inhibits demineralization. Fluorides if present in plaque fluid during the time bacteria produces acids, it will penetrate along with the acids at the subsurface, adsorb to the apatite crystal surface and protect the crystal from dissolution. The coating makes the characteristics of crystal similar to those of fluorapatite, so that no demineralization takes place until the pH reaches 4.5 or less. Fluorides present at low levels along the enamel crystals inhibit dissolution of the minerals by acids. The fluoride incorporated developmentally and systemically into the normal tooth mineral is insufficient to have a measurable effect on its acid solubility. The topical fluorides are effective in achieving resistance to acid solubility.

ii. *Enhancing Remineralization*

Fluoride enhances remineralization when the pH returns to above 5.5. The saliva super-saturated with calcium and phosphate ions help providing minerals back to the tooth. Fluorides adsorb to the surface of partially demineralized crystals and attract calcium ions. The tooth surface preferentially takes up fluorides from the solution surrounding the crystals. Fluorides bring calcium and phosphate ions together on to the tooth surface, which subsequently has a lower solubility. The remineralized surface is more resistant to acid challenges.

iii. *Antibacterial Action* *(inhibiting bacterial activity)*

Fluorides exhibit antibacterial actions by:
- Enzyme inhibition of bacterial cells
- Enhancing proton permeability of cell membrane in the form of hydrogen fluoride

Hydrogen fluoride (HF), formed under acidic conditions, enters the cell due to its high permeability along the bacterial cell membrane. Inside the cytoplasm, hydrogen fluoride then dissociates to ionic forms, viz. H^+ and F^-. This intracellular F^- inhibits glycolytic enzymes, resulting in a decrease acid production from glycolysis. Fluoride ions inhibit a wide range of enzymes, viz. enolase, urease, P-ATPase, F-ATPase, etc. essential for bacterial presence. F^- also lowers cytoplasmic pH, affecting both the acid production and

acid tolerance of *Streptococcus mutans*; however, the antibacterial actions of fluoride are achieved at high concentration of fluoride (3000–9500 rpm). Such high concentration of fluoride in plaque fluid is not achieved by local or systemic use. Moreover, these effects are confirmed in *in-vitro* studies, their *in-vivo* efficacy is under research.

1. SYSTEMIC FLUORIDATION

Systemic fluoridation is widely used in different formats to prevent caries. Let us first understand the concept of prenatal and postnatal fluorides.

Prenatal and Postnatal Fluorides

Use of prenatal fluorides in preventing dental caries has always been a controversial topic. The beneficial effects of prenatal fluorides could not be confirmed.

The permeability of the placenta to fluoride has been questioned due to several observations such as:
- Fluorosis in deciduous teeth is not documented properly.
- High concentration of fluoride in placenta.
- Fluoride concentration of bound tissues of fetus differ in areas with different concentration of fluorides in water.
- Validity of transfer of fluoride from the maternal circulation to the fetal circulation.

It is accepted that primary teeth calcify before birth and fluorides might have limited access to the fetus. Thylstrup (1978) observed that primary teeth of all children in areas where water contained more than 3.5 ppm fluoride exhibited varying degrees of fluorosis (severity of fluorosis was directly proportional to the concentration of fluoride in water). He opined that placenta is permeable to fluoride and the appearance of fluorosis in primary teeth may be affected by enamel thickness.

Fluoride supplements given to pregnant mothers are absorbed primarily in the stomach and to a lesser degree in the small intestine. Fluoride as hydrogen fluoride diffuses across the gastric mucosa and then dissociates in the circulatory system to yield fluoride ions. The maximum plasma fluoride level is achieved within 30–60 minutes, after that the excretion of fluoride from plasma exceeds absorption. Ultimately, most of the fluoride is either taken up by the mineralized tissues or excreted in the urine. Unabsorbed fluoride is excreted in the feces. High fluoride concentration in the placenta has been observed and also that the placenta acts as a barrier to prevent even traces of fluoride from reaching the fetus. Few authors are of the view that fluoride is taken up by the fetal bones and teeth.

Fluoride uptake increases with age of the fetus and is greater in bones than teeth. There is a little significant difference between tissues formed at 1 ppm F and 0.5 ppm F.

A 30–35% reduction in caries was noticed when fluorides were given both prenatally and postnatally. Also fluoride given both prenatally and postnatally was found to be more effective as compared to when it was given only postnatally. Since the results were consistent with the studies of fluorides analysis of fetuses, it was concluded that prenatal exposure to fluoride produced pronounced reduction in dental caries. However, the clinical evidences do not justify prenatal fluoride supplements having any cariostatic effect. The formats of systemic fluoridation are:

A. Water Fluoridation

Water fluoridation can be defined as *the adjustment of the concentration of fluoride ion in public water supply in such a way that the concentration of fluoride ion in water may be consistently maintained at 1 ppm by weight.* In hot climate countries where water consumption is more, slightly less than 1 ppm fluoride (0.7 ppm) level is maintained. In very cold climate, level of 1.2 ppm fluoride is recommended. The optimum fluoride concentration

for a particular community can be calculated by the following equation.

ppm = (Fluoride concentration by weight) = 0.34/K

where K = –0.038 + 0.0062 × Temperature of the area in °F

Water fluoridation requires an efficient and continuous public water supply so that the appropriate effect can be achieved.

Water fluoridation is considered as the best way to reduce caries prevalence. This is being utilized in most of the developing countries. The process is economically reliable, time saving and accepted by the society.

The United States carried out artificial water fluoridation in 1945, whereby children were given water containing 1 ppm fluoride for six years. It was observed that caries prevalence was reduced to half. Subsequent studies also confirmed that 1 ppm fluoride in drinking water was the best source to act as a caries inhibitor. Till date, more than 70 million people all over the world are protected by artificial fluoridation. Unfortunately in India, a water fluoridation project has not been started at the Government level even though around 30% people consume pipe water.

Compounds used in water fluoridation

- Fluorspar.
- Sodium fluoride.
- Sodium silicofluoride.
- Hydrofluorosilicic acid.
- Ammonium silicofluoride.

Advantages

- Effective and reliable.
- Practical and economical.
- Accepted by the society.

B. Fluoride Supplements

Fluoride supplements provide systemic fluoride in areas where water fluoridation is not available. The main supplements used are:

a. Salt Fluoridation

The rationale of using salt fluoridation was that if iodised salt can be helpful in reducing goitre incidence, fluoridated salt can be utilized in reducing caries. The recommended dose of salt fluoridation is 250–350 mg F/kg salt; however, there is no international consensus regarding the concentration of fluoride in salt. 90 mg fluoride/kg salt was used in Switzerland, while 200 mg/kg salt was used in Columbia and Spain. Since the addition of fluoride in salt does not alter its color and taste, it is accepted by all. Various studies reported 20–25% reduction in dental caries after using salt containing 90 ppm fluoride. Toth in his study reported that after 8 years of salt fluoridation (250 mg fluoride/kg salt), there was 41% decrease in dmft in 2–6 years old children; 58% decrease in 7–11 years and 36% in 12–14 years old children. Various other studies substantiated that the addition of fluoride in salt reduces prevalence of caries.

Fluoride is usually added by mixing concentrated solution of sodium fluoride or potassium fluoride in the salt. Premixed granules of NaF and CaF_2 are also added to salt.

Advantages
- Supply of fluoride can be controlled.
- Individual monitoring not required (average consumption 58 gm of salt per day).
- Cariostatic effects are equal to water fluoridation.
- Non-toxic.
- Viable and feasible.
- Cost effective.

Disadvantages
- Daily consumption may not be sufficient.
- Excess intake of salt can be harmful.

b. Fluoridated Sugar
It is accepted that 2–5 ppm fluoride in sucrose solution decreases caries prevalence due to reprecipitation of fluoride rich apatite on the tooth surface.

c. Milk Fluoridation
Milk fluoridation is considered advantageous; however, consumption of milk is not organized especially in developing countries. Various studies have indicated that an addition of 2.5 mg NaF in milk which was served daily to schoolchildren resulted in substantial reduction in caries.

There was a controversy regarding the use of fluoride in milk. One concept was that fluoride binds with calcium and protein making it unavailable for its anticariogenic activity. However, various researchers confirmed that the availability of fluoride four hours after consumption of milk was the same as that of water.

The compounds used in milk are: CaF_2, NaF and disodium monofluoro phosphate (NaF is mainly used). In pasteurized milk, fluoride can be added before or after pasteurization.

d. Fluoride Tablets
The use of fluoride tablets provides dual effect, i.e. systemic effect before mineralization of primary and permanent dentition and topical effect thereafter. The consumption of these tablets is avoided where water supply contains more than 0.5 ppm of fluoride.

Various studies have shown caries reduction in the range of 50–80% when fluoride tablets were administered for a period of 2–3 years. 0.5 mg fluoride tablet is recommended daily for children below three years of age and 1.0 mg thereafter. Most of the studies were conducted using NaF tablets; however few of them used Acidulated phosphate fluoride (APF) tablets.

It is accepted that fluoride must be ingested systemically during the mineralization period in order to exert maximum cariostatic effect.

Commercially, fluoride tablets are available as NaF tablets of 2.2 mg, 1.1 mg and 0.55 mg yielding 1 mg, 0.5 mg and 0.25 mg fluoride respectively. The trade name of these tablets are Fluoroday, Tymaflour and Luride.

Fluoride tablets should be chewed and swallowed to obtain dual benefits of topical as well as systemic effects. This dual role of fluoride tablets is considered an effective tool for caries prevention: The recommended dosage of fluoride tablet is described in Table 12.5.

Combinations of NaF and vitamins in tablet form are also available and can be advised under the following situations:

- Children from deprived families who did not have adequate diet.
- Children suffering from anorexia, poor appetites and poor eating habits.
- Dietary insufficiency in breast-fed infants of malnourished mothers.

Vitamin supplements generally are of no use since there is a little evidence of mineral insufficiency except that of iron. However, total insufficiency of minerals is the major nutritional problem in children especially amongst lower socioeconomic groups.

e. Fluoride Drops

Fluoride drops are recommended in younger children who cannot swallow tablets (below 2 years). A solution of NaF is added by a dropper to the child's drinking water or juice. The method of administering fluoride in drop should be as good as fluoride tablets, but the chances of inaccurate dosage are increased. The intake of higher doses may lead to mottling of teeth.

2. TOPICAL FLUORIDATION

It was demonstrated that fluoride solution when kept in contact with teeth, the fluoride ions bind with the enamel surface and render it less soluble than the original enamel surface. This observation led to the idea of topical fluoridation. Since water fluoridation may have limitations, topical fluoridation can be an effective method, especially in younger population.

A. Sodium Fluoride

Sodium fluoride is the most commonly used topical fluoride agent. Earlier 0.1% NaF was used for topical application; however, 2.0% NaF is being preferred by various authors.

Method of preparation of 2.0% NaF

2.0% Neutral NaF solution can be prepared by dissolving 20 grams of NaF powder in one liter of distilled water (pH 7) in a plastic bottle. It is essential to store fluoride in plastic bottles because if stored in glass containers, the fluoride ion of the solution can react with silica of glass forming Silicon fluoride, thus reducing the availability of free fluoride for anti-caries action.

Knutson's Technique

Knutson and Armstrong (1942) applied NaF 8–15 times in the 1st year of their 3 years study and observed 39.8% reduction after 1st year, 41.4% after 2 years and 36.7% after 3 years.

Knutson in subsequent studies recommended a technique of 4 applications and also recommended 3, 7, 11 and 13 years as specific age groups of NaF application.

Procedure

Prior to a topical fluoride application, the teeth should be cleaned with pumice slurry. The

Age	Fluoride concentration in water (ppm)		
	< 0.3	0.3–0.6	> 0.6
Birth to 6 months	0	0	0
6 months to 3 years	0.25 mg	0	0
3 to 6 years	0.50 mg	0.25 mg	0
6 to at least 16 years	1.00 mg	0.50 mg	0

Table 12.5: Recommended dosage of fluoride tablets

surface debris, etc. should be removed thoroughly, which might interfere with the fluoride uptake and reduce its clinical effectiveness.

The teeth are then isolated with cotton rolls and dried with compressed air. Teeth can either be isolated by quadrant or by half mouth.

Using cotton tip applicator sticks, 2.0% NaF solution is painted on the air-dried teeth so that all surfaces are visibly wet. The solution is allowed to dry for 3–4 minutes. This procedure is repeated for each of the isolated segments until all the teeth are treated.

After completion of treatment, the patient is instructed to avoid eating, drinking or rinsing for 30 minutes so as to prolong the availability of fluoride ions to react with the tooth surfaces.

A second, third and fourth fluoride application, each not preceded by a prophylaxis, is scheduled at intervals of approximately one week. The four-visit procedure is recommended for ages 3, 7, 11 and 13 years, coinciding with the eruption of different groups of primary and permanent teeth. Thus, most of the teeth would be treated soon after their eruption, maximizing the protection afforded by topical application.

One disadvantage of Knutson's technique is that the patient has to visit dental clinic four times.

Mechanism of Action

The efficacy of fluoride treatment in reducing dental caries depends on the ability of fluoride agents to increase the enamel fluoride concentrations, subsequently enhancing remineralization and suppressing the bacterial growth.

When NaF is applied topically, it reacts with hydroxyapatite crystal to form CaF_2, which is the main product of reaction.

$$Ca_{10} (PO_4)_6 (OH)_2 + 20F^- \rightleftharpoons 10CaF_2 +$$
$$6PO_4^{3-} + 2OH^-$$

This is due to the high concentration of fluoride (9,000 ppm) in 2.0% NaF due to which the solubility product of CaF_2 get exceeded and the initial rapid reaction is followed by drastic reduction in its rate and the phenomenon is called choking off. This occurs because once a thick layer of CaF_2 gets formed, it interferes with further diffusion of fluoride from the topical fluoride solution to react with hydroxyapatite.

$$CaF_2 + 2Ca_5 (PO_4)_3 OH \rightleftharpoons 2Ca_5(PO_4)_3F + Ca (OH)_2$$

It is because of this reason, NaF once applied is left to dry for 4 minutes. Further CaF_2 reacts with hydroxyapatite to form fluoridated hydroxyapatite, which increases the concentration of surface fluoride thus making the tooth structure more stable and less susceptible to dissolution by acids. It also interferes with plaque metabolism through antienzymatic action and helps in remineralization of the initial decalcified areas, subsequently showing anticaries effects.

The prolonged retention of reaction products, which form a coating on the enamel surface, may influence both initiation and progression of enamel caries by:
- Acting as a diffusion barrier.
- Reducing enamel solubility.
- Acting as a reservoir for the enamel microenvironment.
- Desorbing proteins and micro-organisms from the enamel surface.

B. Stannous Fluoride

Stannous fluoride is also commonly used topical agent and is considered more effective than sodium fluoride in preventing acidic dissolution of calcium and phosphorus from enamel.

The imbibement of the stannous fluoride produced an enamel surface that was less acid soluble than surface treated with other fluorides including NaF.

Stannous fluoride in concentration of 8% and 10% has been used in routine (10%

solution is usually used for adults and 8% for children). There is no clinical difference between the two concentrations.

Preparation of SnF₂ Solution

Stannous fluoride solution is not stable. Soon after mixing, it becomes cloudy due to the formation of tin hydroxide. The stannous is believed to contribute to the anti-caries benefits of stannous fluoride.

It is recommended that a fresh solution of stannous fluoride be prepared for each patient (aged solutions are considered clinically less effective).

To prepare 8% stannous fluoride solution, the content of one capsule (0.8 gm) is dissolved in 10 ml of distilled water in a plastic container and the solution is shaken briefly. The solution is then applied immediately to the teeth. Usually 10 ml solution is sufficient for the entire dentition. The remaining solution, if any, be discarded and not used again.

Procedure

The application of SnF_2 is carried out following the steps as:

- The tooth surface must be thoroughly cleaned and polished with pumice including the proximal surface (unwaxed dental floss is used because it is believed that waxed floss may coat the tooth surface and adversely affect fluoride uptake).
- The teeth are then isolated with cotton rolls and dried preferably with compressed air.
- Either a quadrant or half of the dentition can be treated at one time. The teeth to be treated should be kept free of saliva; continuous use of saliva ejector is preferred.
- A freshly prepared 8% solution of SnF_2 is applied continuously to the teeth with cotton applicators.
- It is suggested that the solution should be applied for 15–30 seconds (prolonged application for 4 minutes not necessary).
- The recommended frequency of 8% SnF_2 applications is once per year.

It is accepted that second coat of 8% stannous fluoride solution be applied within a day or two after the first application. A few authors, however, reported that four-semi annual application of 10% solution of stannous fluoride applied for 30 seconds produced benefits, after two years, equal to those produced by the traditional four-minute application of 8% solution.

Mechanism of Action

It is established that when stannous fluoride reacts with hydroxyapatite, the tin of stannous fluoride reacts with enamel and forms a new crystalline product (stannous-tri-fluoro-phosphate), which is more resistant to decay than enamel. It is suggested that a freshly prepared SnF_2 solution should be used and the capsules of SnF_2 should be kept in air tight containers, otherwise the stannous form of tin gets oxidized to stannic form, thus making the SnF_2 inactive for anti-caries action.

Infra-red absorption and X-ray diffraction analysis of the reaction of stannous fluoride with hydroxyapatite have shown the formation of following products:

- Tin hydroxyl phosphate $[Sn_2(OH)PO_4]$ when SnF_2 is applied in low concentration.
- Tin trifluorophosphate $[Sn_3F_3PO_4]$ and calcium trifluorostannate $[Ca(SnF_3)_2]$ when SnF_2 is applied high concentration.
- CaF_2 is formed both in low and high concentration.

The reaction at low concentration is:

$$Ca_5(PO_4)_3 OH + 2SnF_2 \longrightarrow 2CaF_2$$
$$+ Sn_2(OH)PO_4 + Ca_3(PO_4)_2$$
(Tin hydroxyl
phosphate)

The reaction at high concentration is:

$$Ca_5(PO_4)_3 OH + 16SnF_2 \longrightarrow CaF_2 +$$
$$4CaF_2(SnF_3)_2$$
(Calcium trifluorostannate)
$$+ 2Sn_3F_3PO_4 \quad + \quad Sn_2(OH)PO_4$$
(Tin trifluorophosphate) (Tin hydroxyl phosphate)

CaF_2 so formed further reacts with hydroxy apatite and small fraction of fluro hydroxy apatite also gets formed.

$$2Ca_5 (PO_4)_3 \ OH + CaF_2 \longrightarrow 2Ca_5(PO_4) \ F + Ca(OH)_2$$

The other end product, tin hydroxy phosphate, gets dissolved in oral fluid and is responsible for the metallic taste after topical application of stannous fluoride. The main end product, which is tin-tri-fluoro phosphate, is responsible for making the tooth structure more stable and less susceptible to decay.

Anti-bacterial Effects

Stannous fluoride (SnF_2) has been shown to be more effective against oral micro-organisms as compared to sodium fluoride (NaF).

SnF_2 selectively inhibits *Streptococcus mutans*, the bacterium most frequently associated with dental caries.

The effects of SnF_2 on oral bacteria have been attributed to:

   i. The divalent cation tin, interacting with the negatively charged plaque components to alter bacterial adhesion/cohesion.

  ii. The oxidization of Thiol groups of bacterial enzymes by tin.

 iii. The alteration of the bacterial metabolism due to uptake of tin by bacteria.

 iv. The naturally low pH of SnF_2 causing HF formation, which is reportedly more anti-bacterial than fluoride (F^-).

The unique anti-bacterial properties of SnF_2 appear to be associated with the observed intracellular retention of tin.

The intracellular tin accumulation appears to disrupt the metabolism of *Streptococcus mutans*, as demonstrated by the reduced growth and acid production. SnF_2 used in concentrations between 0.02 and 1.64% has resulted in a reduction of plaque and subsequently the caries.

Stannous fluoride appears to affect the growth and adherence properties of bacteria rather than being bactericidal.

Disadvantages

- It occasionally causes pigmentation of teeth which has a characteristic light brown color.
- 8% solution is quite astringent and disagreeable in taste (metallic taste).
- Solution causes reversible tissue irritation manifested by gingival blanching.

Stannous Fluoride Gel

To overcome disadvantages of the freshly prepared 8–10% stannous fluoride, a gel containing 0.4% stannous fluoride in a methyl cellulose/glycerin base was developed. Flavored with cinnamon or grape, it remains stable for 15 months. However for the fluoride to be released, the gel should be diluted prior to its application on to the teeth.

This gel has been effective in reducing caries in post-irradiation cancer patients. It can also reduce enamel decalcification around bands in orthodontic patients.

Commercial preparations have been used effectively as self-applied agents.

C. Acidulated Phosphate Fluoride

The researchers, over the years, hypothesized that as the pH of NaF solution was lowered, fluoride was absorbed more effectively into enamel. The concept may have inherent limitations, as lowering of pH of NaF solution may cause decalcification/demineralization of enamel thus obviating the fluoride effect. Acidulated phosphate fluoride (APF) was tried as an alternating topical agent to achieve the benefits of fluorides.

Pomeijer and Brudevold (1963) compared the effectiveness of NaF with APF solution in preventing caries and reported APF to be 50% more effective than neutral NaF.

The practical difficulties of topical application with APF is that the teeth must be kept in solution for four minutes (APF solution being acidic and bitter in taste, the repeated applications necessitates the use of suction, thereby minimizing its effects). To overcome this problem, APF gels were introduced. With the use of gel, fluoride remains in contact with teeth, so re-application is not required and moreover, self-application with gel reduces the cost of application.

The thixotropic gel displays a high viscosity at low shear rates and very low viscosity at the higher shear rates. The inference is that the gel thins out under biting forces and more easily penetrates between the teeth; when it is not under stress, it remains stable in the tray and does not leach down the patient's throat.

APF Foam

Acidulated phosphate fluoride in foam base is used in an attempt to minimize the risk of overdosage of fluoride and to maintain the efficacy of topical fluoride treatment. The advantages of APF foam are:

- It is much lighter than a conventional gel and therefore only a small amount of APF is needed for topical application (4.0 gm of gel/oral cavity while less than 1.0 gm of foam/oral cavity).
- The surfactant in the foaming agent has a cleansing action (lowers the surface tension). This also facilitates the penetration of the material into interproximal surfaces where its action is most needed.
- Since APF foam does not require suctioning, it is preferred for the treatment of young children and disabled persons where saliva evacuation is difficult or may not be feasible.
- Accepted method for home use.

Preparation of APF Solution/gel

APF usually contains 1.23% of fluoride in 0.1M phosphoric acid at a pH of 3 and is stable when stored in opaque plastic bottles. It is prepared by dissolving 20 grams of NaF in one liter of 0.1M phosphoric acid. 50% hydrofluoric acid is added to adjust the pH at 3 (Fluoride concentration at 1.23%).

For the preparation of APF gel, methyl cellulose/hydroxy ethyl cellulose is to be added to the solution (pH adjusted between 4–5).

Procedure

The preferred method of application using aqueous preparation of acidulated phosphate fluoride is the paint-on-technique and for gel, the tray technique.

Acidulated phosphate fluoride is recommended for application at 6 or 12 months intervals.

Prior to the application of APF, the teeth are cleaned, isolated and thoroughly dried with air. The solution is then applied repeatedly with a cotton applicator, so as to keep the teeth moist with the fluoride solution throughout the four-minute period. This means re-application every 15–30 seconds, depending upon the fluoride solution used.

The patient is instructed not to eat, drink or rinse for at least 30 minutes.

APF is stable and need not be freshly prepared for each patient.

The topical application of APF in the form of a viscous gel has advantages over APF solution because the gel adheres to the teeth, eliminating the need for continuous rewetting of enamel surface. In addition, the full mouth can be treated simultaneously, resulting in a substantial reduction in the time of total treatment.

Clinical application of APF gel should be carried out using trays that fit the patients upper and lower dental arches. The foam lined trays are usually preferred.

The interproximal surfaces, their contacts and protected areas are high-risk surfaces. The application of topical fluorides using trays certainly contacts the buccal and lingual surfaces, but may not cover the interproximal sites. The areas below the contact points are not covered with conventional gels. Flossing of the interproximal surfaces with APF gel is beneficial to achieve fluoridation of these areas. This will carry the gel into the inter-proximal sites.

Mechanism of Action

When APF is applied to the tooth surface, it initially leads to dehydration and shrinkage of hydroxyapatite crystals. The crystals further on hydrolysis form an intermediate product called dicalcium phosphate dihydrate (DCPD). This DCPD is highly reactive with fluoride ions when APF is applied, fluoride penetrates more deeply through the openings produced by shrinkage and leads to formation of fluorapatite (FAp).

$$Ca_5(PO_4)_3\,OH + 4H^+ \xrightarrow{OH^-}$$

$$5Ca^{2+} + 3HPO_4^{2-} + H_2O$$

$$Ca^{2+} + HPO_4^{2-} \xrightleftharpoons{OH^-} Ca.HPO_4.\,2H_2O$$
$$\text{(Dicalcium phosphate dihydrate)}$$

$$5Ca.HPO.2H_2O \xrightleftharpoons{F^-} Ca_5\,(PO_4)_3\,F + 2HPO_4^-$$

The amount and depth of fluoride deposited as fluorapatite is dependent on the amount and depth at which dicalcium-phosphate dihydrate is formed. For conversion of whole DCPD into fluorapatite, deeper penetration and continuous supply of fluoride is required. To achieve continuous supply, APF is applied every 30 seconds and the tooth has to be kept wet for 4 minutes.

Because high fluoride concentrations and low pH favor fluoride deposition, acidification of the fluoride solution with phosphoric acid is preferred.

The main advantage of the APF is its ability to deposit fluoride in enamel to a deeper depth than neutral sodium fluoride or stannous fluoride.

Guidelines for Fluoride Application

- Limit the amount (not more than 2.0 ml or 40% of the tray capacity).
- Limit the amount of gel to 5 to 10 drops.
- Seat patient in the upright position with head titled forward.
- Use suction throughout fluoride application.
- Never leave child patient unattended.

D. Fluoride Mouthrinses

Wherever water fluoridation is not feasible, different modalities have been tried. It has been confirmed that using 0.2% NaF mouthrinse would lead to 40–50% reduction of caries. Various authors have observed that both APF and NaF possessed equal cariostatic potential.

Fluoride rinsing is preferred daily; however, twice a week rinsing is also effective. Mouth-rinsing with a fluoride solution twice or thrice a week can be helpful. One tablet of 200 mg NaF can be dissolved in approximately 25 ml of clean water which is sufficient for rinsing for one family.

It is established that frequent use of a low concentration of fluoride (0.05% NaF) is more cariostatic than less frequent use of higher concentration (0.25% NaF). It is reported that rinsing with a diluted solution of fluoride results in rapid elevation of plaque fluoride levels; however, it returns to normal within 24 hours. It is advised that daily rinsing would be superior as compared to once a week rinsing. It is observed that stannous fluoride provides additional cariostatic action because of its antibacterial effect against some plaque micro-organisms. It also inhibits plaque formation by reducing the free energy of enamel.

It is established that low levels of fluorides in the oral fluids are associated with concentrated level of fluorides in plaque. Further, the low concentrations of fluorides are sufficient to inhibit glycolysis and acid production by plaque organisms. In addition, repeated exposure to low concentration of fluoride effectively promotes remineralization of incipient carious lesions.

Various authors opined that optimum preventive results could be achieved by frequent exposure of plaque to low concentrations of fluoride ions.

A few fluoride compounds, viz. amine fluoride, ammonium fluoride, etc. have also been used as mouthrinses, but none of them have shown sufficient cariostatic activity as compared to sodium fluoride and stannous fluoride.

Rinsing with 200 ppm SnF_2 for two years resulted in selective suppression of *Streptococcus mutans*. Chemically, the changes in *Streptococcus mutans* have been associated with the accumulation of tin in these cells. The antimicrobial effects of stannous fluoride mouthrinsing infer inhibiting acid production in plaque for several hours, subsequently increasing the plaque pH, which is not conducive for *Streptococcus mutans*.

Stannous fluoride has long been used without any adverse effects. The tin ions are considered safe even when ingested; however, metallic taste in mouth has been reported in a few cases.

Fluoride mouthrinses are relatively safe, as accidental swallowing of even the full volume of the rinse would result in ingestion of 9 mg F (used weekly) or 2.3 mg F (used daily). This is well below the minimum dose of 120 mg F estimated to be safely tolerated by a 5-year-old-child. Older children have a proportionally greater margin of safety.

Fluoride mouthrinsing appears to be quite successful in reducing caries incidence. It is a simple, safe, well accepted and relatively inexpensive way of preventing caries.

E. Fluoride Dentifrices

The term dentifrice infers 'rubbing the tooth'. The most commonly used dentifrices are NaF and SnF_2; however, sodium monofluorophosphate has also been used.

It is established that organic fluorides were better than inorganic fluorides when used as dentifrices. Dentifrices containing monofluorophosphate at a concentration of 0.76% fluoride with sodium metaphosphate have led to 17–34% reduction in caries prevalence. Monofluorophosphate dentifrices are more effective than SnF_2 because MFP has a neutral pH (6.5) as compared to SnF_2, which has an acidic pH (4.8).

Fluoride containing toothpastes generally have approximately 500–1000 ppm fluoride. Ingestion of toothpaste is a matter of concern to a dental professional. About 8 to 16 mg fluoride per kg body weight is considered safe. The lethal dose of fluoride is 32–64 mg fluoride per kg body weight. It accounts for about 5,000 to 10,000 mg of NaF for a 70 kg adult. So a tube containing 200 gm toothpaste is safe even if all its contents are ingested at once.

The recommended norms for use of fluoride toothpastes are:

- Below 6 years, no fluoride toothpaste.
- 6–10 years, once daily.
- Above 10 years, twice daily.

The fluoride containing and fluoride-free pastes may not have any beneficial effect. It has been established that prophylaxis pastes play no role in the prevention of caries. However, pastes do remove extrinsic stains and help reducing plaque. Whenever teeth are polished, a thin layer of enamel is abraded resulting in loss of fluoride from the tooth surface. Fluoride containing toothpastes may replenish the fluoride abraded by the dentifrice. Since dentifrices do not require specific methods and supervision, their use is considered safe and effective. The common home-use fluorides (concentration, ppm) are given in Table 12.6.

F. Varnish

The topical fluoride agents (NaF, SnF_2, APF in aqueous form) currently in use, have major disadvantage that they remain in contact with the teeth for a very short time and get diluted by saliva. It has also been observed that topical fluoride solutions soon after application, leach away within 24 hours.

The cariostatic effect of topical fluoride agents is related to their ability to deposit

Table 12.6: Topical fluorides (home use)

	Chemical formula	ppm	Concentration
Dentifrice	• NaF	• 1000	• 0.22%
	• SnF	• 1500	• 0.60%
Gel	• NaF	• 1000	• 0.40%
	• APF	• 5000	• 2.0%
	• SnF	• 1500	• 0.60%
Mouthrinse	• NaF	• 230	• 0.05%
	• NaF	• 260	• 0.02%
	• NaF	• 920	• 0.2%
	• NaF	• 200	• 0.044%
	• SnF	• 1500	• 0.63%

fluoride in the enamel superficially and also to their depth of penetration.

To enhance the caries inhibitory property of topical fluoride, researchers were developing methods whereby the contact of fluoride solutions with tooth enamel can be prolonged and also to achieve penetration of fluorides in enamel.

To prolong the action of fluoride in the oral cavity, the teeth were coated with a lacquer containing fluoride (fluoride lacquer), which released fluoride ions for several hours. This led to the concept of fluoride varnish in the caries prevention.

The ingredients commonly used in varnish are:

- *Sodium saccharin:* Used as a sweetener.
- *Flavors:* Different flavors such as raspberry essence, etc.
- *Bees wax and Ethanol:* Forms a gel type structure to stabilize sodium ions.
- *Shellac and mastic:* Provides a flexible permeable hard surface that prevents the varnish dissolving quickly in saliva.
- *Flow enhancer:* Colophonium, which enhances flow.

The types of varnish routinely used are:
a. Duraphat.
b. Fluor Protector.
c. Duraflor.
d. Cavity Shield.
e. Fluoritop.
f. Bifluoride.

a. Duraphat

Duraphat varnish is a formulation of 5.0% sodium fluoride (22,600 ppm) in a viscous colophonium base. The base is saturated in an alcoholic suspension, which evaporates when applied to the tooth surface. One milliliter of the varnish contains 50 mg of NaF (22.6 mg fluoride /ml). It is available as a 10.0 ml tube.

b. Fluor Protector

Fluor protector contains 1.0% difluorosilane in a polyurethane base. Each milliliter of varnish contains 1.0 mg of fluoride (1000 ppm). Fluor protector has a lower pH than Duraphat. Each vial of Fluor Protector contains a 0.4 ml (0.4 mg F) solution. Fluor protector is less viscous than duraphat or duraflor.

c. Duraflor

Duraflor, similar to duraphat, contains 5.0% NaF varnish in an alcoholic suspension. It is supplied as 10 ml tube. One additional ingredient, sweetening agent xylitol, is added in duraflor which may improve taste and patient acceptability. This varnish is less viscous than Duraphat.

d. Cavity Shield

Cavity shield contains 5.0% NaF in a resinous base. Each milliliter contains 50 mg NaF. The difference between cavity shield and other varnishes is that it is a unit-dosed fluoride varnish. Each pouch contains either 0.25 ml (12.5 mg NaF) or 0.4 ml (20 mg NaF).

Cavity shield avoids wastage and is cost-effective. Each patient gets a controlled amount of fluoride, which prevents over-application. It also reduces the chances of over ingestion, subsequently prevents fluoride toxicity.

e. Fluoritop

Fluoritop is manufactured in India (ICPA Health Products Ltd, Mumbai).

It contains 50 mg sodium fluoride per ml equivalent to 22.6 mg of fluoride. It is available in 30 ml plastic bottle.

Various authors have observed reduction in caries prevalence with the use of fluoride varnishes. A single application of duraphat (0.5 ml) contains 11.3 mg F and fluor protector contains 3.1 mg F. The plasma fluoride level for fluor protector has been found to be lower than duraphat owing to low fluoride content.

The plasma fluoride level after 2 hours was found to be 0.180 g/ml after duraphat application and 0.140 g/ml after fluor protector application. A few authors have compared duraphat and fluor protector and have found that caries was significantly reduced by both fluoride varnishes, but duraphat was found to be more effective than fluor protector. However, Groeneveld (1982) has reported no difference in caries incidence after an annual application of fluor protector and duraphat. It has been shown that silane fluoride of fluor protector reacts with water to produce considerable amounts of hydro-fluoric acid (HF), which penetrates enamel more readily than fluoride. Fluorosilanes enhance retention and penetration of fluoride in enamel. It was hypothesized that the acidic condition produced by a reaction between silane fluoride and oral fluids enhances the formation of CaF_2, which leads to slow release of fluoride to the deeper layers. It was also observed that if a sufficient amount of CaF_2 is deposited on the enamel surface for a sufficiently long time, the amount of fluoride in enamel can be increased significantly (Fig. 12.11).

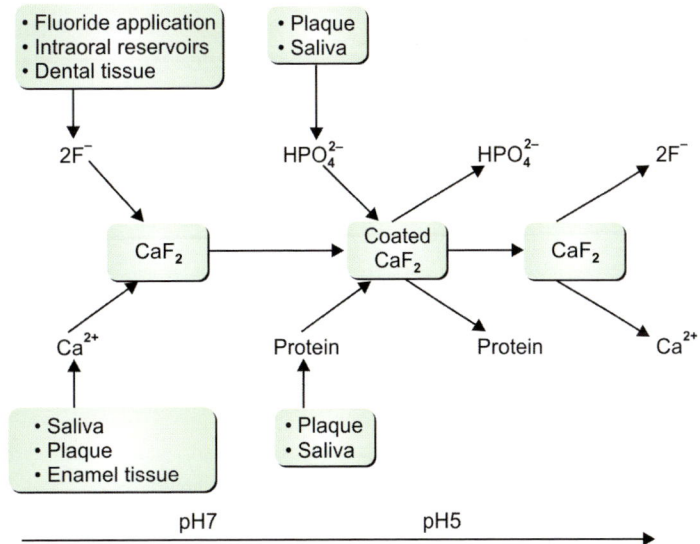

Fig. 12.11: Formation and decomposition of calcium fluoride (Modified from Lussi, 2012)

Procedure

The protocol of fluoride varnish; whether once a week, once a month or four times a year, has not been properly documented. However, twice a year application is considered sufficiently effective. The frequency of fluoride varnish application can be increased depending upon the caries risk of the children. The steps followed are:

- The teeth should be cleaned properly; however, a few authors opined that plaque removal is not critical prior to varnish application.
- The teeth are isolated using cotton rolls. Most varnishes set in the presence of moisture; so drying with air is not necessary.
- Dispense fluoride varnish as per manufacturer's instruction (0.5–1.0 ml is considered adequate for one quadrant).
- Varnish is applied on tooth surface using a disposable brush or cotton applicator. The entire surface of the tooth must be covered. Varnish should not impinge on the soft tissue. The varnish sets in a few seconds leaving a fluoride rich layer (a yellowish brown discoloration) on to the tooth surface.

Children are advised not to brush for at least 12 hours and should avoid solid food (may take liquids).

In order to prevent the deleterious effects of saliva, its flow can be decreased using systemic medicines.

G. Prophylaxis Pastes

The prophylaxis pastes contain a variety of abrasive materials that are helpful in removing extrinsic stains, salivary pellicle and plaque from the tooth surface.

The pastes may and may not contain fluorides. Both types of pastes are helpful in managing plaque, vis-à-vis caries; however, fluoride pastes are considered more effective. Earlier authors confirmed that incorporating fluoride into a prophylaxis paste proved to be an effective cariostatic agent.

Various authors using pumice-hydrogen peroxide slurry containing 1.0% NaF, observed caries reductions ranging from 25–40%.

Two types of fluoride containing prophylaxis pastes (9% SnF_2 with zirconium silicate and 1.23% APF with silicon dioxide) are mainly used.

Various studies conducted on children (age 6–14 years) using these pastes for one year observed substantial decrease in caries prevalence.

Prophylaxis pastes may not play any direct role in the prevention of dental caries. This does not imply that prophylaxis pastes provide no benefit since they do remove extrinsic stains from the teeth. The tooth surface is cleaned so as to facilitate application of fluorides.

REMINERALIZATION

Remineralization infers the restoration of lost dental apatite. Demineralization and remineralization is a continuous process; a disruption in the balance of these two processes could be detrimental to the tooth repair. Incipient carious lesions can be naturally repaired by remineralization (Fig. 12.12). If the lesions are detected at an early stage, the caries development can be avoided. Different strategies that favor remineralization need to be tried to achieve success.

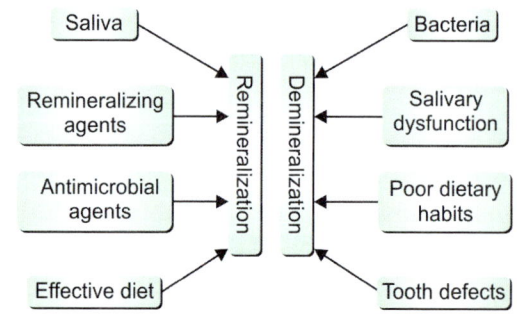

Fig. 12.12: Process of remineralization and demineralization

Requirements of Remineralizing Agents

- Should be safe for human use; be effectively bioactive.
- Should attach itself to the enamel surface and continue its effect for a longer period.
- Should transform into a stable apatite; resistant to subsequent bacterial/acidic attack.
- Should exert a beneficial effect over fluorides.
- Should be active both at the surface and the subsurface of the lesion; can pass through the biofilm and reach the subsurface.

Clinical Effectiveness

The criteria establishing the clinical effectiveness of the remineralizing agents are:

- Should provide additional remineralizing benefit in addition to the natural remineralizing properties of saliva (under most physiological conditions the calcium and phosphate in the saliva and plaque fluid remain supersaturated and favor remineralization over demineralization).
- Must demonstrate better effectiveness over and above the established agents such as fluorides.

The delivery methods of remineralizing agents include toothpastes, mouthrinses, gels, pastes, chewing gums, lozenges, etc.

The commonly employed remineralizing agents are:

i. Fluorides.
ii. Sugar alcohols.
iii. Amorphous calcium phosphate.
iv. Casein phosphopeptides.
v. Bioactive glasses (NovaMin).
vi. Arginine (SensiStat).
vii. Tricalcium phosphate and sodium trimetaphosphate.
viii. Biomimetic remineralization.
ix. Nanohydroxyapatite (nanotechnology).

i. Fluorides

The hard tissues of tooth is made up of hydroxyapatite along with traces of inorganic salts like magnesium, sodium and carbonate, etc.

Hydroxyapatite crystals in presence of fluorides change into fluorapatite crystals which dissolve in the oral environment only at pH lower than 5.0. The critical pH for demineralization process lowers by approximately 0.5–1.0, making the tooth more resistant to demineralization as compared to conventional hydroxyapatite.

It is established that fluorides replaced the hydroxyl ions in the hydroxyapatite lattice. To achieve effective remineralization, fluoride must be constantly present on to the tooth surface.

Dentin is more vulnerable to acid dissolution than enamel due to its chemical composition. The crystal lattice is smaller than the enamel crystals, which means that the surface area is increased, subsequently the crystals are easily attacked. Dentin demineralizes faster and remineralizes slowly than enamel; therefore concentrated fluoride is needed to inhibit demineralization and to enhance remineralization.

Various fluoride preparations (sodium fluoride and strontium fluoride in ppm range 500–5000) have been used as topical agents enhancing remineralization.

Titaniumtetrafluoride (TiF_4) has also shown effectiveness against caries. The interaction of titanium fluoride with the tooth tissues leads to the formation of a resistant coating on the tooth surface, which helps in rapid and higher uptake of fluoride. It is non-irritating, stable and nontoxic solution; however, its high acidity is of concern to the researchers.

It is established that TiF_4 have great advantages as compared to other topically used fluorides. Higher uptake and greater penetration of fluoride and lower acid solubility of the tissues has been observed with TiF_4 as compared to sodium fluoride. In the case of acidulated phosphate fluoride (APF), a considerable uptake and penetration of fluoride has also been observed.

During erosion, the pH drops far below the critical pH of fluorapatite, which explains that the fluorides may not be very effective against erosion lesions.

ii. *Sugar Alcohols*

Sugar is the established 'criminal' in caries process. Various substitutes of sugars have shown better results in managing caries. The bacterial flora do not utilize sugar alcohols as good as sugars, affecting their growth and accumulation in plaque. Artificial sugars like xylitol, etc. are known to induce remineralization of demineralized enamel by facilitating calcium movement. Xylitol chewing gum also increases salivary flow rate, thereby enhancing the protective properties of saliva. The concentration of bicarbonate and phosphate is higher in stimulated saliva; the resultant increase in plaque pH and salivary buffering capacity prevents demineralization of tooth structure. The higher concentration of calcium, phosphate and hydroxyl ions in stimulated saliva enhances remineralization.

iii. *Amorphous Calcium Phosphate*

Amorphous calcium phosphate (ACP) is the initial solid phase that precipitates from a highly supersaturated calcium phosphate solution and can convert readily to stable octacalcium phosphate/other apatites. It acts as a bioapatite precursor, playing a vital role in biomineralization.

The ACP technology was incorporated into toothpastes, viz. Enamelon, Recaldent, etc. It was also used in other topical preparations as White Bleaching Gel, Polishing Paste and Pit and Fissure Sealant.

The ACP technology is a two-phase delivery system. The rationale is to avoid calcium and phosphorus components from reacting with each other before use. Currently two salts are used; calcium sulfate for calcium and dipotassium phosphate for phosphorous. When the two salts are mixed, they rapidly form ACP that can precipitate onto the tooth

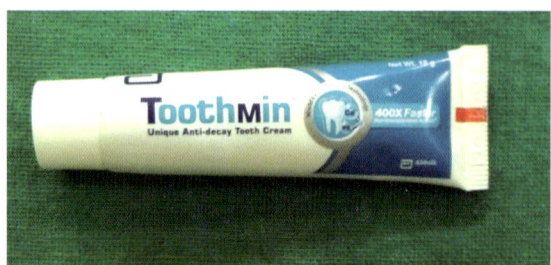

Fig. 12.13: ToothMin tooth cream

surface and help remineralization. Calcium sucrose phosphate (commercial preparation ToothMin) is also being used as a remineralizing agent (Fig. 12.13).

iv. *Casein Phosphopeptides*

Caseins are a heterogeneous family of proteins predominated by α1, α2 and β-caseins. A complex of casein phosphopeptides (CPPs) and amorphous calcium phosphate (ACP) is used having the ability to bind/stabilize calcium and phosphate in oral solutions and also bind plaque and enamel.

The casein phosphopeptides inhibit adherence of oral bacteria to saliva-coated hydroxyapatites. By selectively inhibiting streptococcal adhesion to teeth, the microbial composition of plaque favors establishment of less cariogenic species, viz. actinomyces, etc. They also act as buffering agents, preventing a pH decrease in the oral cavity, the saliva and plaque. The buffering capacity helps preventing the dissolution of hydroxyapatite from the enamel; enamel is remineralized following combined use of CPP-ACP and is more acid-resistant than normal enamel. It is established that CPP-ACP remineralize the interior of the lesions; whereas fluorides remineralize the lesion surfaces only.

v. *Bioactive Glasses (NovaMin)*

Bioactive glasses have long been used in dentistry. NovaMin is one such technology whereby bioactive glass material (less than 20 microns) is used to remineralize tooth tissues.

When NovaMin comes in contact with saliva or any aqueous media, it releases sodium ions, elevating the pH to 7.5–8.5, considered essential for hydroxyapatite formation. The calcium and phosphates are released supplementing the normal levels found in saliva. This increase in ionic concentration and also in pH help forming calcium hydroxy-carbonate apatite, required to remineralize the defective tooth surfaces. NovaMin alone and in combination with fluorides enhance remineralization and prevent demineralization. The antibacterial effect of NovaMin is originated from its sodium and calcium contents followed by high rates of ion release with their associated local changes in pH. It adheres to exposed tooth surface and forms a mineralized layer that is resistant to acid. The release of calcium is continuous over time, maintaining the protective effects on dentin. Commercial products based on NovaMin technology include SootheRx, NUPRO Sensodyne solution, etc.

vi. *Arginine (SensiStat)*

Arginine bicarbonate, an amino acid complex along with particles of calcium carbonate is commonly available in toothpastes (SensiStat). The arginine complex is responsible for adhering the calcium carbonate particles to the dentin or enamel surface. The dissolution of calcium carbonate releases calcium that helps in remineralization of the tooth surface. A combination of arginine bicarbonate and sodium monofluorophosphate has also been tried in dentin hypersensitivity.

vii. *Tricalcium Phosphate and Sodium Trimetaphosphate*

β-tricalcium phosphate (TCP) alone and in combination with fluorides has been tried as a remineralizing agent in topical agents (TCP and 1000–5000 ppm F used in toothpastes). This combination improves remineralization by building stronger, more acid-resistant mineral in eroded tooth tissues. It is also used in treatment of white spot lesions. The commercial products are Cerasorb, Bio-Resorb, etc.

Trimetaphosphate (TMP) ions adsorb on to the enamel surface, causing a barrier coating that is effective in preventing or retarding acidic challenges and hence reducing demineralization.

viii. *Biomimetic Remineralization*

The biomimetic remineralization infers the use of polyanionic molecules to mimic the biological functions of noncollagenous proteins of dentin during the natural biomineralization process. The conventional remineralization techniques differ in two aspects as compared to biomimetic effect.

First, it mimics the dehydration mechanism of natural biomineralization by replacing the free and loosely bound water within a collagen matrix. The polyanions (calcium phosphate nanoprecursors) help in this phenomenon.

Second, the biomimetic mineralization approach proceeds in the absence of apatite crystals in a collagen matrix. Mineralization in the absence of apatite crystals requires alternate pathways for lowering the activation energy barrier for crystal nucleation.

ix. *Nanohydroxyapatite (Nanotechnology)*

Nanohydroxyapatite (nHA) have been used in the paste form showing potential for remineralization (Fig. 12.14). The use of a toothpaste containing nanosized calcium carbonate enabled remineralization of early enamel lesions. The bacteriostatic effects of silver, zinc oxide and gold nanoparticles on

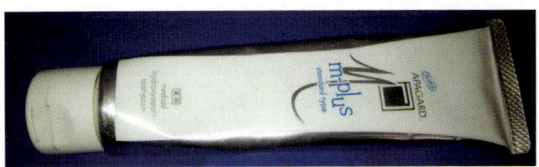

Fig. 12.14: Nanohydroxyapatite paste

Streptococcus mutans has been established. It is reported that silver nanoparticles had an antimicrobial effect even in lower concentrations as compared to other nanoparticles.

Combination of nHA and fluoride enhances the effectiveness of both nHA and fluoride.

PROBIOTICS AND CARIES PREVENTION

The ancient Roman literature has mentioned about food fermented with micro-organisms, which could be used as a therapeutic agent. Earlier authors established that lactic acid producing strain *Lactobacillus bulgaricus* was capable of replacing pathological intestinal microbiota by useful microbes. Elie Metchnikoff in his early studies stated that 'Probiotics are viable bacteria that beneficially affect the host by improving its intestinal microbial balance.'

The term probiotic, meaning *for life*, was first used to describe substances secreted by one micro-organism which stimulates the growth of another. It can be defined as 'Live micro-organisms which when administered in adequate amounts in food or as dietary supplements confer a health benefit on the host'. Food and Agricultural Organization of United Nations has defined Probiotics as *live micro-organisms, principally bacteria, that are safe for human consumption and, when ingested in sufficient quantities, have beneficial effects on human health, beyond basic nutrition*. In dentistry, they help improvement of the flora of oral cavity, subsequently preventing caries.

The term probiotic is to be differentiated from *Prebiotic* and *Synbiotic*. Prebiotics is defined as 'the ingestible food ingredients that beneficially affects the host by stimulating the growth and/or activity of, one or a limited number of bacteria in the colon. Synbiotic term is used when a product contains both prebiotics and probiotics. The food supplement includes both the live cells of the beneficial bacteria and the selective substrate.

In the recent past, there has been a paradigm shift towards an ecological and microbial based approach to understand oral diseases. This led to the possibility of developing novel strategies, may also be through manipulation of the resident oral microbiota and the host immune responses. Dental caries is one of the most common disease affecting people throughout their lifetime. Various approaches are being tried to prevent caries; however, effects of these approaches are still limited. The probiotic bacteria supplements have been successfully used to improve gastrointestinal health, which prompted the researchers to utilize this approach for oral applications.

The oral diseases which can be managed by probiotics include caries, gingivitis/periodontitis, halitosis, oral candidiasis, xerostomia, etc. The main aim is to control and manipulate oral-pharyngeal microbiota.

Requisite Characteristics of Probiotic Bacteria

The vast majority of these bacterial species having probiotic properties are isolated from healthy humans although a few also originate from fermented food.

The requisite characteristics of probiotic bacteria are:

- The bacterial strain and species must easily be identified.
- Should have good growth potential.
- The bacterial strains should be resistant to antibiotics; characterized by their metabolic and hemolytic activities and capacity to produce toxins.
- Should be able to survive the pH changes in the oral cavity and the salivary stress factors.
- Should be able to colonize the sloughing and non-sloughing surfaces of the oral habitat.
- Should be compatible to biofilm microflora.
- Should be non-pathogenic.

- Should not transmit antibiotic resistance genes to other genera.
- Should be isolated from the same species.
- Should have binding capacity, especially on tooth tissues.
- Should minimize inflammatory response.

Probiotic Micro-organisms used in Food Items

Many strains have been used in oral probiotics. The common ones are:

- Lactobacillus strains (*L. rhamnosus* GG, *L. reuteri*, *L. salivarius*, Certain strains of *L. casei* and *L. acidophilus*).
- Bifidobacteria (*B. bifidum*, *B. longum*, *B. breave*, *B. adolescentis*).
- Strains of *Escherichia coli*.
- *Enterococcus faecium* strain (SF68).
- *Saccharomyces boulardi* (yeast).
- Propionibacterium.
- Streptococcus strains (*S. lactis*, *S. salivarius*, *S. thermophilus*).
- *Weissella cibaria*.

The mechanism of action of common probiotic bacteria is:

1. *Lactobacillus rhamnosus:* Hampers growth of oral *Streptococcus mutans*.
2. *Weisella cibaria:* Secretes significant quantity of hydrogen peroxide and bacteriocin that acts against gram-positive bacteria; co-aggregates with *Fusobacterium nucleatum* and forms a barrier, which prevents the colonization of pathogenic bacteria.
3. *Lactobacillus reuteri:* Decreases plaque deposition; effective against *Streptococcus mutans*.
4. *Streptococcus thermophillus and Lactobacillus lactis:* Decreases cariogenic bacterial levels.
5. *Bifidobacterium:* Inhibits growth of *Streptococcus mutans*.

Availability of Probiotics (Figs 12.15a to c)

i. As a culture concentrate added to beverages; for example, fruit juices.

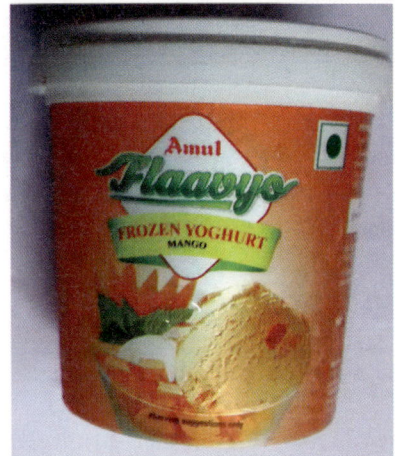

Fig. 12.15a: Probiotic frozen yoghurt

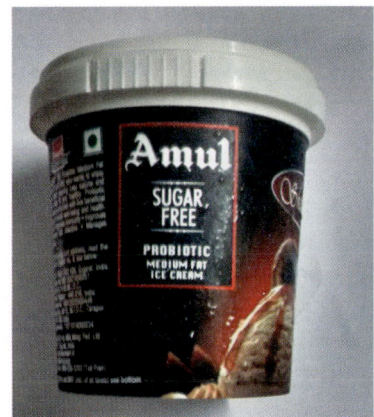

Fig. 12.15b: Probiotic ice cream

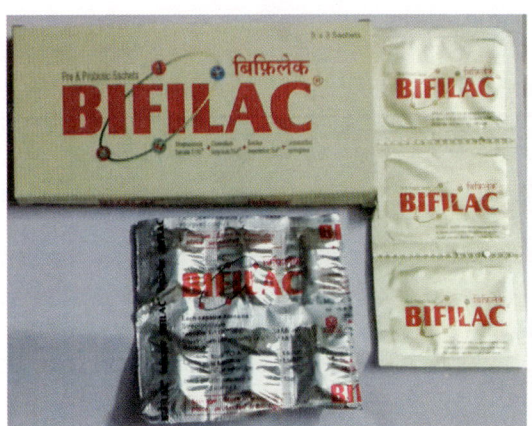

Fig. 12.15c: Probiotic tablet

ii. Inoculated into prebiotic fibres which promote the growth of probiotic bacteria.

iii. Inoculated into milk and milk based foods; for example, milk drinks, yoghurt, ice cream, cheese, etc.

iv. As lyophilized, dried cells packaged as dietary supplements; for example, tablets, chewing gums, etc.

Delivery of Probiotics

Probiotics are administered in the form of sachets or capsules, or even added directly to the food items. The vehicle by which probiotics are ingested and delivered to oral environment affects their colonization in the oral cavity. Probiotics are ingested through fortified foods (Yogurt, cheese, butter milk), lozenges, mouthrinses, etc. The dietary lactobacilli are commonly consumed in milk products, viz. yoghurt, cheese, etc. When lactic acid bacteria are being consumed in milk products, the buffer capacity of the milk will decrease the production of acid. The presence of calcium, calcium lactate and other organic and inorganic compounds in milk are anticariogenic, which could reduce the colonization of the pathogen.

The important factors are the formulations, the vehicles of delivery and the frequency of administration of probiotics. Usually the administration is carried out once or twice daily. The formulation has to be acid/alkali stable while at the same time palatable. The vehicle of delivery should be stable to deliver the appropriate quantity of organism/dose; generally 10^{10} CFU/ml. The dose is considered sufficient if reinforced with proper oral hygiene measures. The most appropriate time of delivery of probiotics is before bedtime, preferably after brushing and flossing.

An early installation and colonization of probiotics in the oral environment is mandatory to achieve its long term effects. Permanent installation of probiotics is usually difficult; however, transient colonization using the probiotic products can be achieved.

Another potential probiotic approach for reducing dental caries involves the use of oral streptococci that are able to metabolise arginine/urea to ammonia. Recently, *Streptococcus oligofermentans*, a bacterium isolated from caries-free humans, was found to metabolize lactic acid into hydrogen peroxide, thus inhibiting the growth of *Streptococcus mutans*.

Mechanism of Action

- Probiotics create a biofilm, which acts as a protective lining minimizing bacterial pathogens to colonize on oral tissues.
- They modify the oral environment by modulating the pH and/or the oxidation-reduction potential, thus compromising the ability of pathogens to colonize.
- These bacteria secrete various antimicrobial substances such as organic acids, hydrogen peroxide and bacteriocins, which act against oral pathogens.
- They compete for adhesion sites with cariogenic bacteria and also for their nutrients.
- Probiotics may provide beneficial effects by stimulating non-specific immunity and modulating the humoral and cellular immune response (enhance production of IgA and defensins) (Flowchart 12.1).

Role of Probiotics in Caries Prevention

The carious process involves acidogenic and acid-tolerating bacterial species in oral cavity. Mutans streptococci and lactobacilli are observed in abundance; however, other bacteria can also be found like *Bifidobacteria*, *Actinomyces* spp., *Propionibacterium* spp., *Veillonella* spp., etc. Use of probiotics and molecular genetics to replace and displace cariogenic bacteria with non-cariogenic bacteria have been tried with varying results.

The probiotics should adhere to dental tissues creating the biofilm. These bacteria compete with the growth of cariogenic bacteria and subsequently preventing their

Flowchart 12.1: Mechanism of action of probiotic bacteria

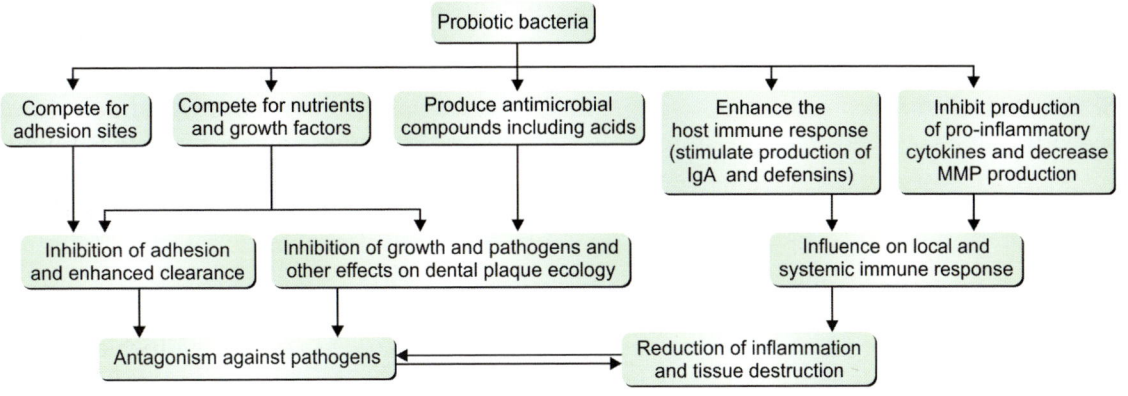

proliferation. The metabolism of sugars by the probiotic should also result in low acid production. It is reported that *Streptococcus thermophilus* and *Lactobacillus lactis* were among the few bacteria having capacity to integrate into the biofilm and interfere with development of the cariogenic microflora.

Recently, it was demonstrated that isolates of *Weissella cibaria* had the capacity to inhibit biofilm formation by *Streptococcus mutans* and to prevent proliferation of this bacterial strain. A few authors have also observed a competition between *Lactobacillus rhamnosus* and *Streptococcus sobrinus*.

It has been established that lactobacillus and Bifidobacterium strains used in commercial probiotic products may affect the oral ecology by specifically preventing the adherence of *Streptococcus mutans* and by modifying the protein composition of the salivary pellicle.

The studies which utilized probiotics adopted the following approaches:
1. Utilizing bacteria that expressed bacteriocins or bacteriocin-like inhibitory substances that specifically prevented the growth of cariogenic bacteria.
2. Probiotic bacteria having ability to colonize teeth and influence the supragingival plaque.
3. Bacterial strains were screened for suitable antagonistic activity against relevant oral bacteria.

4. Recombinant strain of *Streptococcus mutans* expressing urease, which can reduce the cariogenicity of plaque.
5. Genetically modified probiotics, viz. a recombinant strain of Lactobacillus that expressed antibodies targeting adhesions of *Streptococcus mutans* (antigen I/II) and reducing their viable counts, thereby caries.

Several studies have established that regular consumption of yogurt, milk or cheese containing probiotics led to a decrease in the number of cariogenic streptococci in the oral environment. Nikawa, et al (2004) reported that consumption of yogurt containing *Lactobacillus reuteri* over a period of two weeks, reduced the concentration of *Streptococcus mutans* up to 80%. A couple of long term studies on young children have also reported significantly fewer counts of *Streptococcus mutans* and less caries after consuming milk containing probiotics.

Kang, et al (2006) in their study using mouthrinses having *Weissella cibaria* observed that the water soluble polymers produced sucrose by *Weissella cibaria* inhibited the formation of *Streptococcus mutans* biofilm.

Caglar, et al (2006) investigated the effect of probiotic bacteria *Lactobacillus reuteri* on the levels of *Streptococcus mutans* and *lactobacilli* and observed that by using their lozenges, the level of *Streptococcus mutans* was reduced.

Summary of the studies carried out to assess the effects of probiotics strains is tabulated in Table 12.7.

Side Effects and Risks

Side effects of probiotics are usually mild in the form of gas or bloating. Serious side effects have also been observed in a few cases. Probiotics may lead to severe infections that need to be treated with antibiotics, especially in people with compromised health conditions. The probiotic infection may cause unhealthy metabolic activities, too much stimulation of the immune system, or even gene transfer.

Probiotic products usually taken as a dietary supplement are regulated as food and not as drugs. Furthermore, uncertainty about specificity of effects of probiotics and their mechanism of action remains a cause of concern.

Based on the currently available clinical data, it seems that dietary probiotics do not confer a major risk for oral health. However, the possibility of transferring antibiotic resistance from probiotics to virulent micro-organisms needs thorough evaluation. There is a great need to identify and elucidate the role of beneficial bacteria by conducting large-scale studies on the usefulness of probiotics in improving oral health.

Most of the cases of infection occur in the patients with immuno-compromised or underlying diseases such as diabetes, cardiovascular disease, gastrointestinal disorder, malignancies, or organ transplant patients. However, there has not been any reported evidence that consumption of either lactobacilli or bifidobacteria exert increased risk of opportunistic infections among immuno-compromised patients who are more vulnerable to pathogenic bacterial infection or have more risk of opportunistic infections. The safety of probiotics in patients with HIV infection has also been documented.

Precautions and Contraindications

Since probiotics contain live micro-organisms, these preparations may cause pathological

Table 12.7: Studies assessing the effects of probiotic strains			
Author	*Study*	*Probiotic species*	*Inference*
Nase, et al (2001)	594 children, 1–6 years; milk for 7 months	*Lactobacillus rhamnosus* GG	Decreased *S. mutans* count Decreased caries
Cagler, et al (2006)	120, 21–24 years; Tablet for three weeks	*Lactobacillus reuteri*	Decreased *S. mutans* count
Caglar, et al (2007)	80, 21–24 years; Chewing gum for three weeks	*Lactobacillus reuteri*	Decreased *S. mutans* count
Stecksen-Bricks, et al (2009)	248, 1–5 years; capsules in milk for 21 months	*Lactobacillus rhamnosus* LB 21 and fluorides	Decreased caries
Tenzer, et al (2010)	20, 21 days old rats; food supplements	*Lactobacillus paracasei* DSMZ 16671	Inhibited colonization of *S. mutans* and caries in rats
Lexner, et al (2010)	18 adolescents; milk for two weeks	*Lactobacillus rhamnosus* LB 21	No effect
Petersson, et al (2011)	160, 58–84 years; milk for 15 months	*Lactobacillus rhamnosus* LB 21	Reverse primary root caries
Chuang, et al (2011)	78, 20–26 years; Tablets for two weeks	*Lactobacillus paracasei* GM50L-33	Decrease *S. mutans* count

infections, especially in severely immuno-compromised patients. Probiotic strains of Lactobacillus have been reported to cause bacteremia in patients with short-bowel syndrome. Lactobacillus preparations are contraindicated in persons with a hyper-sensitivity to lactose or milk. *Streptococcus boulardii* is contraindicated in patients with a yeast allergy. However, no contraindications have been listed for Bifidobacteria, since most species are considered nonpathogenic and non-toxigenic.

Probiotic Products

The commonly available probiotic products are:

i. Evora Plus/EvoraPro

EvoraPlus/Evora Pro is a probiotic mint that contains the blend of patented beneficial bacteria. This all-in-one product provides naturally fresh breath while gently whitening teeth. The beneficial bacteria inhibit the destructive bacteria from overpopulating and creating imbalances in the oral cavity.

ii. BioGaia

BioGaia is the combination of two complementary strains, *Lactobacillus reuteri* (DSM17938) and *Lactobacillus reuteri* (ATCC PTA 5289), specifically selected for their exclusive synergistic properties in reducing plaque, gingivitis and periodontitis.

iii. BLIS M18

BLIS M18, developed from a specific strain of *Streptococcus salivarius* (a common and beneficial oral bacterium) has shown promising result in improving oral health.

Besides competing for space and nutrients, it also produces three potent antibacterial BLIS molecules: Salivaricin A, Salivaricin 9 and Salivaricin M, which act upon microbes in the oral cavity giving BLIS M18 a wider range of activity, especially its potential to inhibit *Streptococcus mutans*.

iv. Probiotic Mixture (ProBiora 3)

ProBiora 3 contains a proprietary blend of three selected species of naturally occurring oral bacteria, each with a specific function for maintaining a healthy oral environment. These strains include *Streptococcus oralis* (KJ3sm), *Streptococcus uberis* (KJ2sm) and *Streptococcus rattus* (JH145).

A mixture of *Lactobacillus rhamnosus* GG and *Lactobacillus casei* have also reported temporary reduction in *Streptococcus mutans* levels during the period of probiotic treatment.

v. Oraldiet

Oraldiet is an oral probiotic lozenge that contains lactobacillus reuteri. Each pack contains 30 mint lozenges, which is more suitable for vegetarians. It is advised not to brush teeth or rinse after taking Oraldiet.

REPLACEMENT THERAPY

Replacement therapy involves use of an effector strain that is permanently colonized in the particular site of the host. This effector strain is designed to prevent the colonization/growth of a particular pathogen.

Replacement therapy has also been referred to as *modified probiotic therapy*, wherein a natural or genetically modified effector strain is used to intentionally colonize the sites in susceptible host tissues that are normally colonized by a pathogen. The differences of Replacement therapy and Probiotics are tabulated in Table 12.8. If the effector strain is better adapted than the pathogen, colonization/growth of the pathogen will be prevented by blocking the attachment sites or by competing for essential nutrients; may be by other mechanisms. As long as the effector strain persists as a resident of the indigenous flora, the host is protected for an unlimited period of time. It is established that both positive and negative bacterial interactions occur, or by which a specific indigenous micro-organism either promotes or blocks the presence of a pathogen.

Table 12.8: Differences of replacement therapy and probiotics	
Replacement therapy	*Probiotics*
• Effector strain is applied directly on the site of infection	• Generally used as dietary supplements
• Involves long term change in the indigenous microbiota	• Long term change is rare
• Colonization of the site by the effector strain is essential	• Exert beneficial effect without permanently colonizing the site
• Has minimal immunological impact	• Influence the immunological response

In order to achieve optimal remineralization, a genetically engineered 'effector strain' of *Streptococcus mutans* that will replace the cariogenic strain is applied to prevent/arrest caries. Another approach is based on a genetic modification of cariogenic streptococci spp. to create organisms that produce ammonia from urea and arginine. These organisms will reside in dental plaque and the ammonia produced from salivary and dietary substrates will prevent the colonization of cariogenic bacteria.

Implantation of an effector strain should be carried out in children immediately after tooth eruption and before the acquisition of a caries-inducing strain. To prevent over-colonization by cariogenic strains, an effector strain should provide selective advantage to colonization. This would also enable subjects who have already been infected with a caries-inducing strain of *Streptococcus mutans* to be treated by replacement therapy.

Advantages

- Provides lifelong protection by a single application.
- Provides protection via natural transmission of the therapeutic micro-organism within the human population.
- Negligible risk.
- No need for patient education and compliance.
- Low cost.
- Short time of application.

Limitations

The minimum infectious dose has not been determined for this strain or any *Streptococcus*

mutans strain in humans. There is need to perform further studies with larger populations to measure the potential for horizontal transmission. It is presumed that, like cariogenic strains of *Streptococcus mutans*, vertical transmission of BCS3-L1 from mother to child may also occur.

Effector Strains

Streptococcus mutans strain BCS3-L1 is a genetically modified effector strain designed for use in replacement therapy to prevent dental caries. Effector strain must satisfy the following pre-requisites:

- Should be genetically stable.
- Should have a significantly reduced pathogenic potential to promote caries.
- It must persistently colonize the *Streptococcus mutans* sites, thereby preventing colonization by disease-causing strains.
- Should displace indigenous strains of *Streptococcus mutans*, allowing previously infected subjects to be treated with replacement therapy.
- Should be safe and not make the host susceptible to other diseases.

It is established that an LDH-deficient *Streptococcus mutans* strain (BCS3-L1) has significantly reduced pathogenic potential and thus satisfy the first prerequisite for use as an effector strain in replacement therapy. This reduced acidogenic potential of BCS3-L1 has been demonstrated in animal models.

Mutacin 1140 is capable of killing virtually all other strains of mutans streptococci against which it was tested, but it has not been purified to directly test its toxicity. However, the prototype 1 antibiotic, nisin, have extremely low toxicity. Mutacin production by BCS3-L1 and the fermentation products resulting from LDH deficiency could alter plaque ecology and produce another micro-organism with reduced pathogenic potential. The reduced pathogenic potential of the BCS3-L1 probiotic strain, its proven colonization potential and its genetic stability support its potential use as an effector strain for replacement therapy.

Antibacterial Peptides

The antimicrobial peptides interfere mainly with the multiplication of pathogens. Antimicrobial peptides are a new class of antimicrobial therapeutic agents that are also being tried.

The benefits of antimicrobial peptides include:

- Can be used directly.
- Serve as a selective force to maintain a non-pathogenic bacteriocin-producing strain in an effort to prevent establishment of the pathogenic strain.

Mechanism of Action

a. Initial Attraction

The antimicrobial peptides are initially attracted to the cell-wall of micro-organisms by electrostatic interactions between the anionic or cationic peptides on the cell surface.

- *Gram-negative bacteria:* Cationic peptides and the negative charges present on the bacterial envelope interact (the anionic phospholipid and the phosphate group of lipopolysaccharide).
- *Gram-positive bacteria:* The primary relationship occurs between anionic antimicrobial peptides and the cell surface teichoic acid and lipoteichoic acid.

b. Attachment Phase

After the initial attraction, the antimicrobial peptides bind to cell surfaces and initiates the attachment phase. They cross through the outer membrane (lipopolysaccharides in Gram-negative bacteria and teichoic and lipoteichoic acids in Gram-positive bacteria) and interact directly with the bacterial cytoplasmic membrane.

At low peptide/lipid ratios, the anti-microbial peptides are connected parallel to the lipid bilayer. As this ratio increases, the peptides begin to orient perpendicularly to the membrane. When peptide/lipid ratios are high, antimicrobial peptides will start to penetrate the cell membrane, leading to the formation of transmembrane pores that subsequently cause cell death by loss of fluid and disruption of the cell membrane.

SMaRT Replacement Technology

SMaRT Replacement technology (Company-Oragenics) is based on the creation of a genetically altered strain of *S. mutans*, called SMaRT, which does not produce lactic acid. Further they are engineered to have a selective colonization over native *S. mutans* strains. SMaRT also releases lantibiotic that kills the native strains but leaves the SMaRT strain unharmed. Lantibiotics are rare antibiotic compounds having ability to overcome antibiotic-resistant infections. The SMaRT Replacement technology can permanently replace native lactic acid-producing strains of *S. mutans* in the oral cavity, thereby providing lifelong protection against the primary cause of tooth decay. This material will displace the native *S. mutans* strains over a six to twelve months period and permanently occupy that site affording a lifelong prevention of caries.

BACTERIOCIN LIKE INHIBITORY SUBSTANCES (BLIS)

Bacteriocins are bacterially produced natural peptides released by different varieties of bacteria and archea that are active against other bacteria. Bacteriocins are proteins that kill representatives of same species as the producer organism or related species. A large amount of bacteriocins have a relatively narrow spectrum of antibacterial activity, i.e. inhibit growth of only certain species, generally those phylogenetically related to the producer strain. A few bacteriocins exhibit broader spectrum, which includes protozoa, yeast, fungi, etc. Bacteriocins are distinguished from antibodies by two features: (i) bacteriocins are ribosomally synthesized and (ii) have relatively narrow killing spectrum.

Bacteriocin-like inhibitory substances (BLIS) is a new method of caries control which depends upon exploiting the ability of certain bacteria to produce antibiotics like substances. It has been tried through oral administration of the purified BLIS or the genetic modification of existing plaque bacteria. In caries prevention, BLIS is being used to eliminate or de-activate cariogenic flora of the oral cavity, especially *Streptococcus mutans*.

Streptococcus salivarius is considered as the most beneficial bacteria of the oral cavity; however, all strains of *S. salivarius* do not act equally to inhibit other oral microbes. It might be the first oral probiotic, a bacterium shown to colonize the oral cavity and to express a wide variety of anti-competitor molecules, termed BLIS (bacteriocin-like inhibitory substances) capable of targeting oral pathogens.

A few longitudinal studies conducted on Dunedin schoolchildren have observed that *S. salivarius* was the commensal streptococcal species that could express the strongest and wide variety of bacteriocin-like activities, especially directed against *S. pyogenes*.

BLIS produced by *S. salivarius* have the following characteristics:

- Show inhibitory activity against a variety of oral pathogens.
- Exhibit adhesion specificity for oral tissues, subsequently increasing their colonization efficacy and oral retention, thereby resulting in enhanced immune defense against virus infection.
- Exhibit immune reactivity due to interaction with immunocytes or immunologically

responsive oral tissues. Interestingly, strain K12 has been shown to be inhibitory to group B streptococci, the major bacterial pathogen for newborn infants. It is known that during the first year of life, *S. salivarius* establishes within the nasopharynx. Dental caries, being the public health issue for young children, the strain M18 displays greatest potential for modulation of the caries potential of oral flora.

Action: Bacteriocins interact with a sensitive cell and interfere with its multiplication, metabolism or viability. However, they may or may not have to enter a sensitive cell to be effective, not all are bactericidal against their susceptible target cells. They may assist in the elimination of susceptible bacteria in conditions where competition with closely-related bacteria exists.

Bacteriocins Active Against Caries inducing Bacteria

The following bacteriocins are considered active against caries inducing bacteria.

Mutacins: It is the bacteriocin derived from mutans streptococci having definite influence on the composition of plaque. Different forms of mutacin are:

- *MutacinRm10:* This extracellular bacteriocin was isolated from culture supernatants of *Streptococcus mutans* strain Rm10. Mutacin-Rm10 was shown to be active against mutans streptococci of all serotypes, but not against most tested *S. salivarius*. Oral rinsing with this bacteriocin for 20 minutes has shown to reduce the number of viable bacteria.

- *MutacinC3603:* Bacteriocin from *Streptococcus mutans* strain C3603 (serotype c). It reduced the caries score in *in-vivo* studies with gnotobiotic and specific pathogen-free rats infected with *Streptococcus mutans* serotype c.

- *Mutacin MT3791:* Isolated from the *Streptococcus sobrinus* strain MT3791 (serotype g). It is bacteriocidal against sensitive cells inhibiting DNA, RNA and protein synthesis. It selectively inhibits the growth of *Streptococcus mutans* present in antimicrobial peptides (especially plaque active carious lesions in children).

- *Mutacin 6:* Bacteriocin produced by *S. rattus* strain BHT in liquid media. It is active against a wide variety of oral streptococci.
- *Mutacin II, MutacinsC67-1 and Ny266:* Isolated from a strain of *Streptococcus mutans*. Mutacins C67-1 and Ny266 appear to have the most potential for therapeutic use against gram-positive bacteria because of their wide inhibitory spectra, their thermo-resistance and their small molecular masses.
- *MutacinJH1000:* Strain JH1000 of *Streptococcus mutans* (serotype c) was found to produce antibacterial activity beginning during the early stationary phase of growth and active across a broad range of pH.
- *Mutacin JH1001:* Mutacin JH1001 is a *Streptococcus mutans* strain for bacteriocin production. It is a small molecule synthesized in detectable amounts, which inhibited the growth of virtually every other strain of this organism. The strain JH1001 has been found to colonize the human oral cavity for a longer period; even after two and half years later. JH1001 was found to be active against indigenous mutans streptococci.
- *Bacteriocin MT6223:* It is isolated from *Streptococcus sobrinus* MT6223, had some activity against all serotypes (species) of the *Streptococci mutans*, but it was less effective against serotypes d and g. Bacteriocin-treated sensitive cells are characterized by inhibited synthesis of DNA, RNA and proteins.
- *Mutalipocins:* These are lipid-like anti-bacterial, low molecular weight molecules that are soluble in organic solvents. They are characterized by a narrower spectrum of killing activity than other bacteriocins of Gram-positive bacteria. They are widely active against mutans streptococci.

- *Other antimicrobial peptides:* Human Cathelicidins (one-gene peptide), Human Cathelicidin LL-37 (Dermicidin), Human Histacins (Two-gene peptides) and Human Defensins are a few recent mutacins targeting the cells, inhibiting their DNA/RNA synthesis and also the enzymatic activity.

Limitations
- Non-physiological conditions are significantly reduced in biological fluids (plasma, serum or saliva).
- Due to high toxicity and rapid renal excretion of some antimicrobial peptides, it is difficult to use them by parenteral route.
- High cost of production of native peptides.

STAMP (specifically targeted antimicrobial peptides): These molecules are modified to carry peptide to a recognized domain specific for a particular group of micro-organisms; enabling the antimicrobial peptides to affect the specific microbes without changing the indigenous microbial flora.

The goal for achieving successful replacement therapy is to find an effector strain which is a non-pathogenic micro-organism capable of establishing the same ecological niche as the targeted pathogen(s) and which is capable of specific inhibition or replacement of the target pathogen(s). Replacement therapy using a carefully-selected bacteriocin provides an ecologically sound mechanism for the site-specific and also delivery of a specific bacteriocin having activity against a limited range of pathogenic bacterial species. The design of synthetic peptides and specifically targeted anti-microbial peptides have become increasingly viable, considering new developments in protein synthesis and its purification.

BIOTENE AND CARIES PREVENTION

Biotene, a blend of antibacterial enzymes, found naturally in human saliva contains mainly three enzymes, viz. Glucose oxidase, Lactoperoxidase and Lysozyme, which play an important role in boosting and replenishing saliva's own defense system. Their antibacterial and healing properties create a natural protection. Biotene products, available in the form of toothpaste, gel, mouthwash, etc. are generally prescribed to increase salivary flow in patients suffering from xerostomia. The lack of saliva increases the risk of caries and also creates an uncomfortable sensation of dryness. Biotene oral products to treat dry mouth include toothpaste, mouthwash etc., whereas certain mouth spray and gels are helpful in relieving the discomfort associated with xerostomia. Biotene oral balance gel is a saliva replacement gel containing glucose oxidase (inhibits bacterial growth as it has acidic pH). Properly balanced artificial saliva should be of neutral pH and contain electrolytes corresponding approximately to the composition of saliva; however, some artificial salivary products may cause dental caries because of acidic pH.

Biotene products have been tried in caries prevention with varying results. Earlier authors proposed the use of Biotene antimicrobial mouthrinses as a means of reducing the levels of oral bacteria, specifically *Streptococcus mutans.* They opined that mouthwash containing bioactive preparations were most effective in reducing the level of mutans streptococci in plaque.

A few authors investigated the effect of antimicrobial mouthwash containing bioactive enzymes (Lysozyme, Lactoferrin, Glucose oxidase, Lactoperoxidase) in inhibiting the growth of mutans streptococci in dental plaque. They confirmed that mouth rinsing with Biotene has antibacterial efficacy, especially against *Streptococcus mutans*.

Various studies could not endorse the positive observation of early authors. A study evaluated the efficacy of three antiseptic mouthrinses: 0.1% octenidine dihydrochloride, 0.12% chlorhexidine digluconate and Biotene antimicrobial rinse in adults. *Streptococcus mutans* levels in saliva were evaluated according to total number of colony forming unit (CFU) per ml. Compared to other rinses, Biotene showed no effects on *Streptococcus mutans* levels.

In an another double-blind study using oral balance gel and Biotene toothpaste versus placebo in patients with xerostomia following radiation therapy, superior palliative effects of Oral balance gel and Biotene toothpaste as compared to placebo was observed. No effect on oral colonization by cariogenic oral microflora was seen with use of other topical agents.

The effectiveness of Biotene products need to be evaluated using large number of samples and also for longer period of observations.

PLASMA AND CARIES PREVENTION

There are three states of matter: solid, liquid and gas. When a gas is given more energy, particles of gas collide with each other. As a result, electrons and ions are produced and the gas gets electric charge. This state of matter (the fourth state) is called 'plasma', a partially ionized gas.

Plasma can be classified according to the electron temperature and density. At low pressure, the excited electrons maintain their high temperature, while the plasma temperature remains at a lower level. The thermodynamic equilibrium may not establish; the generated plasma is referred to as 'non-local thermodynamic equilibrium plasma (non-LTE plasma). At low temperature it is also called 'cold plasma' or 'non-thermal plasma'. As pressure increases, thermodynamic equilibrium can be established and plasma temperature approaches the electron temperature; the generated plasma is referred to as 'local thermodynamic equilibrium plasma (LTE plasma)' or 'thermal plasma'.

Recently non-thermal effects of plasma are being widely used in dentistry, like modification of surface of titanium implants, modifying surface of polymers, disinfection of root canals and treatment of dental caries.

Sladek, et al (2004) reported feasibility of plasma application to treat dental caries. They developed a 'portable plasma needle' which operated with radio frequency power and the gas flow (He). The temperature increase in the pulpal chamber was 2.3°C during the plasma treatment. They also confirmed the capability of the plasma device for killing bacteria. Another few studies have also confirmed the bactericidal effect of non-thermal plasma on *Streptococcus mutans* and *Lactobacillus acidophilus*, which are major pathogens in dental caries. Since plasma is effective in eradication and deactivating cariogenic microflora, it has definite role in prevention of dental caries in future.

Bibliography

1. Adair PM, Burnside G and Pine CM. Analysis of health behaviour change interventions for preventing dental caries delivered in primary schools. Caries Res.: 2013;47:2–12.

2. Adair SM. The role of fluoride mouthrinses in the control of dental caries: a brief review. Am. Acad. Pediatr. Dent.: 1998;20:101–4.

3. Agrawal V, Kapoor S and Shah N. Role of 'Live Micro-organisms'(probiotics) in prevention of caries: Going on the natural way towards oral health. Indian J. Multidisci. Dent.: 2012;2:491–6.

4. Amaechi BT and Loveren C. Fluorides and non-fluoride remineralization systems. Monogr. Oral Sci.: 2013;23:15–26.

5. Amaechi BT, Porteous N, Ramalingam K, Mensinkai PK, Ccahuana Vasquez RA, Sadeghpour A and Nakamoto T. Remineralization of artificial enamel lesions by Theobromine. Caries Res.: 2013;47:399–405.

6. Amaechi BT, Ramalingam K, Mensinkai PK and Chediieu I. *In situ* remineralization of early caries by a new high-fluoride dentifrice. Gen. Dent.: 2012;60:e186–e192.

7. Ana PA, Bachmann L and Zezell DM. Lasers effects on enamel for Caries Prevention. Laser Physics 2006; 16: 865–75.

8. Anand TD, Pothiraj C, Gopinath RM and Kayalvizhi B. Effect of oil-pulling on dental caries causing bacteria. African J. of Microbiology Res.: 2008;2:63–6.

9. Anderson MH and Shi W. A probiotic approach to caries management. Pediatr. Dent.: 2006; 28:151–3.

10. Attenburger MJ, Schirrmeister JF, Wrbas KT, Klasser M and Hellwig E. Fluoride uptake and remineralization of enamel lesions after weekly application of differently concentrated fluoride gels. Caries Res.: 2008;42:312–8.

11. Autio-Gold J. The role of chlorhexidine in caries prevention. Oper. Dent.: 2008;33:710–6.

12. Azarpazhooh A and Limeback H. Clinical efficacy of casein derivates: a systematic review of literature. J. Am. Dent. Assoc.: 2008;139:915–24.

13. Bader JD, Shugars DA and Bonito AJ. A systematic review of selected caries prevention and management methods. Commun. Dent. Oral Epidemiol.: 2001;29:399–411.

14. Baig A and He T. A novel dentifrice technology for advanced oral health protection: a review of technical and clinical data. Compend. Contin. Educ. Dent.: 2005;26:4–11.

15. Baig AA, Faller RV, Yan J, Ji N, Lawless M and Eversole SL. Protective effects of SnF_2 - Part I. Mineral solubilisation studies on powdered apatite. Int. Dent. J.: 2014;64:4–10.

16. Baysan A and Beighton D. Assessment of the ozone-mediated killing of bacteria in infected dentin associated with non-cavitated occlusal carious lesions. Caries Res.: 2007;41:337–41.

17. Baysan A and Lynch E. Effect of ozone on the oral microbiota and clinical severity of primary root caries. Am. J. Dent.: 2004;17:56–60.

18. Baysan A, Whiley RA and Lynch E. Antimicrobial effect of a novel ozone-generating device on micro-organisms associated with primary root caries lesions *in vitro*. Caries Res.: 2000;34:498–501.

19. Bekeleski GM, McCombs G and Melvin WL. Oil pulling: an ancient practice for a modern time. J. Int. Oral Health: 2012;4:1–10.

20. Bellini HT, Arneberg P and von der Fehr FR. Oral hygiene and caries: a review. Acta. Odontol. Scand.: 1981;39:257–65.

21. Beltran ED and Burt BA. The pre and post-eruptive effects of fluoride on caries decline. J. Public Health Dent.: 1988;48:233–40.

22. Biesbrock AR, Gerlach RW, Bollmer BW, Faller RV, Jacobs SA and Bartizek RD. Relative anti-caries efficacy of 1,100,1,700, 2,200 and 2,800

ppm fluoride ion in a sodium fluoride dentifrice over 1 year. Comm. Dent. Oral Epidemiol.: 2001;29: 382–9.

23. Birardi V, Bossi L and Dinoi C. Use of the Nd:YAG laser in the treatment of Early Childhood Caries. Eur. J. Paediatr. Dent.: 2004;5: 98–101.

24. Bonifait L, Chandad F and Grenier D. Probiotics for oral health: Myth or realilty? JCDA: 2009;75: 585–90.

25. Burt BA. Prevention policies in the light of the changed distribution of dental caries. Acta. Odontol. Scand.: 1998;56:179–86.

26. Burwell AK, Litkowski LJ and Greenspan DC. Calcium sodium phosphosilicate (NovaMin): remineralization potential. Adv. Dent. Res.: 2009;21:35–9.

27. Buzalaf MA, Pessan JP, Honorio HM and ten Cate JM. Mechanisms of action of fluoride for caries control. Monogr. Oral Sci.: 2011;22:97–114.

28. Cagetti MG, Mastroberardino S, Milia E, Cocco F, Lingstrom P and Campus G. The use of probiotic strains in caries prevention: a systematic review. Nutrients: 2013;5:2530–50.

29. Caglar E, Kavaloglu SC, Kuscu OO, Sandalli N, Holgerson PL and Twetman S. Effect of chewing gums containing xylitol or probiotic bacteria on salivary mutans streptococci and lactobacilli. Clin. Oral Investig.: 2007;11:425–9.

30. Caglar E, Sandalli N, Twetman S, Kavaloglu S, Ergeneli S and Selvi S. Effect of yogurt with Bifidobacterium DN-173 010 on salivary mutans streptococci and lactobacilli in young adults. Acta. Odontol. Scand.: 2005;63:317–20.

31. Cavalli V, Cardoso Cde A, Zandonadi Fde. A, Liporoni PCS, Berger SB and Giannini M. Secondary caries inhibition promoted by adhesive systems and bleaching agents with fluoride. Am. J. Dent.: 2012;25:141–5.

32. Chen F and Wang D. Novel technologies for the prevention and treatment of dental caries: a patent survey. Expert Opinion on Therapeutic Patents.: 2010;20:681–94.

33. Chen L, Yuan H, Tang B, Liang K and Li J. Biomimetic remineralization of human enamel in the presence of Polamidoamine Dendrimers *in vitro*. Caries Res. 2015;49:282–90.

34. Chhabra KG, Shetty PJ, Prasad KVV, Mendon CS and Kalyanpur R. The beyond measures: Non-fluoride preventive measures for dental caries. J. Int. Oral Health: 2011;3:1–8.

35. Chu CH and Lo EC and Lin HC. Effectiveness of silver diamine fluoride and sodium fluoride varnish in arresting dentin caries in Chinese pre-school children. J. Dent. Res.: 2002;81:767–70.

36. Chu CH and Lo EC. Microhardness of dentin in primary teeth after topical fluoride applications. J. Dent.: 2008;36:387–91.

37. Chu CH, Mei L and Lo EC. Use of fluorides in dental caries management. Gen. Dent.: 2010;58: 37–43.

38. Chu CH, Mei L, Seneviratne CJ and Lo EC. Effects of silver diamine fluoride on dentin carious lesions induced by *Streptococcus mutans* and *Actinomyces naeslundii* biofilms. Int. J. Paediatr. Dent.: 2012;22:2–10.

39. Clark CD. A review on fluoride varnishes: An alternative topical fluoride treatment. Comm. Dent. Oral Epidemiol.: 1982;10:117–23.

40. Clark DR, Czajka-Jakubowska A, Rick C, Liu J, Chang S and Clarkson BH. *In vitro* anti-caries effect of fluoridated hydroxyapatite-coated preformed metal crowns. Eur. Arch. Paediatr. Dent.; 2013;14:253–9.

41. Cochrane J, Cai F, Huq NL, Burrow MF and Reynolds EC. New approaches to enhanced remineralization of tooth enamel. J. Dent. Res.: 2010;89:1187–97.

42. Cury JA and Tenuta LM. How to maintain a cariostatic fluoride concentration in the oral environment. Advances in Dental Research: 2008;20:13–16.

43. DaSilva LAB, Nelson-Filho P, Saravia ME, De Rossi A, Lucisano MP and DaSilva RAB. Mutans streptococci remained viable on toothbrush bristles, *in vivo*, for 44 h. Int. J. Pediatr. Dent.: 2014;24:367–72.

44. de Baat C, Kalk W and Schuil GR. The effectiveness of oral hygiene programmes for elderly people—a review. Gerodontology: 1993;10:109–13.

45. de Vrese M and Schrezenmeir J. Probiotics, prebiotics and synbiotics. Adv. Biochem. Eng. Biotechnol.: 2008;111:1–66.

46. Do LG and Spencer AJ. Risk-benefit balance in the use of fluoride among young children. J. Dent. Res.: 2007;86:723–8.

47. Donly KJ. Fluoride varnishes. J. Calif. Dent. Assoc.: 2003;31:217–9.

48. dos Santos APP, Oliveira BH and Nadanovsky P. Effects of low and standard fluoride toothpastes on caries and fluorosis: Systematic

review and meta-analysis. Caries Research: 2013;47:382–90.

49. Easteves-Oliviera M, Zezell DM, Mesiter J, Franzen R, Stanzol S, Lampert F, Eduardo CP and Apal C. CO_2 laser (10.6 mm) parameters for caries prevention in enamel. Caries Res.: 2009;43:261–8.

50. Eckert R, He J, Yarbrough DK, Qi F, Anderson MH and Shi W. Targeted killing of *Streptococcus mutans* by a pheromone-guided "Smart" antimicrobial peptide. Antimicrob. Agents Chemother: 2006;50:3651–7.

51. Eckert R, Sullivan R and Shi W. Targeted antimicrobial treatment to re-establish a health microbial flora for long-term protection. Adv. Dent. Res.: 2012;22:94–97.

52. Eckert R. Road to clinical efficacy: challenges and novel strategies for antimicrobial peptide development. Future Microbiol.: 2011;6:635–51.

53. Elouafkaoui F, Bonetti D, Clarkson J, Stirling D, Young L and Cassie H. Is further intervention required to translate caries prevention and management recommendations into practice? Br. Dent. J. 2015, 218.

54. Erdem AP, Sepet E, Avshalom T, Gutkin V and Steinberg D. Effect of CPP-ACP and APF on *Streptococcus mutans* biofilm: A laboratory study. Am. J. Dent.: 2011;24:119–23.

55. Faller RV and Eversole SL. Enamel protection from acid challenge—benefits of marketed fluoride dentifrices. J. Clin. Dent.: 2013;24:25–30.

56. Faller RV and Eversole SL. Protective effects of stannous fluorides—Part III. Mechanism of barrier layer attachment. Int. Dent. J.: 2014;64:16–21.

57. Feathersone JD. Caries detection and prevention with laser energy. Dent. Clin. North Am.: 2000;44: 955–69.

58. Featherstone JD. Prevention and reversal of dental caries: role of low level fluoride. Comm. Dent. Oral Epid.: 1999;27:31–40.

59. Featherstone JD. The caries balance: the basis for caries management by risk assessment. Oral Health Prev. Dent.: 2004;2:259–64.

60. Featherstone JD. The science and practise of caries prevention. JADA: 2000;131:887–99.

61. Featherstone, J.D. Remineralization, the natural caries repair process—the need for new approaches. Adv. Dent. Res.: 2009;21:4–7.

62. Fejerskov O, Thylstrup A and Larsen MJ. Rational use of fluoride in caries prevention: a concept based on possible cariostatic mechanisms. Acta. Odontol. Scand.: 1981;39:241–9.

63. Fraud S, Maillard JY, Kaminski MA and Hanlon GW. Activity of amine oxide against biofilms of *Streptococcus mutans*: a potential biocide for oral care formulations. J. Antimicrob. Chemother: 2005;56:672–7.

64. Giacaman RA, Contzen MP, Yuri JA, Munoz-Sandoval C. Anticaries effect on an antioxidant-rich apple concentrate on enamel in an experimental biofilm-demineralization model. J. Appl. Microbiol.: 2014;117:846–53.

65. Giri S and Singh J : New face in the row of human therapeutics: Bacteriocins. J Microbial Research. 2013;3:71–8.

66. Glacaman RA, Munoz MJ, Ccahuana-Vasquez RA, Munoz-Sandoval C and Cury JA. Effect of fluoridated milk on enamel and root dentin demineralization evaluated by a biofilm caries model. Caries Res.: 2012;46:460–6.

67. Gonzalez-Cabezas, C. The chemistry of caries: remineralization and demineralization events with direct clinical relevance. Dent. Clin. Of North Am.: 2010;54:269–78.

68. Goodis HE, Fried D, Gansky S, Rechmann P and Featherstone JD. Pulpal safety of 9.6 micron CO_2 laser used for caries prevention. Lasers Surg. Med.: 2004;35:104–10.

69. Grender J, Williams K, Walters P, Klukowska M and Reick H. Plaque removal efficacy of oscillating-rotating power toothbrushes: Review of six comparative clinical trials. Am. J. Dent.: 2013;26:68–74.

70. Griffin SO, Regnier E, Griffin PM and Huntley V. Effectiveness of fluoride in preventing caries in adults. J. Dent. Res.: 2007;86:410–415.

71. Groeneveld A, Van Eck AA and Backer Dirks O. Fluoride in caries prevention: Is the effect pre- or post-eruptive? J. Dent. Res.: 1990;69:751–55.

72. Hamada S, Koga T and Ooshima T. Virulence factors of *Streptococcus mutans* and dental caries prevention. J. Dent. Res.: 1984;63:407–11.

73. Hannig M and Hannig C. Nanotechnology and its role in caries therapy. Adv. Dent. Res.: 2012;24:53–57.

74. Hannig M. The protective nature of the salivary pellicle. Int. Dent. J: 2002;52:417–23.

75. He T, Barker ML. Biesbrock AR, Eynon H, Milleman JL, Milleman KR, Putt MS and Wintergerst AM. Digital plaque imaging evaluation of stabilized stannous fluoride

dentifrice compared with a triclosan/copolymer dentifrice. Am. J. Dent.: 2013;26:303–06.

76. He X, Lux R, Kuramitsu HK, Anderson MH and Shi W. Achieving probiotic effects via modulating oral microbial ecology. Adv. Dent. Res.: 2009;21:53–56.

77. Hedberg M, Hasslof P, Sjostrom I, Twetman S and Stecksen-Blicks C. Sugar fermentation in probiotic bacteria—an *in vitro* study. Oral Microbiol. Immunol. 2008;23:482–5.

78. Hicks J and Flaitz C and Westerman GH. Enamel caries initiation and progression following low energy argon laser and fluoride treatment J Clin. Pediat. Dent.: 1995;20:9–13.

79. Hicks J and Flaitz C. Role of remineralizing fluid in *in-vitro* enamel caries formation and progression. Pediat. Dent.: 2004;26:189.

80. Hilgert LA, Leal SC, Mulder J, Creugers NHJ and Frencken JE. Caries-preventive effect of supervised toothbrushing and sealants. J. Dent Res 2015;94:1218–24.

81. Hochbaum AI, Kolodkin-Gal I, Foulston L, Kolter R, Aizenberg J and Losick R. Inhibitory effects of D-amino acids on *Staphylococcus aureus* biofilm development. J. Bacteriol.: 2011; 193:5616–22.

82. Holmes J. Clinical reversal of root caries using ozone, double-blind, randomized, controlled 18-month trial. Gerodontology: 2003;20:106–14.

83. Horst JA, Pieper U, Sali A, Zhan L, Chopra G, Samudrala R and Featherstone JD. Strategic protein target analysis for developing drugs to stop dental caries. Adv. Dent. Res.: 2012;24:86–93.

84. Howden GF. The cariostatic effect of betel nut chewing. PNG Med. J.: 1984;27:123–31.

85. Howlin RP, Fabbri S, Offin DG, Symonds N, Kiang KS, Knee RJ, Yoganantham DC, Webb JS, Birkin PR, Leighton TG and Stoodley P. Removal of dental biofilms with an ultrasonically activated water stream. J. Dent Res 2015;94: 1303–09.

86. Hsu CY, Jordan TH, Dederich DN and Wefel JS. Laser-matrix-fluoride effects on enamel demineralization. J Dent. 2001,80, 1797–801.

87. Huang SB, Gao SS and Yu HY. Effect of nano-hydroxyapatite concentration on remineraliza- tion of initial enamel lesion. Biomed. Mater.: 2009;4:034101.

88. Iijima Y, Cai F, Shen P, Walker G, Reynolds C and Reynolds EC. Acid resistance of enamel subsurface lesions remineralized by a sugar-free chewing gum containing casein phospho-peptide-amorphous calcium phosphate. Car. Res.: 2004; 38:551–6.

89. Ijaz S, Croucher RE and Marinho VC. Systematic reviews of topical fluorides for dental caries: a review of reporting practice. Caries Res.: 2010;44: 579–92.

90. Ivanoff CS, Morshed BR, Hottel TL and Garcia-Godoy F. Fluoride uptake by human tooth enamel: Topical application versus combined dielectrophoresis and AC electroosmosis. Am. J. Dent.: 2013;26:166–72.

91. Kakuda S, Siddhu SK and Sano H. Buffering or non-buffering; an action of pit and fissure sealants. J dent. 2015, (In press).

92. Kallestal C, Norlund A, Soder B, Nordenram G, Dahlgren H, Petersson LG, Langerlof F, Axelsson S, Lingstrom P, Mejare I, Holm AK and Twetman S. Economic evaluation of dental caries prevention: a systematic review. Acta. Odontol. Scand.: 2003;61:341–6.

93. Kang MS, Chung J, Kim SM, Yang KH and Oh JS. Effect of *Weissella cibaria* isolates on the formation of *Streptococcus mutans* biofilm. Caries Res.: 2006;40:418–25.

94. Kargul BN, Ozcan M, Peker S, Nakamoto T, Simmons WB and Falster AU. Evaluation of human enamel surfaces treated with Theobromine: a pilot study. Oral Health Prev. Dent.: 2012; 10:275–82.

95. Karlinsey RL and Pfarrer AM. Fluoride plus functionalized-TCP: a promising combination for robust remineralization. Adv. Dent. Res.: 2012; 24:48–52.

96. Khambe D, Eversole SL, Mills T and Faller RV. Protective effects of SnF$_2$-Part II. Deposition and retention on pellicle-coated enamel. Int. Dent. J.: 2014;64:11–15.

97. Klish AJ, Porter JA and Bashirelahi N. What every dentist needs to know about the human microbiome and probiotics. General Dent.: 2014;62:30–6.

98. Kumar VL, Itthagarun A and King NM. The effect of casein phosphopeptide-amorphous calcium phosphate on remineralization of artificial caries-like lesions: an *in vitro* study. Aust. Dent. J. 2008; 53:34–40.

99. Laheij AM, Strijp AJ and Loveren C. *In situ* remineralization of enamel and dentin after the use of an amine fluoride mouthrinse in addition to twice daily brushings with amine fluoride toothpaste. Car. Res.: 2010;44:260–6.

100. Lee VA, Karthikeyan R, Rawls HR and Amaechi BT. Anti-cariogenic effect of a cetylpyridinium chloride-containing nanoemulsion. J. Dent.: 2010;38:742–9.

101. Lippert F, Churchley D and Lynch RJ. Effect of lesion baseline severity and mineral distribution on remineralization and progression of human and bovine dentin caries lesion. Caries Res. 2015;49:467–76.

102. Liu BY, Lo EC, Chu CH andLin HC. Randomized trial on fluorides and sealants for fissure caries prevention. J. Dent. Res.: 2012;291:753–8.

103. Liu J. Ling JQ, Zhang K, Huo LJ and Ning Y. Effect of sodium fluoride, ampicillin and chlorhexidine on *Streptococcus mutans* biofilm detachment. Antimicrob Agents Chemother: 2012;56:4532–5.

104. Liu YL, Nascimento M and Burne RA. Progress toward understanding the contribution of alkali generation in dental biofilms to inhibition of dental caries. Int. J. Oral Sci.: 2012;4:135–40.

105. Loesche WJ. Clinical and microbiological aspects of chemotherapeutic agents used according to the specific plaque hypothesis. J. Dent. Res.: 1979; 58:2404–12.

106. Lussi A, Hellwig E and Klimek J. Fluorides-mode of action and recommendations for use. Schweiz Monatsscxhr Zahnmed: 2012;122:1030–36.

107. Lynch E and Baysan A. Reversal of primary root caries using a dentifrice with a high fluoride content. Caries Res.: 2001;35:60–4.

108. Lynn Powell G. Prevention of Dental Caries by Laser Irradiation: A Review. J. Oral Laser Applications: 2006;6:255–7.

109. Malhotra N, Rao SP, Acharaya S and Vasudev B. Comparative *in vitro* evaluation of efficacy of mouthrinses against *Streptococcus mutans*, lactobacilli and *Candida albicans*. Oral Health Prev. Dent.: 2011;9:261–8.

110. Maltz M and Beighton D. Multidisciplinary research agenda for novel antimicrobial agent for caries prevention and treatment. Adv. Dent. Res.: 2012;24:133–6.

111. Marinho VC. Evidence-based effectiveness of topical fluorides. Adv. Dent. Res.: 2008;20:3–7.

112. Marino RJ, Khan AR and Morgan M. Systematic review of publications on economic evaluations of caries prevention programs. Caries Res.: 2013;47:265–72.

113. Marquis RE. Antimicrobial actions of fluoride for oral bacteria. Can. J. Microbiol.: 1995;41:955–64.

114. Mei ML, Ito L, Cao Y, Li QL, Lo ECM and Chu CH. Inhibitory effect of silver diamine fluoride on dentin demineralisation and collagen degradation. J. Dent.: 2013;41:809–17.

115. Meurman JH. Probiotics: do they have a role in oral medicine and dentistry? Eur. J. Oral Sci.: 2005;113:188–96.

116. Milicich GW. Caries management in the dental practice. Compend. Contin. Educ. Dent.: 2009; 30:62–66 and 68.

117. Moreno EC. Role of Calcium, Phosphorous and Fluorides in caries prevention: chemical aspects. Int. Dent. J.: 1993;43:71–80.

118. Moynihan P. Foods and dietary factors that prevent dental caries. Quintessence Int.: 2005;38:320–4.

119. Nagayoshi M, Kitamura C, Fukuizumi T, Nishihara T and Terashita M. Antimicrobial effect of ozonated water on bacteria invading dentinal tubules. J. Endod.: 2004;30:778–81.

120. Nascimento MM, Liu Y, Kalra R, Perry S, Adewumi A, Xu X, Primosch RE and Burne RA. Oral arginine metabolism may decrease the risk for dental caries in children. J. Dent. Res.: 2013; 92:604–8.

121. Newbrun E. Topical fluorides in caries prevention and management: A North American Perspective. J. Dent. Educ.: 2001;65: 1078–83.

122. Nikawa H, Makihira S, Fukushima H, Nishimura H, Ozaki Y, Ishida K, Darmawan S, Hamada T, Hara K, Matsumoto A, Takemoto T and Aimi R. *Lactobacillus reuteri* in bovine milk fermented decreases the oral carriage of mutans streptococci. Int. J. Food Microbiol.: 2004;95:219–23.

123. Nordstrom A and Birkhed D. Preventive effect of high-fluoride dentifrice (5,000 ppm) in caries-active adolescents: a 2-year clinical trial. Caries Res.: 2010;44:323–31.

124. Ogaard B. CaF_2 formation: Cariostatic properties and factors of enhancing the effect. Caries Res.: 2001;35:40–4.

125. Ogaard B, Rolla G, Dijkman T, Ruben J and Arends J. Effect of fluoride mouthrinsing on caries lesion development in shark enamel: an *in-situ* caries model study. Scand J Dent Res. 1991;99:372–7.

126. O'Hehir TE. Ozone and Caries. Periodontics: 2003;23:45–60.

127. Okuno A, Nezu T and Tanaka M. A warmed topical fluoride solution enhances KOH-soluble and -insoluble fluoride formation on tooth surfaces *in vitro*. Pediatr. Dent. J.: 2014;24:22–6.

128. O'Mullane DM. Systemic fluorides. Adv. Dent. Res.: 1994;8:181–4.

129. Oshiro M, Yamaguchi K, Takamizawa T, Inage H, Watanabe T, Irokawa A, Ando S and Miyazaki M. Effect of CPP-ACP paste on tooth mineralization: an FE-SEM study. J. Oral Sci.: 2007;49:115–20.

130. Pandit S, Kim JE, Jung KH, Chang KW and Jeon JG. Effect of sodium fluoride on the virulence factors and composition of *Streptococcus mutans* biofilms. Arch. Oral Biol.: 2011;56:643–9.

131. Panich M and Poolthong S. The effect of casein phosphopeptide-amorphous calcium phosphate and a cola soft drink on *in vitro* enamel hardness. J. Am. Dent. Assoc.: 2009;140:455–60.

132. Papas AS, Vollmer WM, Gullion CM, Bader J, Laws R and Fellows J. Efficacy of chlorhexidine varnish for the prevention of adult caries: a randomized trial. J. Dent. Res.: 2012;91:150–5.

133. Park KK, Zitterbart PA and Christen AG. Preventive management of root caries: state of the art. J. Indiana Dent. Assoc.: 1987;66:11–19.

134. Paul S, Shrikrishna SB, Suman E, Shenoy R and Rao A. Effect of fluoride varnish and chlorhexidine-thymol varnish on mutans streptococci levels in human dental plaque: a double-blinded randomized controlled trial. Int. J. Pediatr. Dent.: 2014;24:399–408.

135. Peng JJ, Botelho MG and Matinlinna JP. Silver compounds used in dentistry for caries management: a review. J. Dent.: 2012;40:531–41.

136. Peters MC. Strategies for non-invasive demineralized tissue repair. Dent. Clin. of North Am.: 2010;54:507–25.

137. Petti S, Tarsitani G and Simonetti D'Arca A. Antibacterial activity of yoghurt against viridans streptococci *in vitro*. Arch. Oral Biol.: 2008;53:985–90.

138. Pfarrer AM and Karlinsey RL. Challenges of implementing new remineralization technologies. Adv. Dent. Res.: 2009;21:79–82.

139. Phan TN and Marquis RE. Triclosan inhibition of membrane enzymes and glycolysis of *Streptococcus mutans* in suspensions and biofilms. Can. J. Microbiol.: 2006;52:977–83.

140. Pitchika V, Kokel C, Andreeva J, Crispin A, Hickel R, Kuhnisch J and Heinrich-Weltzien R. Effectiveness of a new fluoride varnish for caries prevention in pre-school children. J. Clin. Pediatr. Dent.: 2013;38:7–12.

141. Pitts NB. Are we ready to move from operative to non-operative/preventive treatment of dental caries in clinical practice? Caries Res.:2004;38:294–304.

142. Rahiotis C, Vougiouklakis G and Eliades G. Characterization of oral films formed in the presence of a CPP-ACP agent: An *in situ* study. J. Dent.: 2008;36:272–80.

143. Reynolds EC, Cai F, Cochrane NJ, Shen P, Walker GD, Morgan MV and Reynolds C. Fluoride and casein phosphopeptide-amorphous calcium phosphate. J. Dent. Res.: 2008;87:344–8.

144. Reynolds EC. Calcium phosphate-based remineralization systems: scientific evidence? Aust. Dent. J.: 2008;53:268–73.

145. Rezaei Y, Bagheri H and Esmaeilzadeh M. Effects of laser irradiation on caries prevention. J. Lasers Med. Sci.: 2011;2:159–64.

146. Rmaile A, Carugo D, Capretto L, Aspiras M, De Jager M, Ward M and Stoodley P. Removal of interproximal dental biofilms by high-velocity water microdrops. J. Dent. Res.: 2014;93:68–73.

147. Rodrigues LKA, dosSantos MN. Pereira D, Assa AV and Pardi V. Carbon dioxide laser in dental caries prevention. J. Dentistry: 2004;32: 531–40.

148. Rosenblatt A, Stamford TCM and Niederman R. Silver diamine fluoride: a caries 'silver-fluoride bullet'. J. Dent. Res.: 2009;88:116–25.

149. Rosin-Grget K and Lineir I. Current concept on the anticaries fluoride mechanism of the action. Coll. Antropol.: 2000;25:703–12.

150. Roveri N, Foresti E, Lelli M and Lesci IG. Recent advancements in preventing teeth health hazard: the daily use of hydroxyapatite instead of fluoride. Recent patents on Biomedical Engg.: 2009;2:197–215.

151. Rugg-Gunn AJ. Dental caries: Strategies to control this preventable disease. Acta. Med. Acad.: 2013;42:117–30.

152. Sanders ME. Probiotics: definition, sources, selection and uses. Clin. Infect. Dis.: 2008;46: 558–61.

153. Santos VE, Filho AV, Ribeiro AG, Flores MAP, Galembeck A, Caldas AF and Rosenblatt A. A new "Silver-Bullet" to treat caries in children-Nano Silver Fluoride: A randomised clinical trial. J. Dent.: 2014;42:945–51.

154. Schaeken MJM, Keltjens HMAM, Vander Hoeven JS. Effects of fluoride and chlorhexidine on the microflora of dental root surfaces and progression of root-surface caries. J. Dent. Res.: 1991;70:150–3.

155. Schafer F. Evaluation of the anticaries benefit of fluoride toothpastes using an enamel insert model. Caries Res.: 1989;23:81–6.

156. Scheie AA and Fejerskov OB. Xylitol in caries prevention: What is the evidence for clinical efficacy? Oral Disease: 1998;4:268–78.

157. Schwendicke F, Dorfer C, Kneist S, Meyer-Lueckel H and Paris S. Cariogenic effects of probiotic *Lactobacillus rhamosus* GG in a dental biofilm model. Caries Res.: 2014;48:186–92.

158. Schwendicke F, Jager AM, Paris S, Hsu LY and Tu YK. Treating Pit and Fissure Caries: A systematic Review and network meta-analysis. J. Dent Res 2015;94:522–33.

159. Seppa L. Fluoride varnishes in caries prevention. Med. Princ. Pract.: 2004;13:307–311.

160. Seppa L. The future of preventive programs in countries with different systems for dental care. Caries Res.: 2001;35:26–9.

161. Shivakumar V, Shanmugam M, Sudhir G and Priyadarshoni SP. Scope of photodynamic therapy in periodontics and other fields of dentistry. J. Interdisciplinary Dent.: 2012;2:78–83.

162. Soukos NS and Goodson JM. Photodynamic therapy in the control of oral biofilms. Periodontol.: 2011;55:143–66.

163. Stamm JW. The value of dentifrices and mouthrinses in caries prevention. Int. Dent. J.: 1993;43:517–27.

164. Steiner M, Helfenstein U and Menghini G. Effect of 1,000 ppm relative to 250 ppm fluoride toothpaste. A meta-analysis. Am. J. Dent.: 2004;17:85–8.

165. Su Nan, Marek CL, Ching V and Grushka M. Caries prevention for patients with dry mouth. J. Can Dent. Assoc.: 2011;77:b85.

166. Sugano N. Biological plaque control: novel therapeutic approach to periodontal disease. J. Oral Sci.: 2012;54:1–5.

167. Tan HP, Lo ECM, Dyson JE, Luo Y and Corbet EF. A randomized trial on root caries prevention in elders. J. Dent. Res.: 2010;89:1086–90.

168. Tavares JG, Eduardo CP, Burnett Jr. LH, Boff TR and deFreitas PM. Argon and Nd:YAG lasers for caries prevention in enamel. Photomed. Laser Surg.:2012;30:433–7.

169. Tavss EA, Boenta CY, Joziak MT, Fisher SW and Campbell SK. High potency sodium fluoride: a literature review. Compound Contin. Edu. Dent.: 1997;18:31–6.

170. ten Cate JM and Featherstone JDB. Mechanistic aspects of the interactions between fluoride and dental enamel. Crit. Rev. Oral Biol. Med.: 1991;2:283–96.

171. ten Cate JM and van Loveren C. Fluoride mechanisms. Dent. Clin. North Am.: 1999;43:713–42.

172. ten Cate JM and Zaura E. The numerous microbial species in oral biofilms: How could antibacterial therapy be effective? Adv. Dent. Res.: 2012;24:108–11.

173. Tenuta LMA and Cury JA. Fluoride: its role in dentistry. Braz. Oral Res.: 2010;24:9–17.

174. Tenuta LMA, Cerezetti RV, Del Bel Cury AA, Tabchoury CPM and Cury JA. Fluoride release from calcium fluoride and enamel deminera-lization. J. Dent. Res.: 2008;87:1032–6.

175. Thaweboon S, Nakaparksin J and Thaweboon B. Effect of oil-pulling on oral micro-organisms in biofilm models. Asia J. Public Health: 2011;2:62–6.

176. Tickle M, Milsom KM, Donaldson M, Killough S, O'Neill C, Crealey G, Sutton M, Noble S, Greer M and Worthington HV. Protocol for Northern Ireland Caries Prevention in Practice Trial (NIC-PIP): A randomized controlled trial to measure the effects and costs of a dental caries prevention regime for young children attending primary care dental services. BMC Oral Health: 2011;11:27.

177. Tsai CL, Lin YT, Huang ST and Chang HW. *In vitro* acid resistance of CO_2 and Nd-YAG laser-treated human tooth Enamel. Cries Res 2002;36:423–9.

178. Tsang P, Qi F and Shi W. Medical approach to dental caries: fight the disease, not the lesion. Pediatr. Dent.: 2006;28:188–91.

179. Tschoppe P, Zandim DL, Martus P and Kielbassa AM. Enamel and dentin reminerali-zation by nano-hydroxyapatite toothpastes. J. Dent.: 2011;39:430–7.

180. Twetman S and Keller MK. Probiotics for caries prevention and control. Adv. Dent. Res.: 2012;24:98–102.

181. Twetman S, Axelsson S, Dahlgren H, Holm AK, Kallestal C, Lagerlof F, Lingstrom P, Mejare I, Nordenram G, Norlund A, Petersson LG and Soder B. Caries-preventive effect of fluoride

toothpaste: a systematic review. Acta. Odontol. Scand.: 2003;61:347–55.

182. Twetman S. Are we ready for caries prevention through bacteriotherapy? Braz. Oral Res.: 2012;26:64–70.

183. Twetman S. Caries prevention with fluoride toothpaste in children: an update. Eur. Arch. Paediatr. Dent.: 2009;10:162–7.

184. Van Loveren C. Sugar alcohols: What is the evidence for caries-preventive and caries-therapeutic effects? Caries Res.: 2004;38:286–93.

185. Vander HC, Engles E, De Vries J and Busscher HJ. Effects of amine fluoride on biofilm growth and salivary pellicles. Caries Res.: 2008;42:19–27.

186. Vilhena FV, Olympio KP, Lauris JR, Delbem AC and Buzalaf MA. Low-fluoride acidic dentifrice: a randomized clinical trial in a fluoridated area. Caries Res.: 2010;44:478–84.

187. Vilhena FV, Olympio KP, Lauris JR, Delbem AC and Buzalaf MA. Low-fluoride acidic dentifrice: a randomized clinical trial in a fluoridated area. Caries Res.: 2010;44:478–84.

188. Vollmer WM, Papas AS, Bader JD, Maupome G, Gullion CM, Hollis JF, Synder JJ, Fellows JL, Laws RL and White BA. Design of the Prevention of Adult Caries Study (PACS): a randomized clinical trial assessing the effect of a chlorhexidine dental coating for the prevention of adult caries. BMC Oral Health: 2010;10:23.

189. Walsh LJ. Preventive dentistry for the general dental practitioner. Aust. Dent. J.: 2000;45:76–82.

190. Wang G: Human antimicrobial peptides and proteins. Pharmaceuticals, 2014;7:545–94.

191. Wefel JS, Jensen ME, Triolo PT, Faller RV, Hogan MM and Bowman WD. De/remineralization from sodium fluoride dentifrices. Am. J. Dent.: 1995;8:217–20.

192. Weinstein P, Spiekerman C and Milgrom P. Randomized equivalence trial of intensive and semiannual applications of fluoride varnish in the primary dentition. Caries Res.: 2009;43:484–90.

193. Weintraub JA, Ramos-Gomez F, Jue B, Shain S, Hoover CI, Featherstone JDB and Gransky SA. Fluoride varnish efficacy in preventing early childhood caries. J. Dent. Res.: 2006;85:172–6.

194. Wennhall I, Hajem S, Ilros S, Ridell K, Ekstrand KR and Twetman S. Fluoridated salt for caries prevention and control—a 2-year field study in a disadvantaged community. Int. J. Pediatr. Dent.: 2014;24:161–7.

195. Westerman GH. Lynn Powell G, Flaitz CM and Hicks MJ. Argon laser and remineralizing solution treatment effects on root surface caries. J. Oral Laser Applications: 2006;6:285–90.

196. Wong MCM, Clarkson J and Glenny AM, et al. Cochrane reviews on the benefits/risks of fluoride toothpastes. J. Dent.Res.: 2011;90:573–9.

197. Wright JT, Hanson N, Ristic H, Whall CW, Estrich CJ and Zenty RR. Fluoride toothpaste: efficacy and safety in children younger than 6 years: a systematic review. JADA: 2014;145:182–9.

198. Xie Q, Li J and Zhou X. Anticaries effect of compounds extracted from Galla chinensis in a multispecies biofilm model. Oral Microbiol. Immunol.: 2008;23:459–65.

199. Yang YM, Jiang D, Qiu YX, Fan R, Zhang R, Ning MZ, Shao MY, Zhang CL, Hong X and Hu, T. Effects of combined exogenous dextranase and sodium fluoride on *Streptococcus mutans* 25175 monospecies biofilms. Am. J. Dent.: 2013; 26:239–43.

200. Yee R, Holmgren C, Mulder J, Lama D, Walker D and van Palenstein Helderman W. Efficacy of silver diamine fluoride for arresting caries treatment. J. Dent. Res.: 2009;88:644–7.

201. Yevlahova D and Satur J. Models for individual oral health promotion and their effectiveness: a systematic review. Aust. Dent. J.: 2009;54:190–7.

202. Young DA, Lyon L and Azevedo S. The role of dental hygiene in caries management: a new paradigm. J. Dent. Hyg.: 2010;84:121–9.

203. Zhan L, Cheng J, Chang P, Ngo M, Denbestan PK, Hoover CI and Featherstone JDB. Effects of xylitol wipes on cariogenic bacteria and caries in young children. J. Dent. Res.: 2012;91:855–905.

204. Zhang W, McGrath C, Lo EC and Li JY. Silver diamine fluoride and education to prevent and arrest root caries among community-dwelling elders. Caries Research: 2013;47:284–90.

205. Zhegova GG, Rashkova MR and Yordanov BI. Perception of Er-YAG laser dental caries treatment in adolescents—a clinical evaluation. J. IMAB: 2014;20:500–3.

13

Caries Immunology

Dental caries is established as a multifactorial infectious disease. The interactions over a given period of time amongst host, diet and micro-organisms on the tooth surface result in dissolution of tooth tissues, subsequently leading to caries. The role of biofilm (a slime layer consisting of millions of bacteria, salivary polymers and food debris) is considered important in the initiation and progress of caries. The organized biofilm provides an excellent site for the colonization and growth of many micro-organisms including the cariogenic ones.

The oral microbiota function as a part of host defense system by acting as a barrier (may create unfavorable conditions to exogenous organisms pathogenic to the host).

Over 700 bacterial species have been found in oral cavity; however, all may not be present in every individual. Most of these species are harmless, but under some environmental conditions, a few of them can cause diseases. An improved understanding of the role of these bacterial species in caries process is mandatory.

It has long been a matter of concern whether caries has any genetic predisposition. The pathogenesis of caries is well understood by now. The caries attack in humans may be a consequence of the following attributes:

- Structural integrity of tooth tissue (enamel, dentin and cementum).
- Functioning of salivary glands.
- Dietary habits and day-to-day nutrition.
- Oral hygiene measures.
- Preventive measures, especially fluoridation

Genetics control the salivary functioning and also the maturation of tooth tissue. Various studies have confirmed that genetics play an important role in determining individual resistance against caries. A few authors could not detect influence of environment factors that might explain the caries susceptibility between caries-free and caries-prone individuals.

Naturally-induced Antibodies in Children

It is accepted that infants and young children develop secretory IgA (sIgA) antibodies against many oral antigens, presumably by the salivary pathway. However, an association between these sIgA antibodies and resistance to dental infection by these pathogens has yet to be authenticated. A few authors could not observe salivary IgA or crevicular IgG corresponding with colonization by cariogenic bacteria. The crevicular IgG antibodies are produced locally and reflect caries experience rather than protection. These observations do not infer that naturally-induced antibodies are unable to interrupt the caries process.

Caries has been correlated with elevated sIgA antibodies and elevated serum IgM antibodies to *Streptococcus mutans*. This may reflect the elevation of antibodies which occurs during and after infections. Such antibodies might not be protective in nature prior to infection.

History of Vaccination

- The Greek historian, Thucydides, as early as 429 BC, observed that the people who survived the smallpox plague in Athens did not become re-infected.
- Chinese in 900 AD used primitive form of vaccination called variolation against smallpox. The trend continued till 17th century.
- Variolation became popular in other countries to fight smallpox epidemic.
- The modern form of vaccination was discovered by Dr. Edward Jenner, a British physician in 1796.
- Vaccination became popular in Europe and USA. Royal Jennerian Institute was founded in 1803.
- Louis Pasteur developed vaccination against rabies in 1880.
- In 1890, Japanese physician Shibasaburo Kitasato discovered the antitoxins of diphtheria and tetanus. By early 19th century vaccination became popular. Vaccines for whooping cough and tuberculosis were available by that time.
- In 1955, polio vaccination was introduced.
- Smallpox eradication was launched by WHO in 1956 and was totally eradicated by 1980.
- Abdul Gaffar and Richard Charles developed caries vaccines from levan producing strains of *Streptococcus mutans* in 1971. Carlo and others in 1980 prepared caries vaccines from polysaccharides of *S. pneumoniae*. Smith and Taubman in 1993 improved upon caries vaccines by using synthetic peptides. They further used

particular immunogenic (subunit) portion of GTF for the development of caries vaccines in 2004.

- In 2006, HPV 2 (human papillomavirus) vaccine, Cervarix was introduced for cervical cancer. Herpes zoster vaccine, zotavax was also introduced in the same year for Shingles.
- In 2007, avian influenza vaccine was introduced against H5N1 virus.
- In 2008, Rotavirus vaccine, rotavix was introduced.
- In 2014, meningococcal vaccine was introduced.
- In 2015, avian influenza vaccine was introduced against H1N1 virus.

CARIES VACCINES

Vaccine is an immuno-biological substance designed to produce specific protection against a specific disease, stimulating the production of protective antibodies and other immune mechanisms. They are prepared from live/inactivated/killed organisms, extracted cellular fractions, toxoids and their combinations, etc. They produce two types of responses, (i) Primary response (when an antigen is administered for the first time, there is a latent period of induction of 3 to 10 days before antibodies appear in the blood, which is entirely of the IgM type) and (ii) Secondary (collaboration of B and T cells is necessary to initiate a secondary response. It involves the production of both IgM and IgG antibodies).

Naturally-induced immunity may not be the same as artificially-induced immunization. Artificially-induced immunization results in the elevation of antibodies to therapeutic or preventive levels against a specific micro-organisms. Generally, the aim of a vaccine is to reduce the numbers of the offending pathogens or to interfere with their metabolic activities. In case of inducing artificial immunization, certain important issues must be considered: (i) the microbial target (the offending pathogen), (ii) component of the immune system to be targeted and (iii) any evidence suggesting effectiveness of vaccine.

Candidate Antigens

Immunization with whole cells of *Streptococcus mutans* was not much effective since the antigen was cross reactive with heart muscles, especially caridolysin of the sarcolemma sheaths. Another reason why whole cell should not be used as an immunogen may be because the whole cells have mechanisms of immune evasion based on which polyclonal B-cells are stimulated regardless of antigen specificity. It was important to use an alternative means of vaccination, such as (i) purification of the candidate antigens and use of subunit vaccine or (ii) using recombinant DNA methods to place virulence factors in non-cariogenic organisms.

Candidate antigens targeting extracellular protein include glucosyltransferase (GTF), dextranases, adhesins and glucan-binding proteins (Table 13.1). The candidate antigens are:

i. Glycosyltransferases

Two types of basic glycosyltransferase exist in *Streptococcus mutans*, (i) GTF-S (synthesize water soluble glucan) and (ii) GTF-1 (synthesize water insoluble glucan); whereas *Streptococcus sobrinus* has three glycosyltransferase, i.e. GTF-S (primer dependent), GTF-S (primer independent) and GTF-1 (synthesize water insoluble glucan). Primer dependency infers that these surfaces require a primer to catalyze glucose polymerization. The immunization with GTF protein or subunit vaccine from one species can induce a measure of protection for the other species.

ii. Adhesins

Adhesins or the surface protein antigens are large proteins constituting 35% of the cell surface protein. The main function of these surface proteins is to facilitate sucrose independent adherence (attachment of organisms to the tooth surface in the absence of sucrose). The adhesins are SAg I/II, of *Streptococcus mutans* and Spa A of *Streptococcus sobrinus*. SAg I/II also possesses a saliva binding region. The antibodies against this saliva binding region protect against the colonization of *Streptococcus mutans* in animals.

iii. Dextranase

Dextranase is a protein enzyme produced by *Streptococcus mutans*, which can break down polymers of glucose, i.e. Dextran, a constituent of early dental plaque. Dextranase may function in sucrose-independent adherence via Spa A, an antigen which can prevent early colonization of the mutans streptococci. Mutans lacking dextranase/Spa A are virulent.

iv. Glucan-binding proteins

Glucans function in plaque accumulation by acting as molecular rein. They may not help in initial colonization; however, they

Table 13.1: List of candidate antigens	
Antigen	Sites
• Glucosyltransferases	• Enzymatic site Glucan binding site
• Adhesins	• Ag I/II (*Streptococcus mutans*) SpaA (*Streptococcus sobrinus*)
• Dextranase	• Enzymatic site Glucan binding site
• Glucan-binding proteins	• Glucan binding site

strengthen the subsequent attachment of the organisms. *Streptococcus mutans* secrete three distinct proteins with glucan-binding activity, i.e. Gbp A, Gbp B and Gbp C. It has been established that only GbpB has shown to induce protective immune response to caries. GbpB has been tried through intranasal route and subcutaneous injection as well.

Streptococcus mutans: Virulence and Cariogenicity

Streptococcus mutans exhibit a set of virulence factors that enable them to adhere and accumulate in oral biofilms. The ability of mutans streptococci to survive acidic environment is regulated by the phenomenon 'quorum sensing' (a cellular communication system of micro-organisms based on the emission of stimuli and responses from the fellow organizer, which play a key role in the development of biofilm).

Four antigens associated with these micro-organisms affect their adhesion and accumulation in the biofilm. These antigens [(glucosyltransferase-(Gtfs), antigen adhesin I/II (Ag I/II), dextranase and glucan-binding proteins-(Gbp)] are the main targets for the development of caries vaccines. The major virulent characteristic of *Streptococcus mutans* is its ability to produce glucosyltransferase (Gtfs), an enzyme that synthesize intracellular and extracellular polysaccharides from sucrose of the diet. Four Gtfs have been identified, viz. GtfA, GtfB, GtfC and GtfD having different affinities to polysaccharides. These polysaccharides enable the aggregation of mutans streptococci to other micro-organisms.

The caries vaccine should target the virulence factors of mutans streptococci. The host immune system influences the caries susceptibility. Saliva contains various components of innate immunity, such as the bacterial proteins, lactoferrin and lysozyme and also lactoperoxidase and agglutinin. Salivary innate immunity may not be effective for caries protection. Components of acquired immunity have a significant role, highlighting stimulation of secretory IgA present in saliva. The IgG and IgM are also involved in defense mechanism of caries, but are less significant than secretory IgA.

Anticaries vaccines operate on the principle of reducing the population of the indigenous bacteria that are associated with the caries disease process.

The development of caries vaccine involves two-steps, (i) the identification of appropriate antigens of mutans streptococci against which protective immune responses could be induced and (ii) the selection of immunization method that will generate sustained levels of salivary antibodies. The antigens involved are streptococcal surface proteins and glucosyltransferases that synthesize adhesive glucans from sucrose.

Mechanism of Action

- The salivary immunoglobulin may act as a specific agglutinin interacting with the bacterial surface receptors and inhibiting colonization and subsequent caries development. The immunoglobulins may inactivate surface glucosyltransferase, which would reduce the synthesis of extra-cellular glucans, leading to reduction in plaque accumulation.
- The salivary glands produce secretory IgA antibodies by direct immunization of the gut associated lymphoid tissue (GALT), from where sensitized B-cells get activated. The salivary IgA antibodies have direct access to the tooth surface; may prevent mutans streptococci from adhering to the tooth surface and may prevent formation of dextran by inhibiting the activity of glucosyltransferase.
- The gingival crevicular mechanism involves all the humoral and cellular components of the systemic immune system. In subcutaneous immunization, mutans are phagocytosed and may

undergo antigenic processing by macrophages.

Routes of Immunization

Several routes have been tried by which an individual can be immunized. Mucosal applications of dental caries vaccines are generally preferred for the induction of secretory IgA antibody in the salivary compartment. The mucosal immune system, whereby antigen is exposed to mucosally associated lymphoid tissue (gut, rectal, bronchial, etc.) is common in dental caries vaccination. Mucosal immunization induces high levels of salivary antibodies that can be sustained for longer periods. Immunizing infants may establish effective immunity against an ensuing colonization by mutans streptococci. It is established that mucosal vaccine antigen delivery have resulted in inhibition of dental caries. The passive administration of antibodies to virulence antigens of *S. mutans* has also shown promise. The routes of immunization are:

a. Oral Route

Most of the earlier studies relied on induction of immunity in the gut associated lymphoid tissues (GALT) orally to elicit salivary IgA antibody response. Daily administration of 10 cells of mutans streptococci in capsules has successfully produced small increase in IgA. An antigen is to be applied by oral feeding, gastric intubation, or in vaccine containing capsules. Various animal studies have observed significant reduction of caries and increased level of salivary IgA antibodies after immunization through drinking water. The drawbacks include, very little increase in secretory antibodies and that too for short duration (even after secondary immunization), immunological memory in secretory IgA responses were limited, detrimental effects of stomach acidity on antigen and also the inductive sites were relatively distantly placed.

b. Intranasal Route

The induction of immunity in mucosal sites anatomically closer to the oral cavity (mainly intranasal) is being tried. Intranasal installation of the antigen, targeting the nasal associated lymphoid tissue (NALT), has been tried to induce immunity to many bacterial antigens including mutans streptococci. It is established that nasal spray route produced better response as compared to oral and tonsillar administration.

c. Tonsillar Route

The application of antigens inducing immune responses has also been tried through tonsils. The tonsillar tissues contain the required elements of immune induction although IgG, rather than IgA dominate the response characteristics. The palatine and the nasopharyngeal tonsils may contribute precursor cells to mucosal effector sites, such as salivary glands. Various animal studies have observed significant success after topically applying the antigens (formalin killed *Streptococcus sobrinus*) subsequently decreasing the infection of these cariogenic bacteria.

d. Rectal Route

The remote mucosal sites, such as rectal route has also been tried. The colon/rectal region has the highest concentration of lymphoid follicles in the lower intestinal tract. Rectal immunization with non-oral bacterial antigens such as *Helicobacter pylori* or *Streptococcus pneumoniae*, may lead to induction of secretory IgA antibodies in distant salivary sites. Preliminary studies have indicated that this route could also be used to induce salivary IgA responses to mutans streptococcal antigens (GTF, etc.).

e. Minor Salivary Gland

Minor salivary glands are present in lips, cheeks and the soft palate. These glands are considered as the potential route for mucosal induction of salivary immune responses as they possess short, broad secretory ducts. The lymphatic tissue aggregate associated with their ducts facilitate retrograde access of bacteria and their products. In a couple of studies, labial GTF significantly proved successful, decreasing the oral streptococci in the whole saliva.

f. Systemic Route of Immunization

Subcutaneous administration of *Streptococcus mutans* in monkeys has successfully elicited antibodies, such as IgG, IgM and IgA. A subcutaneous injection of killed *Streptococcus mutans* in aluminium hydroxide or any other adjuvant has elicited antibodies such as IgG, IgM and IgA.

g. Gingival-crevicular-salivary Route

To limit the potential side effects of other routes and to localize the immune response, gingival crevicular fluid has been used as the route of administration. Immunization with this route led to increased IgA and IgG levels. Lysozyme has been tried into rabbit gingiva eliciting local antibodies. Lesser molecular weight streptococci antigens have resulted in better performance; however, brushing them on the gingiva of monkeys failed to induce antibody development.

Types of Immunization for Caries Vaccines

a. Active Immunization (Stimulation of secretory IgA production)

The secretory IgA prevents adhesion of micro-organisms to the tooth surface, avoiding the onset of bacterial colonization. The active induction of mucosal immune system stimulates production of secretory IgA. The systemic immunization induces production of serum antibodies (IgG), which may reach dental tissues through gingival crevicular fluid. Earlier authors focused on incorporation of purified antigen of mutans streptococci on the mucosal immune system. The rationale was to block the micro-organisms receptors

and to modify the metabolic functions of bacterial enzymes; subsequently affecting biofilm organization and the caries. The antibodies specific for antigen I/II interfere with virulence factor of mutans streptococci and inhibit their adhesion and colonization in the oral biofilm.

Stimulation of secretory IgA has shown promising results in animal studies; whereas the cross-reactivity between surface antigens of mutans streptococci and human tissues make immunization non-viable for human beings.

b. Passive Immunization (addition of specific antibodies)

It involves passive or external supplementation of the antibodies (the antibody remain only for a few hours, making it difficult to maintain sufficient level of inhibition in biofilms). The disadvantage of passive immunization is the repeated applications, as the immunity conferred is temporary. This type of immunization has the advantage of avoiding any risk due to active immunization.

A pre-formed antibody is introduced orally in passive immunization. The source of these antibodies may be:

- Monoclonal antibodies.
- Bovine milk and eggs.
- The cows get systemic vaccination using whole *Streptococcus mutans*; subsequently the bovine milk of the vaccinated cows containing polyclonal IgG antibodies is used.
- Egg-yolk antibodies.
- Extracts of transgenic plants, such as *Nicotiana tabacum*, have been tried in the passive immunization.

These antibodies have been tried to control bacterial colonization and dental caries in humans. Such immunization is believed to be a safer approach for controlling dental caries than active immunization.

c. DNA-based Immunization

A new way of presenting immunogens, the DNA vaccines are being tried in which a specific gene is injected, which generates its products within the organisms. The DNA of *Streptococcus mutans* (encoding gene of the antigen protein), extracted by chemical lysis is used for the development of this type of vaccine. The immune response induced by DNA vaccines is initiated with the activation of antigen-presenting cells. After immunization, DNA vaccines directly transfect somatic cells. The antigen-presenting cells capture these antigens, process them and submit them as peptides to T-lymphocytes where antigen specific T-cells are activated.

Advantages

- Easy preparation and administration.
- Induce an effective immune response.
- Stable in storage.

Disadvantages

- Vaccines in large scales are not produced.
- Costly.

The important studies on caries vaccines are summarized in Table 13.2.

Table 13.2: Important studies on anticaries vaccines		
Author (year) and type of study	Type of vaccine, type of cell/animal (Route of administration)	Inference
Russell Colman (1981) In-vivo	Protein (purified Gtf), Monkeys (subcutaneous)	The serum antibodies level against Gtf was elevated; however, no difference in caries development. The Gtf could not induce specific immune response.
Mitoma, et al (2002) In-vivo	Antibodies (milk immune), Rats (oral)	Animals had significantly less caries development. Because of passive immunization, it does not generate a lasting response.
Fan, et al (2002) In-vivo	Vaccine of DNA pCIA-P, Gnotobiotic rats (intramuscular/submucosa/subcutaneous)	High levels of serum sIgA and IgG observed. Induce immune responses, subsequently low level of caries.
Xu, et al (2005) In-vivo	Vaccine DNA pGJA-P/VAX, Mice (intranasal)	The antibody responses induced by pGJA-P/VAX vaccine had long lasting effect in the cervical lymph nodes (six months or even more). The persistent immune responses act as a booster immunization.
Jia, et al (2006) In-vivo	Vaccine of DNA pGJA-P/VAX, Rabbits and monkeys (intranasal/intramuscular)	The vaccines induced significant increase in salivary IgG and IgA in monkeys. The fusion of vaccines has promising results in caries development.
Xu, et al (2007) In-vivo	Vaccine DNA pGJA-P/VAX, Rats (intranasal)	Improved sIgA response resulted in reduction of lesions caused by *S. mutans* and *S.sobrinus*. The vaccine provides immune response to infection by *S.mutans* and also provides cross-protection against *S.sobrinus* strains.

Contd...

Table 13.2: Important studies on anticaries vaccines (*Contd...*)

Author (year) and type of study	Type of vaccine, type of cell/animal (Route of administration)	Inference and remarks
Zhang, et al (2007) In-vivo/in-vitro	Vaccine DNA pGJA-P/VAX1 pGJA-P pGLUA-P Gnotobiotic hamster/human dendritic cells (intramuscular/intranasal)	Fewer caries lesions observed after immunizing with pGJA-P/vax1 and pGJA-P (induced better response in salivary/serum antibodies). The combination of CTLA-4 associated to DNA vaccine, pGJA-P/vax1 increased the immunogenicity and protective efficacy of the vaccine.
Niu, et al (2009) In-vivo	Vaccine of DNA pGJGAC/VAX and pGJGA-5C/VAX Gnotobiotic rats (Intramuscular intranasal)	Improved form of DNA vaccine was significantly effective against *Streptococcus mutans* and *Streptococcus sobrinus*.
Yang, et al (2009) In-vivo	Vaccine DNA pGJA-P/VAX, Gnotobiotic mice and rats (intranasal)	Increased production of IgG and sIgA and decreased development of caries. The production of anticaries DNA vaccine, pGJA-P/VAX was good. The vaccine showed desired results.
Shi, et al (2012) In-vivo	Vaccine DNA pGJA-P/VAX with FLic protein form salmonella (intranasal)	Increased production of IgA in saliva and inhibit the colonization of *Streptococcus mutans*.
Chen, et al (2013) In-vitro	Vaccine DNA pGJA-P/VAX	The new DNA vaccine induce high level of sIgA. Efficient delivery of immunity.
Su, et al (2014) In-vitro/in- vivo	Vaccine-DNA pCI-IL-6, Rats (intranasal)	Recent DNA vaccine showed less development of caries. Significantly improves immunogenicity.

Vaccines Tried

- A cell surface protein antigen of *Streptococcus mutans* (PAc) involved in the binding of bacteria to the tooth surface is used in the development of vaccines.
- Liposome vaccines containing *Streptococcus mutans* glucosyltransferase (GTF).
- Vaccines prepared from purified antigens of mutans streptococci (proven good in primates but yet to be tested on humans).
- The structural gene for a surface protein antigen of *Streptococcus mutans* serotype c (PAc) has been tried.
- Anti-id (idiotype) vaccines into salivary gland and liposomes lead to increase in salivary immunoglobulins and providing protective immune responses to pathogens of mucosal surfaces.

- Anti-caries DNA vaccines, viz. pGJA-P/VAX derived from GLU fragment of *Streptococcus mutans* gtf B gene and A-P fragment of the *Streptococcus mutans* of PAc gene.
- pGJA-P/VAX encoded with catalytic fragment of *Streptococcus sobrinus* gtf-I to form pGJAC/VAX vaccine. It inhibits the ability of water insoluble glucan synthesis by *Streptococcus sobrinus* and also raises the level of serum IgG and salivary IgA antibody responses.
- pGJA-P/VAX encoded with full length of 1.1 kb CAT fragment of *Streptococcus sobrinus* to form p-GJA-5C/VAX.
- Anticaries DNA vaccine, pGJA-P/VAX recombined with FLIc protein derived from salmonella flagella as a mucosal adjuvant. It increases serum PAc specific IgG and

saliva PAc specific IgA antibody responses as compared with pGJA-P/VAX alone and significantly decreased the colonization of *Streptococcus mutans*.

- Another DNA was tried by using the A-P fragment of PAc from *Streptococcus mutans* (rPAc) at the c-terminus of flagella derived from *E. coli* (designated as KF) to produce single recombinant protein (KF-rPAc). It increases antibodies in serum as well as in saliva and provide protection against caries.

- Caro Rx™ binds to *Streptococcus mutans* and prevents its adherence to *Streptococcus mutans*; however, colonization of other oral bacteria continues. Caro Rx™ has been developed by planet biotechnology and is under clinical trial.

ADJUVANTS AND DELIVERY SYSTEMS

The protective effects of active immunization with dental caries vaccines have not been successfully documented. Mucosal application of these antigens may not effectively result in sustained IgA response. The researchers, over the years, were developing adjuvants (immune modulators) and the delivery system, which could enhance the response to dental caries vaccines. The following approaches have been tried with varied results:

a. *Synthetic peptides:* It is hypothesized that subcutaneous immunization with a synthetic peptide derived from the alanine-rich Ag I/II of *Streptococcus mutans* induced higher level of serum IgA antibodies than synthetic peptides derived from proline-rich Ag I/II of *Streptococcus mutans*. The synthetic peptide is derived from GTF enzymes. These peptides provide antibodies to saliva as well as to gingival crevicular fluid.

b. *Microcapsules and microparticles:* The microcapsules and microparticles made of poly lactide-co-glycolide (PLGA) have been used as local delivery systems because of their ability to control the rate of release of vaccine in the gut lymphoid tissues. These micro particles also evade pre-existent antibody clearance mechanisms and degrade slowly without eliciting any inflammatory response.

c. *Liposomes:* Liposomes are bilayered phospholipids membrane vesicles used to deliver drugs and antigens at the target cells. Liposomes are thought to improve mucosal immune responses by facilitating M cell uptake and delivery of antigen to lymphoid elements of inductive tissue. Various studies have confirmed increased IgA antibody level in humans.

d. *Recombinant vaccines:* Recombinant method is followed whereby fusion of different strains is effectively utilized. It is reported that oral immunization with the recombinant salmonella vaccine was effective in inducing protection against *Streptococcus sobrinus* in rats.

e. *Conjugate vaccines:* The conjugation of protein with polysaccharides enhances the immunogenicity of the T-cell independent polysaccharides. The chemical conjugation of functionally associated protein-peptide components with bacterial polysaccharides (conjugate vaccine) is being tried to interrupt various aspects of mutans streptococci pathogenesis.

f. *Subunit coupling:* It is established that coupling of proteins with subunit of cholera toxin was effective in suppressing colonization of *Streptococcus mutans*. Addition of small amount of cholera toxin or even *E. coli* may enhance mucosal immune responses to the mutans streptococci antigens or to peptide derived from these antigens.

Drawbacks

The drawbacks involved in caries vaccines are:

- Difficulty in convincing parents for vaccination.

- Lack of prioritization of caries vaccines in health administrators.
- Number of contacts required with the primary provider.
- Benefits versus risks of active and passive immunity approaches.
- Acceptance by the dental profession and the public.
- Cost factor.

Risk and Caries Vaccines

Usually caries vaccines carry no risk when administered properly. However, some patients with rheumatic fever may present serological cross-reactivity between heart tissue antigens and certain antigens from hemolytic streptococci. Such cross reactions have been confirmed in animal and human studies. Since caries is a continuous life long process, the vaccine/immune protection should also be long lasting. Immunization prior to infection is the main goal of vaccination. Mutans streptococci colonization occur early in life. The vaccination should be initiated early, at least within 2 years of the child. Question remains, whether eradicating mutans streptococci from oral cavity or making them ineffective would be sufficient to halt caries process, since it is established that mutans streptococci are not the only micro-organisms causing caries. There might be need to create vaccines for other pathogenic micro-organisms.

Bibliography

1. Bao R, Yang JY, Sun Y, Zhou DH, Yang Y, Li YM, Cao Y, Xiao Y, Li W, Yu J, Zhao BL, Zhong MH and Yan HM. Flagellin–PAc Fusion Protein Inhibits Progression of Established Caries. J.Dent.Res.2015;94:955–60.
2. Book I and Grahnen H. Clinical and genetic studies of dental caries. II. Parents and siblings of adult highly resistant (caries-free) proposition. Odont. Rev.: 1953;4:1–52.
3. Boraas JC, Messer LB and Till MJ. A genetic contribution to dental caries, occlusion and morphology as demonstrated by twins reared apart. J. Dent. Res.: 1988;67:1150–5.
4. Borges O, Lebre F and Bento D, Borchard G, Jungingen HE. Mucosal vaccines: recent progress in understanding the natural barriers. Pharm. Res.; 2010;27:211–23.
5. Bowen WH and Koo H. Biology of *Streptococcus mutans* derived Glucosyltransferase: role in extracellular matrix formation of cariogenic biofilms. Caries Research: 2011;45:69–86.
6. Chen L, Zhu J, Li Y, Lu J, Gao L, Xu H, Fan M and Yang XL. Enhanced nasal mucosal delivery and immunogenicity of anti-caries DNA vaccine through incorporation of anionic liposomes in Chitosan/DNA complexes. Plos One:8, e71953 2013.
7. Childers NK, Tong G, Li F, Dasanayake AP, Kirk K and Michalek SM. Humans immunized with *Streptococcus mutans* antigens by mucosal routes. J. Dent. Res. 2002;81:48–52.
8. Coffman RL, Sher A and Seder RA. Vaccine adjuvants: putting innate immunity to work. Immunity: 2010;33:492–503.
9. Crawford JM, Taubman MA and Smith DJ. Minor salivary glands as a major source of secretory immunoglobin A in the human oral cavity. Science 1975;190:1206–9.
10. Cui Z. DNA vaccine. Advances in Genetics: 2005; 54: 257–89.
11. DA Silva DR, DA Silva ACB, Filho RM, Verli FD and Marinho SA. Vaccine against dental caries: an update. Advances in Microbiology 2014;4: 925–33.
12. Danielsson NL, Hernell O and Johansson I. Human milk compounds inhibiting adhesion of mutans streptococci to host ligand-coated hydroxyapatite *in-vitro*. Caries Res. 2009;43: 171–8.
13. Davey ME and O'toole GA. Microbial biofilms: from ecology to molecular genetics. Microbiol. Mol. Biol. Rev.: 2000;64:847–67.
14. Doetzer AD, Brancher JA, Pecharki GD, Schlipf N, Werneck R, Mira MT, Riess O, Bauer P and Trevilatto PC. Lactotransferrin gene polymorphism associated with caries experience. Caries Res. 2015;49:370–7.
15. Enioutina EY, Visic DM and Daynes RA. The induction of systemic and mucosal immunity to protein vaccines delivered through skin sites exposed to UVB. Vaccine: 2002;20:2116–30.
16. Fan MW, Bian Z, Peng ZX, Z hong Y, Chen Z, Peng B, Jia R. A DNA vaccine encoding a cell-surface protein antigen of *Streptococcus mutans* protects gnotobiotic rats from caries. J. Dent. Res. 2002;81:784–7.

17. Gambhir RS, Singh S, Singh G, Singh R, Nanda T and Kakar H. Vaccine against dental caries—an urgent need. J. Vaccines Vaccin: 2012;3:136.

18. George S and Anitha R. Dental Caries Vaccine—A Current Update. Am. J. Pharm Health Res. 2014;2:28–33.

19. Guo JH, Jia R, Fan MW, Bian Z, Chen Z and Peng B. Construction and immunogenic characterization of a fusion anti-caries DNA vaccine against pAc and glycosyltransferase I of Streptococcus mutans. J. Dent. Res. 2004;83:266–70.

20. Hagan T, Shah GR and Caufiled PW. DNA fingerprinting for studying transmission of Streptococcus mutans. J. Dent. Res. 1989;67:407.

21. Hajishengallis G and Michalek SM. Current status of a mucosal vaccine against dental caries. Oral Microbiol. Immunol. 1999;14:1–20.

22. Hamada S and Salde HD. Biology, immunology and cariogenicity of Streptococcus mutans. Microbiol. Rev. 1980;44:331–84.

23. Harris R. Vaccines for dental caries. Aust. Dent. J.: 1983;28:115–6.

24. Hassell TM and Harris EL. Genetic influences in caries and periodontal diseases. Critical Reviews in Oral Biology and Medicine: 1995;6:319–42.

25. Hayashi F, Smith KD, Ozinsky A, Hawn TR, Yi EC and Goodlett DR. The innate immune response to bacterial flagellin in mediated by Toll-like receptor 5. Nature: 2001;410:1099–1103.

26. Haznedaroglu E, Koldemir-Gunduz M, Bakir-Coskun N, Bozkus HM, Cagatay P, Susleyici-Duman B and Mentes A. Association of Sweet Taste Recptor Gene Polymorphism with Dental Caries Experience in Schoolchildren. Caries Res. 2015;49:275–81.

27. Hillman JD, Brooks TA and Michalek SM. Construction and characterization of an effector strain of Streptococcus mutans for replacement therapy of Streptococcus mutans therapy of dental caries. J. Dent. Res. 2000; 68:543-9.

28. Holla LI, Linhartova PB, Lucanova S, Kastovsky J, Musilova K, Bartosova M, Kukletova M, Kukla L and Dusek L. GLUT2 and TAS1R2 Polymorphisms and Susceptibility to Dental Caries.Caries Res. 2015;49:417–24.

29. Huang L, Xu Q, Liu C, Fan M and Li Y. Anti-caries DNA vaccine-induced secretory immunoglobulin A antibodies inhibit formation of Streptococcus mutans biofilms in vitro. Acta. Pharmacol. Sinica.: 2013;34:239–46.

30. Huang L, Xu QA, Liu C, Fan MW and Li YH. Anti-caries DNA vaccine-induced secretory immunoglobulin A antibodies inhibit formation of Streptococcus mutans biofilms in vitro. Acta. Pharmacol. Sin: 2013;34:239–46.

31. HuiMin Y. Salivary IgA enhancement strategy for development of a nasal-spray anti-caries mucosal vaccine. Life Sciences: 2013;56:406–13.

32. Huleatt JW, Jacobs AR and Tang J. Vaccination with recombinant fusion proteins incorporating Toll-like receptor ligants induces rapid cellular and humoral immunity. Vaccine: 2007;25:763–75.

33. Jakubovics NS, Stromberg N, Van Dolleweerd CJ, Kelly CG and Jenikson HF. Differentia binding specificities of oral streptococcal antigen I/II family adhesions for human or bacterial ligands. Molecular Microbiology: 2005;55:1519–1605.

34. Jefferson KK. What drives bacteria to produce a biofilm? FEMS Microbiol. Lett.: 2004;236:163–73.

35. Jespersgaard C, Hajishengallis G, Russell MW and Michalek SM. Identification and characterization of a non-immunoglobulin factor in human saliva that inhibits Streptococcus mutans glucosyl-transferase. Infect. Immun.: 2002;70:1136–42.

36. Jia R, Guo JH, Fan MW, Bian Z, Chen Z and Fan B. Immunologicity of CTLA4 fusion anti-caries DNA vaccine in rabbits and monkeys. Vaccine: 2006;24:5192–200.

37. Koga T, Hamada S, Murakawa S and Endo A. Effect of a glucosyltransferase inhibitor on glucan synthesis and cellular adherence of Streptococcus mutans. Infect. Immun.: 1982;38:882–6.

38. Koga T, Oho T, Shimazaki Y and Nakano Y. Immunization against dental caries. Vaccine: 2002;20:2027–44.

39. Kolenbrander PE. Oral microbial communities: biofilms, interactions and genetic systems. Annu. Rev. Microbiol.: 2000;54:413–37.

40. Krasse B, Emilson CL and Gahnberg L. An anticaries vaccine: report on the status of research. Caries Res. 1987;21:255–76.

41. Kuramitsu HK. Virulence factors of mutans streptococci: role of molecular genetics. Crit. Rev. Oral Biol. Med. 1993;4:159–76.

42. Kurtz J. Memory in the innate and adaptive immune systems. Microbes Infgect.: 2004;6:1410–7.

43. Lam A, Smith D, Barnes L, Clements JD, Wise D and Taubman MA. Alternate routes for dental caries vaccine delivery. J. Dent. Res.: 2001;80:124.

44. Lamont RJ, Demuth DR, Davis CA, Malamud D and Rosan B. Salivary-Agglutinin-Mediated adherence of Streptococcus mutans to early plaque bacteria. Infect. Immun.: 1991;59:3446–50.

45. Lehner T, Russell MW, Caldwell J and Smith R. Immunization with purified protein antigens from *Streptococcus mutans* against dental caries in Rhesus monkeys. Infection and Immunity: 1981;34:407–15.

46. Levine M, Owen WL and Avery KT. Antibody response to actinomyces antigen and dental caries experience: implications for caries susceptibility. Clinical and Diagnostic Laboratorial Immunology: 2005;12:764–9.

47. Li Y, Jin J, Yang Y, Bian Z, Chen Z and Fan MW. Enhanced immunogenicity of an anti-caries vaccine encoding a cell-surface protein antigen of *Streptococcus mutans* by intranasal DNA prime-protein boost immunization. J. Gene Med.: 2009;11:1039–47.

48. Liu C, Fan M, Xu Q and Li Y. Biodistribution and expression of targeted fusion anti-caries DNA vaccine pGJA-P/VAX in mice. J. Gene Med.: 2008;10:298–305.

49. Lycke N. Recent progress in mucosal vaccine development potential and limitations. Nat. Rev. Immunol.: 2012;12:592–605.

50. Mattos-Graner RO and Smith DJ. The vaccination approach to control infections leading to dental caries. Braz. J. Oral Sci.: 2004;3:595–608.

51. Michalek SM and Childers NK. Development and outlook for a caries vaccine. Crit. Rev. Oral Biol. Med.: 1990;1:37–54.

52. Mitoma M, Oho T, Michibata N, Okano K, Nakano Y, Fukuyama M and Koga T. Passive immunization with bovine milk containing antibodies to a cell surface protein antigen-glucosyltransferase fusion protein protects rats against dental caries. Infect. Immunity: 2002;70:2721–4.

53. Mizel SB and Bates JT. Flagellin as an adjuvant: cellular mechanisms and potential. J. Immunol.: 2010;185:5677–82.

54. Monsan P, Bozonnet S, Albenne C, Joucla G, Willemot RM and Remaud-Simeon M. Homopolysaccharides from lactic acid bacteria. Int. Diary J.: 2001;11:675–85.

55. Niu Y, Sun J, Fan M, Xu QA, Guo J, Jia R and Li Y. Construction of a new fusion anti-caries DNA vaccine. J. Dent. Res.: 2009;88:455–60.

56. Ozturk A, Famili P and Vieira AR. The antimicrobial peptide DEFB1 is associated with caries. J. Dent. Res.: 2010;6:631–6.

57. Plotkin SA. Correlates of protection induced by vaccination. Clin. Vaccine Immunol.: 2010;17:1055–65.

58. Rogers AH. Immunization against dental caries. A review. Aust.Dent. J.1982;27:81–5.

59. Russell MW, Childers NK, Michalek SM, Smith DJ and Taubman MA. A caries vaccine? The state of the science of immunization against dental caries. Caries Res.: 2004;38:230–5.

60. Russell MW, Hajishengallis G, Childers NK and Michalek SM. Secretory immunity in defense against cariogenic mutans streptococci. Caries Res.: 1999;33:4–15.

61. Russell RR. Wall-associated protein antigens of *Streptococcus mutans*. J. Gen. Microbiol.: 1979; 114: 109–15.

62. Russell RRB and Colman G. Immunization of monkey (*Macaca fascicularis*) with purified *Streptococcus mutans* glucosyltransferase. Archives of Oral Biology: 1981;26:23–8.

63. Sanui TI and Gregory RL. Analysis of *Streptococcus mutans* biofilm proteins recognized by salivary immunoglobulin A. Oral Microbiol Immunol. 2009;24:361–8.

64. Seemann R, Bizhang M, Kluck I, Loth J and Roulet JF. A novel *in vitro* microbial-based model for studying caries formation—Development and initial testing. Caries Res.: 2005;39:185–90.

65. Seki M, Yamashita Y, Shibata Y, Torigoe H, Tsuda H and Maeno M. Effect of mixed mutans streptococci colonization on caries development. Oral Microbiol. Immunol.: 2006;21:47–52.

66. Shi W, Li YH, Liu F, Yang JY, Zhou DH, Chen YQ, Zhang Y, Yang Y, He BX, Han C, Fan MW and Yan HM. Flagellin enhances saliva IgA response and protection of anti-caries DNA vaccine. J. Dent. Res.: 2012;91:249–54.

67. Sims W. *Streptococcus mutans* and vaccines for dental caries: a personal commentary and critique. Community Dent. Health 1985;2:129–47.

68. Smith DJ and Mattos-Garner RO. Secretory immunity following mutans streptococcal infection or immunization. Curr. Top. Microbiol. Immunol. 2008;319:131–56.

69. Smith DJ and Taubman MA. Emergence of immune competence in saliva. Crit. Rev. Oral Biol. Med.: 1993;4:335–41.

70. Smith DJ and Taubman MA. Ontogeny of immunity to oral microbiota in humans. Crit. Rev. Oral Biol. Med.: 1992;3:109–33.

71. Smith DJ, King WF, Barnes LA, Trantolo D, Wise DL and Taubman MA. Facilitated intranasal induction of mucosal and systemic immunity to mutans streptococci glucosyltransferase peptide vaccines. Infect. Immune.: 2001;69:4767.

72. Smith DJ, King WF, Rivero J and Taubman MA. Immunological and protective effects of diepitopic subunit dental caries vaccines. Infect. Immun.: 2005;73:2797–804.

73. Smith DJ. Caries vaccines for the twenty first century. J. Dent. Educ. 2003;67:1130–9.

74. Smith DJ. Dental caries vaccines: prospects and concerns. Crit. Rev. Oral Biol. Med. 2002;13:335–49.

75. Smith DJ. Dental caries vaccines: prospects and concerns. Expert Review of Vaccines: 2010;9:1–3.

76. Smith DJ. Prospects in caries vaccine development. J. Dent. Res. 2012;91:225–6.

77. Su LK, Yu F, Li Z, Zeng C, Xu QA and Fan MW. Intranasal co-delivery of IL-6 gene enhances the immunogenicity of anti-caries DNA vaccine. Acta Pharmacologica ASinica: 2014;35:592–8.

78. Sun J, Xu Q and Fan MW. A new strategy for the replacement therapy of dental caries. Medical Hypothesis: 2009;73:1063–4.

79. Sun J, Yang X, Xu Q, Bian Z, Chen Z and Fan M. Protective efficacy of two new anti-caries DNA vaccines. Vaccine: 2009;27:7459–66.

80. Taubman MA and Nash DA. The scientific and public-health imperative for a vaccine against dental caries. Nature Reviews Immunology: 2006;6:555–63.

81. Taubman MA, Holmberg C, Smith DJ and Eastcott J. T and B cell epitopes from peptide sequences associated with glucosyltransferase function. Clin. Immunol. Immunopathol.: 1995;76:S95.

82. Taubman MA, Holmberg CL and Smith DJ. Immunization of rats with synthetic peptide constructs from the glucan biding or catalytic region of mutans. Streptococcal glucosyltransferase protect against dental caries infection and immunity: 1995;63:3088–93.

83. Thomas JG and Nakaishi LA. Managing the complexity of a dynamic biofilm. J. Am. Dent. Assoc.: 2006;137:10S–15S.

84. Toda Y, Moro I, Koga T, Asakawa H and Hamada S. Ultrastructure of extracellular polysaccharides produced by serotype c *Streptococcus mutans*. J. Dent. Res.: 1987;66:1364–9.

85. Tsumori H, Minami T and Kuramitsu HK. Identification of essential amino acids in the *Streptococcus mutans* glucosyltransferases. J. Bacteriol.: 1997;179:3391–6.

86. Vieiras AR, Marazita ML and Goldstein-McHenry. Genome-wide scan finds suggestive caries loci. J. Dent. Res.: 2008;87:435–9.

87. Waterhouse JC and Roy RB. Dispensable genes and foreign DNA in *Streptococcus mutans*. Microbiology: 2006;152:1777–88.

88. Wendell X, Wang X and Brown M. Taste genes associates with dental caries. J. Dent. Res.: 2010;89:1198–2002.

89. Wiater A, Choma A and Szczodrak J. Insoluble glucans synthesized by cariogenic streptococci: a structural study. J. Basic Microbiol.: 1999;39:265–73.

90. Xu QA, Yu F, Fan MW, Bian Z, Chen Z, Fan B, Jia R and Guo JH. Immunogenicity and persistence of a targeted anti-caries DNA vaccine. J. Dent. Res.: 2006;85:915–8.

91. Xu QA, Yu F, Fan MW, Bian Z, Chen Z, Peng B, Jia R and Guo JH. Protective efficacy of a targeted anti-caries DNA plasmid against cariogenic bacteria infections. Vaccine: 2007;25:1191–5.

92. Xu QA, Yu F, Fan MW, Bian Z, Guo J, Jia R, Chen Z, Peng B and Fan B. Immunogenicity and protective efficacy of targeted fusion DNA construct against dental caries. Caries Res.: 2005;39:422.

93. Yang YP, Li YH, Bi L and Fan MW. Good manufacturing practices production and analysis of DNA vaccine against dental caries. Acta. Pharamcologica Sinica: 2009;30:1513–21.

94. Younson J and Kelly CG. The rational design of an anti-caries peptide against *Streptococcus mutans*. Molecular Diversity: 2004;8:121–6.

95. Zhang F, Li YH, Fan MW, Jia R, Xu KA, Guo JH, Yu F and Tian KW. Enhanced efficacy of CTLA-4 fusion anticaries DNA vaccines in gnotobiotic hamsters. Acta. Pharmacologica Sinica: 2007;28:1236–42.

96. Zhang Z, Nadezhina E and Wilkinson KJ. Quantifying diffusion in a biofilm of *Streptococcus mutans*. Antimicrobial Agents and Chemotherapy: 2011;55:1075–81.

Resin Infiltration

14

Caries has long been detected at the level of cavitation. The accepted treatment option was to remove the caries, create cavity and to restore that cavity with suitable restorative material. The geometric cavities were created, depending on the retentive properties of the restorative materials to be used. Over the years, the threshold was directed towards detection of caries at an early non-cavitated stage, also called 'white spot' lesion. The proximal caries also pose considerable problem (50% carious lesions in an adult are proximal caries).

Presently, the preventive strategies focus on to reverse the early non-cavitated carious lesions with the use of topical fluorides, remineralizing agents and modifying oral ecology in favor of remineralization, etc. These preventive regimes have shown varying degrees of success but are dependent on patient compliance. These are also time consuming, since the patients need to use these remineralizing agents for months together so as to achieve reversal of the lesions. Moreover, the access of these remineralizing agents into proximal areas might be limited.

Traditionally, the surgical mode of managing caries, being an invasive method, involves losing some sound tooth structure prior to restoration; whereas the preventive strategies are directed for reversal of early carious lesions. Several approaches have been proposed for the non-invasive management of non-cavitated (initial caries) lesions. These include remineralization using fluorides and casein phosphopeptide-amorphous calcium phosphate, use of sealants, use of resorcinol-formaldehyde resin, etc. 60% lesion's pore volume could be occluded using resorcinol-formaldehyde; however, discoloration effect of resorcinol made it clinically unacceptable. Resorcinol-formaldehyde was effective in reducing further acid demineralization.

A novel technique is being tried that involves infiltration of very low viscosity resins into the pores of early non-cavitated carious lesions so as to halt the progression of caries. This concept is called 'Resin Infiltration'. In contrast to sealing carious lesions with sealants (lead to external occlusion of the lesion), the pores get occluded within the entire body in resin infiltration.

Earlier it was debated that bacteria entrapped at the base could trigger and spread caries; however, later it was established that the count of remaining bacteria was low and not detrimental.

Resin infiltration is a micro-invasive treatment regime for arresting early carious lesions. The initial carious lesion is porous due to loss of minerals from the tooth surface.

These porosities can be infiltrated by low viscosity resin (a low viscosity resin with a high penetration coefficient has been developed by Dental Milestones Guaranteed-DMG and is marketed as ICON caries infiltrant), which lead to strengthening of the demineralized tooth surface without any drilling. The infiltration procedure also provides optical blending of the carious lesion with the healthy enamel. The concept of resin infiltration was first developed at the University of Kiel (Germany) to be used for the management of smooth surfaces and proximal non-cavitated carious lesions.

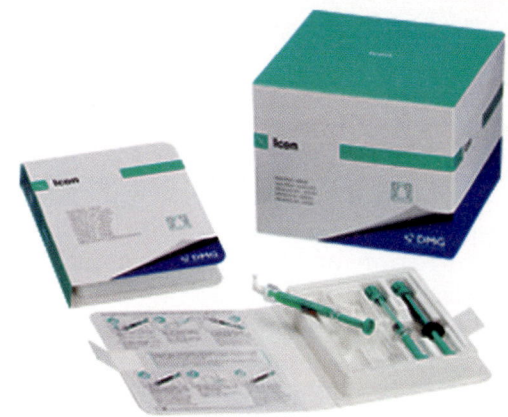

Fig. 14.1: Resin infiltration kit

Requirements of Resin Infiltrant

The requisite characteristics of resin infiltration are:

- Should be hydrophilic, highly surface-active and with low viscosity.
- Should be bacteriostatic.
- Should be non-toxic to oral tissues.
- Easily polymerizable in oral environment.
- Should resist chemical and mechanical challenges of the oral cavity.
- Esthetically pleasing.

Resin Infiltration Kit

The resin infiltration kit is available separately for vestibular and proximal lesions containing three syringes, (i) acid gel (ICON Etch), (ii) drying agent (ICON Dry) and (iii) Resin infiltrant (ICON Infiltrant) along with special applicator tips. The Etchant (acid) gel is composed of 15% hydrochloric acid, water, silica, etc. which effectively etches the tooth surface. Drying agent is ethanol, which removes water retained in micro-porosities. The infiltrant is composed of tri-ethylene glycol di-methacrylate (TEGDMA), a light cure low viscosity resin which penetrates the pores due to capillary action, filling the pores completely (Fig. 14.1).

Development of Resin Infiltrant, Etchant and Drying Agent

The micro-porosities created by demineralization process and subsequently filled with resins have been evaluated since long. Even earlier studies have demonstrated that the penetration of resins into demineralized surfaces inhibited the progress of early caries lesions; even though the resins available at that time might not penetrate effectively deep due to their high viscosity (higher the viscosity lesser is the penetration coefficient). Researchers continued to develop resins of low viscosity capable of penetrating deep into the pores created by demineralization. The resins exhibiting rapid penetration abilities were termed 'Infiltrants'.

The infiltration depth of these resins was evaluated clinically. The infiltration of 'low-viscosity' resins into the natural tooth surface was difficult; might be due to the presence of pseudo-intact layer covering the porous structure hampering the infiltration. The surface layer is formed by precipitation of minerals on the outer surface and has a much lower pore volume compared to the lesion body, thus inhibiting the penetration of the resin.

Conventional phosphoric acid etching was not effective as the penetration of resins remained superficial (phosphoric acid affected only 25 µm of surface). 15% hydrochloric acid for two minutes was tried as an alternative etching protocol. It removed 58 µm of demineralized/normal enamel surface. Etching with 15% HCl gel for 90–120 seconds was found to be more effective than 37% phosphoric acid gel (hydrochloric acid in concentration of 18% has been used in dentistry for micro-abrasion). The erosion depth with hydrochloric acid was more than twice as compared to phosphoric acid when etched for two minutes (Paris, et al 2010). HCl penetrates into deepest part of the lesion, preventing further attacks.

The addition of ethanol application after etchant application significantly increased the penetration of infiltrant due to decrease of viscosity and contact angle. Better penetration was observed using combination of TEGDMA and HEMA as infiltrant along with using 20% ethanol.

Indications for Resin Infiltration

- White spot lesions (early caries).
  - Proximal.
  - Cervical.
  - Occlusal (under trial).
- Fluorosis stains (non-pitted).
- Amelogenesis imperfecta.
- Molar-incisor hypomineralization.

Utilization of Resin Infiltration

Resin infiltration technique is utilized in the following clinical conditions:

i. Masking White Opacities

The process of caries starts with the loss of minerals leading to formation of micro-porosities in the tooth surface. This incipient lesion is usually covered by pseudo-intact layer. The outer surface loses its sheen and appears as chalky white opaque area also referred to as 'white spot' lesion.

The white opacity can be easily appreciated when the tooth surface is dried. Sound tooth

Table 14.1: Refractive index of various objects

Object	Refractive index
Sound tooth	1.62
Water	1.33
Air	1.00
Resin infiltrant	1.52

enamel has a refractive index of 1.62 and the incipient lesions (micro-porosities) usually get filled with salivary fluid (water) having a refractive index of 1.33 (Table 14.1). Since the refractive index of sound tooth and water is nearly the same, it becomes difficult to visualize the white spot lesion by naked eyes. On drying the tooth surface, the water is removed and the pores get filled with air. Since air has refractive index of 1 and due to appropriate difference between sound tooth and air, the white opacity can be visualized with naked eye.

When these micro-porosities are filled with the resin infiltrant having a refractive index of 1.52, the white opacity gets masked, regaining the esthetics of the tooth.

The masking of white spot lesions is based on filling the porosities by resin infiltrant having a similar refractive index as that of sound tooth.

ii. Managing Fluorosis, Traumatic Hypoplasia and Molar-incisor Hypomineralization

Fluorosis is a condition of enamel hypo-mineralization which can lead to surface and subsurface porosities. Mild form of fluorosis may appear as loss of translucency on cuspal tips (usually premolars), incisal border of anterior teeth, white flecks/striations on labial surfaces, etc.

The traumatic hypoplastic teeth behave similar to inactive caries lesions (results are not as esthetically pleasing as in case of active lesions).

Molar-incisor hypomineralization infers hypomineralization of systemic origin that can affect one to all first permanent molars along with permanent incisors. Clinically, it appears as white/yellow/brown opacities which are well demarcated compared to normal enamel. Molar-incisor hypominera-lized molars are fragile and more prone to caries. The esthetics is compromised in both the conditions.

Several techniques have been tried to improve the appearance of such lesion, viz. micro-abrasion, bleaching and other invasive techniques ranging from composite restoration to tooth veneers. These techniques warrant compromising large amount of enamel, which may lead to postoperative sensitivity. Resin infiltration is considered as an accepted alternative approach for managing these lesions.

Mild to moderate type of such lesions can be effectively treated with resin infiltration technique; however, the limitations of this technique is the need to diagnose and distinguish between developmental and non-developmental opacities, since infiltration may not be effective in case of developmental defects.

iii. *Managing Orthodontic Scars*

The patients who have undergone fixed orthodontic treatment may exhibit white opacities on labial/buccal surfaces. These opacities are termed orthodontic scars. The orthodontic treatment compromises oral hygiene maintenance, increasing the risk of subsequent enamel demineralization. Resin infiltration technique is helpful in improving esthetics of the affected tooth.

Types, etiology and treatment options of white spots are tabulated in Table 14.2.

iv. *Infiltration in Primary Dentition*

It is established that ultrastructure and mineral content of primary enamel is different (less mineralized and more porous and aprismatic as compared to permanent enamel). Since the proximal surface layer is less mineralized in primary molars, the rate of caries progression is significantly higher in primary molars.

The conventional etching with 15% HCl for 40–60 seconds resulted in considerable erosion of the mineralized surface layer. The penetration of resin is better in primary teeth than permanent teeth even with shorter duration of application.

Ekstrand, et al (2010) compared caries progression clinically and radiologically, after treating with resin infiltration and fluoride varnish cover and fluoride varnish only on

Table 14.2: White spots: Types, etiology and treatment option(s)		
Types of white spots	*Etiology*	*Treatment option(s)*
• Single white spots (diameter less than 0.5 mm)	• Natural occurrence in maxillary incisors	• Whitening only
• Mottled enamel (white specks)	• During development (less chances)	• Whitening and microabrasion
• Brown/white discolorations	• Fluorosis (multiple lesions)	• Whitening and microabrasion
• White patches	• Trauma to the primary dentition	• Whitening, followed by resin infiltration
• White spots covered with yellow layer	• Bleeding during traumatic injury, which might have seeped into the areas of mineralization	• Whitening and resin infiltration
• Faint white lesions; black edges around	• Demineralization lesions after removal of orthodontic brackets	• Resin infiltration/whitening/ micro-abrasion, depending on the size
• Enamel defects in deciduous incisors and molars	• Molar incisor hypoplasia	• Resin infiltration of the anterior lesions; GIC filling in posterior
• Enamel hypoplasia	• Preterm birth/developmental problem	• Whitening/microabrasion/resin infiltration

proximal surfaces of deciduous molars. They reported that proximal caries in deciduous molars treated with resin infiltration and fluoride varnish progressed significantly less (23%) than those treated with fluoride varnish only (61%).

In a study conducted by Martignon, et al (2006), the rate of failure of resin infiltration in non-cavitated proximal lesions after 1, 2 and 3 years of follow-up was 15.8%, 24.3% and 32.4% respectively. The failure rates obtained in the control group (placebo) were 47.4%, 62.2% and 70.3% for the same follow-up periods. Meyer-Leuckel, et al (2008), however observed only 4% (42% in the control group) after 3 year follow-up.

The observable differences between these results and those obtained by Martignon, et al (2012) and Ekstrand, et al (2010) may possibly be explained by a higher proportion of dentin lesions that were infiltrated by them and consequently a higher rate of its progression and reduced efficacy of infiltration.

The results of various studies conducted in order to define an effective resin infiltration protocol show that a higher rate of inhibition of caries progression occurs with the application of a 15% hydrochloric acid gel for 2 minutes in order to dissolve the superficial hypermineralized enamel surface and to allow a greater penetration of resin. This layer reflects the remineralization that characterizes the dynamics of tooth decay and, if not removed, it behaves as a barrier to resin infiltration.

v. Preventing Caries Progression

The development of caries is the net result of demineralization and remineralization cycle; a constant process occurring at the tooth-biofilm interface. The tooth surface becomes susceptible to caries if biofilm is frequently exposed to environment that lower the pH; whereas, it becomes protective and helps in remineralization if frequently exposed to carioprotective agents. The caries process

should stop automatically if the nutrition supply to the organisms is cut off, i.e. sealing the early lesion by an external agent. Early studies have observed that sealing off the early lesion with the use of composite resin, prevent progression of caries.

Clinically it is difficult to flow the resins into the pores created by the early caries. The flow of resin is dependent on various factors, especially penetration coefficient of the resin. It is impossible to infiltrate viscous solution into the pores. The penetration coefficient of early resins was in the range of 350 cm/second. Different combinations of resin monomers having variable penetration coefficient were tried with varying success. The monomer mixtures with penetration coefficient of 50 cm/second, termed 'infiltrants' were practically successful. These infiltrants flowed into the pores created by caries process and acted as physical barrier.

Advantages of Resin Infiltration

- Improve aesthetics.
- Occlusion of microporosities (up to certain depth).
- Obturation of deeply porous demineralised areas.
- Arrest/retardation of lesion progression.
- Minimizes risk of secondary caries.
- Mechanical stabilisation of demineralised enamel.
- Preservation of tooth tissue.
- No risk of postoperative sensitivity.
- Pulpal reactions are negligible.
- Restorative intervention can be delayed.
- Time and cost effective.
- Reduced risk of gingivitis and periodontitis.

Procedure for Vestibular Treatment

The extent of the lesion is to be assessed before proceeding to infiltration. Radiographs are also helpful. Resin infiltration can effectively be used, if the radiolucency is confined up to the outer third of the dentin with no cavitation. Enamel caries can be divided into two halves and designated as E1 and E2; whereas dentin caries can be divided in three halves categorizing as D1, D2 and D3. Infiltration therapy is indicated for lesions extending from E1 to D1. The resin infiltration is tried in vestibular as well as in proximal surfaces (occlusal areas are not tried; resin infiltration of occlusal areas is under development). The steps followed in vestibular treatment (Fig. 14.2a to f) are:

i. Place the rubber dam to ensure a dry working field and also to protect the soft tissues.

ii. The tooth/teeth to be treated is thoroughly cleaned using appropriate modalities.

iii. The icon etchant syringe is twisted to release the etchant (15% HCl), which is applied to the tooth surface for two minutes. After etching, rinse the tooth (at least 30 seconds) with clean water. Then dry the surface with oil free air (preferably chip syringe). If after etching there is a lack of or absence of chalky white appearance, the etching procedure must be repeated.

iv. 99% ethanol supplied in the cannula (DMG ICON DRY) is applied on the tooth surface for 30 seconds. The residual ethanol is dried with air without oil. The ethanol removes the water retained in microporosities of the lesion. The drying

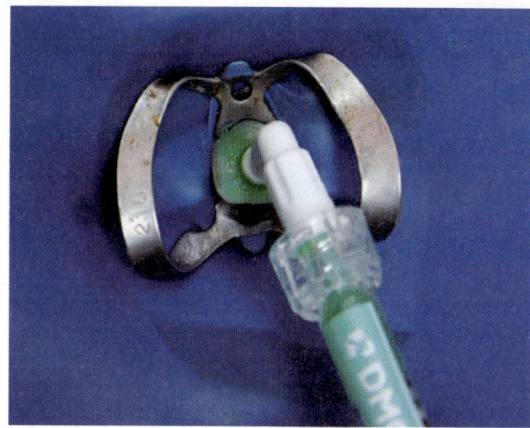

Fig. 14.2b: Application of ICON etchant

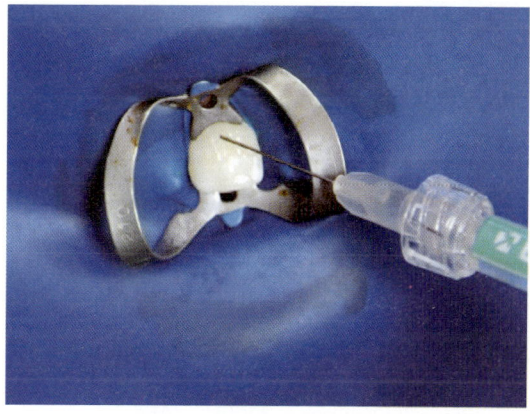

Fig. 14.2c: Application of ICON dry

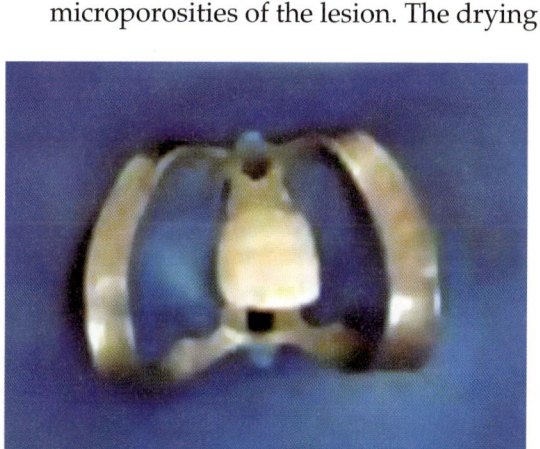

Fig. 14.2a: Application of rubber dam

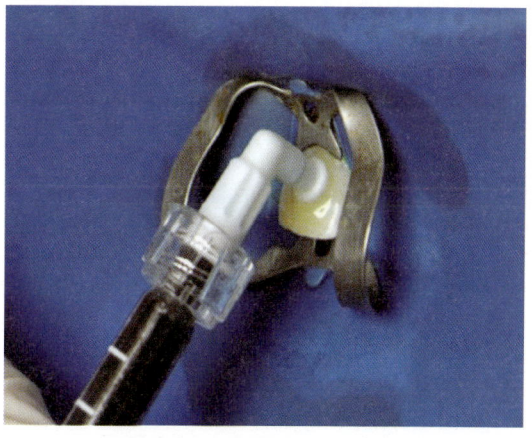

Fig. 14.2d: Application of ICON infiltrant

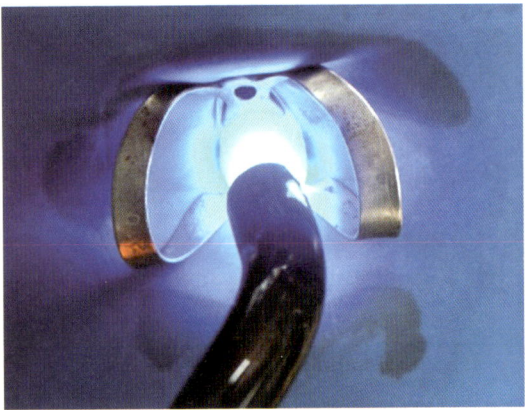

Fig. 14.2e: Light curing the infiltrant

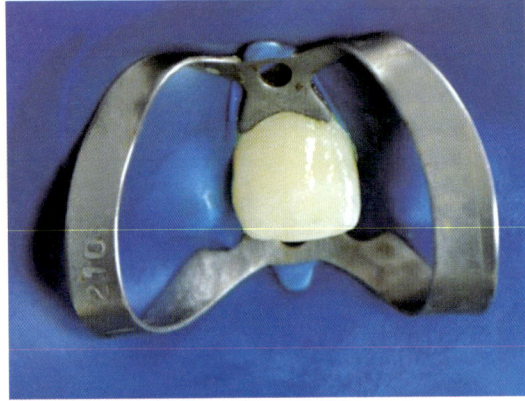

Fig. 14.2f: Post treatment

of tooth surface leads to accentuated picture of white porosities.

v. After drying, the lesion is checked visually after applying water (may be twice or thrice). At this stage, the spot should have almost disappeared; if not, the etching step is to be repeated.

vi. Apply ample amount of ICON infiltrant on the surface so prepared and let it be there for three minutes to allow the penetration of infiltrant deep into the lesion.

vii. The infiltrant soaked surface is light cured (the unit should have an output of 450 nm and light intensity of at least 800 mW/cm² for 40 seconds. Repeat application of resin infiltration and light

cure again for one minute (second application of resin is beneficial occluding the space generated by the first application).

viii. The excess resin is removed and the surface is polished. Polishing improves the stability of masking effect, likely due to reduction in surface porosity and the possible removal of oxygen inhibition layer.

Procedure for Proximal Treatment

The steps followed in proximal treatment (Fig. 14.3a to g) are:

i. The proximal surface of the affected and the adjacent tooth is cleaned with dental floss. Dental wedge can be inserted to improve upon the access.

ii. Rest of the procedures, rubber dam application, etching, drying, priming with ethanol, infiltrating resin and finally curing are the same as for vestibular surfaces.

All erosive patients are informed about the ease of the treatment vis-a-vis managing the erosive cavity. The limitation of achieving partial success in severe cases is also informed.

Erosion infiltration is usually delayed for two weeks if the patient has undergone bleaching with carbamide peroxide (resin is not permeable to carbamide peroxide). Bleaching usually facilitates attenuation of the white spots visibility. If the lesion is not visible even after etching/bleaching, microabrasion may be tried. Care should be taken using icon etch (15% HCl), which is higher than usual concentration (6% HCl) used in microabrasion.

CLINICAL EFFICACY

Various studies have observed successful efficacy of resin infiltration technique. A clinical study was conducted on 22 young adults, with 29 pairs of interproximal lesions (radiological extension into inner half of enamel or outer 1/3rd of the dentin) dividing

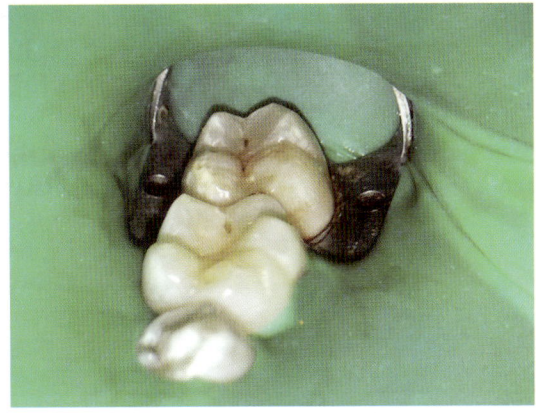

Fig. 14.3a: Initial clinical situation

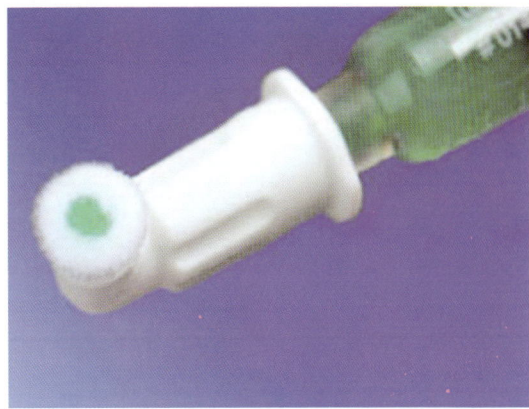

Fig. 14.3d: Special proximal applicator for etching

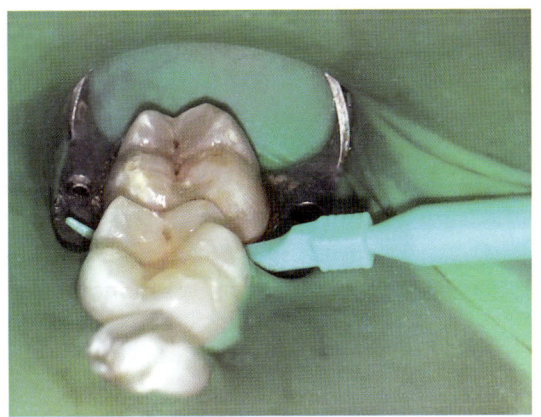

Fig. 14.3b: Separation with dental wedge

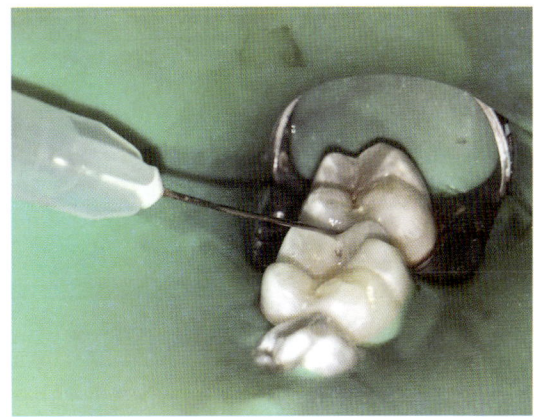

Fig. 14.3e: Drying the tooth using ICON dry

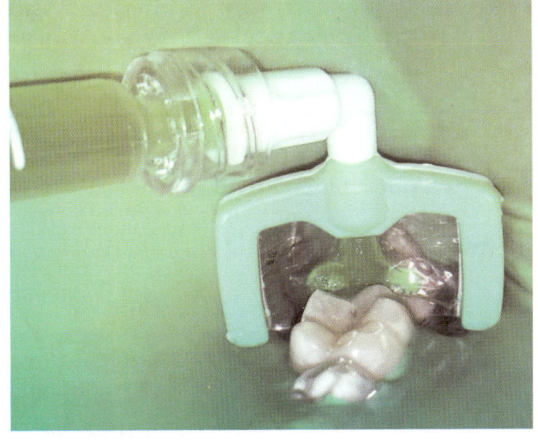

Fig. 14.3c: Etching using special proximal applicator

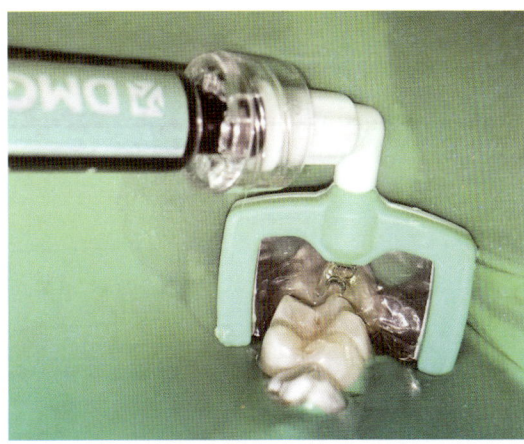

Fig. 14.3f: Applying ICON infiltrant

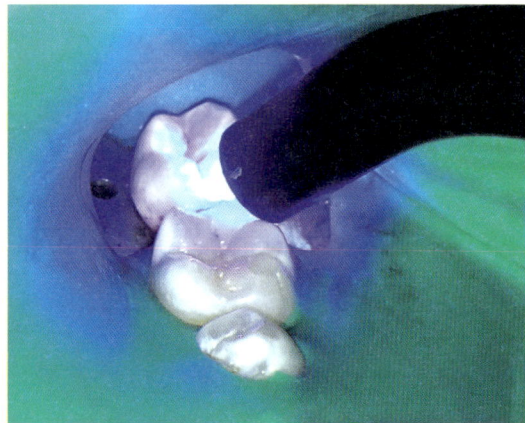

Fig. 14.3g: Light curing the infiltrant

into two groups. One group was treated with DMG ICON and the other group was kept as control. All participants received instructions for diet, flossing and fluoridation. After 18 months, the lesions were evaluated using digital subtraction radiography. 37% lesions showed progression in experimental group; whereas, only 7% showed progress in control group. It signifies that infiltration of the inter-proximal carious lesions is an effective method in reducing caries progression.

A few authors opined that depending upon the size of the lesion, bleaching prior to resin infiltration provides better results. Clinically the masking of the white spots have shown better results after bleaching.

Resin infiltration technique may not be successful in every white spot lesion. Various studies have concluded that the masking effect might be dramatic in some cases and partial for others. The long term clinical studies may improve upon the recommendations as regard choice of the resin and also whether to carry out bleaching prior to resin infiltration or not.

Limitations of Resin Infiltration Therapy

Though resin infiltration is successful and effective technique, yet inefficient isolation, depth and inactivity of the lesion, presence of cavitation, incomplete resin polymerization

and difficulty in controlling the amount of resin being infiltrated are some areas to be looked into.

It is established that greater the depth of carious lesion, the lower the probability of achieving a complete infiltration. Extensive lesions may lead to polymerization shrinkage of the resin and subsequent appearance of porosities/cracks. The infiltration of cavitated lesions may not be satisfactorily achieved because of the weak capillary action of the resin in these lesions. The presence of air bubbles within the cavitation may also hinder the infiltration of the resin.

It is demonstrated that incompletely infiltrated lesions are more susceptible to progression of demineralization. It is also established that pit and fissure sealants are effective not because of infiltration, but due to their isolation from the acidic oral environment.

Bibliography

1. Altarabulsi MB, Alkilzy M and Splieth CH. Clinical applicability of resin infiltration for proximal caries. Quint. Int.: 2013;44:97–104.
2. Azizi Z. Management of white lesions using resin infiltration technique: A review. Open J. Dent. And Oral Medicine: 2015;3:1–6.
3. Basaran G, Veli I and Basaran EG. Non-cavitated approach for the treatment of white spot lesions: A case report. Int. Dent. Res.: 2011;1:65–9.
4. Bullio Fragelli CM, Jeremias F, feltrin de Souza J, Paschoal MA, de Cassia Loiola Cordeiro R and Santos-Pinto L. Longitudinal evaluation of the structural integrity of teeth affected by molar incisor hypomineralisation. Caries Res. 2015; 49:378–83.
5. Crombie F, Manton D, Palamara J and Reynolds E. Resin infiltration of developmentally hypo-mineralized enamel. Int. J. Pediat. Dent.: 2014;24:51–5.
6. Domejean S, Ducamp R, Leger S and Holmgen C. Resin infiltration of non-cavitated caries lesions: a systematic review. Med. Princ. Pract.: 2015;24:216–21.
7. Ekstrand KR, Bakhshandeh A and Martignon S. Treatment of proximal superficial caries lesions on primary molar teeth with resin infiltration and

fluoride varnish versus fluoride varnish only: efficacy after one year. Caries Res.: 2010;44:41–6.

8. Greenwall L. White lesion eradication using resin caries infiltration. Int. Dent.: 2013;3:54–62.

9. Gugnani N, Pandit IK, Gupta M and Josan R. Caries infiltration of non-cavitated white spot lesions: a novel approach for immediate esthetic improvement. Contemp. Clin. Dent.: 2012;3:S199–202.

10. Hammad SM, El Banna M, El Zayat I and Mohsen MA. Effect of resin infiltration on white spot lesions after debonding orthodontic brackets. Am. J. Dent.: 2012;25:3–8.

11. Huang TTY, He LH, Darendeliler MA and Swain MV. Nano-indentation characterisation of natural carious white spot lesions. Caries Research: 2010;44:101–7.

12. Kielbassa AM, Ulrich I, Treven L and Mueller J. An updated review on the resin infiltration technique of incipient proximal enamel lesions. Medicine in Evolution: 2010;16:3–15.

13. Kugel G, Arsenault P and Papas A. Treatment modalities for caries management, including a new resin infiltration system. Compend. Contin. Educat. Dent.: 2009;30:1–10.

14. Lasfargues JJ, Bonte E, Guerrieri A and Fezzani L. Minimal intervention dentistry: part 6. Caries inhibition by resin infiltration. Br. Dent. J.: 2013;214:53–9.

15. Liu Y, Ge L, Chen H and Chi X. A study on the penetration abilities of natural initial caries lesions with resin infiltration. West China J. Stomato.: 2012;30:483–6.

16. Martignon S, Bakhshandeh A and Ricketts DNJ. The non-operative resin treatment of proximal caries lesions. Dent. Update: 2012;39:614–22.

17. Martignon S, Ekstrand KR, Gomez J, Lara JS and Cortes A. Infiltrating/sealing proximal caries lesions: A 3-year randomized clinical trial. J. Dent. Res.: 2012;91:288–92.

18. Meyer-Lueckel H and Paris S. Improved resin infiltration of natural caries lesions. J. Dent. Res.: 2008;87:1112–6.

19. Meyer-Lueckel H and Paris S. Progression of artificial enamel caries lesions after infiltration with experimental light curing resins. Caries Res.: 2008;42:117–24.

20. Meyer-Lueckel H, Paris S, Mueller J, Colfen H and Kielbassa AM. Influence of the application time on the penetration of different dental adhesives and a fissure sealant into artificial subsurface lesions in bovine enamel. Dental Mater.: 2006;22:22–8.

21. Meyer-Lueckel H, Paris S and Kielbassa AM. Surface layer erosion of natural caries lesions with phosphoric and hydrochloric acid gels in preparation for resin infiltration. Caries Res.:2007; 41:223–30.

22. Mueller J, Meyer-Lueckel H, Paris S, Hopfenmuller W and Kielbassa AM. Inhibition of lesion progression by the penetration of resins in vitro: influence of the application procedure. Oper Dent.: 2006;31:338–45.

23. Munoz MA, Arana-Gordillo LA and Gomes GM. Alternative esthetic management of fluorosis and hypoplasia stains: blending effect obtained with resin infiltration techniques. J. Esthet. Restor. Dent.: 2013;25:32–9.

24. Nainar SMH. Resin infiltration technique for proximal caries lesions in the permanent dentition: A contrarian viewpoint. Oper. Dent.: 2014;39:1–3.

25. Nainar SMH. The evidence is lacking to support resin infiltration for primary molar proximal lesions. Pediat. Dent.: 2014;36:201.

26. Paris S, Bitter K, Naumann M, Dorfer CE and Meyer-Lueckel H. Resin infiltration of proximal caries lesions differing in ICDAS codes. Eur. J. Oral Sci.: 2011;119:182–86.

27. Paris S, Dorfer CE and Meyer-Lueckel H. Surface conditioning of natural enamel caries lesions in deciduous teeth in preparation for resin infiltration. J. Dent.: 2010;38:65–71.

28. Paris S, Hopfenmuller W and Meyer-Lueckel H. Resin infiltration of caries lesions: An efficacy randomized trial. J. Dent. Res.: 2010;89:823–826.

29. Paris S, Meyer-Lueckel H and Kielbassa AM. Resin infiltration of natural caries lesions. J. Dent. Res.: 2007;86:662–6.

30. Paris S, Meyer-Lueckel H, Colfen H and Kielbassa AM. Resin infiltration of artificial enamel caries lesions with experimental light curing resins. Dent. Materials J.: 2007;26:582–8.

31. Paris S and Meyer-Lueckel H. Masking of labial enamel white spot lesions by resin infiltration—a clinical report. Quint. Int.: 2009;40:713–8.

32. Paris S and Meyer-Lueckel H. Inhibition of caries progression by resin infiltration in situ. Caries Reviews.: 2010;44:47–54.

33. Paris S and Meyer-Lueckel H. Infiltrants inhibit progression of natural caries lesions in vitro J. Dent. Res.: 2010;89:1276–80.

34. Paris S, Schwendicke F, Keltsch J, Dorfer C and Meyer-Leuckel H. Masking of white spot lesions by resin infiltration in vitro. J. Dent.: 2013;41:28–34.

35. Paris S, Schwendicke F, Seddig S, Muller WD, Dorfer C and Meyer-Leuckel H. Micro-hardness and mineral loss of enamel lesions after infiltration with various resins: influence of infiltrant composition and application frequency *in vitro*. J. Dent.: 2013;41:543–8.

36. Peters MC. Strategies for non-invasive demineralized tissue repair. Dent. Clinic N. America: 2010;54:507–25.

37. Robinson C. Filling without drilling. J. Dent. Res.: 2011;90:1261–3.

38. Schmidlin PR, Zehnder M, Pasqualetti T, Imfeld T and Besek MJ. Penetration of a bonding agent into de- and remineralized enamel *in vitro*. J. Adhes. Dent.: 2004;6:111–5.

39. Shivanna V and Shivakumar B. Novel treatment of white spot lesions: A report of two cases. J. Conserv. Dent.: 2011;14:423–6.

40. Soviero VM, Paris S, Leal SC, Azevedo RB and Meyer-Leuckel H. Ex vivo evaluation of caries infiltration after different application times in primary molars. Caries Res.: 2012;47:110–6.

41. Subramanian P, Babu G and Lakhotia D. Evaluation of penetration depth of a commercially available resin infiltrate into artificially created enamel lesions: An *in-vitro* study. J. Conserv. Dent.: 2014;17:146–9.

42. Freitas T, Santos LF, Chagas Rego HM, Buhler Borges A, Pucci CR and Rocha Gomes TC. Efficacy of bleaching treatment on demineralized enamel treated with resin infiltration technique. World J. Dent.: 2012;3:279.

43. Tirlet G, Chabouis HF and Attal JP. Infiltration, a new therapy for masking enamel white spots: a 19-month follow-up case series. Eur. J. Esthet. Dent.: 2013;8:180–90.

44. Torres CRG, Rosa PCF, Ferreira NS and Borges AB. Effect of caries infiltration technique and fluoride therapy on microhardness of enamel carious lesions. Oper. Dent.: 2012;37:363–9.

45. Wiegand A, Stawarczyk B, Kolakovic M, Hammerie CH, Attin T and Schmidlin PR. Adhesive performance of a caries infiltrant on sound and demineralized enamel. J. Dent.: 2011;39:117–21.

46. Yazicoglu O and Ulukapi H. The investigation of non-invasive techniques for treating early approximal carious lesions: an in vivo study. Int. Dent. J.: 2014;64:1–11.

15

Caries Excavation

The term "caries excavation" has long been used as a synonym for "cavity preparation". The excavation of enamel caries is considered relatively easy, since it does not cause any problem to the patient; however, the excavation of dentin caries may pose problems as the odontoblastic processes connect dentin to the pulp. Caries excavation is the basic and mandatory step to finally prepare a tooth to receive the filling material. Preparation of tooth implies excavation of caries along with extension of the cavity if need be and giving definite form suitable for the final restoration.

Various techniques and methods have been tried to effectively excavate caries without any damage. The requirements of an effective technique/method are:

- Comfortable to both operator and the patient.
- Ease of use in the clinical environment.
- The ability to remove diseased tissue only.
- Painless to patient.
- Minimal vibration or heat during excavation.
- Cost effective.

It is established that caries in dentin is presented in two layers. The 'outer' layer is contaminated with bacteria. The bacterial actions have damaged the collagen matrix in such a way that the remineralization is not possible; therefore, this layer is to be removed completely. The 'inner' layer is less contaminated (bacteria may be few or even nil). In case the bacterial by-products are removed, this layer of dentin can be remineralized.

The methods/techniques used for caries excavation from time to time are:

a. Caries Excavation with Excavators (Mechanical non-rotary devices)

Excavators with different shapes (discoid, cleoid, spoon) have been used for caries excavation. Excavators are also used for refinement of the internal parts of the cavity preparation. The extensively used spoon excavators are usually the paired instruments categorized into three varieties depending upon the sizes.

- Small (approximately 1.0 mm diameter) is used in smaller cavities for caries removal.
- Medium (about 1.5 mm diameter) is used in larger cavities for caries removal.
- Large excavator (about 2.0 mm diameter) is used mainly for excavation of filling material.

The direction of movement for the spoon excavator is from periphery to centre of cavity to avoid the pulp exposure. Excavators are better suited for removal of softened dentin; whereby they leave the healthy dentin alone.

Advantages

- Simple and gentle ease of use.
- Low pressure exerted.
- No thermal irritation.
- Low cost.
- Effective removal of caries.

Disadvantages

- Usually cannot be re-sharpened.
- Time consuming.
- May lead to incomplete excavation.

b. Excavation with Burs (Mechanical rotary devices)

Various burs used are:

i. Carbon-steel/Tungsten-carbide Burs

Carbon-steel burs have the same caries-removing properties as tungsten-carbide burs and are less expensive; however, carbon-steel burs are much more prone to corrosion. Therefore, carbon-steel burs were replaced with hard tungsten-carbide burs. The burs are available in different shapes and sizes. The most commonly used is the rose-head bur.

The caries excavation starts from the periphery towards the center of the lesion in order to minimize the risk of infection in case of accidental pulp exposure. Larger burs are recommended for caries removal to minimize the risk of infection. The burs are rotated in low-speed contra-angle handpieces. The use of burs is considered to be the most efficient method to excavate caries in terms of time; the burs being the most widely used caries-excavation method.

Advantages

- Effective work rate.
- Ease of use.
- Cost effective.

Disadvantages

- Vibrations.
- Danger of overexcavation.
- Danger of thermal damage.

ii. Polymeric Burs

A variety of plastic rotary burs were introduced, which consist of a polyamide/imide polymer. These burs possess lower mechanical properties than sound dentin. If the bur touches sound or caries-affected dentin, it quickly becomes dull and produces undesirable vibration, making further cutting impossible. The bur blades are designed to remove the carious dentin by plowing during which the carious dentin is first locally compressed and then the compressed softened carious dentin is pushed along the more sound dentin surface. The loosened caries fragments are carried to the surface and removed.

SmartPrep and Smart Bur (SSWhite, USA) consist of polyether-ketone-ketone, a polymer having hardness of 50 KHN. The hardness of these burs was higher than the hardness of carious dentin (0 to 30 KHN), but lower than that of sound dentin (70 to 90 KHN). SmartPrep burs are available in three ISO sizes, 010, 014 and 018. As opposed to conventional carbide burs, their cutting edges were not spiral but straight. For caries excavation, it starts from the center to the periphery in order to avoid contact with sound tooth tissues, otherwise the bur would be prematurely and irreversibly damaged. The plastic cutting blades wear away immediately when they come in contact with harden material and become unusable. These burs are self-limiting and are intended for single use only.

Smart Bur is available with different blade configuration, claiming to be better than SmartPrep. The disadvantage of SmartPrep was that it could not remove the caries completely.

iii. Ceramic Burs

A new variety of burs made of ceramic materials is now available for excavation of caries. The CeraBurs (Komet-Brasseler; Germany) are all-ceramic round burs consisting of alumina-yttria stabilized zirconia and are available in four different diameter sizes (10, 14, 18 and 23 mm). The ceramic burs have high cutting efficiency in infected, soft dentin and also provide tactile sensation, subsequently reducing preparation time. However, the caries-removal efficiency and efficacy did not show any significant difference between the ceramic and conventional tungsten-carbide burs.

The rotary burs are universally used; however, there are certain problems that need to be improved upon. The problems are:

- The sensitivity of vital dentin, causing pain during excavation.
- Mechanical pressure on the tooth.
- Noise and vibration (more with air-turbine handpiece).
- High temperatures at the cutting end.

c. Chemo-mechanical Excavation

The conventional caries excavation methods usually induce pain and fear in patients, especially the children. To make the caries removal painless, selectively soften the carious lesion facilitating the removal by excavation without any pressure. The chemical agents (Fig. 15.1) used are:

i. Sodium Hypochlorite-based Agents

5.0% Sodium hypochlorite has been used to soften carious lesions. Later, the use of 5.0% sodium hypochlorite was observed to be toxic to adjacent healthy tissues. A new solution, GK-101 was developed, which consists of sodium hydroxide, sodium chloride and glycine in addition to 5.0% sodium hypochlorite. GK-101 was more effective than the hypochlorite alone; however, the carious softening effect was very slow.

Caridex, a commercial preparation, consists of sodium hypochlorite solution buffered with an amino acid containing mixture of amino butyric acid, sodium chloride and sodium hydroxide. The ability of sodium hypochlorite to selectively soften carious lesion is attributed to the buffering effect of the amino acids, which enhances disrupting effect on the degenerated collagen of the carious dentin. The resultant friable collagen fibrils can be easily removed with excavators.

Caridex was not fully successful in clinical practice because of the need of a specific apparatus to deliver the solution into the cavity, short shelf-life, longer treatment time and higher treatment cost.

Another caries removing chemical agent based on sodium hypochlorite was introduced in the name of Carisolv. It is available in the form of a gel. It consists of two components, one is transparent liquid containing 0.5% w/v sodium hypochlorite and the other component contain an amino acid mixture (glutamic acid, leucine and lysine), sodium carboxymethyl cellulose to enhance the viscosity, sodium hydroxide providing pH of 11 and water to act as vehicle.

The chemical composition and microstructure of dentin after excavation with Carisolv remained unchanged. The calcium and phosphorus content remain similar after excavation; however the hardness values of residual dentin was same as for sound dentin. The etch pattern of dentin in Carisolv-excavated lesions is deeper than caries removed with a conventional bur. Carisolv excavated dentin shows better bonding characteristics, viz. patent dentinal tubules, not covered by smear layer, irregular surface

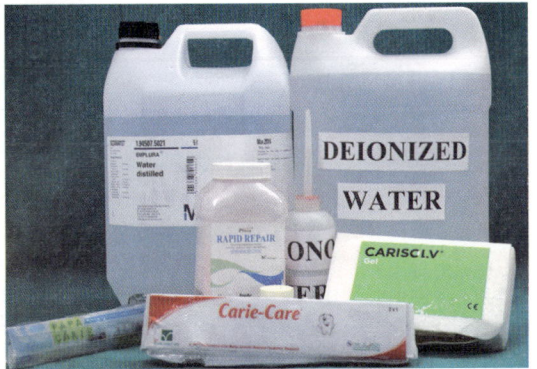

Fig 15.1: Chemical agents

and the improved wetting potential. Carisolv has superior property in reducing the counts of viable bacteria in residual dentin, as compared to conventional bur excavation. Carisolv has bactericidal activity due to formation of chloramine compounds. The disadvantages include its high cost and need of special instruments. Children usually dislike the chlorine taste and odor.

The procedure of excavation of caries using Carisolv is depicted in Fig. 15.2a to c. The process is repeated until no turbidity of the applied gel is seen.

ii. Pepsin-based Caries Excavation

An enzyme pepsin in a phosphoric acid/ sodium bisphosphate buffer has also been tried as a chemical agent softening caries. SFC-VIII (3M ESPE, Germany) is the commercially available pepsin based agent. The advantage of this new pepsin based agent is that it acts on more specific denatured collagen than the sodium hypochlorite-based agents. The phosphoric acid dissolves the inorganic component of carious dentin, while at the same time pepsin gets access to the organic part of the carious mass, selectively dissolving the denatured collagen. SFC-VIII gel should be used along with an excavator having hardness between that of sound and infected dentin for caries removal. The limitation of SFC-VIII excavation is that the heavily pigmented and arrested dentin caries pose problem in pepsin digestion.

Papacarie

Papacarie (Sao Paulo-Brazil) is another chemomechanical caries removing agent, which contains papain, chloramines, toluidine blue and certain salts. Papain is a proteolytic enzyme similar to pepsin. Papain comes from latex of leaves and fruits of green adult papaya, carica papaya. Papacarie is available in syringes having 3.0 ml gel. The papacarie gel is allowed to act in a cavity for 60 seconds.

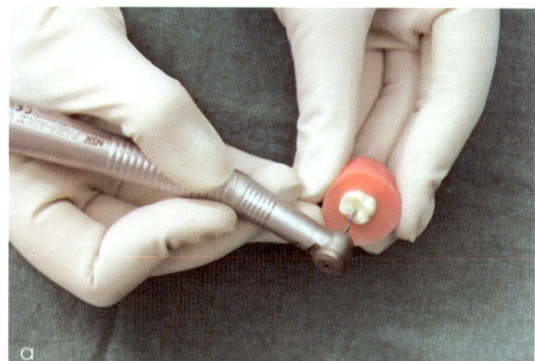

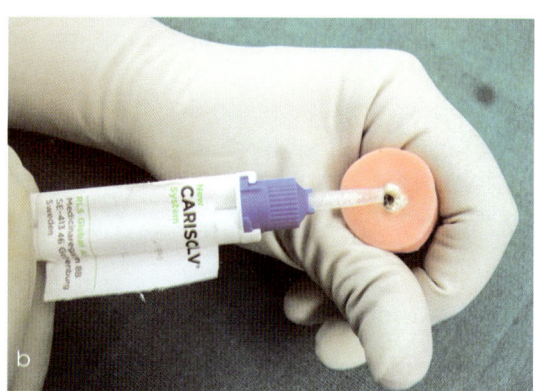

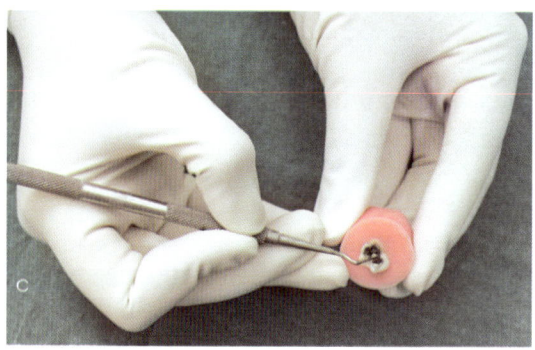

Fig. 15.2a to c: Caries excavation with Carisolv: (a) Exposing caries, (b) Applying Carisolv gel, (c) Excavating caries

As the collagen fibrils gel dissolved the clear gel becomes dark in color. The papain digests dead cells and breaks the partially degraded collagen molecules, contributing to the degradation of the collagen fibrils formed by the carious process.

The procedure of excavation of caries using Papacarie is explained in Fig. 15.3a to c.

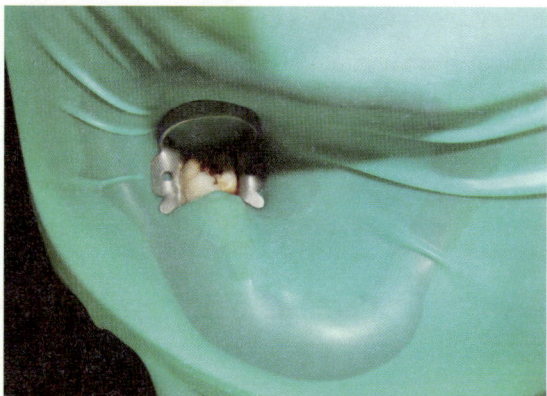

Fig. 15.3a: Rubber dam application

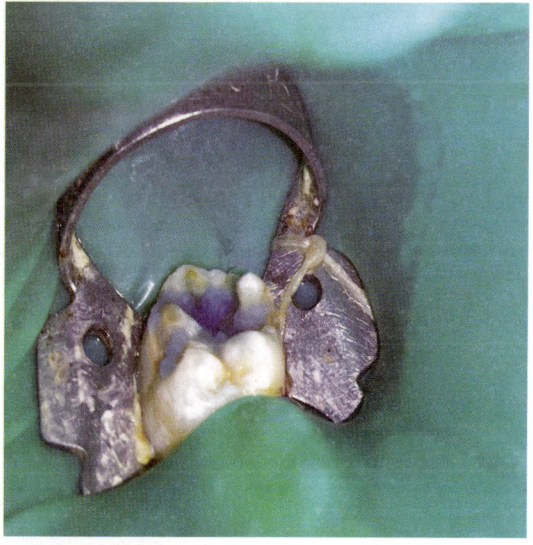

Fig. 15.3b: Application of Papacarie

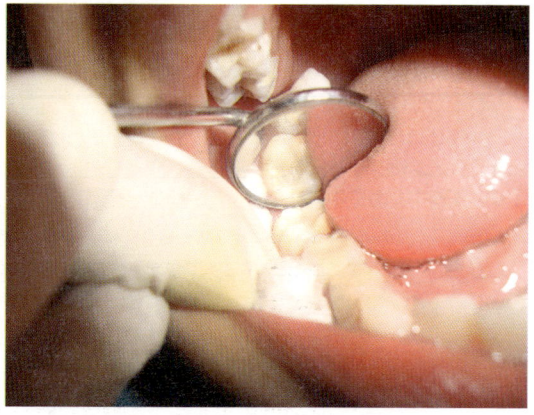

Fig. 15.3c: Caries excavated

Carie-Care

It is an enzyme derived from Papaya plant, "the Carica Papaya". It is composed of papaya extract, therapeutic essential oil, coloring gel, sterile water, chloramines and sodium chloride.

Carie-care (papain) acts on the carious tissue, which lacks alpha-anti-trypsin (a plasmatic anti-protease system), which inhibits proteolysis. The absence of anti-protease allows papain to act on the partially degraded collagen by breaking the peptide bonds. In addition to papain, the chloramines dissolve carious dentin by means of chlorination of the partially degraded collagen. The gel also contains therapeutic oils (clove oil), which induce analgesic and antiseptic action. It minimizes pain sensation and has a pleasant taste acceptable by the children and adults as well.

d. Ultrasonic Excavation

Ultrasonic energy with a 25 kHz oscillating frequency has been tried in cavity preparation. It is used with thick aluminium oxide and water slurry, resulting in the cutting action of tooth. The kinetic energy of water molecules is transferred to the tooth surface through the high speed oscillations of the cutting tip. The disadvantage of ultrasonic excavation is that it is unable to remove soft, carious dentin; whereas, the leathery, deeper layer are more susceptible to ultrasonic action.

Excavation by Sono-abrasion

It is based on the use of ultrasonic cutting tips along with sonic air-scaler handpieces under water cooling. The handpiece oscillates in the sonic region (< 6.5 kHz), while the tips perform an elliptical motion. A requisite torque (2-N) is mandatory, otherwise the cutting efficiency is reduced.

The advantage of this technique is that no chemical or structural changes were observed in dentin. Sono-abrasion excavation using diamond-coated tips appeared as efficient as conventional hand excavation using excavators.

Cariex system (Kavo Dental, Germany), includes two sets of cutting tips; two diamond-coated tips with different diameters for enamel preparation and two tungsten-carbide tips with different diameters for dentin excavation.

e. Air-abrasion Excavation

Air-abrasion, developed by RB Black (1945) involves bombarding the tooth surface with high-velocity particles, conventionally aluminium oxide, carried in a stream of air. Other particles, viz. spherical glass beads, Polycarbonate resin powder, alumina and hydroxyapatite (ratio 3:1) and bioactive glass powder have also been tried. Pure aluminium oxide particles have been preferred as the abrading agent because of their high cutting effectiveness, chemical stability, low cost, low affinity for water and neutral color. This method reduces heat generation, vibration and other mechanical stimulation as compared with the dental drill. Disadvantages include loss of tactile sensation because the nozzle does not touch the surface of the tooth, creating risks of over-preparation of the cavity and inadequate removal of the caries. Cavities produced in sound tooth are deeper than carious surface because carious surface absorbed the impact due to its soft consistency resulting in reduction of the cutting ability in carious dentin.

Following factors affect the caries excavation:

- Type of particle.
- Size of particle.
- Particle speed.
- Angle of surface approach.

It is established that 27 µm alumina particles result in better removal of carious dentin than particles with larger dimensions (50 µm and more).

Air-polishing

Air polishing has been tried in caries excavation at the end of cavity preparation. Water soluble particles of sodium bicarbonate are added to tricalcium phosphate (0.08% by weight) to improve the flow characteristics. The mixture is then applied onto a tooth surface under continuous water jet and air pressure.

f. Fluorescence-aided Caries Excavation (FACE)

Fluorescence technique was basically used to clinically differentiate between infected and affected carious dentin. The fluorescence of the carious dentin was based upon the fact that several oral micro-organisms produce orange-red fluorophores as by-products of their metabolism (porphyrins); the infected carious tissue fluoresce in the red fraction of the visible spectrum due to the presence of proto- and meso-porphyrins. This facilitates continuous visual detection of orange-red fluorescence and thereby caries excavation.

Slow-speed handpiece with a fiber-optic violet light source (370 to 420 nm) is used for caries excavation. During caries removal, areas exhibiting orange-red fluorescence can be selectively identified and removed with the bur. This method showed the highest sensitivity, specificity and predictive values for residual caries detection. It was proved to be efficient and less time consuming.

Steps used for Caries Excavation

- *Preparation of the cavity:* In case the carious dentin is not fully accessible, a large cavity should be prepared prior to caries excavation.
- *Diagnosis and excavation of the residual caries:* After the cavity preparation, the extent of caries is evaluated. Carious dentin areas exhibit a red fluorescence, which is differentiated from the green fluorescence of non-carious areas. The residual caries can be removed with a bur or excavators.

- *End point of caries excavation:* The red-fluorescing dentin areas must be completely excavated so that as little infected dentin as possible is left behind.

In areas that are away from the pulp, the complete removal of red-fluorescing (severe bacterial infection) dentin is recommended for a tight restoration margin and a secure retentive or adhesive margin.

A small amount of red-fluorescing dentin may be left in the areas close to the pulp cavity in order to avoid the root canal procedure. These areas must be covered with a calcium hydroxide type material before the restoration of the cavity.

g. Laser Excavation

The erbium yttrium-aluminium-garnet (Er:YAG—wavelength 2.78 mm) and the erbium-chromium-yttrium-scandium-gallium-garnet (Er,Cr:YSGG—wavelength 2.94 mm) lasers are currently used in cavity preparation and caries excavation.

The mechanism by which enamel and dentin are removed consists of explosive subsurface expansion of water interstitially trapped in the dental hard tissues. During irradiation, the water molecules absorb the incident radiation, causing sudden heating and water evaporation. As a result, a high-stream pressure is formed, inducing a violent expansion and ejection of dental hard tissues. Er-Cr-YSGG laser system delivers photons through air-water spray straight on to the target tissue. The micro-explosive forces turning into water droplets, contribute to the hard-tissue removal.

Laser ablation provides more comfort to the patient due to the absence of vibration and a lower pain sensation. It has definite role in the prevention of recurrent caries. The major drawbacks are:

- Time consuming; the time required for a complete excavation is twice that with rotary instruments.

- It can induce irreversible chemical and structural alteration of dentin and even damage the pulp.
- It produces an undefined and irregular excavation pattern in dentin.
- The irregular dentin surface left after laser ablation hinders tactile sensation.
- Laser may change the organic matrix component of dentin, thereby impairing the adhesive treatment.

Stepwise Excavation in Deep Caries Lesions

The excavation of deep caries in steps was suggested as the preferred way of removal of deep carious tissue in an effort to avoid pulp exposure.

The stepwise excavation technique is recommended for teeth with deep caries lesions, where the removal of carious tissue in a single step would lead to pulp exposure. The technique is recommended especially for young patients, having broad pulp chamber. The teeth with incomplete apices, also pose problems during caries excavation risking for pulp exposure. As the age advances, the pulp gradually becomes more fibrous with a reduction in volume due to the physiological production of dentin and reduction in blood supply and regeneration capacity.

Method

After gaining access to the dentinal caries, the extent of caries is analyzed. The carious dentin is excavated slowly with sharp curettes. The process is repeated until the patient feels pain. The remaining carious dentin is left on the pulp wall. Rest of the carious lesion is covered with calcium hydroxide. A period of 60 to 90 days would be sufficient for the dentin hardening and tertiary dentin deposition. The tooth is isolated and the temporary sealing is removed. The caries is again excavated slowly. The underlying dentin is evaluated. If it presents a dark color, with a hard consistency on probing (arrested caries), the restoration is placed accordingly; otherwise residual caries if any, is to be removed repeating the pulp protecting regime. Final restoration can be placed in the subsequent visit.

Bibliography

1. Ahmed AA, Garcia-Godoy F and Kunzelmann KH. Self limiting caries therapy with proteolytic agents. Am. J. Dent.: 2008;21:303–12.

2. Allen KL, Salgado TL, Janal MN and Thompson VP. Removing carious dentin using a polymer instrument without anesthesia versus a carbide bur with anesthesia. J. Am. Dent. Assoc.: 2005; 136, 643–51.

3. Banerjee A, Kidd EA and Watson TF. *In vitro* evaluation of five alternative methods of carious dentin excavation. Caries Res.: 2000;34:144–50.

4. Banerjee A, Watson TF and Kidd EA. Dentin caries excavation: A review of current clinical techniques. Br. Dent. J.: 2000;188:476–82.

5. Beeley JA, Yip HK and Stevenson AG. Chemo-mechanical caries removal: A review of the techniques and latest developments. Br. Dent. J.: 2000;188:427–30.

6. Boston DW. New device for selective dentin caries removal. Quintessence Int.: 2003;34:678–85.

7. Bussadori SK, Castro LC and Galvao AC. Papain gel: a new chemomechanical caries removal agent. J. Clin. Pediatr. Dent.: 2005;30:115–9.

8. Celiberti P, Francescut P and Lussi A. Performance of four dentin excavation methods in deciduous teeth. Caries Res.: 2006;40:117–23.

9. Clementino-Luedemann TN, Dabanoglu A, Ilie N, Hickel R and Knuzelmann KH. Micro-computed tomographic evaluation of a new enzyme solution for caries removal in deciduous teeth. Dent. Mater. J.: 2006;25:675–83.

10. Dammaschke T, Vesnic A and Schafer E. *In vitro* comparison of ceramic burs and conventional tungsten carbide bud burs in dentin caries excavation. Quintessence Int.: 2008;39:495–9.

11. Dammascke T, Rodenberg TN, Schafer E and Ott KH. Efficiency of the polymer bur SmartPrep compared with conventional tungsten carbide bur in dentin caries excavation. Oper. Dent.: 2006;31:256–60.

12. Eberhard J, Bode K, Hedderich J and Jepsen S. Cavity size difference after caries removal by a fluorescence-controlled Er:YAG laser and by conventional bur treatment. Clin. Oral Invest.: 2008;12:311–8.

13. Eberhard J, Eisenbeiss AK, Braun A, Hedderich J and Jepsen S. Evaluation of selective caries removal by a fluorescence feedback-controlled Er:YAG laser *in vitro*. Caries Res.: 2005;39:496–504.

14. Ekstrand KR, Ricketts DN and Kidd EA. Do occlusal carious lesions spread laterally at the enamel-dentin junction? A histopathological study. Clin. Oral Invest.: 1998;2:15–20.

15. Ericson D, Zimmerman M, Raber H, Gotrick B, Bornstein R and Thorell J . Clinical evaluation of efficacy and safety of a new method for chemo-mechanical removal of caries: A multi-centre study. Caries Res.: 1999;33:171–7.

16. Foley J, Evans D and Blackwell A. Partial caries removal and cariostatic materials in carious primary molar teeth: a randomized controlled clinical trial. Br. Dent. J.: 2004;197:697–701.

17. Ganesh M and Parikh D. Chemomechanical caries removal (CMCR) agents: review and clinical application in primary teeth. J. Dent. and Oral Hygiene: 2010;3:34–45.

18. Goldman M and Kronman JH. Preliminary report on a chemo-mechanical means of removing caries. J. Am. Dent. Assoc.: 1976;93:1149–53.

19. Gulcin B, Osman Z, Cemal E and Haken B. Effect of Carisolv on the human dental pulp: a histological study. J. Dent.: 2004;32:309–14.

20. Horiguchi S, Yamada T, Inokoshi S and Tagami J. Selective caries removal with air abrasion. Oper. Dent.: 1998;23:236–43.

21. Hosoya Y, Taguchi T and Tay FR. Evaluation of a new caries detecting dye for primary and permanent carious dentin. J. Dent.: 2007;35:137–43.

22. Huda EA and Al-Rubaye. Evaluation of Carisolv in the chemico-mechanical removal of carious dentin in primary molars (*in vivo* study). Tikrit Journal for Dent. Sci.: 2013;61–70.

23. Kidd EA, Ricketts DN and Beighton D. Criteria for caries removal at the enamel-dentin junction: A clinical and microbiological study. Br. Dent. J.: 1996;180:287–91.

24. Kotb RM, Abdella A, Kateb MA and Ahmed AM. Clinical evaluation of Papacarie in primary teeth. J. Clin. Pediatric. Dent.: 2009;34:117–23.

25. Lager A, Thornqvist E and Ericson D. Cultivatable bacteria in dentin after caries excavation using rose-bur or Carisolv. Caries Res.: 2003;37:206–11.

26. Lennon AM. Fluorescence-aided caries excavation (FACE) compared to conventional method. Oper. Dent.: 2003;28:341–5.

27. Lennon AM, Buchalla W, Rassner B, Becker K and Attin T. Efficiency of four caries excavation methods compared. Oper. Dent.: 2006;31:551–555.

28. Maltz M, Alves LS, Jardim JJ, Moura MS and Oliveira EF. Incomplete caries removal in deep lesions: a 10-year prospective study. Am. J. Dent.: 2011;24:211–4.

29. Maragakis GM, Hahn P and Hellwig E. Clinical evaluation of chemo-mechanical caries removal in primary molars and its acceptance by patients. Caries Res.: 2001;35:205–10.

30. Motisuki C, Lima LM, Bronzi ES, Spolidorio DM and Santos-Pinto L. The effectiveness of alumina powder on carious dentin removal. Oper. Dent.: 2006;31:371–6.

31. Nadanovsky P, Carneiro CF and Mello SF. Removal of caries using only hand instruments: A comparison of mechanical and chemo-mechanical methods. Caries Res.: 2001;35:384–9.

32. Neves AA, Coutinho E, Cardoso MV, Lambrechts P and Meerbeek BV. Current concepts and techniques for caries excavation and adhesion to residual dentin. J. Adhes. Dent.: 2011;13:7–22.

33. Okamoto K, Aoki S and Tamura Y. Comparisons of discomfort among cutting instruments for removal of carious dentin in children. Pediatr. J: 2014;24:46–52.

34. Phonghanyudh A, Phantumvanit P, Songpaisan Y and Petersen PE. Clinical evaluation of three caries removal approaches in primary teeth: a randomized controlled trial. Comm. Dent. Health: 2012;29:173–8.

35. Pitts NB. Are we ready to move from operative to non-operative/preventive treatment of dental caries in clinical practice? Caries Res.: 2004;38: 294–304.

36. Rafique S, Fiske J and Banerjee A. Clinical trial of an air abrasion/chemo-mechanical operative procedure for the restorative treatment of dental patients. Caries Res.: 2003;37:360–4.

37. Ricketts DN, Kidd EA, Innes N and Clarkson J. Complete or ultraconservative removal of decayed tissue in unfilled teeth (review). The Cochrane 2006 Database System Rev 3: CD003808.

38. Schwendicke F, Meyer-Lueckel H, Dorfer C and Paris S. Failure of incompletely excavated teeth– a systematic review. J. Dent.: 2013;41:569–80.

39. Schwendicke F, Schweigel H, Petrou M, Santamaria R, Hopfenmuller W, Finke C and Paris S. Selective or stepwise removal of deep caries in deciduous molars: study protocol for a randomized controlled trial. Trials: 2015;16:1–10.

40. Silva NR, Carvalho RM, Pegoraro LF, Tay FR and Thompson VP. Evaluation of a self-limiting concept in dental caries removal. J. Dent. Res.: 2006;85:282–6.

41. Yazicioglu O and Ulukapi H. The investigation of non-invasive techniques for treating early approximal carious lesions: an *in vivo* study. Int. Dent. J.: 2014;64:1–11.

42. Yazici AR, Atilla P, Ozgunaltay G and Muftuoglu S. *In vitro* comparison of the efficacy of Carislov and conventional rotary instrument in caries removal. J. Oral Rehab.: 2003;30:1177–82.

43. Yip HK and Samaranayake LP. Caries removal techniques and instrumentation: A review. Clin. Oral Invest.: 1998;2:148–54.

44. Zheng L, Hilton JF, Habelitz S, Marshall SJ and Marshgall GW. Dentin caries activity status related to hardness and elasticity. Europen J. Oral Sci.: 2003;111:243–52.

Early Childhood Caries

Early childhood caries (ECC) implies caries amongst pre-school children, toddlers and infants. The accepted age for early childhood caries (neonatal—up to four weeks, infants— up to one year, toddler—up to three years and pre-school children—up to five years) has been described as 6 months to 5 years. Early caries usually affects maxillary primary incisors and the first primary molars, reflecting the pattern of eruption. Such caries pattern differs from caries pattern at other age groups. These type of caries have also been designated as 'bottle caries', 'baby bottle tooth decay', 'nursing caries', 'night bottle mouth', etc.

Dr. Ellias Fass (1962) first documented caries in infants, which he termed, "nursing bottle mouth". He observed that children were put to sleep with a bottle of milk or a sugar containing beverage. He further opined that the carbohydrate containing liquid provided an excellent culture medium for acidogenic micro-organisms and development of caries. Evidences, later suggested that use of sugar containing liquid in a bottle might be an important etiological factor; however, not necessarily the only one. Simultaneously many studies contradicted this belief and reported that a small proportion of children on bottle feeding actually develop caries. The studies from developed countries also suggested that high caries prevalence in infants and toddlers cannot be attributed to bottle feeding only. The studies further observed that communities where bottle feeding was rare, showed high caries rate, especially in primary maxillary incisors.

Breastfeeding, especially during sleep, has also been associated with early childhood caries. Various studies have correlated prolonged or night time breastfeeding with caries of maxillary anterior teeth.

In 1994 the "Center for Disease Control and Prevention" recommended the use of a specific term, 'Early childhood caries (ECC)'; since the association between bottle habits and caries was not absolute. Children experiencing caries in early age have a much greater probability of subsequent caries in both primary and the permanent teeth. Apart from affecting teeth, ECC may lead to widespread health issues. Infants with ECC grow at a slower pace than caries-free infants. Some young children with ECC may be severely underweight because of associated pain and their disinclination to eat. A few authors have associated ECC with iron deficiency also.

Nomenclature and Definitions

Ellias Fass (1962) first coined the term "nursing bottle mouth" to describe early caries pattern. Winter (1966) described the pattern of dental decay in young children due to prolonged and improper nursing habits and named the condition as 'nursing caries'.

Shelton (1977) termed early caries as "nursing bottle syndrome" and described the condition as devastating that may render young children dentally crippled. Dilly (1980) named it "night bottle syndrome".

Croll (1984) defined it as a destructive carious process which can affect infants and toddlers and named it "baby bottle mouth". The term "baby bottle tooth decay" was also proposed.

Tsamtsouris (1986) termed the pattern "nursing bottle caries" and defined it as caries caused by a prolonged use of a bottle filled with any liquid other than the water. Later Moss (1996) shifted the emphasis from the bottle to the need for cleaning and called the disease process "tooth cleaning neglect".

Horowitz (1998) emphasized the importance of the age group affected by the disease and the rapidity of its development and termed the condition "Rampant infant and early childhood dental decay".

The American Academy of Pediatric Dentistry in 2002 defined early childhood caries (ECC) as the presence of one or more decayed (non-cavitated or cavitated), missing (due to caries), or filled tooth surfaces in any primary tooth in a child 71 months of age or younger. The academy also specified that in children younger than 3 years of age, any sign of smooth-surface caries is indicative of severe early childhood caries (S-ECC). From the ages of 3 through 5, one or more cavitated, missing (due to caries) or filled smooth surfaces in primary maxillary anterior teeth or a decayed, missing or filled score of ≥4 (age 3); ≥5 (age 4) or ≥6 (age 5) surfaces constitute S-ECC.

Classification

Wyne (1999) classified early caries into three types:

Type 1 (mild to moderate)

The existence of isolated carious lesion(s) involving molars and/or incisors (Fig. 16.1a).

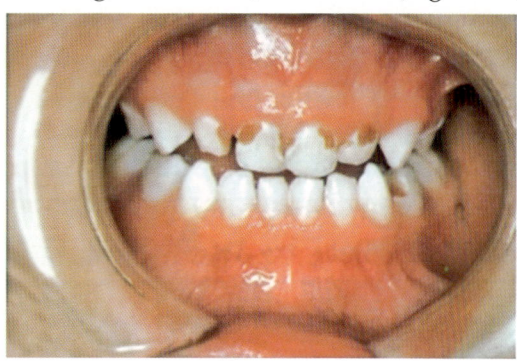

Fig. 16.1a: Type 1 (mild to moderate)

Type 2 (moderate to severe)

Carious lesions affecting maxillary incisors (labio-lingual), with or without affecting molars depending on the age of the child and stage of the disease. The mandibular incisors remain unaffected (Fig. 16.1b).

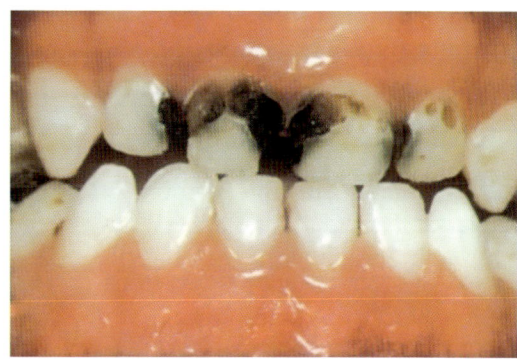

Fig. 16.1b: Type 2 (moderate to severe)

Type 3 (severe)

Carious lesion affecting almost all the teeth including the lower incisor. The condition is rampant and involves tooth surfaces which are usually unaffected by caries (Fig. 16.1c).

ETIOLOGY

Caries is the result of an ecological imbalance in the oral cavity that is illustrated in Flowchart 16.1. The basic process involves action of cariogenic micro-organism on

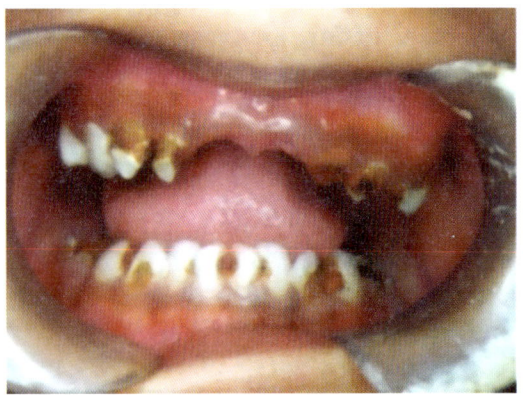

Fig. 16.1c: Type 3 (severe)

fermentable carbohydrates producing acids, which act on susceptible tooth surface causing demineralization.

It has been established that carbohydrates along with cariogenic plaque bacteria play an important role in the development of caries.

The carious lesion develops as the result of dynamic, complex interaction of cariogenic bacteria and the host defense mechanism. The source of carbohydrates may be breast milk and the sugars in the liquid/solid food consumed by the infant. The carbohydrate fermentation lead to production of acids, which may lead to demineralization of enamel. Buffers such as ammonia produced by plaque bacteria and salivary buffers may neutralize the acids produced in plaque.

The causative factor and biologic mechanisms involved in ECC are basically the same as in other type of coronal caries. For details, refer to Chapter 5.

However, the etiology of early childhood caries differs mainly in some biological respect; the bacterial flora and host defense system in young infants are in the process of being established. In addition, the tooth surfaces are newly erupted and immature and may show hypoplastic defects.

The associated factors responsible for caries development are:

A. TOOTH FACTORS

The factors involving tooth tissues are:

a. Tooth Maturation and Defect

It is established that the period immediately after eruption and prior to final maturation is when the tooth is most susceptible to caries.

Even after eruption, newly exposed enamel surface undergo final stages of post-eruptive maturation and hardening. During this period, ions such as fluoride are incorporated into the enamel surface.

In infants, the immature enamel in an environment of cariogenic flora and fermentable carbohydrates becomes susceptible to caries. The improper maturation of enamel

Flowchart 16.1: Etiology of early childhood caries

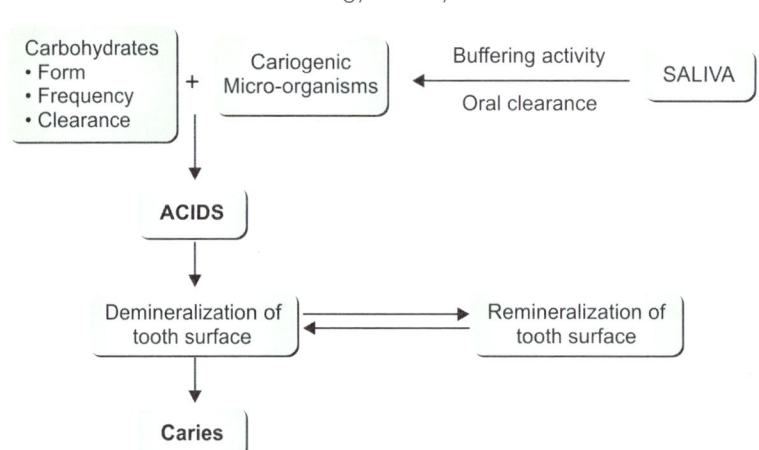

and the defects thereof are the major components of caries etiology in younger teeth.

b. Developmental Defects of Enamel

It is established that in addition to improper maturation, the presence of developmental structural defects in enamel may increase the caries risk. Developmental defects of enamel may be manifested as partial or total loss of enamel or a change in its translucency.

Lai (1997) observed a variety of causes for generalized enamel defects, ranging from hereditary diseases to acquired prenatal, perinatal and postnatal conditions such as birth prematurity and low birth weight infections, malnutrition, metabolic disorders and chemical toxicity. Milgram (2000) later added local trauma and infection as the localized defects.

In the primary dentition, enamel defects are common. Their overall prevalence ranges from 13 to 39% in normal full term infants and over 60–62% in preterm babies born with very low birth weight.

c. Enamel Hypoplasia

Surface irregularities such as pits and grooves or in any other form predispose to plaque retention and increased bacterial colonization, minimizing oral clearance of the carbohydrates. In severe cases, total loss of enamel may expose the dentin, which provides low resistance to acid attack. The patients with linear enamel hypoplasia present a form of rampant decay in primary dentition, known as odontoclasia.

Li (1996) observed association of enamel hypoplasia with malnutrition in under privileged population. He further reported that in linear enamel hypoplasia, the location of hypoplastic line between the neonatal line and the gingival margin of the maxillary primary incisors suggested disturbance of enamel formation in newly erupted teeth. Since the resistance of teeth had been decreased significantly from loss of enamel integrity, the bacterial attack becomes easier.

It is observed that the frequency of enamel hypoplasia is much less in developed communities. Enamel hypoplasia definitely renders children more susceptible to developing early caries than others having similar oral environment.

B. DIETARY FACTORS

The main dietary factors affecting caries in children are:

a. General Cariogenicity of Sugars

Carbohydrates, utilized by oral micro-organisms, especially *Streptococcus mutans* form a sticky film enabling the micro-organisms to adhere to the tooth surfaces. The carbohydrates further serve as metabolites in the production of organic acids, which subsequently demineralize the teeth.

It has been established that sucrose is the preferred substrate used for the generation of dextrans, which are essential for bacterial adherence. These features facilitate the growth of cariogenic bacteria in the oral cavity. Monosaccharide like glucose and fructose are also able to cause fall in pH and demineraliza-tion of enamel. Starches, though lead to marginal fall of pH, may not be much effective in cariogenic process.

b. Frequency of Consumption

The increased frequency of sucrose consumption undoubtedly enhances the establishment of aciduric mutans streptococci, subsequently increasing the cariogenic ability of plaque. The consumption of sugary drinks in between the meals by young children increases the caries activity.

Van Houte (1994) observed that increased time of sugar retention in the oral cavity increases the potential for enamel demineralization, leaving inadequate time for remineralization by saliva; subsequently demineralization prevails, leading to caries.

c. Oral Clearance

The amount of time the carbohydrates remain in oral cavity is an important parameter for the development of caries. Oral clearance of carbohydrate depends on the salivary flow and the stickiness of the food material. It is established that the consumption of sugar is common among infants, especially during sleep time. The low salivary flow during sleep decreases oral clearance of sugars and increases the length of contact time between plaque and the substrate; subsequently, increasing the cariogenic potential.

The oral clearance of carbohydrates varies at different intraoral sites. This might be related to difference of velocity of saliva at different sites in the oral cavity. It is established that the oral clearance is slow on labial surfaces of the maxillary incisors and buccal surfaces of mandibular molars. This difference explains the characteristic distribution of the carious lesions in early childhood caries.

d. Milk and Milk Formula Drinks

Milk and milk formula drinks are common in early ages. The various types and their effects are:

i. Bovine Milk

A widely used drink in childhood and also in adults, milk, remains a subject of interest as regard to its cariogenic potential. Milk contains calcium, phosphorus and other ingredients in addition to potentially cariogenic lactose.

The calcium and phosphorus in milk are bound to organic and inorganic molecules and are also present in ionic form; hence, contributing to the remineralization of enamel. Moreover, milk contains a number of proteins, including casein (a milk phospho-protein) that may provide a protective organic coating on the enamel surface, thereby inhibiting adherence of *mutans streptococci*.

Lactose is present in bovine milk at a concentration of around 4.0% and in human milk at around 7.0%. Although potential demineralization from fermentation of lactose has been shown in a few studies; however, none of studies could confirm pH less than 6.0. It demonstrates low demineralization potential of milk.

The cariogenicity of bovine milk could not be established; on the contrary, there are reasons to accept that milk is cariostatic.

ii. Human Milk

Human milk has comparatively lower mineral content, higher concentration of lactose, less protein and low mineral content.

It is established that prolonged and excessive breastfeeding is associated with early childhood caries in infants. The child who feeds for long periods may develop habit of interrupted sucking, leading to stagnation of milk on teeth for long periods of time, subsequently developing caries. According to Babcely (1989), the severity of early caries, depends upon the frequency and duration of the time the child was exposed to breastfeeding.

It is accepted that oral hygiene practice of the child is an important factor for development of early childhood caries. Various authors have observed a direct correlation between poor oral hygiene practice and development of ECC with same feeding pattern.

Shantinath (1996) studied relation of early childhood caries and child's sleeping habit. A greater incidence of ECC was observed in children who fell asleep with contents of the bottle unfinished than in the children who finished the content, discarded the bottle and fell asleep.

A few authors, however, disagreed to this concept reporting that many children who have taken bottle of milk to bed did not develop caries of anterior teeth. The authors were of the view that social and biological factors coupled with inappropriate use of bottle might be responsible for initiation of caries. Other factors such as heredity, fluoride usage, oral hygiene and dietary practice may also be associated with the development of caries.

Many studies have observed that breast-feeding if given for a prolonged period of time might not be deterrent as long as hygiene measures are adopted.

Dini (2000) and others observed a significant association between social class, mother's education and age at which breast-feeding is terminated with early childhood caries. They opined that appropriate infant feeding, both breast and bottle, should not be discouraged.

iii. *Milk Formulas*

In order to make milk more palatable the manufacturers add additional nutrients like vitamins, minerals, chocolate, etc.

The added sugar to the flavored products leads to increased acid production. Conventional milk showed pH decrease of 0.75 from resting plaque; whereas chocolate milk showed pH decrease up to 2.5.

It is established that the relative cariogenicity of food is dependent on variations in composition, solubility, retentiveness and ability to stimulate flow of saliva. Since the development of dental caries is food related, the related features associated with intake of food play an important part in progress of caries.

Dodds (1988) ranked the reference foods, viz. apple drink, caramel, chocolate, cookie, skimmed milk powder, snack cracker and wheat flake according to their plaque pH response. He observed skimmed milk powder to be the lowest ranked reference food. Bowen (1997) determined the cariogenic potential of many commonly used infant formulae and observed high caries scores in the animals receiving sucrose water; negligible to low in animals on milk and lactose-free infant formulae, mild to moderate with baby formulae with soya, moderate to severe seen with low-iron infant formulae. The nutrient content of milk and milk formulas are tabulated in Table 16.1.

A few authors advocated that iron added to sugar products could reduce incidence of smooth surface caries and also prevents anemic conditions. Further, the combination of iron and fluoride reduces caries in interproximal surfaces. The cariostatic effects of iron have been attributed to formation of an acid insoluble layer, which can absorb calcium and phosphate ions.

e. Acidic Fruit Drinks

Non-carbonated soft drinks and juices are being popularized amongst youngsters. Dental health professionals feel concerned fearing that these drinks may encourage parents to give inappropriate beverages to their children. These beverages contain mainly sugar and have negligible nutritional values.

Many authors have suggested that acids present in these beverages might significantly decrease the oral pH, making tooth surfaces prone to demineralization. Ismail (1984) reviewed the effects of cariogenic soft drinks and reported that the amount and frequency of consumption of soft drinks between meals were significantly associated with high DMFT scores. The greater increase in DMFT was associated with frequency of consumption of these drinks rather than the quantity.

Table 16.1: Nutrient contents of different milk sources					
Milk type	Protein (gm)	Fat (gm)	Lactose (gm)	Calcium (mg)	Phosphorus (mg)
Human	1.2	3.8	7.0	36	18
Bovine	3.3	3.7	4.0	120	95
Milk formula	1.8	3.6	7.0	40	20
Soya-formula	2.0	3.5	0.0	60	50

Smith (1987) opined that, loss of enamel could occur due to excessive consumption of fruit drinks in children. The pH values of undiluted baby fruit juices were acidic and even dilution of juices resulted in an acidic pH.

Risk Factors

The risk factors are categorized as:

a. *Microbiological Risk Factors*

Vertical transmission of mutans streptococci from caregiver to child has been established. The child acquires mutans streptococci from mother during early period. The infant colonization of maternally transmitted mutans are generally related to the magnitude of inoculums and the frequency of inoculations. Mothers with dense salivary reservoirs are at high risk of transmitting bacteria to their infants. Horizontal transmission (through siblings and other family members) is also of concern. The father-to-child transmission has also been reported. Transmission of microbes also occurs from *Ayas* and nurses, etc. in the early period.

Neonatal factors may also increase the risk for early acquisition of *Streptococcus mutans* via vertical transmission. Infants delivered by cesarean section acquire mutans streptococci earlier than conventionally delivered infants although it is reverse for other types of micro-organisms. It is hypothesized that conventional delivery may expose newborns to numerous bacteria earlier and with great intensity, thereby affecting a particular microbial pattern. Cesarean infants are delivered in an aseptic manner, resulting in an atypical microbial environment that may increase susceptibility to subsequent early colonization of mutans streptococci.

The time span between bacterial colonization and caries development is approximately 13–16 months. In high-risk children (preterm and/or low-birth-weight infants, with hypomineralized teeth), the duration may be much shorter. It is accepted that malnutrition/ undernutrition during the prenatal and perinatal periods causes hypoplasia. A consistent association has been reported between enamel hypoplasia and early childhood caries.

b. *Dietary Risk Factors*

Children with early childhood caries usually have frequent and prolonged consumption of sugar beverages. Sugar beverages are readily metabolized to organic acids, leading to demineralization of enamel. The use of nursing bottles enhances exposure to such beverages.

Cow milk, once thought to be the primary causative agent in the development of early childhood caries, has been reported to have negligible cariogenicity. Indeed, cow milk is essentially non-cariogenic because of its mineral content and low level of lactose. The presence of a sugary treat during sleep may promote the cariogenic potential of the infant's diet, since saliva production decreases during sleep.

The human milk or the breastfeeding for longer than one year and particularly at night has been associated with an increased prevalence of caries, since human milk was significantly more cariogenic than cow milk. An epidemiological study however, demonstrated that breastfeeding and its duration were independently associated with an increased risk for early childhood caries.

c. *Environmental Risk Factors*

The microbiological risk factors in early childhood caries can be compensated by good oral hygiene practice. Development of oral hygiene habits may be sensitive to the environmental factors which include caregivers' social status, poverty and literacy, etc. Despite the widespread decline in caries prevalence in developed countries, disparities remain and many children still develop dental caries. This relatively new area of research has been designated as "life-course epidemiology". The life-course concept for investigating the chronic diseases proposes that advantages and disadvantages are accumulated throughout life; generating health differentials throughout the life, subsequently leading to large effects during lifetime.

Children whose primary caregiver have severe dental caries, are regarded as being at increased risk for the disease. A cross-sectional study in Japan contradicted the view and reported that dental caries in 3-year-old children was more strongly associated with child related behaviors than mother-related factors. The risk factors are summarized as:

- Bottle feeding, especially during sleep or prolonged use of 'sippy cup'; flow of saliva decreased during sleep, subsequently slowing down the oral clearance.
- Level of fluoride on the tooth surfaces; low level of fluoride reduces chances of remineralization.
- Children with early caries are at high risk for developing future caries.
- Flow of saliva below 0.7 ml/minute is considered insufficient to wash off carbohydrates from the tooth surfaces. Low salivary buffering capacity reduces potential to neutralize acids in the plaque; thereby increasing the chances of caries.
- Low socio-economic status; poor oral hygiene measures and ineffective diet are potential for caries development.

MICROFLORA OF EARLY CHILDHOOD CARIES

It has been established that *Streptococcus mutans* is the principal micro-organism responsible for coronal caries in humans. Microbial studies have reported that one of the variables necessary for caries initiation and progression (i.e. micro-organisms) can be present in infant's oral cavity immediately after the eruption of their first primary teeth.

As more and more teeth erupted in oral cavity, the *Streptococcus mutans* level increased quantitatively. By the age of 5 years, almost all children harbor *Streptococcus mutans* in sufficient quantity.

A few authors in their studies have failed to isolate *Streptococcus mutans* from the infant's oral cavity. Edwardsson and Mejare (1978) found *Streptococcus mutans* in samples obtained from a 3-month-old infant. The established hypothesis is that, although *mutans streptococci* can contaminate the mouth transiently in infancy, these organisms require a non-shedding surface for their persistent oral colonization. Various studies have established that *Streptococcus mutans* colonize after the eruption of primary teeth.

The *Streptococcus mutans* scores of mother and infant (11–22 months old) with nursing caries is tabulated in Table 16.2.

Most studies have reported increased prevalence of *mutans streptococci* with age, correlating with the number of teeth present in the infant's oral cavity; probably reflects the increasing number of retentive sites for bacterial colonization.

Grindefjord (1996) studied the age of microbial acquisition vis-à-vis caries formation and observed that, age at which mutans streptococci were first acquired in

Table 16.2: The *Streptococcus mutans* scores of mother and infant younger than two years old with nursing caries [Ripa, 1988]

Age (in months)	Number of erupted teeth	Number of carious surface	Streptococcus mutans score	
			Infant	Mother
11	6	4	High	Moderate
12	6	4	Moderate	High
13	4	2	High	High
19	16	3	High	High
22	16	13	Low	Moderate

infants influenced their susceptibility to caries. The aciduricity of *Streptococcus mutans* encourages their accumulation in plaque, which is directly responsible for its cariogenicity. If during the eruption of the tooth the depth of fissures become colonized by *Streptococcus mutans*, the probability of caries development increases. Hence, any factor that interferes with the colonization of the tooth by *S. mutans* can greatly reduce the incidence of caries in man.

Various authors opined that the mean age at which mutans streptococci colonize in the oral cavity coincided with time of emergence of incisors. However, Caufield, et al (1993) observed that the mean age of initial acquisition of *Streptococcus mutans* was 26 months, ranging from 9 to 31 months, which coincide with the emergence of primary molars.

Micro-organisms responsible for dental caries can be transmitted from one individual to another. It is accepted that the transmission of *Streptococcus mutans* to human infants is usually from their mothers.

A mother with high numbers of *Streptococcus mutans* in her saliva is a source of infection to the child. It is established that mothers used spoon if taken to child's mouth, several hundreds of micro-organisms are transmitted to the child. Berkowitz, et al (1981) observed that the frequency of infants infection was approximately nine times greater when maternal salivary level of organism exceeds 10^5 CFU/ml, relative to as observed when maternal salivary reservoirs were less than 10^3 CFU/ml. The authors further observed significant relationship between *Streptococcus mutans* counts of mothers and infants and also between *S. mutans* counts and number of erupted primary teeth.

Kohler, et al (1983) demonstrated that infant infection could be prevented or at least delayed by clinically suppressing maternal reservoirs of mutans streptococci.

Lin Y (2001) evaluated the transmission of pathogenic bacteria of rampant caries from mother to child and observed that mothers were probably the main source of infection with *S. mutans*. Rampant caries in children also has been associated with levels of *Streptococcus sobrinus* in saliva of mothers.

Various studies have reported that about 10–15% caries-active subjects may not have detectable level of *Streptococcus mutans*, inferring that certain other species might be associated with caries activity. It was hypothesized that bacterial etiology of caries involve other potential and producing species, some of which might not have been cultivated. The species associated with severe early childhood caries include *Streptococcus mutans*, *Veillonella parvula*, *Streptococcus cristatus* and *Actinomyces gerensceriae*. A new species, *Scardovia wiggsiae* (Tanner, et al 2011) has been found to be associated with severe early childhood caries. *S. wiggsiae* has been observed in those children in whom *Streptococcus mutans* was not detected. A few authors have detected *Scardovia wiggisiae* in advanced dentinal caries of adults and occlusal carious lesions of children. Recently *S. wiggsiae* has been detected in white spot lesions. *S. wiggsiae* and *Streptococcus mutans* in combination has been associated with childhood caries, as confirmed by various authors. The ecology of micro-organisms specific to sites is tabulated in Table 16.3.

The commonly found micro-organisms in early childhood caries are:

- *Streptococcus gordonii.*
- *Streptococcus mutans.*
- *Streptococcus sobrinus.*
- *Streptococcus cristatus.*
- *Streptococcus intermedius.*
- *Streptococcus mitis.*
- *Streptococcus sanguis.*
- *Lactobacillus gasseri.*
- *Veillonella atypical.*
- *Veillonella dispar.*

Table 16.3: Site-specific micro-organisms in early childhood caries

Intact enamel	White-spot lesion	Dentin lesion	Deep-dentin lesion
Actinomyces spp.	*Veillonella* spp.	*Veillonella* spp.	*Streptococcus mutans*
Veillonella spp.	*Streptococcus sanguis*	*Streptococcus mutans*	*Veillonella* spp.
Leptotrichia spp.	*Leptotrichia* spp.	*Streptococcus sanguis*	*Actinomyces* spp.
Streptococcus sanguis	*Streptococcus cristatus*	*Streptococcus salivarius*	*Lactobacillus* spp.
Streptococcus mitis	*Capnocytophaga sputigena*	*Capnocytophaga sputigena*	*Streptococcus salivarius*
Streptococcus salivarius	*Capnocytophaga granulosa*	*Streptococcus mitis*	*Streptococcus mitis*
Streptococcus sanguis	*Streptococcus mutans*	*Selenomonas* spp.	*Selenomonas* spp.
	Actinomyces gerenseriae	*Leptorichia* spp.	
		Actinomyces gerenseriae	

- *Dialister invisus.*
- *Selenomonas dianae.*
- *Selenomonas infelix.*
- *Selenomonas noxia.*
- *Leptotrichia hofstadii.*
- *Leptotrichia buccalis.*
- *Leptotrichia wadei.*
- *Actinomyces naeslundii.*
- *Actinomyces gerenseriae.*
- *Actinomyces dentalis.*
- *Bifidobacterium dentium*
- *Neisseria* spp.
- *Scardovia wiggsiae.*

PREVALENCE OF EARLY CHILDHOOD CARIES

The dental health of preschool children has been largely ignored. The relatively inaccessibility of preschool children might be the reason why the dental health of preschool children has not been studied extensively.

Many studies have recognized that, infant feeding practices are influenced by cultural, ethnic and socio-economic factors. The methodological problems have complicated determination of the prevalence of nursing caries in general public at large.

Prevalence Globally

The global prevalence of early childhood caries is tabulated in Table 16.4. Goose (1967) selected 309 children from two locations in England and reported a nursing caries prevalence of 6.8 percent. Goose and Gittus (1968) further studied 5549 randomly selected 1–2 years old children from 72 locations in England and reported 5.9% prevalence. In both studies the examiners were not qualified. The children's labial surfaces of maxillary incisors were photographed and categorized as mild and advanced.

Preschool children who attended maternal and child welfare clinics in London were examined for nursing caries in studies of Winter (1971), Holt (1982), Hot (1988) and reported a decline in prevalence of nursing caries from 8 to 3% (1971 to 1982) and 8 to 4% (1973 to 1988). Higher prevalence was more clearly associated with unemployment, single parenting and lower socioeconomic status.

Wendt, et al (1991) found a nursing caries prevalence of 7.7% in group of 632, 1 and 2 years old children from Sweden. Immigrant children had much higher prevalence of nursing caries than Swedish children.

Paunio, et al (1993) in Finland selected 1018, 3-year-old children by means of a stratified cluster sampling and reported 6% nursing caries prevalence.

Constante HM, et al (2014) studied the distribution of caries in schoolchildren from Brazil and found that the prevalence of dental caries decreased from 98% in 1971 to 36.9% in 2011. The Gini coefficient was 0.624 in 2002 but increased to 0.725 in 2011; the Lorenz curve showed that 70–75% of dental caries

Table 16.4: Global prevalence

Authors (Year) Place	Sample size	Criteria adopted	Prevalence
Goose (1967) England	Random selection of 309 1–2-year-old children in two countries	Comparison of child's labial surfaces of maxillary incisors by photographs categorizing the children in mild and advanced stages	6.8%
Goose and Gittus (1968) England	Random selection of 5549, 1–2-year-old children from 72 locations in England	Comparison of child's labial surfaces of maxillary incisors by photographs categorizing the children in mild and advanced stages	5.9%
Winter, et al (1966) England	One hundred, 1–5-year-old children, attending a welfare center	Visual examination by dentist; rampant caries recorded when labial or palatal surfaces of two or more maxillary incisors involved	12.0%
Winter, et al (1971) England	601, 12–60-month-old children from all social classes in London	Visual examination by dentist; rampant caries recorded when labial or palatal surfaces of two or more maxillary incisors	8.0%
Silver (1973) England	263, 3-year-old children representing 78% of all 3-year-old in Bishop's Storford	Rampant caries recorded if involvement of labial/palatal surfaces of two or more maxillary incisors	2.0%
Silver (1981) England	252, 3-year-old children representing 78% of all 3-year-old in Bishop's Storford	Rampant caries recorded if involvement of labial/palatal surfaces of two or more maxillary incisors	3.0%
Holt, et al (1982) England	555, 12–60-month-old children from all social classes in London	Visual examination by dentist; rampant caries recorded when labial or palatal surfaces of two or more maxillary incisors involved	12–23 mths 3% 24–35 mths 3% 36–47 mths 4% 48–59 mths 4% Overall 7%
Holt, et al (1988) England	565, 12–60-month-old children attending maternal and child welfare clinics in Camden	Visual examination by dentist; rampant caries recorded when labial or palatal surfaces of two or more maxillary incisors involved	12–23 mths 0% 24–35 mths 9% 36–47 mths 10% 48–59 mths 16% Overall 7%
Silver (1989) England	230, 3-year-old children representing 61% of all 3-year-old in Bishop's Storford	Rampant caries recorded if involvement of labial or palatal surfaces of two or more maxillary incisors	4.0%
Wendt, et al (1991) Sweden	632, 12–14-month-old children living within the area of four child welfare centers in Jonkoping	Presence or absence of initial demineralization and cavitation	Incisors only 0.5%

Contd...

Table 16.4: Global prevalence (*Contd...*)

Authors (Year) Place	Sample size	Criteria adopted	Prevalence
Paunio, et al (1993) Finland	1018, 3-year-old children selected by means of a stratified cluster sampling	Extent of caries recorded for maxillary incisors alone or in combination with canines/molars; initial caries excluded	6.0%
Brown, et al (1985) Australia	112 children, less than 2 years old, attending maternal and child health clinics in lower middle-class suburbs of Brisbane	Nursing caries pattern	5.4%
Aldy, et al (1979) Indonesia	100 children, less than 5-year-old, who visited a hospital	Caries on labial surface of one or more maxillary incisors	48.0%
Cleaton-Jones, et al (1978) South Africa	499, 1–5-year-old white children in Johannesburg	Labial surfaces caries on one or more maxillary incisors	11.4%
		Labial surface caries on two or more maxillary incisors	8.6%
Cleaton-Jones, et al (1978) South Africa	439 rural and 192 urban black children, 1–5 years old	Labial surface caries affecting one or more maxillary incisors or canines	Rural 13.7% Urban 3.1%
Richardson, et al (1981) South Africa	437 rural black, urban, 250 urban black, and 468 urban white children, 1–6-year-old	Labial surface caries affecting one or more maxillary incisors or canines	Black rural 11.7% Black urban 4.0% White urban 12.0%
Salako (1985) Nigeria	560, 3–7-year-old children, presented to the school of Dental Science in Lagos	Visible cavitation or sticking of probe in carious lesion	38.4%
Matee, et al (1992) Tanzania	442 infants, 1–2½ years old, who attended maternal and child health clinics in Mwanza and Morogoro	At least two maxillary incisors exhibiting caries. (Presence of linear hypoplasia in association with nursing caries pattern)	Rural regions: Negerengere 1.8% Bukumbi 5.9% Kizuka 17.3% Turiani 22.2% Urban regions: Makongoro 9.8% Overall: 10.6%
Raadal, et al (1993) Sudan	275, 3½–5½ years old pre-school children in Khartoum city	Caries involving labial or lingual surfaces of two or more maxillary incisors	5.5%
Paes, et al (2004) Brazil	369 randomly selected aged 36 to 71 months from a low-income population	A 24-hour recall diary was used to assess data about infant feeding practices and dietary habits. The data were statistically analyzed.	36%
Peressini, et al (2004) Ontario	All children aged 3 and 5 years in seven first Nations communities in the Manitoulin District.	Children with caries on two or more primary maxillary incisors or canines or those having a total decayed,	52%

Contd...

Table 16.4: Global prevalence (*Contd...*)

Authors (Year) Place	Sample size	Criteria adopted	Prevalence
		missing, filled primary teeth (dmft) score of 4 or greater	
Simin Z, et al (2006) Tehran	504 children aged 1–3 years from 18 public health centres in Tehran	Mothers were interviewed about their child's birth, gender, primary caregiver, the mother's age and the educational level of both parents. Dental examination carried out according to the WHO criteria. Early childhood caries (ECC) was defined as the presence of any dmf teeth.	Prevalence in 12–15 months (dt) was 3%, being 9% for 16- to 19- and 14% for 20–25 months and 33% for the 26–36 month-old
Martha, et al (2009) Boston	1–3 years old 787 children, 610 children from BMC and 177 children from NEMC	787, 1- to 3-year-old children from two urban Boston medical centers compared with US children surveyed as part of NHANES III.	Boston children 3.0% US children 6.3%

attacks was restricted to 30% of the population in 2011. A reduction of 41.2% in the mean SiC index was observed between 2002 (3.4) and 2011 (1.9). An effective decline in the prevalence and severity of dental caries in schoolchildren was observed throughout 40 years of monitoring.

Mantonanbaki M, et al (2013) studied the dental caries and use of dental services experience in 5-year-old children attending public kindergartens in Greece. The prevalence of dental caries was 16.5%. Caries index was 32% and dental visits were reported for the 84% of the children. Medium socioeconomic level (SEL) was associated with no detectable caries. High socioeconomic level was related to decreased decayed, missing, filled teeth values, while female gender and rented houses had the opposite effect. The age of the mother (35–39 years) and the higher SEL were related to higher levels of dental services use.

In Indonesia, Aldy, et al (1979) reported prevalence of 48% in 100 children younger than 5 years of age who visited a local hospital.

Brown, et al (1985) reported a prevalence of 5.4% caries in 112 Australian children less than 2-year-old who attended maternal and children health clinics.

Many African societies, especially developed societies, promote breastfeeding because it is safe, economical and nutritious. Several studies from South Africa revealed that although the majority of black infants were breastfed in contrast to white infants who were bottle fed, nursing caries occurred most often in blacks.

Salako (1985) reported 38.4% nursing caries prevalence among 560 Nigerian children of 3–7 years, who visited school of dental sciences in Lagos.

On the basis of clinical appearance of primary teeth and nursing history of the child, Powel (1976) identified 40 Los Angeles children with nursing caries among 4000 children of study group. Currier and Glinka (1977) reported prevalence of 5% in predominating black children who attended maternal and child health clinics, in Virginia.

Johnson, et al (1984) studied 200 children of 3.5 to 5 years old living in Fluorinated communities in Ohio and reported a prevalence of 11%. Kelly and Bruerd examined 3–5 years old American Indian and Alaska Native children who were attending Head start programs in 18 rural locations in Oklahoma and Alaska. The range of nursing caries in nine Alaska sites was 44–85%, whereas range for Oklahoma sites was 17–60%. The reason may be due to economical and cultural difference. Further Broderjet (1989) in a large study of 1607, 3–5 years old children of Navago and Cherokee reported overall 72% of prevalence in Navago and 55% prevalence in Cherokee children.

Branes (1992) studied nursing caries prevalence among four ethnic groups of Head Start children—White, black, hispanic and Native American, among 1230 children of 3–5 years age group and found that, native American children had a significantly higher prevalence (35%) than Hispanic (23.8%) white (22.2%) and black (20.5%) children. Rural children were twice as likely to develop nursing caries on their non-rural counterparts (34.1% vs 16.6%). High prevalence of nursing caries among Aboriginal children in Canada and Native American children in the United States could be explained by the lack of access to dental care or behavioural, social or cultural conditions as yet unidentified.

Studies from several urban setting in Canada and United States show wide variation in prevalence of nursing caries. Derkson and Ponts reported a prevalence of 3.2% among 594 randomly selected children, 9 month to 6 years of age, on the other hand, Budoroski reported a prevalence of 7.4% among 302 children, 9 month to 5 years of age from 10 day care center in Toronto.

Wyne A, et al (2001) evaluated the prevalence of nursing caries in Saudi preschool children. They reported mean DMFT 6.7 at the age of 2 years, 6.9 at 3 years, 8.5 at 4 years, 9.2 at 5 years and 9.3 at 6 years of age.

The teeth most affected by caries were maxillary central incisors and the least affected were mandibular canines. The probability of bilateral molar caries was very high; 86.2% for maxillary first molars, 88.1% for maxillary second molars, 94.7% for mandibular first molars and 93.4% for mandibular second molars.

Prevalence in India

India is the seventh largest country in world (in terms of area) and second largest (in terms of population). It comprises 29 states and seven union territories. The majority of the population (72%) in this country lives in rural areas (the number of villages approximately 5.5. lacs). The literacy rate as of 2012 consensus is 74.04%.

A few investigations, evaluating dental caries status of the children below 5 years have been carried out in India. This might be due to difficulty to get the samples at a common place, un-cooperative behaviour of young children, varied number of erupted teeth and lack of accepted single criteria for evaluating young children. The studies conducted in the past, their results and the criteria adopted are tabulated in Table 16.5.

The prevalence of dental caries is very low in the first year of life (1–1.5%), thereafter as the teeth erupt with age, caries prevalence increases. At 3 years of age (all primary teeth erupted), almost half the primary teeth are reported to be carious. At 5 years of age almost half of the children are affected. The caries prevalence from Karnataka as found to be as high as 66.3% (deft 2–9) at 4–5 years of age in urban population and 58.4% (deft 2–3) in rural areas. Sarkar reported 25.9% prevalence in Calcutta. Ashima reported a prevalence of 48% in 5-year-old children in Chandigarh with socioeconomic status having negative association with caries status.

Kuriakose (1999) reported prevalence of dental caries in preschool children to be 57% among 600 children examined in Trivandrum.

Sudha and Kammar (2000) reported prevalence of 65% caries among pre-school

Table 16.5: Indian prevalence

Authors, (Year) Place	Index used	Total number	Prevalence (%)	Mean dmft/dmfs
Virjee Shanker (1987) Bangalore	Johnson (1984)	673	66.3	2.9
Sarkar & Chowdary (1992) West Bengal	WHO (1971)	40	25.5	–
Sethi & Tandon (1996) Udupi	William (1994)	404	65.5	–
Goyal, et al (1997) Chandigarh	WHO (1983)	154	19.4	0.4 (0.7)
Kuriokose (1999) Kerala	WHO	600	57	2.28 (4.10)
Babu, et al (2003) Kerala	Modified WHO criteria(1997)	530	12	1.84 ± 2.87
Priyadarshini, et al (2011) Bangalore	Gruebell's criteria	566	37.3	1.90±3.38
Prashanth, et al (2012) Bangalore	Modified WHO criteria (1997)	1500	27.5	0.854
Shilpi, et al (2012) Bangalore	Gruebell's criteria	717	40	1.89+3.3
Subramanium, et al (2013) Bangalore	WHO criteria 1997	1500	27.5	0.854
Gaidhane, et al (2013) Wardha	WHO Oral Health Assessment Form 1997	330	33.48	–
Shrutha, et al (2013) Kanpur	WHO criteria 1997	2000	48	2.03±2.99
Kuriakose (2015) Trivandrum	Gruebell's criteria	1329	54	2.3±3.2
Shah, et al (2015) Srinagar	Gruebell's criteria	466	39.9	1.80±3.38
Stephen, et al (2015) Salem	WHO Oral Health Assessment Form 1997	2771	16	5.23 ± 1
Kaikure, et al (2015) Bylakuppe	WHO Oral Health Assessment Form 1997	500	92.2	6.15 (10.27)

children of Hubli-Dharwad. They observed higher prevalence in low socioeconomic group families.

Kramer M, et al (2007) studied the effect of prolonged and exclusive breastfeeding on dental caries in early school-age children and found no beneficial or harmful effect on dental caries.

Shrutha SP, et al (2013) assessed the caries experience in 3–5-year-old children and evaluated the relationship with their mothers' practices regarding feeding and oral hygiene habits in Kanpur and observed high caries prevalence among those who were breastfed for longer duration, during nighttime, those falling asleep with bottle and those fed with additional sugar in milk.

Kaikure MK, et al (2015) demonstrated high prevalence of ECC in children with bottle feeding, addition of sugar to bottle content and to regular food, in-between meal snacking habits and increase intake of sweets like chocolate, candies and toffees, lesser frequency of brushing and child brushing unassisted/unsupervised.

Stephen Λ, et al (2015) evaluated the prevalence of ECC in preschool children in the age group between 18 and 72 months and its relationship with parent's education and socioeconomic status of the family and observed higher prevalence of ECC in children of working mothers, lower parental education and lower socioeconomic groups.

DIAGNOSTIC CRITERIA

The criteria used to evaluate early childhood caries vary in different studies. Mostly visual experimentation has been the criteria adopted in early studies. The presence of cavitation or 'stickiness' of one or more, two or more, or three or more decayed or filled maxillary incisors has been the accepted criteria. A few authors have not specified the criteria used in their respective studies. The main criteria used are:

- Visual examination (staining, cavitation).
- Probing ('sticking' probe).
- WHO criteria (cavitation).
- Radike/NIDR criteria (cavitation).

The WHO criteria used natural or artificial light, dental mirror and sickle probes (No. 23). The Radike/NIDR criteria mainly had three different scores; these include:

0   No visible evidence of caries or restoration.

1   At least one maxillary incisor showed visual evidence of caries or restoration.

2   Subject could not be examined (could not distinguish between stained or carious teeth).

Initially, the early carious lesions were diagnosed, when examiner noticed "loss of translucency" or "chalky appearance" without microscopic loss of tooth structure. Caries was also diagnosed when an explorer "got stuck" in a carious lesion in a couple of studies.

Epidemiological evidences have indicated that non-cavitated caries are more prevalent than cavitation during first 18 months of life. Hence investigators might not be able to detect early lesions, especially in population with severe childhood caries, because most children might have been examined at an age when caries had already advanced into dentin.

The lack of agreement on diagnostic criteria for dental caries in preschool aged children hinders evaluation protocol, subsequently the prevalence of dental caries in the selected population.

Drury, et al (1999) suggested the following point for diagnosing early childhood caries, which are to be emphasized during evaluation process:

a. Should the diagnostic criteria be based entirely on the presence of one or more cavitated or non-cavitated lesion on any tooth surface; or should the diagnostic criteria be based both on inclusion and exclusion criteria?

b. Should the palatal surface of maxillary second primary molar or buccal surface of mandibular second primary molar be considered smooth surface or pit and fissure surface? If these surfaces are considered as smooth surfaces, is there any condition under which can be considered pit and fissure surfaces?

c. Considering that the diagnostic criteria used in past and future studies, have been or will be, based on manifestational criteria; what kind of studies need to be considered to explore the feasibility of going beyond manifestational criteria to a consideration of etiological criteria as a basis for diagnosis.

The diagnostic criteria should be assessed as regard to their ease of use, requirements for training and calibration, examiner reliability and also their predictive validity.

Also the research programs are needed for new diagnostic tools for dental caries that are more predictive for evaluation of preventive and treatment interventions.

CLINICAL APPEARANCE

Early childhood caries, especially when associated with the feeding bottle habit, has been characterized as first affecting the primary maxillary anterior teeth, followed by involvement of primary molars and then canines. The longevity of the caries process affects the severity of caries in incisors and involvement of other teeth.

It is established that mandibular incisors are more resistant to caries because of their close proximity to secretions of submandibular salivary glands as well as the cleansing action of the tongue during the process of sucking the bottle. It has been documented that the reason for unequal severity of lesion between incisors and other teeth is related to the following three factors.

- The chronology of primary tooth eruption.
- The duration of deleterious habit.
- Muscular pattern of infant sucking.

A dull white demineralization areas along the gum line of maxillary incisors that usually goes undetected by parents is the common observation in early caries. As condition progresses, the white area develops into cavities encircling the cervical collar. In advanced cases, the crowns of all maxillary incisors may be destroyed completely leaving decayed brownish-black root stumps. It is reported that the primary canines and second molars are usually minimally affected by nursing caries, since they erupt by the time the children have left the use of bottle.

It is accepted that higher prevalence of oral *Streptococcus mutans* in association with poor oral hygiene, may lead to severe form of early childhood caries involving almost all the teeth including mandibular incisors.

Clinically, severe form of early caries can also be seen in children who have a greatly reduced salivary flow as a result of radiotherapy for the treatment of cancer of the head and neck region or as a result of surgical removal of neoplasms in the oral cavity.

Clinical Patterns

Clinically, early childhood caries may exhibit fairly distinct patterns. The clinical appearance of the teeth in childhood caries follows a definite pattern. There is early carious involvement of the maxillary anterior teeth, the maxillary and mandibular first primary molars and sometimes, the mandibular canines.

The pattern of progress of caries is summarized as:

- Initial caries begins at the palatal surface of the maxillary incisors followed by involvement of the facial (along the cervical margin of teeth) and proximal surface; subsequently may lead to the loss of the entire crown.
- Then there is involvement of the occlusal surface of the maxillary and mandibular first primary molars followed by their proximal surface.

The severe form of caries depicts involvement of facial surfaces of the mandibular incisors, further progressing to maxillary and mandibular canines. The child is categorized and assigned one of the specific caries patterns according to the following features:

A. Carious Lesions Associated with Developmental Defects

a. *Pit and fissure:* One or more lesion at sites of pit and fissure enamel defects in primary molars, occlusal surface of any molar, palatal surface of maxillary second molar and buccal surface of mandibular second molar.

b. *Hypoplasia:* A detectable rough enamel surface with altered contour and darkened enamel or dentin; caries adjacent to areas of hypoplasia and on mesial aspect of labial surface of primary canine.

B. Smooth Surface Lesions

a. *Faciolingual:* One or more lesion on facial or lingual surface of any tooth or on proximal surface of an incisor tooth.

b. *Proximal:* One or more lesions on the proximal surface of the primary molars or distal surface of primary canines.

c. *Faciolingual proximal:* One or more of both types of smooth surface lesions.

C. Rampant Caries

14 out of 20 primary teeth having carious lesion, including at least one mandibular incisor.

Complications

The common complication of early childhood caries is pain and unesthetic looks. The associated infection affects pharynx, lungs and so on. As the caries remain untreated, the complications like loss of weight, psychological problems, speech problem and malnutrition affects the overall development of the child.

Early childhood caries affects general health of the child. The potential for increased glucocorticoid production in response to pain, decreased sleep patterns and the overall increased metabolic rate during the course of infection may lead to retarded growth and development in such children.

It is established that the timely treatment of nursing caries may preserve the overall health of the children. The caries at an early age need to be prevented or at least diagnosed and treated on time so as to minimize the effect on general health.

i. Effects on Nutrition and Body Weight

Children inflicted by caries in young age mostly avoid frequent meals, which lead to inadequate nutrition, thereby adversely affecting the growth of the child.

Acs (1992) studied the effect of nursing caries on body weight and stated that, 8.7% of the children with nursing caries weighed less than 80% of their ideal weight, compared to only 1.7% of children in control group with low weight. Also the children with nursing caries who had lower percentile weight categories were significantly older than children at or above their ideal weight.

Ayhan (1996) studied the effect of early caries on height and body weight in 126 children, aged 3–5 years and observed that mean weight fell between 25th and 50th percentile and that 7.1% weighed less than 90% of their ideal weight. The height and weight of the control group showed a higher percentile category than the rampant/nursing caries group inferring that rampant/nursing caries may adversely affect the growth of the children.

Thomas (2002) observed that children with early caries, who received complete rehabilitation demonstrated significant improvement in their quality of the life.

ii. Psychological Problems

Children with early caries commonly are restless, fussy and ill-tempered. These children may not complain of pain; only convey by decreased appetite, increased irritability and sleeplessness. These problems may lead to poor behavior in school and negative self esteem.

A few authors, however, reported that there was no difference in temperament between the group of children with caries and the group without caries.

iii. Effect of Early Caries on Future Caries

The children with early childhood caries are always at risk of developing future caries of primary molars and also in permanent dentition. It is established that the children with early caries are more susceptible to lesions of proximal surfaces of primary molars than caries-free children.

A few authors contradicted this and observed that, children with labial or lingual caries of incisors (ECC classification) had less risk for caries in permanent dentition; whereas, children having two or more decayed incisor surfaces (ECC classification) were at higher risk of caries in permanent dentition.

When children with maxillary anterior caries were compared with increased risk of caries in other primary teeth, O'Sullivan (1993) observed that these children were three times at greater risk of developing molar caries than children without anterior caries.

O'Sullivan (1994) further studied the association of early dental caries pattern (at mean age 3 years) with caries incidence in preschool children (2 years later) and reported that, children who presented with maxillary anterior caries or pit and fissure caries at base line had a mean posterior dmfs seven and four times greater respectively, than that of children who were caries-free at baseline.

A few authors, considering condition of primary incisors, age of initial examination, gender, use of sealants and age when last dental examination was conducted, reported that children with early caries have shown twice DMFT rate in permanent dentition than those without caries. Also increased age is a risk factor for higher DMFT and regular recalls and sealants were found to be protective factors.

PREVENTIVE PROTOCOL

The caries is reported to be declining in global scenario; however, the children from developing countries and also from some of the developed countries experience early caries affecting the primary dentition.

The preventive programs need to be evaluated on the basis of the following key issues:

a. The preventive regime should be based on scientific studies that have evaluated the efficacy and effectiveness of the interventions used to prevent a disease.

b. The preventive regime should be based on objective and valid definition of the problems targeted for prevention. Usually the problem targeted is only on one habit, i.e. baby bottle use, disregarding other determinants of the disease.

c. The prevention of early caries should be based on a comprehensive rather than a restricted understanding of the condition. All factors responsible for early caries may be looked into.

Preventive Methods

The preventive methods are depicted in Flowchart 16.2. The community based strategy

Flowchart 16.2: Prevention of childhood caries

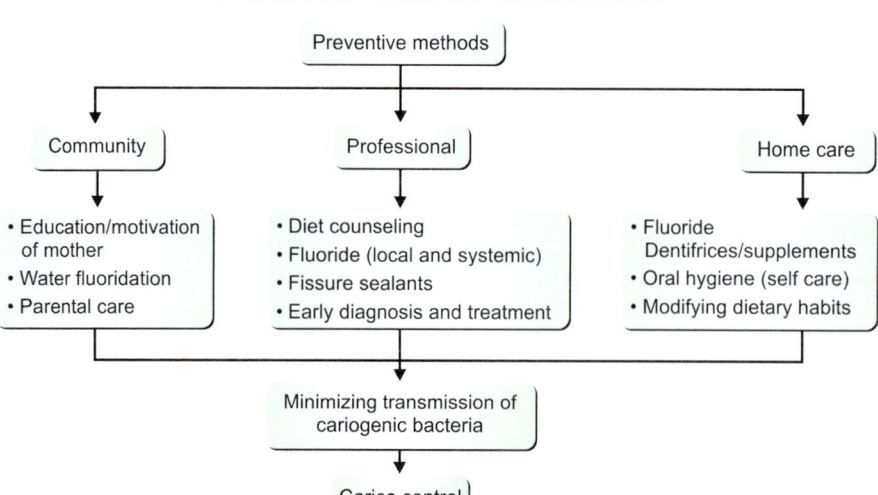

mainly relies on educating and motivating the mother. The water fluoridation of that area can also be improved. The professional care includes diet counseling, fluoride/sealant applications followed by home care means of dietary control and self-care hygiene habits. At every level, the transmission of cariogenic bacteria is to be minimized.

Income and education are strong determinants of dental caries, especially in primary dentition and improvement in these factors have a definite impact on the health of infants and toddlers, provided other social and behavioral factors improve as well.

It is established that children from families of low socioeconomic status or those living in native communities are at a higher risk of developing early caries than low-risk children. The infants with early signs of dental caries, heavy plaque accumulation and high mutans streptococci levels have been categorized as 'high-risk group'.

According to American Academy of Pediatric Dentistry, infant's oral cavity should be examined at an early stage categorizing them in high or low caries risk groups and appropriate preventive strategies be implemented accordingly.

a. Preventive regime of low-risk children.
  - Fluoridated dentifrice.
  - Modification of dietary habits and oral hygiene practices.
b. Preventive regime of high-risk children.
  - Fluoride (local and systemic).
  - Dietary counseling.
  - Chlorhexidine varnish.
  - Fissure sealants.

The routinely employed methods of preventive regimes are:

i. Education and Motivation

The goal of education is to increase the knowledge of mother about early caries, subsequently improving the dietary and nutritional habits of infants and the mothers. It is accepted that an increase in knowledge of mother and caregivers influence the dietary and oral hygiene habits of infants leading to prevention of early caries.

Many mothers lack knowledge about the determinants of early caries, viz. allowing infants to sleep with the bottle and the time when baby should be weaned off the bottle. The educational status is inversely associated with the mean number of decayed, missing and filled (dmft) teeth, at least up to three years of age.

A few authors have suggested that, knowledge may be a prerequisite for healthy behavior, but it is not sufficient to influence a change in non-healthy behavior. They found 40% of mother of infants with early caries admitted knowing about the potential harmful effects that may result from putting infant to bed with a bottle containing milk or a sugary solution, yet they continued the practice.

Mothers are being educated only on the misuse of milk bottles, etc. and not on the other factors affecting early caries. Matee (1994) in his study observed that not all children with early caries use baby bottle and also those children who have constantly used baby bottle did not have caries.

Al-Dashti (1995) opined that children who inappropriately use baby bottle at night might also be having frequent sugar during the day, making it difficult to identify the exact source of sugar causing early caries.

The mother and others in the family should be motivated to use the supervised tooth brushing with fluoridated dentifrice for preventing early caries. Mothers are the primary promoters of oral hygiene practices and have a major influence on the dietary habits and food choices of infants, toddlers and children. It is established that the change in oral health status of infants are linked to changes in the oral health behaviors and dietary practices of their mothers.

The educational programs must involve the participation of caregivers along with mothers. The caregivers should also be educated and motivated to recognize caries and its risk factors at an early age. Health care professionals should motivate parents and caregivers to clean their infant's teeth with a soft brush or moist cloth as soon as the teeth erupt. The parents should be educated to analyze the color variation of infants teeth by routinely lifting the lip and observing. The parents should also be educated as regard to relationship between feeding practices and good oral health. Dieticians, nutritionists and other health care professionals can recommend food, beverages, etc. that promote good oral health.

ii. Water Fluoridation

All infants and toddlers, regardless of their risk status could benefit from water fluoridation. This has been highly effective technique in preventing caries in primary dentition.

A 40–60% reduction in caries by water fluoridation in children below 5-year age has been reported. Further, water fluoridation is more beneficial for children from low socioeconomic groups than those from high socioeconomic groups.

Water fluoridation provides the only means of prevention that does not require a dental visit or parental motivation. Studies support water fluoridation as an effective preventive protocol especially in primary dentition.

iii. Fluoride Dentifrices/Supplements

Fluorides in various forms have been used in caries prevention. The current view is that fluoride present in the plaque fluid, slows down the dissolution of enamel and supports the precipitation phase. After topical application, calcium fluoride depots are formed on the tooth surfaces controlling the pH of the acidic attack.

The basic principle to apply fluoride is that it should always be present in the plaque-enamel interface. This effect can be accomplished by frequent application of low concentrate fluoride source (fluoridated water, fluoride toothpastes, fluoride drops or sucking fluoride tablets) or less frequent treatments with highly concentrated preparations causing calcium fluoride deposit in or on the enamel acting as a slow releasing system (fluoride varnishes). It is established that, the fluoride exposure should be matched against the caries activity; that is, greater the cariogenic challenge, the more intense the fluoride treatment.

When instituting schedules for fluoride application to infants, it is important to look at the feasibility, the risk for dental fluorosis and the individual's caries risk. Apart from water fluoridation, the use of fluoride varnishes is considered to be the most suitable and documented fluoride regimes for the infants.

According to American Academy of Pediatric Dentistry (manual 2002), the dose for fluoride supplements is tabulated in Table 16.6. The fluoride treatment for early caries is tabulated in Table 16.7.

Table 16.6: Dietary fluoride supplementation schedule			
Age	Less than 0.3 ppm F	0.3–0.6 ppm F	More than 0.6 ppm F
Birth–6 months	0	0	0
0–3 years	0.25 mg	0	0
3–6 years	0.50 mg	0.25	0

Table 16.7: Fluoride treatment for children with early childhood caries

Type of fluoride	0–2 years	2–3 years	3–13 years
Dietary fluoride supplements	Not indicated	0.25 mg F daily	0.5 mg F daily
Operator applied fluoride	APF topical solution or gel 1.23% F applied few times a year	APF topical solution or gel, 1.23% F applied four times a year	APF topical solution or gel, 1.23% F applied four times a year
Self-applied topical fluoride	Not indicated	Not indicated	Self application of gel tray daily for approximately 4 weeks; thereafter, continue with a daily F rinse (0.05% NaF)
Fluoride dentifrice	Brush with F containing dentifrice	Brush with F containing dentifrice	Brush with F containing dentifrice

iv. *Modifying Dietary Habits*

The successful management of early (rampant) caries necessitates severe dietary modification. A protocol of slow change over a long period is more acceptable to the parents and the child as well.

The first step is the counseling. Counseling should be carried out in a separate room by the dentist or the nutritionist. The counselor should encourage the parents involvement in discussion so that the child (depend upon age) and the parents understood the importance of diet in maintaining the oral health of the child.

A few authors have opined that, counselor should ask the parents to keep a five-day food diary of the child. An average of these days' food habits serve as a record of the child's routine food intake.

It has been reported that, once the child or the parents come to know about the role of food in dental caries development, they will opt for a self prescribed less cariogenic and more nutritious diet. The parents can decide what to add, delete or substitute from the diet of the child.

v. *Oral Hygiene (self-care)*

The role of oral hygiene as caries preventive measure in young children is not definite; however, the effectiveness depends on the attention and awareness by the caregivers. It is important that parents, especially mothers should know about the importance of tooth cleaning. It is advisable to instruct mother that tooth brushing be carried out before the child goes to bed; thereafter no cariogenic food or drink be consumed.

The oral cavity of the child should be observed regularly, since any change in color of teeth can be indicative of caries. It has been emphasized that good oral hygiene enhances the effect of fluoride supplements; they remain ineffective on tooth surface with poor oral hygiene.

A small soft-bristle toothbrush should be recommended. Professional tooth cleaning should be considered for infants and toddlers with proven caries susceptibility as an effective measure to control the cariogenic challenge.

vi. *Minimizing Transmission of Cariogenic Bacteria*

There is definite evidence that cariogenic bacteria are transmitted from mothers to their infants. The Genotypes of mutans streptococci in infants have been found to be identical to those of the mother.

The preventive programs suppressing the transmission of mutans streptococci help in reducing the infection of the infants and prevent dental caries.

Dabanayake (1993) contradicting the statement observed that the effectiveness of six applications of an iodine sodium fluoride solution to the mothers during tooth eruption of their infants did not find a significant impact on colonization with mutans streptococci. Further, the caries incidence between treatment group and control group remained almost same.

The search is now focused on genetically altering the mutans streptococci so as to inactivate their influence on the infant's oral cavity.

It is established that preventive interventions within the first years of life are critical. This may be best implemented with the help of medical providers who are trained to provide oral screenings, apply preventive measures, also motivate parents and for dental care.

To decrease the risk of developing early childhood caries, the AAPD encourages professional and at-home preventive measures that include:

1. Reducing the parent's/sibling(s)' *Streptococcus mutans* levels to decrease transmission of cariogenic bacteria.
2. Minimizing saliva-sharing activities (e.g. sharing utensils) to decrease the transmission of cariogenic bacteria.
3. Implementing oral hygiene measures as soon as the first primary tooth erupts. Tooth brushing should also be performed for children by the parent, using a soft toothbrush. In children with moderate or high caries risk under the age of 2, fluoridated toothpaste should also be used.
4. Within 6 months of eruption of the first tooth and no later than 12 months of age, the caries risk is assessed providing parental education including guidance for prevention of diseases.
5. Avoiding high frequency consumption of liquids and/or solid foods containing sugar. In particular:
   - Sugar-containing beverages (e.g. juices, soft drinks, sweetened tea, milk with sugar added) in a baby bottle or no-spill training cup should be avoided.
   - Infants should not be put to sleep with a bottle filled with milk or liquids containing sugars.
   - Breastfeeding should be avoided after the first primary tooth begins to erupt and other dietary carbohydrates are introduced.
   - Parents should be encouraged to have infants drink from a cup as they approach their first birthday. Infants should be weaned from the bottle between 12 and 18 months of age.
6. Ensuring all infants and toddlers having access to dental screenings, counselling and preventive procedures (working with medical providers).

Treatment

The treatment options depend on parent's motivation towards dental treatment, the extent of the decay and the age and cooperation of the child. All these features should be analyzed prior to planning treatment for early caries.

It is agreed that the restorative aspect need cyclic repetitions, subsequently becomes costly. The phenomenon of repeated restorative cycles has been established.

It is clarified that the cycle starts with caries diagnosis. The clinicians usually do not distinguish between an active and an arrested lesion, which need different treatment options.

In children, especially the toddlers, the restorative failures are quite common, mostly because of un-cooperative behavior. The replacement of the failed restoration remains the only choice of the operator. The repeated restoration perpetuates the basic error producing a new restoration encountering the same problems.

The tooth structure becomes weaker by the multiple repetitions, which lead to a general deterioration of the child's dentition.

Provisional Restorations

The clinicians usually get discouraged when restoring one tooth at a time; he/she observes new carious lesion developing rapidly, disturbing proper restoration protocol.

A few authors have preferred gross excavation of all the carious lesion in one or two sittings. Gross excavation as an initial approach in the control of early caries has several advantages. The removal of the superficial caries and filling the cavity with some soothing material may temporarily arrest the caries process and prevent its rapid progression. The operator can have sufficient time to take history etc. to determine the cause of rapid destructive process.

Twetman (1999) observed that the dressing of zinc oxide and eugenol not only arrests the caries process but also aids in the stabilization of remaining carious material and also reduces the inflammation of pulp.

The elimination of gross caries coupled with elimination of food debris results in a reduction in the number of oral micro-organisms, which plays an important role in the progress of the caries lesions.

Bibliography

1. Aas JA, Griffen AL, Dardis SR, Lee AM, Olsen I, Dewhirst FE, Leys EJ and Paster BJ. Bacteria of dental caries in primary and permanent teeth in children and young adults. J. Clin. Microbiol.: 2008;46:1407–17.

2. Abbasoglu Z, Tanboga I, Kuchler EC, Deeley K, Weber M, Kaspar C, Korachi M and Vieira AR. Early Childhood caries is associated with Genetic Variants in Enamel Formation and Immune Response Genes. Caries Res. 2015; 49:70–7.

3. Abbey LM. Is breast feeding a likely cause of dental caries in young children? JADA: 1979;98: 21–3.

4. Acs G, Lodolini G, Kaminsky S and Cisneros GJ. Effect of nursing caries on body weight in a pediatric population. Pediat. Dent.: 1992;14: 302–5.

5. Alalnusua S. Early plaque accumulation—a sign for caries risk in young children. Com. Dent. Oral Epidemiol.: 1994;22:273–6.

6. Alaluusua S and Renkonen OV. *Streptococcus mutans* establishment and dental caries experience in children from 2 to 4 yrs. Scand. J. Dent. Res.: 1983;91:453–7.

7. Alm A, Fahraeus C, Wendt LK, Koch G, Andersson-Gare B, Birkhed D. Body adiposity status in teenagers and snacking habits in early childhood in relation to approximal caries at 15 years of age. Int. J. Paediatr. Dent.: 2008; 18:189–96.

8. Alm A, Isaksson H, Fahraeus C Koch G, Andersson-Gare B, Nilsson M, Birkhed D and Wendt LK. BMI status in Swedish children and young adults in relation to caries prevalence. Swed. Dent. J.: 2011;35:1–8.

9. Al-Malik, Holt RD, Bedi R. Erosion, caries and rampant caries in preschool children in Yeddah. Com. Dent Oral Epidemiol.: 2002;30:16–23.

10. Al-Shalan TA, Pamela Erikson, Nancy AH. Primary incisor decay before age 4 as a risk factor for future dental caries. Ped. Dent.: 1997;19:37–41.

11. American Academy of Pediatric Dentistry. Policy on early childhood caries (ECC): classifications, consequences and preventive strategies. Pediat. Dent.: 2012;34:50–52.

12. Aminabadi NA, Ghoreishizadeh A, Ghorei-shizadeh M, Oskouei SG and Ghojazadeh M. Can child temperament be related to early childhood caries? Caries Res.: 2014;48:3–12.

13. Armfield JM and Spencer AJ. Quarter of a century of change: caries experience in Australian children, 1977–2002. Aust. Dent. J.: 2008;53:151–9.

14. Ayhan H Suskane, Yildirims S. The effects of nursing or rampant caries on height, body weight and head circumference. Clin. Ped. Dent.: 1996;20:209.

15. Batchelor PA and Sheiham A. Grouping of tooth surfaces by susceptibility to caries: a study in 5–16 years old children. BMC Oral Health: 2004;4:2.

16. Becker MR, Paster BJ, Leys EJ, Moeschberger ML, Kenyon SG and Galvin JL, Boches SK, Dewherst FE, Griffen AL. Molecular analysis of bacterial species associated with childhood caries. J. Clin. Microbiol.: 2002;40:1001–9.

17. Berkowitz R. Etiology of nursing caries—a microbiologic perceptive. J. Public Health Dent.: 1996;56:51–4.

18. Berkowitz RJ, Turner J and Hughes C. Microbial characteristics of the human dental caries

associated with prolonged bottle-feeding. Arch. Oral Biol.: 1984;29:949–51.

19. Berkowitz RJ. Causes, treatment and prevention of early childhood caries: a microbiologic perspective. J. Canad. Dent. Assoc.: 2003;69: 304–7.

20. Berkowitz RJ. Early establishment of *Streptococcus mutans* in mouth of infants. Arch. Oral Biol.: 1975;20:171-4.

21. Bonecker M and Cleaton-Jones P. Trends in dental caries in Latin American and Caribbean 5–6 and 11–13 years old children: a systematic review. Comm. Dent. Oral Epidemiol.: 2003;31: 152–7.

22. Booth M, Dobbins t, Okely A, Denney-Wilson E and Hardy L. Trends in the prevalence of overweight and obesity among young Australians, 1985-1997 and 2004. Obesity: 2007; 125:1089–95.

23. Buzalaf MA, Vilhena FV, lano FG, Grizzo L, Pessan JP, Sampaio FC and Oliveira RC. The effect of different fluoride concentrations and pH of dentifrices on plaque and nail fluoride levels in young children. Caries Res.: 2009;43: 142–6.

24. Camacho I, Perez S and Perez G. Relationship between severe early childhood caries, mother's oral health and mutans streptococci in a low income group: changes from 1996 to 2007. J. Clin. Pediatr.: 2009;33:241–6.

25. Carino KMG, Shinada K and Kawaguchi Y. Early childhood caries in northern Philippines. Dent. Oral Epidem.: 2003;31:81–89.

26. Casamassimo PS, Thikkurissy S, Edelstein BL and Maiorini E. Beyond the dmft: the human and economic cost of early childhood caries. J. Am. Dent. Assoc.: 2009;140:650–7.

27. Chosack A. Caries prevalence and severity in the primary dentition and *Streptococcus mutans* levels in saliva of preschool children in South Africa. Com. Dent. Oral Epidem.: 1988;16:289–91.

28. Christina SB and Anna KH. Dental caries in Swedish 4-year-old children. Swed. Dent. J.: 1989;13:39–44.

29. Cinar AB and Murtomaa H. Interrelation between obesity, oral health and life-style factors among Turkish schoolchildren. Clin. Oral Investig.: 2011;15:177–84.

30. Cinar AB, Christensen LB and Hegde B. Clustering of obesity and dental caries with lifestyle factors among Danish adolescents. Oral Health Prev. Dent.: 2011;9:123–30.

31. Clarke M, Locker D, Berall G, Pencharz P, Kenny DJ and Judd P. Malnourishment in a population of young children with severe early childhood caries. Pediat. Dent.: 2006;28:254–9.

32. Colak H, Dulgergil CT, Dalli M and Hamidi MM. Early childhood caries update: a review of causes, diagnoses and treatments. J. Nat. Sci. Biol. Med.: 2013;4:29–38.

33. Constante HM, Bastos JL and Peres MA. Trends in dental caries in 12 and 13-year-old school-children from Florianopolis between 1971 and 2009. Braz. J. Oral Sci.: 2010;9:410–4.

34. Constante HM, Souya ML, Bastos JL, Peres MA. Trends in dental caries among Brazilian school children: 40 years of monitoring (1971-2011). Int. Dent. J.: 2014;64:181–6.

35. Corby PM, Lyons-Weiler J, Bretz WA, Hart TC, Aas JA and Boumenna T. Microbial risk indicators of early childhood caries. J. Clin. Microbiol.: 2005; 43:5753-9.

36. Costacurta M, Di Renzo L, Bianchi A, Fabiocchi F, De Lorenzo A and Docimo R. Obesity and dental caries in a paediatric patients. A cross-sectional study. Eur. J. Paediatr. Dent.: 2011;12: 112–6.

37. Curzon MEJ and Preston AJ. Risk groups: nursing bottle caries/caries in the elderly. Caries Res.: 2004;38:24–33.

38. Cynthia KY. Management of rampant caries in children. Quintessence Int.: 1992;23:159–68.

39. Damle SG, Vidya I, Yadav R, Bhattal H and Loomba A. Quantitative determination of inorganic constituents in saliva and their relationship with dental caries experience in children. Dentistry: 2012;2:1–5.

40. David M. Association of early dental caries patterns with caries incidence in preschool children. J. Pub. Health Dent.: 1996;56:81–3.

41. Davies GM, Blinkhorn FA and Duxbury JT. Caries among 3-year-old in greater Manchester. Br. Dent. J.: 2001;190:381–4.

42. Dilley GJ, Dilley DH and Machen JB. Prolonged nursing habit: A profile of patients and their families. ASDC J. Dent. Child: 1980;47:102–8.

43. D'Mello G, Chia L, Hamilton SD, Thomson WM and Drummon BK. Childhood obesity and dental caries among paediatric dental clinic attenders. Int. J. Paediatr. Dent.: 2011;21:217–22.

44. Dolg and Spencer AJ. Risk-benefit balance in the use of fluoride among young children. J. Dent. Res.: 2007;86:723–8.

45. Douglas JM. Caries prevalence and pattern in 3–6 years old Beijing children. Com. Dent. Oral Epidemiol.: 1995;23:340–3.

46. Du MQ, Tai BNJ, Jiang H, Lo ECM, Fan MW and Bian X. A two-year randomized clinical trial of chlorhexidine varnish on dental caries in Chinese preschool children. J. Dent. Res.: 2006;85:557–9.

47. Dye BA, Shenkin JD, Ogden CL, Marshall TA, Levy SM and Kanellis MJ. The relationship between healthful eating practices and dental caries in children aged 2–5 years in the United States, 1988-1994. J. Am. Dent. Assoc.: 2004;135: 55–66.

48. Edwardsson ID and Mejare B. Streptococci milleri and *Streptococcus mutans* in mouth of infants before and after tooth eruption. Arch. Oral Biology: 1978;811–4.

49. Erickson PR and Mazhari E. Investigation of the role of human breast milk in caries development. Pediatr. Dent.: 1999;21:86–90.

50. Eronat N. A comparative study of some influencing factors of rampant or nursing caries in preschool children. J. Clin. Ped. Dent.: 1992;16: 275–9.

51. Febres C, Echeverri EA. Parental awareness, habits and social factors and their relationship to baby bottle tooth decay. Ped. Dent.: 1997;19:22–7.

52. Figueiredo MJ, de Amorim RG, Leas SC, Mulder J and Frencken JE. Prevalence and severity of clinical consequences of untreated dentin carious lesions in children from a deprived area of Brazil. Caries Res.: 2011;45;435.

53. Fomon SJ, Ekstrand J and Zeigler EE. Fluoride intake and prevalence of dental fluorosis: trends in fluoride intake with special attention to infants. J. Pub. Health Dent.: 2000;60:131–9.

54. Foster T, Perinpanayagam H, Pfaffenbach A and Certo M. Recurrence of early childhood caries after comprehensive treatment with general anesthesia and follow-up. J. Dent. Child.: 2006;73:25–30.

55. Gao X, Stepher Hsu CY, Loh T, Hwarng B and Koh D. Role of microbiological factors in predicting early childhood caries. Pediatric Dent.: 2013;36:348–54.

56. Gerdin EW, Angbratt M, Aronsson K, Eriksson E and Johansson I. Dental caries and body mass index by socioeconomic status in Swedish children. Comm. Dent. Oral Epidemiol.: 2008;36: 459–65.

57. Granville-Garcia AF, de Menezes VA, de Lira PI, Ferreira JM and Leite-Cavalcanti A. Obesity and dental caries among preschool children in Brazil. Rev. Salud Publica. (Bogota):2008;10:788–95.

58. Graves CE, Berkowitz RJ, Proskin HM, Chase I, Weinstein P and Billings R. Clinical outcomes for early childhood caries: influence of aggressive dental surgery. J. Dent. Child.: 2004;71:114–7.

59. Grindefjord M, Dahllof G and Modeer T. Caries development in children from 2.5 to 3.5 years of age: A longitudinal study. Caries Res.: 1995;29: 449–54.

60. Gussy MG, Waters EG, Walsh O and Kilpatrick NM. Early childhood caries: Current evidence for aetiology and prevention. J. Paediatr. Child Health: 2006;42:37–43.

61. Hallett KB and O'Rourke PK. Early childhood caries and infant feeding practice. Community Dent. Health: 2002;19:237–42.

62. Hallett KB, O'Rourke P. Pattern and severity of early childhood caries. Comm. Dent. Oral Epidemiol.: 2006;34:25–35.

63. Hallonsten AL. Dental caries and prolonged breast feeding in 18 months old Swedish children. Int. J. Ped. Dent.: 1995;5:149–55.

64. Harris R, Nicoll AD, Adair PM and Pine CM. Risk factors for dental caries in young children: a systematic review of the literature. Comm. Dent. Health: 2004;21:71–85.

65. Harrison R, Wong T, Ewan C, Contreras B and Phung Y. Feeding practices and dental caries in an urban Canadian population of Vietnamese preschool children. ASDC J. Dent. Child.: 1997;64:112–7.

66. Hart CN, Raynor HA, Jelalian E and Drotar D. The association of maternal food intake and infants' and toddlers' food intake. Child. Care Health Dev.: 2010;36:396–403.

67. Hilgers KK, Kinane DE and Scheetz JP. Association between childhood obesity and smooth-surface caries in posterior teeth: a preliminary study. Paediatr. Dent.: 2006;28: 23–8.

68. Holve S. An observational study of the association of fluoride varnish applied during well child visits and the prevention of early childhood caries in American Indian children. Maternal and Child Health J.: 2008;12:564–67.

69. Hong L, Ahmed A, McCunniff M, Overman P and Mathew M. Obesity and dental caries in

children aged 2–6 years in the United States: National health and nutrition examination survey 1999–2002. J. Public Health Dent.: 2008;68:227–33.

70. Hong L, Levy SM, Warren U, Broffitt B. Infant breast-feeding and childhood caries: a nine-year study. Pediatric Dent.: 2014;36:342–7.

71. Hooley M, Skouteris H, Boganin C, Satur J and Kilpatrick N. Body mass index and dental caries in children and adolescents: a systematic review of literature published 2004 to 2011. Systematic reviews: 2012;1–8.

72. Hujoel PP. Vitamin D and dental caries in controlled clinical trials: systematic review and meta-analysis. Nutr. Rev.: 2013;71:88–97.

73. Iida H, Auinger P, Billings RJ and Weitzman M. Association between infant breastfeeding and early childhood caries in the United States. Pediatrics: 2007;120:944–52.

74. Ipa LW. Nursing caries: A comprehensive review. Ped. Dent.: 1988;10:268–82.

75. Irigoyen ME, Mejia-Gonzalez A and Zepeda-Zepeda MA. Dental caries in Mexican school children: a comparison of 1988–89 and 1998–2001 surveys. Med. Oral Patol. Oral Cir. Bucal: 2012; 17:825–32.

76. Ismail AI and Hasson H. Fluoride supplements, dental caries and fluorosis: trends in fluoride intake with special attention to infants. J. Pub. Health Dent.: 2008;139:1457–68.

77. Ismail AI and Sohn W. A systematic review of clinical diagnostic criteria of early childhood caries. J. Public Health Dent.: 1999;47:102–8.

78. Ismail AI, Sohn W, Lim S and Willem JM. Predictors of dental caries progression in primary teeth. J. Dent. Res.: 2009;88:270–5.

79. Ismail AI. Prevention of early childhood caries. Comm. Dent. Oral Epid.: 1998;26:49–61.

80. Jabbarifar SE, Ahmady N, Sahafian SA, Samei F and Soheillipour S. Association of parental stress and early childhood caries. Dent. Res. J.: 2009;6:65–70.

81. James P, Parnell C and Whelton H. The caries-preventive effect of chlorhexidine varnish in children and adolescents: a systematic review. Car. Res.: 2010;44:333–40.

82. Jin BH, Ma DS, Moon HS. Paik DI, Hahn SH and Horowitz AM. Early childhood caries: Prevalence and risk factors in Seoul, Korea. J. Public Health Dent.: 2003;63:183–8.

83. Johnson DC. Susceptibility of nursing caries children to future proximal molar decay. Ped. Dent.: 1986;8:168–70.

84. Jose B and King NM. Early childhood caries lesions in preschool children in Kerala, India. Pediatr. Dent.: 2003;25:594–600.

85. Juarez-Lopez MLA and Villa-Ramos A. Caries prevalence in preschool children with overweight and obesity. Rev. Invest. Clin.: 2010;62:115–20.

86. Kaikure MK, Thomas A , Shetty SB , Jose T, Pidamale R and Kaikure SL. The Prevalence of Early Childhood Caries (ECC) and Its Associated Risk Factors Among Immigrant Tibetan Pre-School Children in Bylakuppe, Mysore, India. Science Journal of Public Health: 2015;3:384–90.

87. Kagihara LE, Niederhauser VP and Stark M. Assessment, management and prevention of early childhood caries. J. Am. Acad. Nurse Pract.: 2009;21:1–10.

88. Kansai E, Dewhirst FE, Chalmers NI, Kent R, Moore A and Hughes CV. Clonal analysis of the microbiota of severe early childhood caries. Caries Res.: 2010;44:485–97.

89. Kantovitz KR, Pascon FM, Rontani RMP and Gaviao MBD. Obesity and dental caries—a systematic review. Oral Health Prev. Dent.: 2006; 4:137-44.

90. Kaste LM, Marians D,Chong R, Phipps KR. The assessment of nursing caries and its relationship to high caries in permanent dentition. J. Public Health Dent.: 1992;89:20–4.

91. Kawashita TY, Fukuda H and Kawasaki K. Pediatrician-recommended use of sports drinks and dental caries in 3-year-old children. Comm. Dent. Health: 2011;28:29–33.

92. King N, Anthonappa R and Itthagarun A. The importance of the primary dentition to children—Part 1: Consequences of not treating carious teeth. Hong Kong Pract.: 2007;29:52–61.

93. Kohlder B and Andreen I. Mutans streptococci and caries prevalence in children after early maternal caries prevention: A follow-up at eleven and fifteen years of age. Caries Res.: 2010;44:453–8.

94. Kramer MS, Vanilovich I, Matush L, Bogdano-vich N, Zhang X, Shishko G, Muller-Bolla M and Platt RW. The effect of prolonged and exclusive breast-feeding on dental caries in early school-age children. New evidence from a large randomized trial. Caries Res.: 2007;41:484–8.

95. Kumar P and Hegde AM. Lead exposure and its relation to dental caries in children. J. Clin. Pediatr. Dent.: 2013;38:71–4.

96. Kuriakose S. Caries prevalence and its relation to socioeconomic status and oral hygiene practices in 600 preschool children of Kerala (India). J. Indian Soc. Ped. Prev. Dent.: 1999;17: 97–100.

97. Li Y, Caufield PW, Dasanayake AP, Weiner HW and Vermund SH. Mode of delivery and other maternal factors influence the acquisition of *Streptococcus mutans* in infants. J. Dent. Res.:2005;84:806–11.

98. Li Y, Ge Y, Saxena D and Caufield PW. Genetic profiling of the oral microbiota associated with severe early childhood caries. J. Clin. Microbiol.: 2007;45:81–7.

99. Li Y, Narra JM, Bron JY. Caries experience in deciduous dentition of rural Chinese children 3–5 years old in relation to the presence or absence of enamel hypoplasia. Caries Res.: 1996;30:8–15.

100. Ling Z, Kong J, Jia P, Wei C, Wang Y and Pan Z. Analysis of oral microbiota in children with dental caries by PCR-DGGE and barcoded pyrosequencing. Microb. Ecol.: 2010;60:677–90.

101. Llena C and Fomer L. Dietary habits in a child population in relation to caries experience. Caries Res.: 2008;42:387–93.

102. Lopez Z, Berkowitz R, Spiekerman C and Weinstein P. Topical antimicrobial therapy in the prevention of early childhood caries: a follow-up report. Pediatric Dent.: 2002;24:204–06.

103. Manarelli MM, Delbem ACB, Lima TMT, Castilho FCN and Pessan JP. *In vitro* reminera-lizing effect of fluoride varnishes containing sodium trimetaphosphate. Caries Res.: 2014; 48:299–305.

104. Mantonanaki M, Koletsi-Kounari H, Mamai-Homata E and Papaioannou W. Prevalence of dental caries in 5-year-old Greek children and the use of dental services: evaluation of socio-economic, behavioural factors and living conditions. Int. Dent. J.: 2013;63:72–9.

105. Marshall TA, Eichenberger-Gilmore JM, Broffitt BA, Warren JJ and Levy SM. Dental caries and childhood obesity: roles of diet and socioeconomic status. Comm. Dent. Oral Epidemol.: 2007;35:449–58.

106. Marshall TA, Levy SM and Broffitt B. Dental caries and beverage consumption in young children. Pediatrics: 2003;112:184–91.

107. Mattila ML. Caries in five years old children and association with family related factors. J. Dent. Res.: 2000;79:875–81.

108. Matto S, Graner RO, Rontami RMP and Gariao DMB. Caries prevalence in 6–36 months old Brazilian children. Com. Dent. Health: 1996;13: 96–8.

109. Milgrom P, Riedy CA, Weinstein P, Tanner ACR, Manibusan L and Brass J. Dental caries and its relationship to bacterial infection, hypoplasia, diet and oral hygiene in 6 to 36 months old children. Comm. Dent. Oral Epid.: 2000;28:295–306.

110. Milgrom P, Zero DT and Tanzer JM. An examination of the advances in science and technology of prevention of tooth decay in young children since the Surgeon General's Report on Oral Health. Acad. Pediatr.: 2009;9: 404–9.

111. Milgrom P. Dental caries and its relationship to bacterial infection, hypoplasia, diet and oral hygiene in 6 to 36 months old children. Com. Dent. Oral Epidemiol.: 2000;28:295–306.

112. Milgrom P. Response to Reisine and Douglass: psychosocial and behavioral issues in early childhood caries. Comm. Dent. Oral Epidem.: 1998;26:45–8.

113. Milnes AR. Description and epidemiology of nursing caries. J. Public Health Dent.: 1996;56: 38–50.

114. Misra S, Tahmassebi JF and Brosnan M. Early childhood caries: a review. Dent. Update: 2007;34:556–8.

115. Muylligan R, Seirawan H and Faust S, et al. Dental caries in under-privileged children of Los Angeles. J. Health Care Poor Underserved: 2011;22:648–662.

116. Narvey A and Shwart L. Early childhood dental disease—what's in a name? J. Canad. Dent. Assoc.: 2007;73:929–30.

117. Nunn ME, Braunstein NS, Krall Kaye EA, Dietrich T, Garcia RI and Henshaw MM. Healthy eating index is a predictor of early childhood caries. J. Dent. Res.: 2009;88:361–6.

118. O'Sullivan DM and Tinanoff N. Social and biological factor contributing to caries of maxillary anterior teeth. Ped. Dent.: 1993;15:41–4.

119. O'Sullivan DM. Maxillary anterior caries associated with increased caries risk in other primary teeth. J. Dent. Res.: 1993;72:12:1577–80.

120. Ohlund I, Holgerson PL, Backman B, Lind T, Hernell O and Johansson I. Diet intake and caries prevalence in four-year-old children living in a low-prevalence country. Caries Res.: 2007;41:26–33.

121. Oulis CJ, Tsinidou K and Vadiakas G. Caries prevalence of 5, 12 and 15-year-old Greek children: a national pathfinder survey. Community Dent. Health: 2012;29:29–32.

122. Palmer CA, Kent R, Loo CY, Hughes CV, Stutius E, Pradhan N, Dahlan M, Kanasai E, Arevalo Vasquez SS and Tanner AC. Diet and caries associated bacteria in severe early childhood caries. J. Dent. Res.: 2010;89:1224–9.

123. Peressini S, Leake JL, Mayhall JT, Maar M and Trudeau R. Prevalence of early childhood caries among First Nations children, District of Manitouline, Ontario. Int. J. Paediatr. Dent.: 2004;14:101–10.

124. Peretz B. Preschool caries as an indicator of future caries: a longitudinal study. Ped. Dent.: 2003;25:116–8.

125. Pessan JP, Al-Ibrahim NS, Buzalaf MA and Toumba KJ. Slow-release fluoride devices: a literature review. J. Appl. Oral Sci.: 2008;16:238–46.

126. Pessan JP, Toumba KJ and Buzalaf MA. Topical use of fluorides for caries control. Monogr. Oral Sci.: 2011;22:115–32.

127. Qin M, Li J, Zhang S and Ma W. Risk factors for severe childhood caries in children younger than 4 years old in Beijing, China. Pediatr. Dent.: 2008;30:122–8.

128. Quinonez R, Santos R, Wilson S and Cross H. The relationship between child temperament and risk factors for early childhood caries. Pediatr. Dent.: 2001;23:5–9.

129. Quinonez RB, Keels MA, Vann WF Jr, McIver FT, Heller K and Whitt JK. Early childhood caries: Analysis of psychosocial and biological factors in a high-risk population. Caries Res.: 2001;35:376–83.

130. Rajab LD and Hamdan MA. Early childhood caries and risk factors in Jordan. Community Dent. Health: 2002;19:224–9.

131. Ramezani GH, Norozi A and Valael N. The prevalence of nursing caries in 18 to 60 months old children in Qazvin. J. Indian Society of Pedodontics and Preventive Dent.: 2003;21:19–26.

132. Ramos-Gomez F, Crystal YO, Ng MW, Tinanoff N and Featherstone JD. Caries risk assessment, prevention and management in pediatric dental care. Gen. Dent.: 2010;58:505–17.

133. Ramos-Gomez FJ, Tomar SL, Ellison J, Artiga N, Sintes J and Vicuna G. Assessment of early childhood caries and dietary habits in a population of migrant Hispanic children in Stockton, California. ASDC J. Dent. Child.: 1999;66:395–403.

134. Ramos-Gomez FJ, Weintraub JA, Gansky SA, Hoover CI and Featherstone JD. Bacterial, behavioral and environmental factors associated with early childhood caries. J. Clin. Pediatric Dent.: 2002;26:165–73.

135. Ramos-Gomez FJ. Bacterial, behaviour and environmental factors associated with early childhood caries. J. Clin. Ped. Dent.: 2002;26:165–73.

136. Ramos-Jorge J, Alencar BM, Pordeus IA, Soares MEC, Ramos-Jorge ML and Paiva SM. Impact of dental caries on quality of life among preschool children: emphasis on the type of tooth and stages of progression. Eur. J. Oral Sci.: 2014;1–8.

137. Ripa LW. Nursing caries: A Comprehensive review. Pediat. Dent.: 1988;10:268–82.

138. Rosenblatt A and Zarzar P. The prevalence of early childhood caries in 12 to 36 months old children in Recife, Brazil. ASDC J. Dent. Child.: 2002;69:319–24.

139. Ruiz-Rodriguez S, Lacavex-Aguilar V, Pierdant-Perez M, Mandeville P, Santos-Diaz M. Garrocho-Rangel A and Pozos-Guillen AJ. Colonization levels of Streptococcus mutans between mother and infant: a postnatal prospective cohort study. J. Clin. Pediatr. Dent.: 2014;38:197–200.

140. Sadeghi M, Darakhshan R and Bagherian A. Is there an association between early childhood caries and serum iron and serum ferritin levels? Dent. Res. J.: 2012;9:294–8.

141. Sadeghi M, Lynch, CD and Arsalan A. Is there a correlation between dental caries and body mass index-for-age among adolescents in Iran? Comm. Dent. Health: 2011;28:174–7.

142. Sampaio-Maia B and Monteiro-Silva F. Acquisition and maturation of oral microbiome throughout childhood: An update. Dent. Res. J.: 2014;11:291–301.

143. Sanchez-Perez L, Irigoyen M and Zepeda M. Dental caries, tooth eruption timing and obesity: a longitudinal study in a group of Mexican schoolchildren. Acta. Odontol. Scand.: 2010;68:57–64.

144. Schroth R, Jeal N and Kliewer E. The relationship between vitamin D and severe early childhood caries: a pilot study. Int. J. Vitam. Nutr. Res.: 2012;82:53–62.

145. Schroth RJ, Brothwell DJ and Moffatt ME. Caregiver knowledge and attitudes of preschool oral health and early childhood caries (ECC). Int. J. Circumpolar Health: 2007;66:153–67.

146. Schroth RJ, Levi JA, Sellers EA, Friel J, Kliewer E and Moffattr ME. Vitamin D status of children with severe early childhood caries: a case-control study. BMC Pediatrics: 2013;13:174.

147. Schroth RJ, Pang JL, Levi JA, Martens PJ and Brownell MD. Trends in pediatric dental surgery for severe early childhood caries in Manitoba, Canada. J. Can. Dent. Assoc.: 2014;80: e65.

148. Schwartz SS, Rssivack RG, Michelatti P. A child's sleeping habit as a cause of nursing caries. J. Dent. Child.: 1993;22–25.

149. Seow WK, Clifford H, Battistutta D, Morawska A and Holcombe T. Case-control study of early childhood caries in Australia. Caries Res.: 2009;43:25–35.

150. Sethi B and Tandon S. Caries pattern in preschool children. J. Indian Dent. Assoc.: 1996; 67:141–5.

151. Shantinath SD. The relationship of sleep problems and sleep associated feeding to nursing caries. Ped. Dent.: 1996;18:375–8.

152. Sheller B, Churchill SS, Williams BJ and Davidson B. Body mass index of children with severe early childhood caries. Pediatr. Dent.: 2009;31:216–21.

153. Shrutha SP, Balarama G, Gupta V, Giri KY and Alam S. Feeding Practices and Early Childhood Caries: A Cross-Sectional Study of Preschool Children in Kanpur District, India ISRN Dentistry: Volume 2013 (2013), Article ID 275193

154. Si Y, Ao S, Wang W, Chen F and Zheng S. Magnetic Bead-Based Salivary Peptidome Profiling Analysis for Severe Early Childhood Caries. Carie Res.: 2015;49:63–9

155. Skies MS, Espelid I, Skaare AB and Gimmestad A. Caries patterns in an urban pre-school population in Norway. Eur. J. Paediat. Dent.: 2005;6:16–22.

156. Spitz AS, Gasparoni KW, Kanellis MJ and Qian F. Child temperament and risk factors for early childhood caries. J. Dent. Child.: 2006;73:98–104.

157. Stephen A , Krishnan A, Ramesh M, Kumar V.S. Prevalence of early childhood caries and its risk factors in 18–72 months old children in Salem, Tamil Nadu. J Int. Soc. Prevent Comm. Dent.: 2015;5:95–102.

158. Straetemons MME. Colonization with mutans streptococci and lactobacilli and the caries experience of children after the age five. J. Dent. Res.: 1998;77:1851–5.

159. Suhonen J, Aaltonen AS and Tenovuo J. Prevention of caries from 2 to 3.5 years age in children after having used a prophylactic lozengel in a slow release pacifier at bedtime. J. Dent. Res.: 1997;76:337.

160. Tanaka K, Hitsumoto S, Miyake Y, Okubo H, Sasaki S, Miyatake N and Arakawa M. Higher vitamin D intake during pregnancy is associated with reduced risk of dental caries in young Japnese children. Annals of Epidemiology. 2015;25:620–5.

161. Tanaka K, Miyake Y, Sasaki S and Hirota Y. Dairy products and calcium intake during pregnancy and dental caries in children. Nutrition Journal: 2012;1–8.

162. Tanner ACR, Mathney JMJ, Kent RL, Chalmers NI, Hughes CV, Loo CY, Pradhan N, Kanasi E, Hwang J, Dahlan MA, Papadopolou E and Dewhirst FE. Cultivable anaerobic microbiota of severe early childhood caries. J. Clin. Microbiol.: 2011;49:1464–74.

163. Tanzer JM, Livingston J and Thompson AM. The microbiology of primary dental caries in humans. J. Dent. Educ.: 2001;65:1028–37.

164. Tewari S and Tewari S. Caries experience in 3–7 years old children in Haryana (India). J. Indian Soc. Pedod. Prev. Dent.: 2001;19:52–6.

165. Thakib A. Primary incisor decay before age 4 as a risk factor for future dental caries. Ped. Dent.: 1997;19:37–41.

166. Tham R, Bowatte G, Dharmage SC, Tan DJ, Lau M, Dai X, Allen KJ and Lodge CJ. Breastfeeding and the risk of dental caries: a systematic review and meta-analysis. Acta Paediatr. 2015, doi: 10.1111/apa.13118.

167. Thenisch NL, Bachmann LM, Imfeld T, Leisebach MT and Steurer J. Are mutans streptococci detected in pre-school children a reliable predictive factor for dental caries risk? A systematic review. Caries Res.: 2006;40:366–74.

168. Thitasomakul S, Piwat S, Thearmontree A, Chankanka O, Pithpornchaiyakul W and Madyusoh S. Risks for early childhood caries analyzed by negative binomial models. J. Dent. Res.: 2009;88:137–41.

169. Tinanoff N, Kanellis MJ and Vargas CM. Current understanding of the epidemiology,

mechanisms and prevention of dental caries in preschool children. Pediatric Dentistry: 2002;24:6.

170. Tramini P, Molinari N, Tentscher M, Demattei C and Schulte AG. Association between caries experience and body mass index of 12-year-old French children. Caries Res.: 2009;43:468–73.

171. Tsai AI, Chen CY, Li LA, Hsiang CL and Hsu KH. Risk indicators for early childhood caries in Taiwan. Community Dent. Oral Epidemiol.: 2006;34:437–45.

172. Tulunoglu O, Demirtas S and Tulunoglu I. Total antioxidant levels of saliva in children related to caries, age and gender. Int. J. Paediatr. Dent.: 2006;16:186–91.

173. Twetman S, Garcia Godoy F and Gekpferd SJ. Infant oral health care. Dent. Clinic of North America: 2000;44:487.

174. Vadiakas G. Case definition, aetiology and risk assessment of early childhood caries (ECC): A revisited review. Eur. Arch. Paediatr. Dent.: 2008;9:114–25.

175. Valaitis R, Hesch R, Passarelli C, Sheehan D and Sinton J. A systematic review of the relationship between breastfeeding and early childhood caries. Canad. J. Public Health: 2000;91:411–7.

176. Valeria de Abreu da Silva Bastos, Freitas-Fernandes LB, da Silva Fidalgo TK, Martins C, Mattos CT, Ribeiro de Souza IP and Maia LC. Mother-to-child transmission of *Streptococcus mutans*: A systematic review and meta-analysis.J.Dent. 2015;43:181–91.

177. Van Everdinglen T. Parents and nursing bottle caries. J. Dent. Child.: 1996;271–4.

178. Van Palenstein, Helderman WH, Soe W and van't Hof MA. Risk factors of early childhood caries in a Southeast Asian population. J. Dent. Res.: 2006;85:85–8.

179. Vazquez-Nava F, Vazquez-Rodriguez EM, Saldivar-Gonzalez AH, Lin-Ochoa D, Martinez-Perales GM and Joffre-Velazquez VM. Association between obesity and dental caries in a group of preschool children in Mexico. J. Public Health Dent.: 2010;70:124–30.

180. Von Everdingen T, Ejekmon MA,Hoogstraten J. Parents and nursing bottle caries. J. Dent. Child: 1996;274–91.

181. Wan AKL, Seow WK, Purdie DM, Bird PS, Walsh LJ and Tudehope DI. A longitudinal study of *Streptococcus mutans* colonization in infants after tooth eruption. J. Dent. Res.: 2003; 82:504–8.

182. Wei SHY, Holm AK, Odont LS and Yuen SW. Dental caries prevalence and related factors in 5 years old children in Hong Kong. Pediatr. Dent.: 1993;15:116–9.

183. Weintraub JA: Prevention of ECC: A public health perspective. Com. Dent. Oral Epidemiol. 1998; 26:Suppl.1:62–6.

184. Weintreaub JA, Ramos-Gomez F, Jue B, Shain S, Hoover CI, Featherstone JD and Gansky SA. Fluoride varnish efficacy in preventing early childhood caries. J. Dent. Res.: 2006;85:172–6.

185. Willershausen B, Moschos D, Azrak B and Blettner M. Correlation between oral health and body mass index (BMI) in 2071 primary school pupils. Eur. J. Med. Res.: 2007;12:295–9.

186. Winstein P, Harrison R and Benton T. Motivating parents to prevent caries in their young children: One-year findings. J. Am. Dent. Assoc.: 2004;135:731–8.

187. Yasin Harnekar S. Nursing caries—A review. J. Clin. Prevent. Dent.: 1998;10:3–8.

188. Zenter M and Bates JE. Child temperament: an integrative review of concepts, research programs and measures. Eur. J. Dev. Sci.: 2008; 21:7–37.

189. Zhang Q, Zou J, Yang R and Zhou X. Remineralization effects of casein phospho-peptide-amorphous calcium phosphate crème on artificial early enamel lesions of primary teeth. Int. J. Paediat. Dent.: 2011;21:374–81.

190. Zohoori FV, Duckworth RM, Omid N, O'Hare WT and Maguire A. Fluoridated toothpaste: usage and ingestion of fluoride by 4 to 6-year-old children in England. Eur. J. Oral Sci.: 2012; 120:415–21.

17

Root Caries

Root caries, also known as cemental/senile caries, is a common problem among the elderly. It involves cementum of exposed root surfaces. It is the soft progressive lesion of the root surfaces usually having ill-defined saucer like appearances.

Katz (1980) defined root caries as soft, progressive and destructive lesion, either totally confined to root surface or involving undermining of enamel at the cemento-enamel junction (clinically the lesion initiated at the root surfaces).

As the name indicates, root caries starts at the cementum or cemento-enamel junction and appears only when the cementum is exposed. Root caries most often occurs supragingivally, at or close to (within 2.0 mm) the cemento-enamel junction (CEJ). The nature of CEJ facilitates the caries process at that site. The location of root caries has been positively associated with age and gingival recession. 'Location' refers to the area on the tooth and/or root surface where the lesion must be located in order to be classified as root caries. The location implies that the lesion must be predominantly on the root (wholly on the root surface or at the cemento-enamel junction or that at least half the lesion must be on the root and the origin of the lesion appears to be on the root). Root caries gets initiated adjacent to the crest of the gingiva where dental plaque accumulates. It can occur on any tooth surface but mandibular molars are most susceptible.

The term 'primary root caries' implies development of new carious lesions on the root surface, which are not associated with any restoration. 'Secondary (recurrent) root caries' refers to caries occurring adjacent to existing restoration.

Clinical Signs and Symptoms

Root caries, unlike the situation with coronal caries, do not present typically with any symptoms of pain or discomfort. Sometimes, it might be felt in advanced lesions.

Generally, root caries have been described as having a distinct outline and presenting with a discolored appearance in relation to the surrounding non-carious root. Many root caries lesions are cavitated, although that is not necessarily the case with early lesions. The base of the cavitated area can be soft, leathery or hard to probing. Probing of root caries lesions with a sharp explorer using controlled, modest pressure, however, may create surface defects that prevent complete remineralization of the lesion.

Root caries frequently is observed near the cemento-enamel junction, although lesions can appear anywhere on the root surface. Lesions usually occur near (within 2.0 mm) the crest of the gingival margin. The distinction between an active and an arrested lesion further complicates clinical detection of root caries. The color of root lesions has been used as an indication of lesion activity. Active lesions have been described as yellowish or light brown in color, whereas arrested lesions appear darkly stained.

The presence of cavitation (loss of surface integrity) associated with a root caries lesion does not necessarily imply lesion activity. Non-cavitated (early) root caries lesions almost universally are considered to be active. A cavitated lesion, however, may be either active or arrested. The clinical and the radiographic view of root caries are depicted in Figs 17.1 and 17.2.

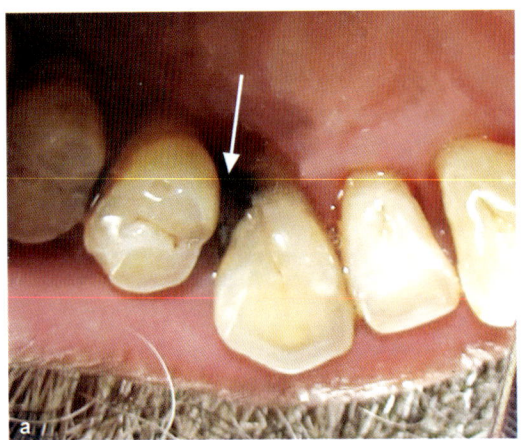

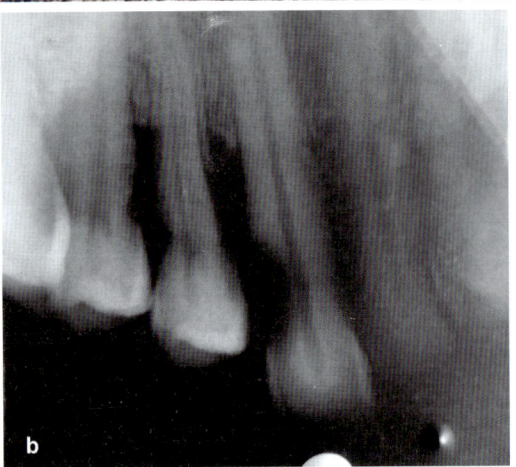

Fig. 17.1: (a) Root caries present on distal surface of upper canine (clinical view), (b) Radiographic view

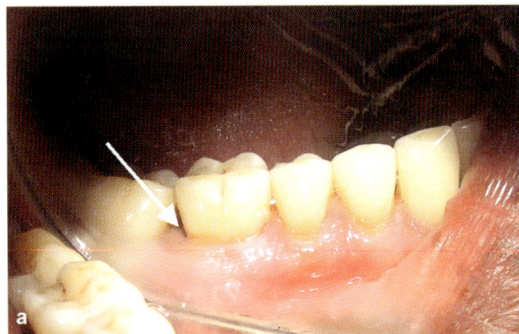

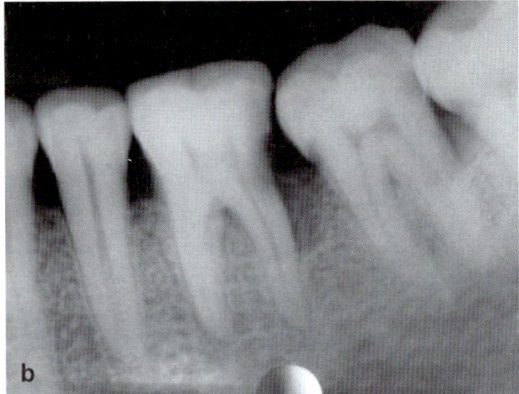

Fig. 17.2: (a) Root caries in lower first molar (clinical view); (b) Radiographic view

3D view of CBCT images of root carries is depicted in Figs 17.3 and 17.4.

The texture of a root caries lesion also has been linked to lesion activity. Active lesions have been described as soft or leathery compared to arrested lesions that have a hard texture. Root caries lesions that occur closely adjacent to (within 2.0 mm) the crest of the gingiva are considered to be active, whereas lesions that occur on the root surface more distant from the gingival crest are more likely to be arrested. There is microbiological evidence to support this clinical observation [Beighton, et al 1993].

CLASSIFICATION OF ROOT CARIES

a. Billing's Classification

Billing's classification of root caries is based on extent of lesion (Fig. 17.5 and Table 17.1):

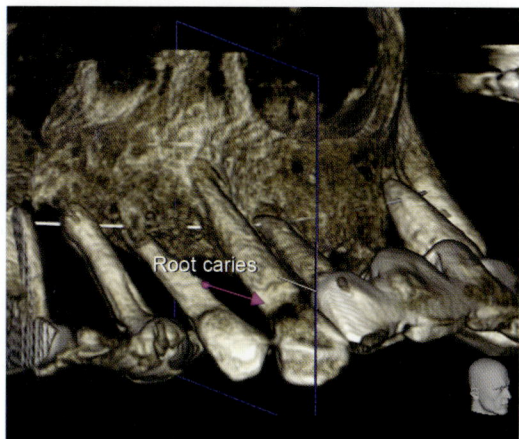

Fig. 17.3: 3D view of CBCT images of root caries

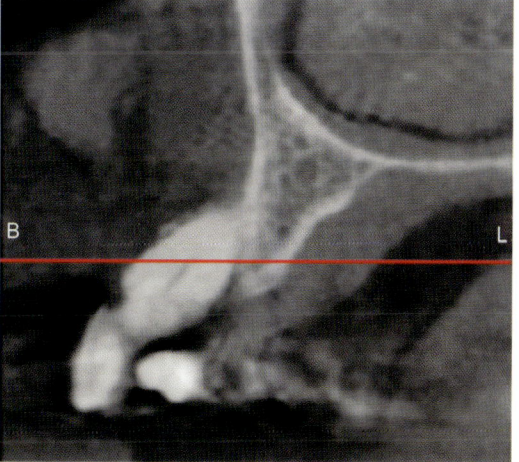

Fig. 17.4: 3D view of CBCT images of root caries

Grade 1 (Incipient)

1. Light brown to tan in color on visual inspection.
2. No surface defect seen.
3. Surface texture is soft and the surface of caries can be disrupted with the pointed tip of dental explorer.

Grade 2 (Shallow)

1. Dark brown to variable tan in color.
2. Surface defect is seen which can be less than 0.5 mm in depth.
3. Surface texture is soft, irregular, rough which can be penetrated with the pointed tip of dental explorer.

Grade 3 (Cavitation)

1. Light brown to dark brown in color which is variable.
2. Surface texture is similar to Grade 1 which is soft and penetrated with a dental explorer.
3. The lesion is penetrating and cavitation is more than 0.5 mm without pulpal involvement.

Grade 4 (Pulpal)

1. It is similar in color to Grade 3 type root caries which is dark brown.

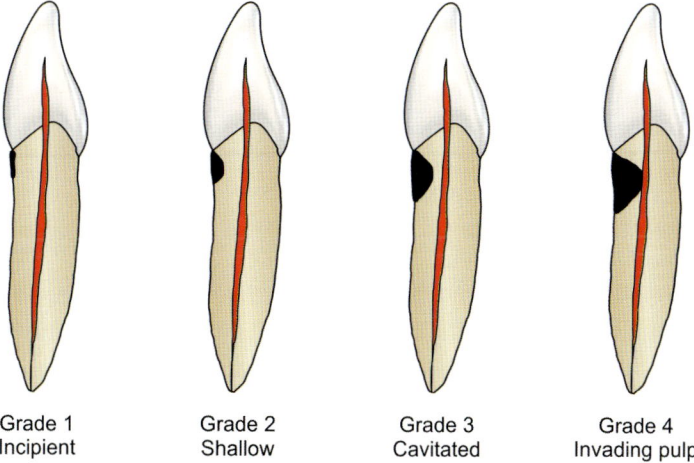

| Grade 1 | Grade 2 | Grade 3 | Grade 4 |
| Incipient | Shallow | Cavitated | Invading pulp |

Fig. 17.5: Billing's classification of root caries

Table 17.1: Billing's classification of root caries

Grade	Description
Grade I	White or light brown; surface cannot be penetrated
Grade II	Light brown; 0.5–1.0 mm penetration
Grade III	Dark brown; penetration equal to or greater than 1.0 mm but not extending to pulp
Grade IV	Brown or black; penetration into dental pulp

2. The surface of lesion is cavitated and the lesion has pulpal involvement extending up to the root canal.

b. Nyvad and Fejerskov Classification

1. Active or inactive.
2. With or without cavitation.
3. According to texture (soft, leathery, hard) and color (yellow, light brown, dark brown black).

Epidemiology of Root Caries

Root caries was common in ancient cultures, ancient skulls and primitive communities have also shown evidence of root caries. Root caries were found in isolation as well as along with coronal caries. Anthropological studies have indicated that root surface caries was dominant as compared to coronal caries in ancient population. There are not enough epidemiological surveys estimating the magnitude and distribution of root caries and the potential sites at risk. Although a decline is being observed in coronal caries in industrialized countries, there is relatively high prevalence of root caries in older adults. Banting (1986) has comprehensively reviewed studies conducted over last 70 years on root caries. A couple of other authors, viz. Katz (1985), Seichler (1987), Levy (1988) and Hunt (1989) have also reviewed root caries.

The definition of what constitutes root caries and the issue of diagnostic criteria lacked consistency amongst the authors undertaking epidemiological studies. Most of the surveys lacked consistency regarding lesion shape, method of probing, personal absence of recession and whether the lesion is only on cementum or both on cementum and enamel.

Later, universally acceptable clinical criteria were adopted modifying probe for exploration, using intra-oral video camera and also the enzyme assays.

An overall estimate of the prevalence of root caries for healthy adults was 20–40%; whereas for chronically ill, institutionalized elders, it was 90%. This was only the crude measurement; however, a more meaningful measure of root caries includes exposed root surfaces as one parameter. Root caries index, already described, usually increases with age; however, in older age groups (70+ and 75+ years), the index is decreased. This might be because the increase in number of root surfaces at risk may not be accompanied by the increase in decayed-filled root surfaces. The root caries index assumes a linear relation, which might not be correct under circumstances where gingival recession does not precede caries. Although recession is an important parameter of root caries, decayed-filled surfaces may not correlate with surfaces at risk; therefore, root caries index varies.

It is also possible that there might be 'maturation' effect once a root surface is exposed to environment. In case root caries do not occur within stipulated years after the root is exposed, it may never occur. Most of the studies do not consider this maturation phenomenon and the incidence is expected to increase with advancing age.

Prevalence of root caries implies that only 15% of all teeth with gingival recession were attacked by caries, with mean number of teeth per person was 2.8. Most of the studies have shown an increase in prevalence of root caries with age.

The Vipeholm dental caries study showed that the incidence of cemental caries in the age group (greater than 37 years) was 0.51 lesion/person/period. Banding, et al (1985) found that 36% residents of a hospital developed root lesions over 34 months period. The incidence rate was 0.25 lesion/person/year. The elderly are usually more prone to root caries; because higher the age, greater is the exposure to risk factors and subsequently the caries. It has been reported that 47% individuals between the age of 65 and 75 years have experienced root caries. The percentage is even higher in 75-plus age group individuals. One study (Hellger, et al 1990), however, reported prevalence of 88.4% in 55 years and above individuals. In one such study, Sikri (1994) observed increase in root caries index rates with advancing age. However, it was maximum in the age group of 60–69 years and then it declined. Definite correlation of age and root caries has been reported by many workers (Banting 1980, Katz 1982). One of the primary etiologic factor for the elderly patients is their use of systemic medicines. Most of such medicines lead to dry mouth (less salivary flow). The subsequent reduction in buffering capacity resulting from decreased salivary flow is responsible for the increase in root caries in elderly individuals.

RCI rate was more for males than females in all groups. This is in concurrence with the findings of Wallace, et al (1988) who have reported significantly greater RCI rates in males. Similar views have also been expressed by Beck, et al (1985). The reasonable explanation for this may be the higher utilization of dental services by females and also the females are usually more conscious towards their dental problems. However, Gustausen, et al (1988) in their survey of Norwegian adults, have reported higher RCI rate in females. The extent and severity of periodontal diseases, vis-a-vis root caries, have also been shown to vary between sexes.

Most authors used either the proportion of the population with decayed (D), decayed and filled (DF), or both D and DF teeth or surfaces. Others reported mean scores of D and DF teeth or surfaces and some have computed age, sex and race specific rates.

Differences in prevalence rates across studies may be accounted for by any one of several population differences or by design differences. It is difficult to compare data from the Brustman study (1986) with other studies reporting DF rates, since Brustman studies were limited to mandibular anterior teeth. Banting, et al (1980) study examined predominantly older, chronically ill, hospitalized patients and indicated a high experience with disease. As expected the mean D and DF rates for the Banting et al (1985) study were higher; perhaps indicating a link between general health and root caries. The prevalence rates have been from 43 to 63% in most of the studies. The Jensen and Kohbut (1988) study (conducted in low fluoride Iowa communities and using radiographs), showed higher rates. Katz, et al (1982) (using a wider range of ages) reported a prevalence rate of 42% and Wallace, et al (1988a), reported a baseline rate of 69%. Differences in population characteristics or design differences should also be considered in instances where different studies report similar prevalence rates. In the Iowa (middle class, white, rural) and Piedmont (all socioeconomic strata, black and white urban and rural) studies, which used similar designs, decay (D) was found in about 25% of the people. In studies encompassing a wider range of ages, Vehkalahti (1987) (in a Finnish population) and Burt, et al (1986) (in a New Mexico Community with 1 ppm fluoride in the water supply) have reported 24% decay. The Locker, et al (1989) study involving suburbanites aged 50 and over reported DF prevalence rates similar to NIDR (1987) rates for people aged 65+ who attended multi-purpose senior centres. It was established that the prevalence of root caries is relatively stable in overall age groups studies, or that differences in populations and designs had somehow produced similar results.

Root caries prevalence within the oral cavity (say one person) have been shown to get influenced by several factors, viz. number and types of teeth remaining and also the teeth surfaces with recession. Katz, et al (1982) have observed that mandibular molars were maximally affected, followed by premolars and incisors. Maxillary anterior teeth, however, have higher root caries index rates than mandibular ones. The exact cause of difference could not be authenticated; however, the proportion of root surfaces at risk (recession etc.) was found to correlate with the findings. Most of the studies suggested that buccal/facial or proximal surfaces are primarily affected followed by lingual surfaces.

Katz (1982) study detected the likelihood of different root surfaces becoming carious. The buccal surfaces of mandibular molars were found to be twice as likely to depict caries as lingual or proximal surfaces; whereas lingual surfaces of maxillary molars were five times more susceptible than buccal surfaces. Mandibular molars have shown the maximum RCI and the mandibular incisors the least. However, RCI of canines is maximum in maxillary arch and is comparable to mandibular molars. Root caries index (RCI) rates for different tooth surfaces were presented as:

Mesial > Distal > Buccal > Lingual

Sumney (1973), however, has reported that mandibular premolars have the highest RCI rate.

Prevalence and intraoral distribution of root surface caries in older adults (residing in Amritsar city and adjoining villages) was studied by Sikri and Sikri in 1994. 760 patients were selected from the Outpatient Department of Punjab Govt. Dental College and Hospital, Amritsar. The criteria for selection were:

- Patient's age should be fifty years or above.
- There should be at least fifteen teeth present in both the arches.

For the convenience, study was divided into four age groups:
- Patient's between 50 and 59 years of ages.
- 60–69 years of age.
- 70–79 years of age.
- 80 years and above.

293 (38.55%) of the total 760 were males while 467 (51.45%) were females.

The diagnosis of caries was based on the visual findings of darkened/discolored lesion and tactile criteria of leathery feel upon probing. An area softer and darkened than the surrounding teeth surfaces, with or without a cavity was taken as carious.

When both coronal and root surfaces were effected by a single carious lesion, only, its most likely site of origin was scored as decayed. A root surface was considered at risk if cemento-enamel function (CEJ) was visible.

RCI rate was calculated as described by Katz.

The average age of patients in the study was 64.6 + 5.7 and the average number of teeth present were 22.5 + 4.1.

As the age advanced, the RCI rate increased. However, it was maximum in the age group of 60–69 years and then it declined. Definite correlation of age and root caries has been reported by many workers (Banting 1980, Katz 1982). The decline in RCI after 70 years of age may be due to a small number of samples in these age groups. RCI rate was more for males than females in all groups.

The RCI rates in mandibular molars were 16 times more than mandibular incisors, comparing the surfaces at risk of both the teeth. These findings should lead to enquiries and further research to evaluate the controlling factors which determine the preferential oral attack. The percentage of missing teeth increased slightly with age, with a maximum in 70–79 years of age group and again decline at 80 years and above age group.

A limited data is available as regard to prevalence studies on root caries of different countries amongst different populations. The available data of some countries is described as follows:

Root Caries in Older individuals from East Sussex

The prevalence of root caries in a selected older population, living in the community and attending a general dental practice in East Sussex was reported, wherein a total of 146 non-institutionalized people, aged at least 55 years having at least 12 teeth were examined. Most of the subjects (88.4%) had evidence of root caries, males and denture wearers had more lesions than females and non-denture wearers, respectively. Active coronal caries was present in only 11.6% of the subjects, whereas active (soft/leathery) root caries lesions were present in 31.5% of the subjects. The teeth and surfaces most commonly affected by root caries were found to be similar to those seen in previous epidemiological survey. The majority of active root caries lesions were within 1.0 mm of the gingival margin, while inactive lesions tended to be greater than or equal to 1.0 mm from the gingival margin. Color of root caries lesions was not diagnostic of caries activity.

Root Caries in Older Individuals from Sri Lanka

Kularatne and Ekanayake (2007) studied the prevalence and factors associated with root surface caries in older individuals from Sri Lanka. The study provided much needed data on root surface caries for older individuals in Sri Lanka. The results showed that 89.7% of the sample had at least one root surface caries lesion. The mean number of root surfaces with decay/filling was 3.8; whereas, mean root caries index was 25.0%. The root caries prevalence was higher in urban population. This prevalence was higher than that reported for elderly from other Asian countries. Shah and Sundaram (2004) reported a prevalence of 67% for elderly from Indian while for older Thai (Nicolau, et al 2000) and Chinese individuals (Lin, et al 2000), the prevalence of

root surface caries was 18% and 37% respectively. The mean RCI for the sample was 25%, which means that on the average 25% root surfaces/person showed caries. Steele, et al (2001) reported 26% RCI for British older adults; whereas in Pomerania, the RCI was low, ranging between 4.6 and 10.6% (Splieth, et al 2004).

It was also observed that betel chewing was negatively associated with development of root surface caries. Why betel chewers had less caries may be because the betel stains on root surfaces act as a chemical/physical barrier against caries attack. Moreover, it has also been reported that *Streptococcus mutans* was not found in betel chewers. This suggests that betel has antibacterial properties that may protect individuals from dental caries. With regard to age, those over 80 years were less likely to have root surface caries compared to 60 to 70 years old when controlled for number of remaining teeth, number of surfaces with recession and betel chewing. In very old subjects, teeth affected by disease may have been extracted or lost and whatever remaining teeth, irrespective of the number, may be those that are resistant to decay. Hence it is possible that the risk of root surface caries is reduced in very old subjects. In contrast, a positive association between root caries and age has been observed in some studies (Zue and Zickert, 1990; Slade and Spencer, 1997), but it is noteworthy that in the analysis, the authors did not control for the influence of confounding variables such as the number of retained teeth and the number of surfaces with recession. Therefore, it was difficult to ascertain whether the age dependent increase in root caries observed in these studies was due to the effect of age. In conformity with the findings of several studies, gingival recession emerged as the strongest predictor of root surface caries. A positive association was established between root surface caries and the number of root surfaces with recession.

Another finding of importance was that the number of retained teeth was negatively associated with the presence of root caries which is consistent with the findings of other authors.

One limitation of this study is that caries was assessed only on two surfaces of the root. Approximal root surfaces were not considered, as clear visualization of these surfaces was difficult.

The study revealed that prevalence of root surface caries in older individuals in Sri Lanka was very high. Moreover, chewing betel, age, number of retained teeth and the number of root surfaces with recession were identified as significant predictors of root caries. Though the use of fluorides is an effective method of preventing and controlling dental caries, it was evident that only about 50% of this population used fluoride toothpaste. Therefore, older individuals should be to educated as regard to use of fluorides in preventing dental caries and also encouraged to brush their teeth with fluoride toothpaste to alleviate the problem of dental caries.

Root Caries in Older individuals from Finland

Vehkalahti, et al (1983) investigated the prevalence of root caries related to age and sex and the number of teeth in the adult Finnish population. The root caries prevalence was much higher in North America than Finland, which might be due to cultural variations.

The difference in the prevalence of lesions between sexes could have been caused by many factors, e.g. the subject's oral hygiene and oral health habits and the frequency of dental visits. Women may clean their teeth better than men and may be more willing to have their affected teeth treated. According to previous reports, from the same population, women have better gingival condition and less retained roots than men and the mean number of teeth is consistently 1–2 teeth lower for women than for men.

However, the differences in the prevalence of root caries between the sexes was presented after adjusting the number of retained teeth.

The prevalence of root caries, related to age have been reported earlier but the prevalences reported have been higher than in their study. The differences between earlier results and their findings were due in part to variations in sampling methods, sample sizes, age and sex distribution to the criteria used in defining root caries in different studies. It can be expected that in the future, aged people will retain more teeth than nowadays. This may lead to a changing dental disease pattern through the increasing number of surfaces at risk to root caries.

Root Caries in Older individuals from Brazil and Benghazi

Marques, et al (2013) conducted a comprehensive study on 9564 adults (age 35–44 years) and 7509 elderly individuals (age 65–74 years) in various cities of Brazil. The prevalence of root caries observed was 16.7% in adults and 13.6% in the elderly. The root caries index of decayed/filled root surfaces was 0.42 for adults and 0.32 for the elderly. In adults, root caries index ranged from 1.4% in Aracaju to 15.1% in Salvador (north region of Brazil). Among the elderly, this index ranged from 3.5% in Porto Velho to 23.9% in Plamas (north region). Root caries were more prevalent in men than women in both the age groups.

Hassan and Omar (2000) conducted study on 420 Benghazi individuals, varying in the age group of 16–70 years. The percentage of root caries observed was: 7.5% in 16–25 years, 48.8% in 26–35, 52.5% in 36–45, 50% in 46–55 and 56.3% in 56–70 years age group. The study does not concur with earlier studies observing root caries to be a problem of elderly.

Clinical Implications of Epidemiological Studies

The current information on root caries could provide guidance as regard to clinical management and prevention of root caries. It has been established that there are some special group of individuals who are at higher risk of root caries than others and this criteria should form the primary focus for screening and preventive programs.

Various studies have confirmed root caries being tooth surface specific, affecting given population after certain age. These special subgroups within the population would be appropriate target for preventive programs. The accessibility of these people might be difficult, since they may include elderly population in homes for aged, chronic hospitals, senior citizen apartments, etc.

Understanding the distribution, etiology and natural history of root caries is mandatory in developing programs that provide access to the activities aimed for these population. Attention is much more focused on adults recently than in the past. Anti-caries agents are being applied both by the private and the government systems. The educational and motivational programs are also necessitated to curb the disease at initial diagnostic level.

CRITERIA FOR CODING OF ROOT CARIES

The lesions are coded so as to facilitate the detection and classification of root caries.

The facial, mesial, distal and lingual root surfaces of each tooth are classified in codes (One score is assigned per root surface).

Code E

The root surface, which cannot be visualized directly as a result of gingival recession/by gentle air-drying, is excluded. Surfaces covered entirely by calculus can be excluded or the calculus is removed and the root surface is evaluated.

Code 0

The root surface does not exhibit any unusual discoloration that distinguishes it from the surrounding surface nor does it exhibit a surface defect either at the cemento-enamel

junction or wholly on the cemental surface (the root surface has a natural anatomical contour), or

The root surface may exhibit a definite loss of surface continuity that is not consistent with the caries process. This loss of surface integrity may be associated with abrasion or erosion. Abrasion is characterized by a clearly defined outline with a sharp border, whereas erosion has a more diffuse border (neither condition shows discoloration).

Code 1

There is a clearly demarcated area on the root surface or at the cemento-enamel junction (CEJ) that is discolored (light/dark brown, black) and there is no cavitation (loss of anatomical contour <0.5 mm) present.

Code 2

There is a clear discolored (light/dark brown, black) demarcated area on the root surface or at the cemento-enamel junction (CEJ) or there is cavitation (loss of anatomical contour ≥ 0.5 mm) present.

i. Primary caries on Root Surface

Flowchart 17.1 serves as a decisive tool for coding of root caries.

ii. Caries Associated with Root Restorations

When a root surface is filled and there is caries adjacent to the restoration, the surface is scored as caries. The criteria for caries associated with restorations on the roots of teeth are the same as those for caries on non-restored root surfaces.

Flowchart 17.2 serves as a tool for coding caries adjacent to restorations on root surfaces.

iii. Root Caries Activity

The characteristics of the base of the discolored area on the root surface can be used to determine whether or not the root caries lesion is active or not. These characteristics

Flowchart 17.1: Decision tree for primary caries on the root surface

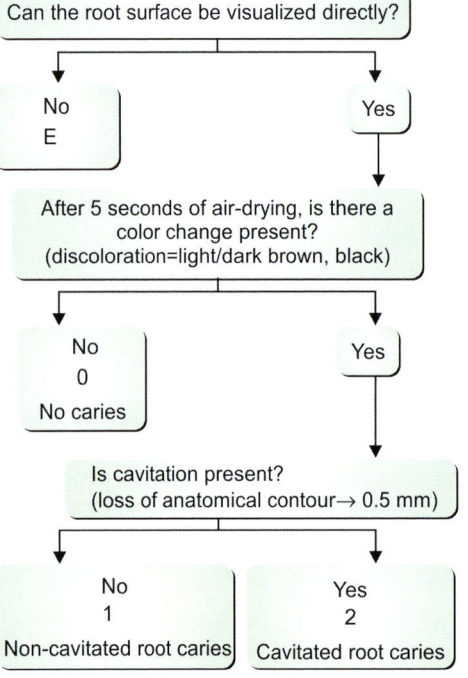

Flowchart 17.2: Decision tree for caries associated with root restorations

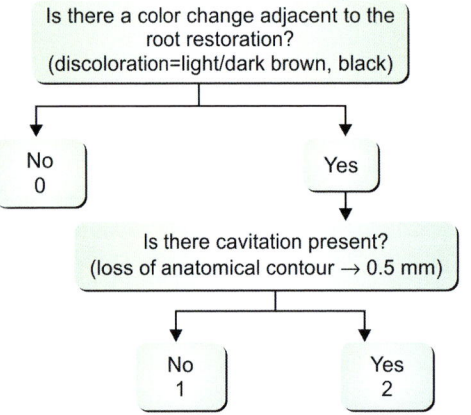

Flowchart 17.3: Decision tree for root caries activity

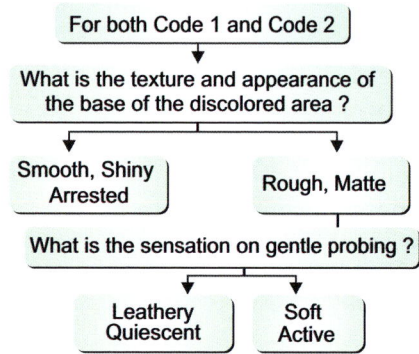

Flowchart 17.3 serves as a tool for coding the activity of root caries.

Special Considerations

Whenever both coronal and root surface are affected by a single carious lesion that extends at least 1.0 mm past the cemento-enamel junction in both the incisal and apical directions, both surfaces should be scored as caries; however, for a lesion affecting both crown and root surfaces that does not meet the criteria of 1.0 mm involvement, only the coronal or root surface that involves the greater portion (more than 50%) of the lesion should be scored as caries. When it is impossible to invoke the 50% rule (i.e. when both coronal and root surfaces appear equally affected), both surfaces should be scored as caries.

When a carious lesion on a root surface extends beyond the line angle of the root to involve at least 1/3rd of the distance across the adjacent surface, that adjacent surface also should be scored as caries.

If more than one lesion is present on the same root surface, the most severe lesion is scored.

Non-vital teeth are scored same as the vital teeth.

Risk Factors

Root caries aetiology is multifactorial involving physical, medical, behavioral and

include texture (smooth, rough), appearance (shiny or glossy, matte or non-glossy) and perception on gentle probing (soft, leathery, hard). Active root caries lesions are usually located within 2.0 mm of the crest of the gingival margin.

social factors. Systemic conditions and their medical treatment affects oral cavity, which in turn may alter patients ability to maintain adequate oral hygiene. Social factors also play an important part in progress of caries. Various studies using multivariate techniques have found significant association between root caries and variety of systemic, behavioral and social variables. Association of root caries and age might not always be true indication; older adults with good hygiene develop a few root caries lesions.

Teeth with gingival recession are considered more susceptible to root caries; however, recession and root caries are more or less tooth specific. Posterior teeth are more likely to develop root caries than anterior teeth. An association between coronal and root caries has also been established, suggesting that factors implicated in the onset of coronal caries are likely to be the same in the onset of root caries.

The number of teeth remaining in oral cavity is inversely related to root caries, i.e. the more the teeth remaining, less is the risk of developing root caries. Older individuals with natural teeth are less susceptible to root caries unless they become victim of other social and medical variables. It is speculated that root caries may involve a change in general health status, may be change in immune system resulting in occurrence of multiple conditions, one could be root caries.

One certain risk factor associated with high prevalence of root caries is the combined effect of carbohydrate and old age. Use of refined carbohydrates alone has also been found to be associated with root caries, especially in females.

Use of medications having potential of producing xerostomic effects is considered as the risk factor. However, Beck, et al (1988) in his study could not observe any correlation with root caries and drugs producing xerostomia. This might be because the individuals using those drugs did not develop side effects producing xerostomia. It is established that xerostomic individuals are at high risk of caries.

A few authors confirmed the association between low salivary flow rate and prolonged clearance time, especially in lower vestibule area. That can be considered as the explanation why mandibular molars are the most susceptible teeth for developing root caries.

It has been documented that smokers are more susceptible to root caries. Smokers usually have more recession areas, periodontal pockets, higher plaque score and deviated salivary secretions and its buffering effect. However, it is not confirmed whether this effect is because of direct biochemical process or indirectly affecting general oral hygiene.

High levels of salivary lactobacilli and streptococci have also been correlated with root caries susceptibility. The root caries incidence was observed to be twice as high for individuals with both high salivary lactobacilli and streptococci, as compared to individuals with only high lactobacilli count. However, Candida levels did not correlate with root caries.

Banting, et al (1985) reported 6.3 root lesions per 1000 tooth surface at risk. The incidence of root caries may be quite high in teeth with gingival recession. A few studies reported approximately half of the population had one or more new carious lesions. The caries increments were remarkably similar even in different population and with different methods of evaluation. Risk factors include:

- Periodontal problems leading to root exposure.
- Decreased flow of saliva.
- Use of medication which diminishes salivary flow.
- Certain medical conditions such as diabetes, Alzheimer disease, etc.
- Improper prosthesis, especially partial dentures with clasps.

- Head and neck radiations.
- Decreased manual dexterity (unable to brush properly); poor oral hygiene.
- Cognitive deficits due to mental illness or autoimmune disease (Sjögrens' syndrome).

Any factor can be considered as a 'risk factor', if it is associated with influencing the disease in a clinical trial. Various studies have been carried out to analyze the potential risk factors associated with the root caries. Summarizing these studies, the factors which influence root caries are:

- Age (elders more prone).
- Sex (males more prone).
- Attachment loss (more prone).
- Drugs leading to xerostomia.
- Smoking and use of tobacco.
- Sugary diet.
- Anxiety.

- Family history.
- Use of fluorides decrease chances of root caries.

Various epidemiologic studies on root caries has led to the following observations:

- The factors identified in root caries include medical, mental, behavioral and social conditions (Table 17.2).
- Comparisons of incidence and prevalence data among studies are hampered by lack of standardization of diagnostic criteria. The differences in diagnostic criteria affect either prevalence estimates or the more sensitive incidence studies.
- Rarely both incidence and prevalence rates are remarkably consistent when roughly similar studies are compared.
- The prevalence rates indicate that a large proportion of the adult population has been affected by root caries.

Table 17.2: Risk indicators and risk factors in root caries

Factor	Effects
A : Social	
• Age	• With increasing age
• Literary level	• More in less educated
• Income	• More in low income group
B : Demographic	
• Race	• More in white
• Gender	• More in males
C : Medical	
• Medication	• More with medications having xerostomic side effects
• Chronic illness	• More (less dexterity for oral hygiene)
• Disability	• More (compromised oral hygiene)
D : Behavioral	
• Oral hygiene (toothbrushing, use of fluorides etc.)	• Less with good oral hygiene measures
• Sugary diet	• More
• Use of tobacco/cigarette	• More
E : Oral cavity	
• *Streptococcus mutans*, lactobacilli, Actinomyces	• Positively correlated (more)
• Candida	• Not confirmed
• Salivary flow, buffering	• More with decreased flow
• Oral health status	• More with gingival recession, periodontal pockets, coronal caries

- Only a few studies through risk assessment methods identify people at high risk of root caries.
- Risk indicators derived from prevalence studies may not be substantiated as risk factors.

Effect of Saliva on Root Caries

A few authors studied the effect of physical nature of saliva and also its fluoride contents on caries development independent of the flow rate. The authors reported that saliva composition affects mineral loss, lesion depth and inorganic content of the surface layer in experimental root caries. The unstimulated saliva composition was considerably more important for this relation than the stimulated saliva composition. Most of these findings are in accordance with the earlier studies evaluating the effect of saliva on caries development.

The significant correlations were obtained with the unstimulated saliva phosphate and protein concentration. High concentration of these constituents was protective against initiation of caries. As the day to day variation for these salivary variables was relatively low, the authors assumed that the salivary constituents remained constant throughout the experimental period. Phosphate can act as a buffer, increase the degree of saturation and decrease the critical pH. Proteins can also function as buffers and also form the acquired pellicle.

It is established that higher buffer capacity protects the teeth against caries development. The qualitative and quantitative saliva protein analysis have revealed correlations between the unstimulated salivary amylase and caries lesion development.

Genetics, Immunity and Root Caries

Studies have shown that one's preference to sweet carbohydrates may put one at risk for caries. This preference may be determined by socioeconomic status but may also be under genetic control. Lui (2003) and a few authors examined genetically determined taste sensitivity to 6-n-propylthiouracil demonstrating that individuals with low taste sensitivity develop less caries than those with high testing sensitivity. TAS1R2 (Taste receptor type 1, member 2) is a member of sweet taste receptor family and guanine nucleotide-binding protein subunit alpha-3 (GNAT 3), which mediates taste receptors in the taste buds. A certain component of taste receptor, type 2, member 38 (TAS2R38) were protective for caries while others were associated with caries risk. The (TAS2R38) single nucleotide polymorphism that were found to be protective for caries cause amino acid changes in the taste receptors that are associated with better sensitivity.

Enamel proteins such as ameloblastin and tuftelin are crucial for enamel formation. Single nucleotide polymorphism markers were genotyped in selected genes (ameloblastin, amelogenin, enamelin, tuftelin etc.) that influence enamel formation. One component of rare amelogenin was associated with increase age related caries experience.

Immune response genes have also been considered as candidate genes to caries susceptibility. Three single nucleotide polymorphisms in DEFB1 (defensin 1) were tested in a cohort of unrelated adult individuals. Carrying a copy of variant allele of DEFB1 marker rs11362 increased the DMFT and DMFS scores more than five fold.

Age related differences in salivary secretion have been studied by various authors. The level of serum immunoglobulins G (IgG) and IgM were significantly reduced in older individuals, whereas not much reduction in the level of IgA with age was observed. The studies demonstrated decline in immunoglobulin concentration with increased age, which might contribute to the increased susceptibility of older adults to caries.

Age related differences in salivary gene expression have been studied in parotid glands of mice. The majority of mice exhibited decreased expression in elderly mice. The effect of age on specific gene expression in human saliva may provide knowledge of morphological changes in oral cavity, vis-à-vis dental caries. Age has a significant influence on the expression of genes associated with reduced protein biosynthesis of salivary gland secretion. Specific genes may be most affected by aging. The expressions of both HLA-DQ1 and HLA-DQB1 genes involved in immunoresponse were decreased in parotid gland in elderly. Chemokine ligand 10 also showed lower expression in the aged population.

Mungia, et al (2008) examined stimulated and unstimulated salivary flow and different proteins (lactoferrin, Secretory IgA, albumin, mucin, etc.) and observed significant association between age, caries and specific salivary flow. Specific genes have been found to be affected by aging (Srivastava, et al 2008), since age is associated with reduced biosynthesis of salivary gland secretion. Complex remodeling of the immune system occurs during process of aging, which may contribute to systemic diseases in the older adults. Certain autoimmune disease and neoplastic pathologies in aged individuals make them susceptible to caries by dysregulation of immune function. Geriatric pathologies and the salivary gland functions are worth evaluating in the elderly as a caries risk factor.

Histopathology of Root Caries

The histopathology of root caries is described as caries of cementum and caries of root dentin. The detailed text is explained in Chapter 9.

Microbiology of Root Caries

The creation of low pH on root surfaces by oral micro-organisms aids in the demineralization of cementum. Once the acidic environment is established, mutans strepto-cocci and other aciduric bacteria may promote lesion formation by sustaining the acidic environment. The detailed text is explained in Chapter 8.

Bibliography

1. Allen AY, McNally ME, Fure S and Birkhed D. Assessment of caries risk in elderly patients using the Cariogram model. J. Can. Dent. Assoc.: 2006;72:459–65.

2. Anusavice KJ. Dental caries: risk assessment and treatment solutions for an elderly population. Compend. Contin. Educ. Dent.: 2002;23:12–20.

3. Baca P, Clavero J, Baca AP, Gonzalez-Rodriguez MP, Bravo M and Valderrama MJ. Effect of chlorhexidine-thymol varnish on root caries in a geriatric population: a randomized double-blind clinical trial. J. Dent.: 2009;37:679–85.

4. Banting DW. Epidemiology of root caries. Gerodontology: 1986;5:5–11.

5. Banting DW. Diagnosis and prediction of root caries. Adv. Dent. Res.: 1993;7:80–86.

6. Banting DW, Ellen RP and Fillery ED. Prevalence of root surface caries among institutionalized older persons. Comm. Dent. Oral Epidemiol.: 1980; 8:84.

7. Banting DW, Ellen RP and Fillery ED. A longitudinal study of root caries baseline and incidence data. J. Dent. Res.: 1985;64:1141.

8. Bardow A, Hofer E, Nyvad B, Ten Cate, Kirkeby, Moe and Nauntofte. Effect of saliva composition on experimental root caries. Caries Research: 2005;39:71–77.

9. Beck JD. The epidemiology of root surface caries. J. Dent. Res.: 1990;69:1216–21.

10. Beck JD. The epidemiology of root surface caries: North American studies. Adv. Dent. Res.: 1993;7:42–51.

11. Bizhang M, Chun YH and Heisrath D, Purucker P, Singh P, Kersten T, Zimmer S. Microbiota of exposed root surfaces after fluoride, chlorhexidine and periodontal maintenance therapy: a 3-year evaluation. J. Periodontology: 2007;78:1580–89.

12. Brailsfordl SR, Shah B, Simons D, Gilbert S, Clark D, Ines L, Adams SE, Allison C and Beighton D. The predominant aciduric microflora of root-caries lesions. J. Dent. Res.: 2001;80:1828–1833.

13. Davies RM. The rational use of oral care products in the elderly. Clin. Oral Investig.: 2004;8:2–5.

14. Donovan T and Swift EJ. Protocol for the prevention and management of root caries. University of North Carolina: 2008;20:405.

15. Dorita P, Ingar O, Tiril W, Susan KB, Sean LC, Bjorn G and Bruce JP. Microarray Analysis of the Microflora of Root Caries in Elderly. Eur. J. Clin. Microbiol. Infect. Dis.: 2009;28:509–517.

16. Du MQ, Jiang H, Tai BJ, Wu B and Bian Z. Root caries patterns and risk factors of middle-aged and elderly people in P.R. China. Comm. Dent. Oral Epid.:2009;37:260–6.

17. Ettinger RL. Oral health and the aging population. J. Am. Dent. Assoc.: 2007;138:5S–6S.

18. Fure S and Zickert I. Prevalence of root surface caries in 55, 65 and 75 years old Swedish individuals. Comm. Dent. Oral Epid.: 1990;18: 100–5.

19. Gati D and Vieira AR. Elderly at greater risk for root caries: A look at the multifactorial risks with emphasis on genetics susceptibility. Int. J. Dent.: 2011;1–6.

20. Griffin SO, Griffin PM, Swann JL and Zlobin N. Estimating rates of new root caries in older adults. J. Dent. Res.: 2004;83:634–8.

21. Hamasha AA, Warren JJ, Hand JS and Levy SM. Coronal and root caries in the older Iowans: 9 to 11 years incidence. Spec. Care Dentist: 2005;25: 106–10.

22. Hand JS, Hunt RJ and Beck JD. Coronal and root caries in older Iowans: 36 months incidence. Gerodontics: 1988;4:136–9.

23. Heijnsbroek M, Paraskevas S and Vander Weijden GA. Fluoride Interventions for Root Caries: A Review. Oral health Prev. Dent.: 2007;5: 145–52.

24. Hellyer PH, Beighton D, Heath MR and Lynch EJ. Root caries in older people attending a general dental practice in East Sussex. Br. Dent. J.: 1990;169:201–6.

25. Hellyer PH and Lynch E. The diagnosis of root caries: a review. Gerodontology: 1990;9:95–102.

26. Holm-Pedersen P, Avulund K and Morse DE, Stoltze K, Katz RV, Vütanen M, Winbla B. Dental caries, periodontal disease and cardiac arrhythmias in community-dwelling older persons aged 80 and older: is there a link? J. Am. Geriatrics Soc.: 2005;53:430–7.

27. Hunt RJ. Recent data on the prevalence and incidence of root caries. J. Dent. Res.: 1989;68 (spl. Issue):177.

28. Johnson G and Almqvist H. Non-invasive management of superficial root caries lesions in disabled and infirm patients. Gerodontology: 2003;20:9–14.

29. Katz RV. Root caries—is it the caries problem of the future? J. Canad. Dent. Assoc.: 1985;51: 511–4.

30. Katz R. The Clinical Identification of Root Caries. Gerodontology: 1986;5:21–24.

31. Katz R. Clinical Signs of Root Caries: Measurement Issues from an Epidemiologic Perspective. J. Dent. Res.: 1990;69:1211–1226.

32. Katz RV, Hazen SP, Chilton NW and Mumma RD. Prevalence and intraoral distribution of root caries in an adult population. Caries Res.: 1982;16: 265–71.

33. Kobayashi S, Kamino Y, Hiratsuka K, Kiyama-Kishikawa M and Abiko Y. Age-related changes in IGF-1 expansion in submandibular glands of senescence-accelerated mice. J. Oral Sci.: 2004;46: 119–25.

34. Kularatne S and Ekanayake L. Root surface caries in older individuals from Sri Lanka. Caries Res.: 2007;41:252–6.

35. Leske GS and Ripa LW. Three-year root caries increments: an analysis of teeth and surfaces at risk. Gerodontology: 1989;8:23–26.

36. Lin HC, Wong MC, Zhang HG, Lo EC and Schwartz E. Coronal and root caries in Southern Chinese adults. J. Dent. Res.:2001;80:1475–9.

37. Lin BP. Caries experience in children with various genetic sensitivity levels to the bitter taste of 6-n-propylthiouracil (PROP): a pilot study. Pediat. Dent.: 2003;25:37–42.

38. Locker D. Incidence of root caries in an older Canadian population. Comm. Dent. Oral Epidemiol. 1996;24:403–407.

39. Marinova-Takorova, M. Incidence of secondary root caries lesions in patients referred for treatment in the faculty of dental medicine - Sofia. J. IMAB: 2014;20:537–41.

40. Mojon P, Favre P, Chung JP and Budtz-Jorgensen, E. Examiner agreement on caries detection and plaque accumulation during dental surveys of elders. Gerodontology: 1995;12:49–55.

41. Mungia R, Cano SM, Johnson DA, Dang H and Brown JP. Interaction of age and specific saliva component output on caries. Aging-Clinical and Experimental Research: 2008;20:503–8.

42. Newbrun E. Prevention of root caries. Gerodontology: 1986;5:33–41.

43. Nicolau B, Srisilapanan P and Marcenes W. Number of teeth and risk of root caries. Gerodontology: 2000;17:91–96.

44. Powell LV, Leroux BG, Persson RE and Kiyak HA. Factors associated with caries incidence in an elderly population. Comm. Dent. Oral Epidemiol.: 1998;26:170–176.

45. Qasim AA. Association of root caries, oral hygiene and gingival health among adult population in Baghdad and Mosul city center (A comparative study). Al-Rafidain Dent. J.: 2009;9: 238–45.

46. Ravald N, Hamp SE and Birkhed D. Long term evaluation of root surface caries in periodontally treated patients. J. Clin. Periodontol.: 1986;13:758–767.

47. Ritter AV, Shugars DA and Bader JD. Root caries risk indicators: a systematic review of risk models. Community Dent. Oral Epidemiol.: 2010;38:383–97.

48. Sadowsky JM, Bebermeyer RD and Gibson G. Root caries - a review of the etiology, diagnosis, restorative and preventive interventions. Texas Dent. J.: 2008;125:1070–82.

49. Schamschula RG, Keyes PH and Hornabrook RW. Root surface caries in Lufa, New Guinea; 1. Clinical observations. J. Am. Dent. Assoc.: 1972;85:603–8.

50. Schupbach P, Guggenheim B and Lutz F. Histopathology of root surface caries. J. Dent. Res.: 1990;69:1195–1204.

51. Scully C and Ettinger RL. The influence of systemic diseases on oral health care in older adults. J. Am. Dent. Assoc.: 2007;138:75–145.

52. Seichter U. Root surface caries: A critical literature review. J. Am. Dent. Assoc.: 1987;115:305–10.

53. Shaeken MJM, Keltjens HM and Vander Hoeven JS. Effects of fluoride and chlorhexidine on the microflora of dental root surfaces and progression of root surface caries. J. Dent. Res.: 1991;70:150–3.

54. Shaker RE. Diagnosis, prevention and treatment of root caries. Saudi Dental Journal: 2004;16:84–92.

55. Splieth CH, Schwahn CH, Berhardt O and John U. Prevalence and distribution of root caries in Pomerania. North-East Germany. Caries Res.: 2004;38:333–40.

56. Srivastava A, Wang J, Zhou H, Melvin JE and Wong DT. Age and gender related differences in human parotid gland gene expression. Archives of Oral Biology: 2008;53:1058–70.

57. Steele JG, Sheiham A, Marcenes W, Fay N and Walls AWG. Clinical and behavioral indicators for root caries in older people. Gerodontolgy: 2001;18:95–101.

58. Sugihara N, Maki Y, Okawa Y, Hosaka M, Matsukubo T and Takaesu Y. Factors associated with root surface caries in the elderly. Bull. Tokyo Dent. Coll.: 2010;51:23–30.

59. Sugihara N, Maki Y, Kurokawa A and Matsukubo T. Cohort study on incidence of coronal and root caries in Japanese adults. Bull Tokyo Dent. Coll.: 2014;55:125–30.

60. Sumney DL, Jordan HJV and Englander HR. The prevalence of root surface caries in selected populations. J. Periodontology: 1973;44:500–4.

61. Surmount PA and Martens LC. Root surface caries: An update. Clin. Prev. Dent. 1989;11:14–20.

62. Takano N, Ando Y, Yoshihara A and Miyazaki H. Factors associated with root caries incidence in an elderly population. Comm. Dent. Health: 2003;20:217–22.

63. Vander Veen MH, Tsuda H, Arends J and ten Bosch JJ. Evaluation of sodium fluorescin for quantitative diagnosis of root caries. J. Dent. Res.: 1996;75:588–93.

64. Van der Veen MH and ten Bosch JJ. A fiber-optic setup for quantification of root surface demineralization. Eur. J. Oral Sci.: 1996;104:118–22.

65. Vehkalahti M, Rajala M, Tuominen R and Paunio I. Prevalence of root caries in the adult Finnish population. Comm. Dent. Oral Epid.:1983;11:188–90.

66. Vehkalahti MM. Relationship between root caries and coronal decay. J. Dent. Res.: 1987;66:1608–10.

67. Vehkalahti MM and Paunio IK. Occurrence of root caries in relation to dental health behavior. J. Dent. Res.:1988;67:911–4.

68. Wallace MC, Retief DH and Bradley EL. Prevalence of root caries in a population of older adults. Gerodontics: 1988;4:84–9.

69. Wallace MC, Retief DH and Bradley EL. Incidence of root caries in older adults. Hawaii Dent. J. 1988;19:8.

70. Walter R, Miguez PA, Arnold RR, Pereira PNR, Duarte WR and Yamauchi M. Effects of Natural Cross-Linkers on the Stability of Dentin Collagen and the Inhibition of Root Caries *in vitro*. Caries Res.: 2008;42:263.

71. Walter R and Swift EJ Jr. Critical appraisal, root caries. J. Compilation: 2007;19:120–4.

72. Warren JJ, Cowen HJ, Watkins CM and Hand JS. Dental caries prevalence and dental care

utilization among the very old. J. Am. Dent. Assoc.: 2000;131:1571–9.

73. Wefel JS, Clarkson BH and Heilman JR. Natural root caries: a histologic and microradiographic evaluation. J. Oral Pathol.: 1985;14:615.

74. Wierichs RJ and Meyer-Lueckel H. Systematic review on noninvasive treatment of root caries lesions. J Dent Res 2015;94:261–71.

75. Wilkinson SC, Higham SM, Ingram GS and Edgar WM. Visualization of root caries lesions by means of a diazonium dye. Adv. Dent. Res.: 1997; 11:515–22.

76. Wyatt C. Elderly Canadians residing in long-term care hospitals: Part II. Dental Caries Status. J. Can. Dent. Assoc.: 2002;68:359–63.

77. Wyatt CC, Wang D and Aleksejuniene J. Incidence of dental caries among susceptible community-dwelling older adults using fluoride toothpaste: 2-year follow-up study. J. Can. Dent. Assoc.: 2014;80:e44.

78. Yoshihara A, Takano N, Hirotomi T, Ogawa H, Hanada N and Miyazaki H. Longitudinal relationship between root caries and serum albumin. J. Dent. Res.: 2007;86:1115–9.

18

Radiation Caries

Radiation is a process in which electromagnetic waves travel through vacuum or matter-containing media. Radiation is also recognized as energy travelling through space. Radiation may be ionizing and non-ionizing. Non-ionizing radiation in limits are generally essential to life; whereas ionizing radiation may destabilize molecules within cells and lead to tissue damage.

Radiobiology is the study of action of ionizing radiation on living objects (also known as radiation biology). Radiation therapy (radiotherapy, or radiation oncology) is the medical use of ionizing radiation, used to control or kill malignant cells.

Ionizing radiations are utilized in treating cancer patients. The radiations form ions (electrically charged particles) in the cells of the tissues they pass through, by removing electrons from atoms and molecules. This can kill cells or change genes so the cells stop growing. The non-ionizing radiations such as radio waves, microwaves and light waves usually do not have as much energy and are not able to form ions.

Some types of ionizing radiation have more energy than others. The higher the energy, the more deeply the radiation can penetrate the tissues. The energy of radiation is important in planning radiation treatments. The radiation oncologist depending upon the need of depth of penetration selects the type and energy of radiation that is suitable for particular type and location of cancer.

Radiation absorbed dose is a measure of the energy deposited in a medium by ionizing radiation per unit mass, which may be measured as joules per kilogram when it is represented by the equivalent SI unit (International System of unit), Gray (Gy). The non-SI unit is rad.

Conversions from the SI units to older units are as follows:
- 1 Gy = 100 rad
- 1 mGy = 100 mrad

In radiation therapy, the amount of radiation varies depending on the type and stage of cancer being treated. For curative cases, the typical dose for a solid epithelial tumour ranges from 60 to 80 Gy, while lymphomas are treated with 20 to 40 Gy. Preventive doses are around 45–60 Gy in 1.8–2 Gy fractions (for breast, head and neck cancers). The salivary glands and tear glands have a radiation tolerance of about 30 Gy in 2 Gy fractions; this dose is exceeded by most radical head and neck cancer treatments, potentially causing dryness of these glands.

RADIATION MECHANISM AND PROTOCOL

Radiation energy (photons, viz. γ-radiations and X-rays, particle radiations, viz. α and β, particles, electrons, protons, neutrons, etc.) damages the DNA of cancerous cells. This damage is either direct or indirect ionization of atoms. Indirect ionization happens as a result of the ionization of water, forming free radicals (hydroxyl radicals) which damage the DNA.

In photon therapy, most of the radiation effect is through free radicals. Because cells have mechanisms for repairing single-strand DNA damage, double-stranded DNA damage is the most significant technique to cause cell death. Single-strand DNA damage is passed through cell division; dismantle cancer cells, DNA accumulates, leading to their death or slow reproduction.

Charged particles such as protons, borons, carbons and neon ions can cause direct damage to cancer cell DNA through high-LET (linear energy transfer).

Two basic protocols are being followed in radiotherapy. External beam radiotherapy is the most common, followed by interstitial or implant seed radiotherapy (neutron beam radiotherapy, the third one, is now rarely used).

External Beam Radiotherapy

The radiations are usually administered with machines called linear accelerators, which produce high-energy external radiation (usually cobalt-60 radiations) beams. This beam of radiation penetrates the tissues and delivers the radiation dose deep in the cancer tissues.

Interstitial Radiotherapy/Brachytherapy

In this method, the radiations are delivered by the use of implants. The radioactive implants are needles or tubes containing a radioactive substance. Such implantations, if carefully performed, are effective, safe and have a low risk of complications. With brachytherapy, high radiation doses may be delivered to specific cancer cells, without damaging adjacent normal tissues. Brachytherapy can be a useful addition to external beam irradiation in the treatment of patients with head and neck cancer.

GENERAL COMPLICATIONS OF RADIOTHERAPY

Tiredness: Fatigue is one of the most common side effects of radiotherapy, which may increase over time. It usually lasts from three weeks to three months. Anemia, stress, depression, etc. may contribute to fatigue.

Nausea and vomiting: Radiotherapy may cause nausea within two to six hours after the radiation and may lasts for about two hours.

Weight loss: Radiation can induce changes in taste, subsequently decrease in intake of food and weight loss.

Skin damage: Radiations can cause a sunburn-like damage (radiation dermatitis) to the skin, which can be further aggravated by chemotherapy.

Hair loss: Radiotherapy may lead to hair loss in the treatment area. Hair usually begins to fall out after 2–3 weeks.

Pharyngoesophageal stenosis: Pharyngoesophageal stenosis is delayed complication leading to narrowing in the pharynx or esophagus. The narrowing makes it difficult to swallow.

Lymphedema: Obstruction of the cutaneous lymphatics results in lymphedema.

Hypothyroidism: Radiotherapy is almost always associated with hypothyroidism.

Ototoxicity: Radiation around ear may result in serous otitis. High doses of irradiation can cause sensory neural hearing loss.

Damage to neck structures: Radiotherapy may lead to neck edema and fibrosis. The edema may harden, leading to neck stiffness after some time.

Secondary cancer: Even though radiation is used to treat cancer; however, it may result in new local and systemic cancer.

Radiation Effects on Oral Tissues

Radiations affect almost all tissues depending upon their intensity and longevity. Even stray radiations do affect human tissues, though at low scales. During head and neck radiations, the main tissues susceptible to get affected are:

i. *Taste buds:* Alteration in taste is an early response to radiation. Bitter and acid flavors are more susceptible to impairment than salt and sweet flavors. Radiations may damage the taste buds or their innervating nerve fibres. The reduction in salivary flow rate also affects loss of taste, which is usually transient. Taste gradually returns to normal or near-normal levels within one year after radiotherapy; however, in certain cases, it may take longer.

ii. *Oral mucosa:* Radiation mucositis (the reactive inflammation of the oral and oropharyngeal mucous membrane during radiotherapy) is quite common after radiations. The etiopathogenesis of radiation mucositis consists of four phases, i.e. inflammatory/vascular phase, epithelial phase, bacterial phase and the healing phase. The first clinical signs of mucositis appear after first week of conventional radiotherapy. Around the third week of radiotherapy, more severe symptoms of mucositis, such as the formation of pseudomembranes and ulceration, may appear. Mucositis is most severe in the soft palate, followed, by mucosa of the floor of the mouth, cheek, tongue, lips and dorsum of the tongue. Candidiasis is the most common infection in the oral cavity shortly after radio-therapy.

iii. *Muscles and joints:* Trismus (limited jaw opening) may develop as the result of radiotherapy of temporomandibular joint (TMJ) area. Generally, trismus develops within three to six months after radiotherapy. Trismus is attributed to muscle fibrosis and scarring in response to radiations as well as to fibrosis of the ligaments around the TMJ. The limited jaw opening interferes with oral hygiene, speech and nutritional intake. The dental treatment also becomes difficult.

iv. *Bone:* The effect of radiations on the bone matrix is relatively slow. Whether the altered bone remodelling activity is the result of direct irradiation injury to the cells or the indirect result of irradiation-induced vascular injury, or a combination of both has not been documented. The initial changes in bone may be the result from injury to the remodelling system (osteoblasts are usually more radio-sensitive than osteoclasts). One of the major complications of bone irradiation is osteoradionecrosis (bone death secondary to radiotherapy). The incidence of osteoradionecrosis of the mandible is much higher than that of the maxilla (because mandible is less vascular than maxilla).

The sequence of changes in osteoradio-necrosis is:

- The ability of bone to replace normal collagen loss or normal cellular loss is severely compromised because of hypoxia, hypocellularity and hypo-vasularity of tissue.
- Collagen lysis and cell death exceed synthesis and cellular replication
- In non-healing wound, the oxygen and the metabolic demands exceed the supply.

v. *Salivary gland:* The quantity and composition of saliva gets affected after radiotherapy. The radiation causes direct damage to the secretory and ductal cells of salivary gland tissue. Four phases of changes have been recognized. The first phase (0–10 days) is characterized by a rapid decline in flow rate without changes in amylase secretion or acinar cell number. The second phase (10–60 days) shows decrease in amylase secretion. The third phase (60–120 days) exhibits the same flow rate, acinar cell number and amylase secretion. The fourth phase (120–240 days) demonstrates further deterioration of gland function.

Radiation results in reduction in amount of saliva as well as change in its composition. Saliva turns into a very viscous, yellow, or brown fluid. The average pH decreases from about 7.0 to 5.0. The buffering capacity is reduced which may be due to the reduction of bicarbonate concentration especially in parotid saliva.

The radiation-induced hyposalivation leads to:

- Dryness of the mouth.
- Burning sensation.
- Difficulties in oral functioning.
- Alterations of mucous membranes.
- Difficulties in accepting artificial prosthesis.
- Changes in the quantity of oral microflora.
- Oral discomfort, especially during night
- Mucus accumulation.
- Periodontal disease.
- Radiation caries.

vi. *Periodontium:* Radiations may lead to decreased vascularity, thickening and disorientation of Sharpey's fibres of the periodontal ligament. The cementum appears completely acellular and its capacity for repair and regeneration is severely compromised. The risk of periodontal infection is increased due to hyposalivation, increased plaque accumulation and shift in oral microflora.

vii. *Dentition:* Radiations effect the development and eruption of teeth. If the radiation precedes the morphodifferentiation and calcification, tooth bud may be destroyed. Irradiation at later stage may alter cellular differentiation causing malformation or arrested growth.

Effects of radiation on developing teeth: The effects of radiations on developing teeth include microdontia, delayed tooth formation, altered morphology of teeth, shortness and tapering of teeth,

narrowing of pulp spaces and widening of periodontal ligament.

Effects of radiation on developed teeth: Radiations lead to changes in organic components of dentin promoting instability in dentino-enamel junction, subsequently may lose its capacity to support enamel. The decrease in circulation to pulp tissue after radiation may lead to pulpal fibrosis, hyalinization and calcification.

Many patients after radiotherapy experience an increased sensitivity to sweet and temperature changes. This might be related to the loss of the protective layer of saliva (because enamel acts as a semi-permeable membrane that allows the passage of fluids and salivary content is not able to plug the channels).

RADIATION CARIES

The most common complication of radiation of head and neck region is radiation-related caries. Radiation caries is a highly destructive form of dental caries which has a rapid onset and progression. Dental caries become evident within three months following the initiation of radiotherapy.

Besides the rapid onset and progression, radiation caries is most commonly found on tooth surfaces that are relatively immune to dental caries. The areas just below the contact points usually are not affected by radiation caries. Furthermore, the mandibular anterior teeth (normally resistant to caries), are equally affected by radiation caries (Fig. 18.1).

Etiology and Pathogenesis of Radiation Caries

The mechanisms involved are as follows:

A. Direct effect of radiations on tooth tissues
   a. Effect of radiations on enamel.
   b. Effect of radiations on dentin.
   c. Effect of radiations on pulp.

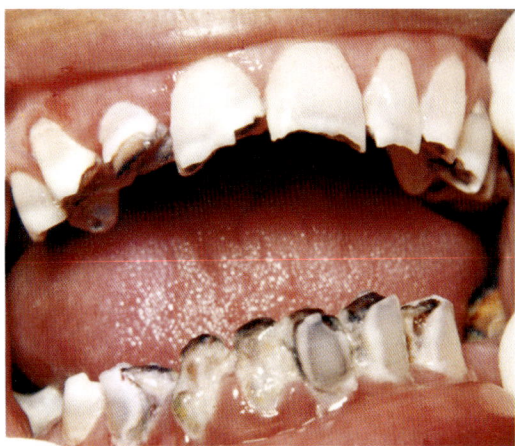

Fig. 18.1: Radiation caries involving both maxillary and mandibular teeth. Note the eroded and worn-out incisal surfaces

B. Indirect effect of radiations on other tissues.

    a. Altered salivary glands secretions.

    b. Deficient oral hygiene.

A. Direct Effect of Radiations on Tooth Tissues

Radiations affect almost all tissues of teeth. 31.5 Gy of radiation is sufficient for the destruction of collagen fibres present in the enamel, dentin and pulp. The effects can be described as follows:

a. *Effect of radiation on enamel:* Enamel becomes less resistant to acid attack. Application of fluorides can substitute hydroxyl ions, making fluorapatite, which is less susceptible to dissolution. The prismatic structures of enamel are lost after irradiation. The organic matrix interacts with apatite crystals leading to electrostatic binding of collagen. The fluorapatite crystal matrix decreases the space filled by the organic matrix which is affected by radiation. The dentin is not altered by the fluorides is the common belief. The application of sodium fluoride showed elevated fluoride levels in the dentin layers, especially the intertubular diffusion of fluoride into dentin, where more organic matrix is present.

b. *Effect of radiation on dentin:* The dentino-enamel junction, the natural connector between enamel and dentin plays a critical role in maintaining the biomechanical integrity of the tooth. Changes in the organic components of dentin may lead to instability at the dentino-enamel junction, thereby making the dentin unable to support enamel.

Radiotherapy activates organic proteins within the dentin matrix causing degradation of the collagen fibril network that connects dentin to enamel leading to enamel fracture. As the enamel is lost, (partially or totally), the underlying dentin is then exposed to the oral cavity, leading to bacterial and enzymatic degradation.

Dentin contains sufficient amount of water, which generally increases at dentino-enamel junction. Water exhibits several chemical reactions to absorption of radiations leading to formation of free radicals. The free hydrogen radicals denatures the organic components of teeth. Organic molecules such as collagen fibres can be held partly responsible for the binding of enamel and dentin. Radiations destroy the organic matrix, compromising the anchoring between enamel and dentin. It also reduces the inner stability of dentin. Chlorhexidine binds specifically to the collagen fibrils and maintain the morpho-logical properties of dentin and prevent degradation of its collagen.

c. *Effects of radiations on pulp:* Radiations destroy the collagen within the pulp leading to fibrosis and decreased vascularity, thereby impairing the odontoblastic metabolism. The dentin tubules are obliterated, preceded by a degeneration of the odontoblast processes. The overall decrease in the circulation of pulp may promote caries initiation.

B. Indirect Effects of Radiations on Other Tissues

a. *Altered salivary gland secretions:* Radiation has definite effect on the salivary glands. The saliva becomes thicker/viscous leading to difficulties in chewing and speaking. In irradiated patients, alterations in salivary composition include changes in its antibacterial properties and ionic concentration, with consequent reductions of buffering capacity and the pH. The average post-irradiation pH falls from about 7.0 to 5.0, which is definitively cariogenic. The buffering capacity of saliva is responsible for increasing pH and switching the demineralization/remineralization equilibrium towards remineralization. Because of the lowered pH and buffering capacity, the minerals of enamel and dentin can easily dissolve following radiotherapy. Artificial saliva can manage tissue lubrication, hydration, pH neutralization; however, it may not affect the colonization by cariogenic micro-organisms. The use of artificial saliva proves promising against radiation induced xerostomia but its efficacy in preventing radiation caries remains debatable.

b. *Deficient oral hygiene:* The side effects of radiations such as mucositis, etc. contribute to changes in the oral environment which indirectly effect food intake. The nutrition status is further deteriorated because of pain during mastication and swallowing, loss of appetite, nausea and physical discomfort. The change in taste may affect susceptibility to caries, since intake of carbohydrates is usually increased.

Radiation Caries and Shift of Microflora

Radiation-induced xerostomia is accompanied by pronounced shifts in specific microflora; whereas total bacterial concentrations remained relatively unchanged. There may be increase in *Streptococcus mutans, Lactobacillus species, Candida* (primarily *C. albicans*) and Staphylococci and decrease in *S. sanguis, Neisseria* species and *Fusobacterium.* The loss of the buffering, antibacterial, lubricating and cleansing properties of saliva, coupled with

rearrangement of the food consumption patterns of the patients treated with radiotherapy lead to such changes.

Pattern of Radiation Caries

Radiation caries is most commonly observed on tooth surfaces that are relatively immune to dental caries. The areas just below the contact points might be least affected. Furthermore, the mandibular anterior teeth, normally most resistant to caries are equally affected by radiation caries. Incisors were the predominant teeth (42%) followed by molars (31%) and canines (17%). Brown discolorations are mandatory signs in irradiated patients and should be considered and treated as incipient caries.

Clinically, three different patterns of caries lesions have been identified. One, two or all the patterns can be observed within the same individual. Rarely any acute pain is associated with radiation caries; even in severe manifestations, though the progress is rapid.

1st pattern: The first pattern is a frequently observed lesion that starts at the cervical third of the labial surface of incisors and canines. Initially, the lesion extends superficially around the entire cervical area of the tooth and then progresses inward. It may involve the complete crown. In molars, involvement of complete crown is rare; however, the caries tend to spread over all surfaces. The tooth may become friable and break.

2nd pattern: The second pattern exhibits generalized superficial defect that first affects the buccal surface followed by affecting the lingual/palatal surfaces on the tooth crowns. The proximal surfaces are less affected. The lesion begins as a diffuse and punctuate effect, progressing to generalized, irregular erosion of the tooth surfaces. The decay is usually localized at the incisal or occlusal edges.

3rd pattern: The third pattern is less frequently observed. It exhibits heavy brown-black discoloration of the entire tooth crown, accompanied by wearing away of the incisal and occlusal surfaces.

DENTAL MANAGEMENT AFTER HEAD AND NECK RADIOTHERAPY

The head and neck cancer patient should be managed with clearly defined goals. The goals are categorized into the following three phases:

a. Phase I: Pre-treatment Goals

- Counsel patient about complications of radiotherapy.
- Control potential sources of infection.
- Provide preventive modalities.

b. Phase II: Goals during Cancer Therapy

- Manage mucus membrane inflammation.
- Manage xerostomia and its implications.
- Prevent trismus.

c. Phase III: Post-treatment (long-term) Goals

- Care of xerostomic patients.
- Prevent trismus and manage trismus related problems.
- Manage radiation related caries.
- Prevent post-radiation osteonecrosis.
- Early detection of recurrence, if any.

Preventive Dental Care

The patient likely to receive radiotherapy or under treatment should be examined frequently to reduce the risk and severity of oral complications. Full mouth X-rays are adjunct to clinical examination. Oral hygiene is monitored in routine. The dentition, periodontium and oral soft tissues are also examined frequently. The preventive features during and after radiotherapy are:

  i. Stents are used to shield the lateral side when unilateral radiotherapy is required. Another technique, which limits radiation to salivary gland is intensity modulated irradiation technique (IMRT). This technique targets the lesion while sparing the major salivary glands from radiation. These measures minimize xerostomia and other related problems.

  ii. The residual salivary flow is stimulated by gustatory, mechanical or pharmaceutical means. Salivary substitutes can also be used. Sugar-free gums may be used to stimulate salivary flow. Addition of xylitol to chewing gum can also be beneficial in preventive caries.

  iii. Artificial saliva helps in tissue lubrication, hydration, salivary clearance and pH neutralization. It is also capable of inhibiting the bacterial growth and stabilizing the oral environment. Inorganic ions such as calcium, phosphates and fluorides, when added to artificial saliva reduce the solubility of apatite, subsequently preventing caries.

  iv. Systemic sialogogues can also be used to stimulate salivary flow, thereby reducing the risk of radiation caries. Systemic medications may induce potential adverse reactions and the effect may be lost once the drug is withdrawn. Systemic therapy should only be initiated in patients with high caries risk and severe hyposalivation.

  v. Patient should be encouraged to maintain an adequate fluid intake and keep oral cavity hydrated to prevent secondary infections.

  vi. Tongue coatings in xerostomic patients impair the taste. The tongue should be cleaned two or three times daily using bicarbonate soda solution (1–2 tsp(s) of baking soda and ½ tsp of salt with one quarter of water) followed by plain water rinse.

  vii. Alcohol should be avoided; may have irritating effects.

  viii. Along with routine tooth brushing, patients may be advised to use chlorhexidine gluconate rinse to suppress bacterial colonization. Sticky foods such as chocolates and pastries should be avoided. Sugar-free candies can also be used.

ix. Patient's medication regime should be adjusted keeping in view the timings of decline in salivary flow (usually at night). So taking a medication that reduces flow in the morning or dividing medication doses may improve oral comfort and reduce xerostomia.

x. Topical fluoride application helps in the prevention of radiation caries. The presence of fluoride ions enhances the teeth's ability to uptake calcium and phosphate ions; however, fluorides rinse do not provide adequate protection from demineralization. Acidulated forms of fluorides have the advantage of increased uptake by surface enamel; however, low pH may result in significant mucosal irritation, burning pain, erythema and ulceration. Neutral (sodium fluoride) or slightly acidic forms of fluoride gel are preferred, since they are well tolerated by patients.

xi. Casein derivatives alongwith calcium phosphate can also be used in routine.

Therapeutic Dental Care

Pre-radiation Care

The patients likely to receive radiotherapy be educated and motivated as regard to probable complications of the treatment.

A thorough dental prophylaxis should be performed. The patient should be motivated to follow preventive home care instructions. Conservative restorations are preferred, avoiding indirect restorations. Fixed prosthesis is substituted with removable ones, thereby diminishing the likelihood of recurrent caries.

Teeth with questionable prognosis are preferably extracted. Questionable prognosis includes:

- Advanced caries lesions with questionable pulpal involvement.
- Extensive periapical lesions.
- Advanced periodontal/bone loss and/or furcation involvement.

- Impacted or incompletely erupted teeth, particularly third molars that are not fully covered by alveolar bone.
- Teeth close to tissues being irradiated.

These teeth should be extracted at least two weeks prior to radiotherapy to allow for proper healing, so that during radiotherapy there should be no naked sockets.

Post-radiation Care

The irradiation can result in mucositis, candidiasis, xerostomia with difficulties in speaking, eating and swallowing, subsequently caries. The shift in cariogenic micro-organisms leads to the rapid progress of carious lesions. The poor oral hygiene consequent to oral discomfort and/or trismus may help in caries progression.

Managing caries: Use of topical fluorides in combination with remineralizing pastes and chewing gum is helpful in controlling the progress of caries. If the lesion is limited, it may not require placement of a temporary restoration, otherwise temporary restoration be placed after excavating the caries. Once caries has been controlled, the temporary restorative material is replaced with permanent restoration. Amalgam is preferred since these restorations can be extended if recurrent decay develops. Also, amalgam restorations are less sensitive to moisture contamination.

During cavity preparation moisture control is less than optimal due to difficulty in controlling gingival hemorrhage. In small lesions glass ionomer cements may be preferred. Fluoride releasing glass-ionomers or fluoride application prior to restoration can be helpful. Casein phosphopeptide-amorphous calcium phosphate nanocomplexes have been incorporated in glass-ionomers to enhance the remineralizing ability of teeth. Erosion due to low pH induced by hyposalivation is the main drawback of glass-ionomers. The erosion is due to formation of hydrofluoric acid (fluorides released from GIC and H^+ ions from saliva).

Due to extensiveness of caries, unsupported enamel may not be removed. Pulp capping is not recommended due to the poor reparative potential of the irradiated dental pulp. Trauma of any kind, especially trauma of gingival tissues is avoided during treatment.

In large class V restorations, restore approximately one half of the gingival area at the first appointment and restore the remaining gingival portion subsequently. Clinically, the lesion at the base of the crown (wrap around caries) which often results in amputation of the crown is the most difficult to treat.

The teeth with radiation caries may and may not respond to pulp vitality testing. Vitality is a matter of blood supply and not of nerve innervations. Because nerves are the most radiation-resistant tissues and pulpal nerve endings arise from cells in the gasserian ganglion, the tooth with radiation caries may have a responsive pulp; however, it behaves non-vital due to necrosis of the vascular pulpal tissues.

In case of pulpitis, root canal treatment under antibiotic coverage is considered. Periapical radiolucency may not get resolved because of decreased bone vitality.

Root canal treatment can be carried out safely in patients undergoing radiotherapy. There has been no incidence of osteoradionecrosis resulting from root canal treatment. If the dose to bone is above 55 Gy, endodontic therapy is a viable alternative to extraction because it minimizes the risk of bone exposure.

Isolation with rubber dam is difficult due to extensive caries. Throat screen is commonly used. The root canal files, etc. should have thread for easy retrieval because oropharyngeal refluxes are compromised after radiation. When access is limited by trismus, files can be bent to increase the working space. Coronal amputation can also be helpful in locating and preparing root canals. Short files are better than long files to prevent the trauma of periapical tissue. If extraction is contraindicated, then crown is amputated at or below the gingival level before or after the endodontic treatment. Later the coronal end is filled with appropriate material to prevent the leakage.

Bibliography

1. Andrews N and Griffiths C. Dental complications of head and neck radiotherapy: Part 2. Aust. Dent. J.: 2001;46:174–82.
2. Bonan PR, Pires FR, Lopes MA and Di Hipolioto, O. Jr.. Evaluation of salivary flow in patients during head and neck radiotherapy. Braz. Oral Res.: 2003;17:156–60.
3. Brown LR, Dreizen S, Handler S and Johnston DA. Effect of radiation induced xerostomia on human oral microflora. J. Dent. Res.: 1975;54:740–50.
4. Chambers MS, Mellberg JR, Keene HJ, Bouwsma OJ, Garden AS, Sipos T and Fleming TJ. Clinical evaluation of the intraoral fluoride releasing system in radiation-induced xerostomic subjects. Part 2: Phase I study. Oral Oncol.: 2006;42:946–53.
5. Davis WB. Reduction in dentin wear resistance by irradiation and effects of storage in aqueous media. J. Dent. Res.: 1975;54:1078–81.
6. Deng J, Jackson L, Epstein JB, Migliorati CA and Murphy BA. Dental demineralization and caries in patients with head and neck cancer. Oral Oncol. 2015, S1368-8735(15)00256-0
7. Eliasson L, Carlen A, Almstal A, Wikstrom M and Singstrom P. Dental plaque pH and micro-organisms during hyposalivation. J. Dent. Res.: 2006;85:334–8.
8. Gabrielle PA, Bruno CJ, Claudia SM, Luis GS and Addah RF. A review of the biological and clinical aspects of radiation caries. J. Contemp. Dent. Pract.: 2009;10:1–10.
9. Goho C. Chemoradiation therapy: effect on dental development. Pediat. Dent.: 1993;15:6–12.
10. Hannig M, Dounis E, Henning T, Apitz N and Stoser L. Does irradiation affect the protein composition of saliva? Clin. Oral Investig.: 2006;10:61–5.
11. Heimdahl A. Prevention and management of oral infections in cancer patients. Support Care Cancer: 1999;7:224–8.

12. Kielbassa AM, Beetz I, Schendera A and Elmar H. Irradiation effects on microhardness of fluoridated and non-fluoridated bovine dentin. Eur. J. Oral Sci.: 1997;105:444–7.

13. Kielbassa AM, Attin T, Schaller HG and Hellwig E. Endodontic therapy in a post irradiated child: Review of the literature and report of a case. Quint. Int.: 1995;26:405.

14. Lee DP, Espejo-Trung LC, Simionato MRL, Alves FA, Novelli MD and Luz MAA. The effects of ionizing radiation on the development of human caries lesions *in vitro*. Clin. Lab. Res. Den.: 2014;20:46.

15. Meng L, Liu J, Penq B, Fan M, Nie M, Chen Z, Gan Y and Bian Z. The persistence of *Streptococcus mutans* in nasopharyngeal carcinoma patients after radiotherapy. Caries Res.: 2005;39:484–9.

16. Narmin M, Seyendnejad F, Oskoee PA, Oskoee SS and Chaharom MEE. Evaluation of radiation-induced class V dental caries in patients with head and neck cancers undergoing radiotherapy. JORDD: 2008;2:82–4.

17. Pamela JH, Joel BE and Sadler GR. Oral and dental management related to radiation therapy for head and neck cancer. J. Can. Dent. Assoc.: 2003;69:585–90.

18. Papas A, Russell D, Singh M, Kent R, Triol C and Winston A. A caries clinical trial of a remineralizing toothpaste in radiation patients. Gerodontology: 2008;25:76–88.

19. Pioch T, Golfels D and Staehle HJ. An experimental study of the stability of irradiated teeth in the region of the dentino-enamel junction. Endod. Dent. Traumatol.: 1992;8:241–4.

20. Seto BG, Beumer J, Kagawa T, Klokkevold P and Wolinsky L. Analysis of endodontic therapy in patients irradiated for head and neck cancer. Oral Surg., Oral Med., Oral Pathol.: 1985;60:540.

21. Silva ARS, Alves FA. Antunes A, Goes MF and Lopes MA. Patterns of demineralization and dentin reactions in radiation-related caries. Caries Res.: 2009;43:43–9.

22. Souza MR, Watanabe I, Azevedo LH and Tanji EY. Morphological alterations of the surfaces of enamel and dentin of deciduous teeth irradiated with Nd:YAG, CO_2 and diode lasers. Int. J. Morphol.: 2009;27:441–6.

23. Spack CJ, Johnson G and Ekstrand J. Caries incidence, salivary flow rate and fluoride gel treatment in irradiated patients. Caries Res.: 1994;28:388–93.

24. Springer IN, Niehoff P, Warnke PH, Bocek G, Kovacs G, Suhr M, Wiltfanq J and Acil Y. Radiation caries -radiogenic destruction of dental collagen. Oral Oncol.: 2005;41, 723-8.

25. Turssi CP, Lima RQ, Faraoni-Romano JJ and Serra MC. Rehardening of caries-like lesions in root surfaces by saliva substitutes. Geodontology: 2006;23:226–30.

26. Vissink A, Jansma J, Spijkervet FK, Burlage FR and Coppes RP. Oral sequelae of head and neck radiotherapy. Crit. Rev. Ora Biol. Med.: 2003;14: 199–212.

27. Vuotila T, Ylikontiola L, Sorsa T, Luoto HJ, Hanemaaijer R, Salo T and Tjaderhane L. The relationship between MMPs and pH in whole saliva of radiated head and neck cancer patients. J. Oral Pathol. Med.: 2002;31:329–38.

28. Whitmyer CC, Waskowski JC and Iffland HA. Radiotherapy and oral sequelae: preventive and management protocols. J. Dent. Hyg.: 1997;71: 23–9.

19

Future of Cariology

Dental caries is disease that has affected the mankind since its evolution. There has been a plethora of changes in its detection strategies, prevention principles and management approaches. Dental caries has always been the subject of interest amongst clinicians, teachers and researchers. The worldwide emphasis is on to prevent this wide spreading disease so as to minimize its overall detrimental effects. The researchers are conceiving newer strategies to change the behavior of children and adults as well towards preventive measures to make the future generations caries-free. Is it really possible to achieve this goal—is still a question. Over the years our knowledge as regard to microbiology and the factors associated with causation of caries has improved; however, detecting caries at its inception or even prior to it needs improvement. The factors involved in caries process is summarized in Fig. 19.1.

The global caries initiative, conceived in 2008 was mainly to address the global public health challenges of dental caries. After a couple of deliberations in association with federation of dental education, the outcomes of the initiative are:

- Prioritization of 0–3 years age group children.
- Eradication of early childhood caries.
- Prioritizing preventive protocols and health promotion for caries management.

- Need for consensus for caries terminology.
- Need to establish a common language for caries classification and management protocol.

Caries Diagnosis

Caries diagnosis is one of the most important and basic skills that dental professionals must learn and be thorough with. Caries diagnosis has traditionally been carried out using visuo-tactile methods and radiographs have been used as an adjunct to its diagnosis. However, with the change in our understanding about the caries progression, there has been a thrust on the detection of caries in its most incipient stages [white spot lesions]. The use of modern diagnostic tools has also ushered to detect caries in its incipient stages.

These modern diagnostic tools are based on a simple principle that there occurs a detectable change in the physical properties of the early carious enamel as compared to the sound tooth. The pores formed due to early caries alter the electrical, optical and fluorescence properties of enamel and this deviation is usually detected by these modern diagnostic tools. These can be categorized as fluorescence-based diagnostic tools like QLF, DIAGNOdent, etc. Tools based on measuring the difference in electrical conductivity include Electronic Caries Meter (ECM) and its

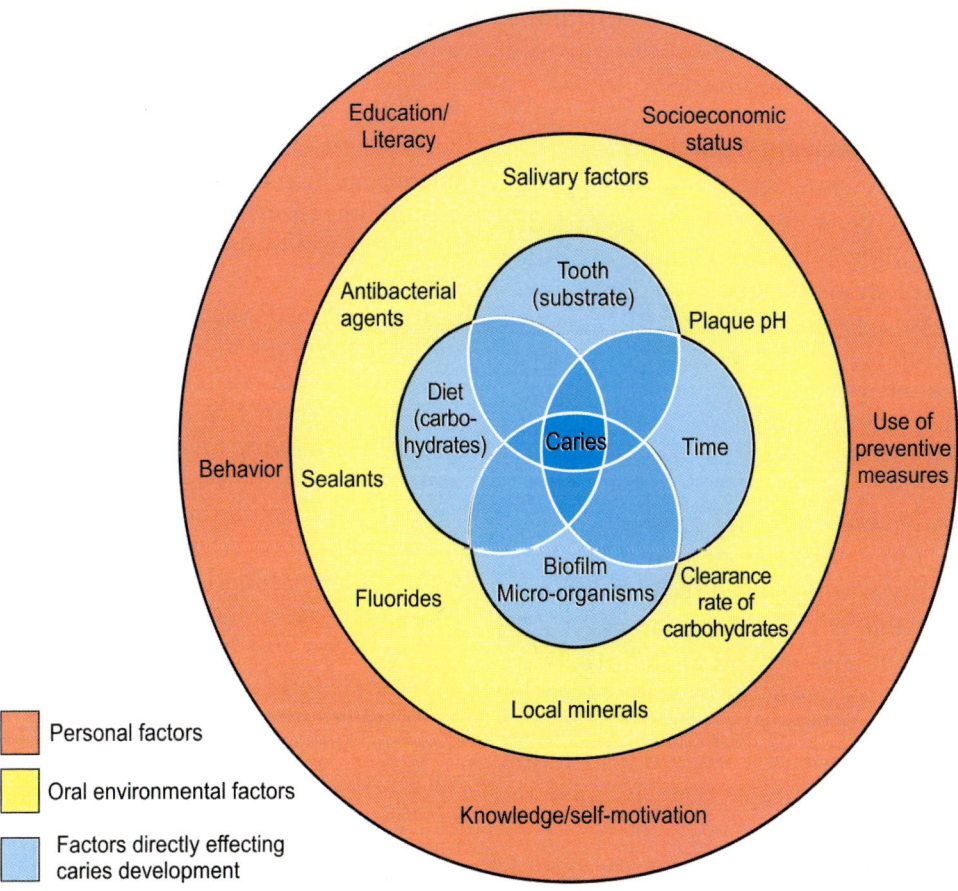

Fig. 19.1: Factors involved in caries process

modified forms etc. while the optical based instruments include FOTI, DIFOTI, DIAGNOcam, etc.

However, all these tools have shown a limited success rate and the future holds in improvement of such diagnostic tools which will have high sensitivity and specificity, cost effectiveness and easy to use. The day is not far when the caries detection tools will be able to detect caries in its most incipient stages and also longitudinally monitor the progression and regression of the lesions.

Research is continuously improving the fluorescence-based equipment. A novel device available as hand held attachment for an SLR camera is quantitative light induced fluorescent digital bi-illuminator (QLF-D). This is an upgraded version of QLF device

(Inspektor research systems, Netherlands) which is also based on photo-fluorescence of teeth. It not only helps to detect mineral loss due to early caries (depicted as loss of green fluorescence) but is also able to detect endogenous porphyrins produced by oral bacteria (depicted as red fluorescence) and thus is helpful in predicting the future caries risk. Researchers are trying to apply the infrared technology to detect early caries.

One of the other techniques that is on the verge of breakthrough is optical coherence tomography (OCT). It is a non-ionizing imaging technique that can produce cross-section images of biological tissues. It has been established that the OCT images can be correlated with the degree of demineralization and lesion severity. The future use of OCT may lead to hand held devices that would be helpful in detecting primary caries as well as caries beneath the restorations.

Recording/Classifying Dental Caries

Traditionally only the cavitated carious lesions have been detected and recorded in literature. However, the change in understanding of etiopathogenesis of dental caries has led to detect and record the caries in continuum. Over the years a number of classification systems have been composed to detect and record both cavitated and non-cavitated caries. Due to the heterogeneity in the previous systems, a new system which is universally acceptable and designed to meet the needs of epidemiology, clinical research and practice was proposed recently.

This system is called International Caries Detection and Assessment System (ICDAS). It records the caries in all its stages (starting from white spot lesion to pulpal exposures). The caries is recorded in continuum, including the recording of caries at non-cavitated and cavitated stages.

Recently, the ICDAS caries detection/recording system has been extended to include objective decision making for caries treatment. This new system is International Caries Classification and Management System (ICCMS). This system seeks to improve decision making and enable improved long-term caries outcomes.

The International Caries Classification and Management System (ICCMS) deliberately incorporated a range of options designed to accommodate the needs of different users across the ICDAS domains of clinical practice, dental education, research and public health.

There are four ICCMS elements, which depict that caries management pathway is cyclical as each element follows in turn. The cycle restarts after each risk based recall interval.

The future holds in widespread usage of such objective classification systems that allow the dentists to take a similar decision, in any given situation.

Remineralizing Agents

The caries-prevention protocols should encourage use of agents affecting the de-/remineralization balance so as to promote the remineralization and reversal of non-cavitated lesions.

In recent years there has been thrust on the use of remineralization agents that aims upon increasing bio-availability of calcium and phosphate onto the tooth surface. As the dentistry is moving towards detection of early carious lesions, there is a need to promote the usage of remineralizing agents.

Fluoride has always been a pivot for remineralization and prevention of caries. It has also shown great success both in reducing dental caries and in promoting the reversal of early lesions.

Various agents have been and are being used to achieve remineralization. The one such preparation, milk-derived CPP-ACP, is a widely used formulation, in which the milk has been modified to form nanocomplexes that are then applied intraorally. This has been shown to remineralize the incipient caries.

The CPP-ACP complexes are stable in the presence of fluoride and have been shown to inhibit demineralization and promote remineralization in a range of clinical trials, *in-situ* models and in *in-vitro* studies.

A new functionalized β-tricalcium phosphate (β-TCP) has shown promise by increasing remineralization when used along with fluorides. In contrast to other calcium-based approaches that seem to rely on high levels of calcium and phosphate to drive remineralization, β-TCP is a low dose system designed to fit within existing topical fluoride preparations.

These agents are not alternative to fluoride, given the significant actions of this ion; however, it must be remembered that the limiting factor for remineralization of existing lesions will be calcium availability.

Ozone, a gas composed of three atoms of oxygen, acts by attacking thiol groups of cysteine amino acid and destroys the cellular membrane of carious bacteria. Ozone allows remineralization by shifting microflora from acidogenic and aciduric micro-organisms to normal commensals. Heal Ozone, a remineralizing solution containing xylitol, fluoride, calcium and phosphate is currently used for caries prevention (2100 ppm ozone + 5% flow rate of 615 cc/minute when used for 60 seconds can produce antibacterial effect against *Streptococcus mutans* even after eight weeks).

Theobromine, a recently introduced remineralizing agent, is a white crystalline powder, an alkaloid readily available in cocoa (240 mg/cup) and chocolate (1.89%). Theobromine is an active ingredient in Rennou™, the patented chocolate extract used in Theodent toothpastes. Rennou increases the size of the surface unit crystals of enamel by four times. Larger unit crystals make teeth less susceptible to bacterial acid demineralization. Kargul, et al (2012) and Amaechi (2013) have suggested that Theobromine can be used as an effective remineralizing agent. They also proposed Theobromine, a nontoxic compound, as an alternative to fluoride with its cariostatic role via induced large crystal formation and increased microhardness of the enamel surface (comparable to that of fluoride).

Toothpastes containing n-Hap (nano-hydroxy-apatite) has revealed better remineralizing effects as compared to amine fluoride toothpastes, both in dentin and enamel.

The widespread use of remineralization agents is on the cards; which would be fast acting, least dependent on patient compliance, reverse the lesions and mask the opacities.

Micro-invasive Dentistry

This era is of minimal invasive dentistry; however, the current modalities for the treatment of early lesions are either invasive or non-invasive in nature. The non-invasive therapies should be preferred, but due to dependency on patient's compliance and incomplete success rates, use of such strategies is restricted.

In the recent past, the concept of Resin infiltration (ICON, DMG Germany) has been introduced which is an attempt to abolish gap between the non-operative and operative modalities. This treatment optically blends lesion with healthy enamel. Resin infiltration is a micro-invasive technique that fills, reinforces and stabilizes demineralized enamel without drilling or sacrificing healthy tooth structure.

Partial and Stepwise Caries Removal *vs* No Caries Removal

The management of dental caries has traditionally involved removal of all soft demineralized dentin prior to restoration. However, the benefits of complete caries removal have been questioned because of concerns about the possible adverse effects of removing all soft dentin from the affected tooth. Three groups of studies have challenged the protocol of complete caries removal and recommended the sealing of dentinal caries using three different techniques. The first technique removes caries in stages (two visits, some months apart), allowing time to the pulp to lay down reparative dentin (the stepwise excavation technique). The second removes part of the dentinal caries and seals the residual caries into the tooth permanently (partial caries removal) and the third technique does not remove dentinal caries prior to sealing or restoring (no dentinal caries removal).

Sealing infected demineralized dentin with a restoration that provides a good peripheral seal, deprives the micro-organisms of nutrients from the oral cavity. The bacteria reduce in numbers and the caries process arrests. Not only do the bacteria reduce in numbers, but also the microbial diversity becomes less complex. It is established that only those micro-organisms capable of breaking down glycoproteins of pulpal tissue are able to survive. A couple of other authors [Fejerskov and Kidd (2008), Thompson (2008)] have supported this theory.

The progressive reduction in the number of micro-organisms and a change to a less cariogenic microflora within sealed carious dentin, leads to a gradual reduction in lesion activity and hence lesion progression. This allows time for the pulp-dentin complex to laydown tertiary dentin and peri-tubular dentin leading to tubular sclerosis and reduces the permeability of the remaining dentin. This reduction in pulpal exudate further depletes the nutrient source for the bacteria. In stepwise excavation, the provisional restoration is removed after a period of time to allow further caries removal. The tertiary dentin formed within that time provides further protection to the pulp. Avoidance of carious pulpal exposures is critical to the long term outcome of the success, as management of such exposures is generally associated with a poor prognosis for maintaining a vital pulp.

Partial caries or no dentinal caries removal techniques also have the potential to reduce cavity size and hence preserve tooth structure. However, a consequence of such techniques is that the restoration does not have a sound foundation. The modality is still debated, although it may not be an important issue, especially in the long term for primary teeth as they exfoliate.

Computer-assisted FACE for Minimal-invasive Caries Excavation

Over the years, methods using light-induced fluorescence have effectively detected bacteria remaining in the tooth's hard tissues. However, methods controlling the complete removal of infected dentin have not been validated. Ganter, et al (2014) evaluated the degree of carious dentin excavated using a camera and software-based device as a guide for fluorescence-aided caries excavation

(FACE) in comparison to visual-tactile inspection and a dye-staining method and observed FACE to be a better modality.

Despite the paradigm of minimal-invasive dentistry, the degree of dentin that has to be removed from a cavity is still a matter of discussion and it is still an unsolved problem for the practitioner.

The future holds in having knowledge about 'when to stop excavation'. The operators have been using subjective parameters like color, consistency and texture as a guide to stop the excavation. However, the future is of 'objective parameters' like fluorescence tools, improved caries detector dyes, etc. The future might not be of restorative dentistry, but definitely is of conservative. These conservative excavation procedure are in accordance with the principles of minimal invasive dentistry, the need of the future.

Nanotechnology

Nanotechnology has promoted the development of bio-inspired routes for caries prevention and biomimetic strategies for enamel repair. The biomimetic nano-technological approaches (biomimetic carbonate hydroxyl apatite nano-particles) for caries therapy are available. Many approaches have been tested *in-vitro*; however, clinical validation is still lacking. Analysis of recent *in-vitro* data indicates that apatite nano-particles might be quite effective in reversing lesion progression in the outer part of artificial white-spot lesions; whereas, remineralizing effects in the deeper areas of the caries lesions seem doubtful.

Nanomaterials are being used in biofilm management (carried out by products that contain bioinspired apatite nanoparticles). Nanomaterials are tried in biomimetic synthesis of enamel and repair of microcavities (amelogenin and β sheet peptide based upon glutamic acid and glutamine help increase remineralization).

The clinical applications of the nano-technological approaches for caries management are not yet conceivable. A facile and controllable strategy to develop apatite nanorods into large-size prism-like structures similar to that of human enamel still remains a major challenge for biomimetic synthesis of enamel.

In the future, nanodentistry may provide comprehensive oral care by employing tissue engineering, biomaterials and ultimately nanorobotics. The researchers are trying to simulate the natural biomineralization process to create the hardest tissues in the body, the enamel, by using organized units of nanorod-like calcium hydroxyapatite crystals arranged approximately parallel to each other.

Genetic Factor and Dental Caries

'Inheritance' of traits from the ancestor and modification of traits to suit the changing environment called 'evolution' is the process, which is controlled by the genes. It is established that dental caries is associated with genetic factors. This disease or its susceptibility can be inherited from the ancestor through genes. One more dimension of complexity is associated with caries; however, it also provides another dimension through which this disease can be controlled or prevented. Research can be aligned with gene modifications and gene therapies to prevent the occurrences of dental caries. As oral microflora is the dominant factor in determining the different levels of caries cavity, more genetic researches are oriented towards altering the genetic activities of the caries pathogens.

It has also been found that saliva contains acidic and basic proline-rich proteins (PRPs). The PRP alleles are located in each of six genes of chromosome 12. There is considerable evidence for the basic PRPs providing a genetic element of protection from caries susceptibility as their allelic phenotypes have a three-fold greater frequency in caries-free adults than in those with severe caries. These proteins can attach to acid-producing streptococci and neutralize their acid production from carbohydrates *in situ*. Levine (2011) suggested that sequencing the exons of the PRP genes along with those for cathepsin H and cystatins C and S is practicable and may ultimately provide a new method for identifying young children susceptible to caries.

Oral bacteria are also genetically engineered to produce alkali environment. Strains of streptococci are altered to produce alkali, which play a vital role in pH homeostasis in oral biofilms, subsequently effecting caries progression.

Keep 32—A New Molecule

Chilean researchers, after a decade long research, have found a molecule that could significantly reduce tooth decay. The molecule is named 'Keep 32', because incorporating into toothpastes and dental care products may help reduce cavities and keep all 32 teeth healthy.

Streptococcus mutans, the main culprit in caries process, is resistant to removal by conventional methods. The potential for reduction in caries can be excellent as this particular species be eliminated or made biologically inactive. In rare instances this bacteria can enter blood stream, subsequently leading to endocarditis (heart valves inflammation). So, it becomes furthermore necessary to manage *Streptococcus mutans*.

The researchers are continuously monitoring the effect of this molecule. Initial findings indicate that the molecule can eliminate *Streptococcus mutans* in 60 seconds, thereby reducing caries and cavities.

The Keep-32 molecule is still in its developing stage. It may take another couple of months before the product can be cleared for incorporation into dental products, such as toothpaste, mouthwash and chewing gum.

Camellia sinensis and Caries

Three major types of tea are derived by boiling *Camellia sinensis* leaves (green, black and oolong). The catechin compound found in these leaves has the potent antioxidant effect. A couple of other flavinoids, viz. saponins, have also been extracted from these leaves.

A cup of green tea contains three times as many catechins than a cup of black tea. Oolong tea is in between the two. Green and black tea leaves have been found to prevent salivary amylase in *Streptococcus mutans*. The catechins in black tea *epigallocatechin gallate (EGCG)* are more detrimental to amylase activity. EGCG is considered effective in breakdown of bacterial membrane. The catechins are also helpful in eradicating toxins generated by *Escherichia coli* in the intestine. The verotoxin of *E. Coli*, causing gastroenteritis, is countered by the catechins of tea leaves.

Conclusion

Comprehensive caries-prevention protocols, early detection with highly sensitive and specific detections tools, using risk-assessment as a daily routine measure for each patient, improved use of remineralizing agents, micro-inavise dentistry using resin infiltration concept and minimal excavation techniques hold the true future of clinical cariology and a correct combination of all these procedures shall be a breakthrough in this field.

The coming days will be the days of 'wonders'. The bright future lies ahead in overall dentistry, especially cariology; but we all will have to work hard to make certain dreams a reality.

Bibliography

1. Chang H, Lynch, E. And Grootveld, M. Oxidative consumption of oral biomolecules by therapeutically-relevant doses of ozone. Adv. In Chem. Engg. And Sci.: 2012;2:238–45.
2. Cohen KL and Day SE. Caries-free communities: Is this for real? Global health through oral health: 2009;30:484.
3. Hannig M and Hannig C. Nanomaterials in preventive dentistry. Nature Nanotech.: 2010;5:565–9.
4. Jager DH, Vissink A, Timmer CJ, Bronkhorst E, Vieira AM and Huysmans MC. Reduction of erosion by protein-containing toothpastes. Caries Res. 2013;47:135–40.
5. Jeon J G, Rosalen P L, Falsetta M L and Koo H: Natural products in Caries Research: Current (Limited) knowledge, challenges and future perspective. Caries Res. 2011;45:243–63.
6. Jhaver HM. Nanotechnology: The future of dentistry. J. Nanosci. Nanotech.: 2005;5:15–7.
7. Levine M: Susceptibility to dental caries and the salivary proline-rich proteins. Int. J Dent. Article ID 2011;953412.
8. Malhotra N, Kundabala M and Acharya S. Current strategies and application of tissue engineering in dentistry—a review. Part 1. Dent. Update: 2009;36:577–9.
9. Mallanagouda P, Singh DP and Sowjanya G. Future impact of nanotechnology on medicine and dentistry. J. Ind. Soc. Periodontol.: 2008;12: 34–40.
10. Moezizadeh M. Future of dentistry, nano-dentistry, ozone therapy and tissue engineering. J. Dev. Bio. And Tissue Engg.:2013;5:1–6.
11. Nall, R. No more cavities? New molecule may provide a cavity-free future. www.everyday-health.com/0712/ new molecule.
12. Pitts N, Amaechi B, Niederman R, Acevedo AM, Vianna R, Ganss C, Ismail A and Honkala E. Global oral health inequalities: dental caries task group—research agenda. Adv. Dent. Res.: 2011; 23: 211–20.
13. Pretty IA, Ellwood RP, Lo EC, Macentee MI, Miller F, Rooney ER, Thomson WM, Van der Putten G, Ghezzi EM and Walls AW. The Seattle Care Pathway for securing oral health in older patients. Gerodontology: 2014;31:77–87.
14. Singh A and Purohit BM. Addressing geriatric oral health concerns through national oral health policy in India. IJHPM: 2015;4:39–42.
15. Tjaderhane L, Buzalaf MAR, Carrilho M and Chaussain C. Matrix mettaloproteinases and other matrix proteinases in relation to cariology: the era of single 'Dentin Degradomics'. Caries Res. 2015;49:193–208.
16. Thomson WM and Ma S. An ageing population poses dental challenges. Singapore Dent. J.: 2014; 35:3–8.
17. Vieira AR, Modesto A and Marazita ML: Caries: Review of human genetics research. Caries Res. 2014;48:491–506.

Index